Thieme

Seven Cavernomas

Tenets and Techniques for Resection

Michael T. Lawton, MD
President and CEO
Department of Neurosurgery Chair
Robert F. Spetzler Endowed Neuroscience Chair
Chief of Neurovascular Surgery
Barrow Neurological Institute
St. Joseph's Hospital and Medical Center
Phoenix, Arizona, USA

Illustrated by
Peter M. Lawrence, MS, CMI - Senior Medical Illustrator
Kristen Larson Keil, MS, CMI - Manager/Senior Medical Illustrator
Danielle VanBrabant, MSMI, CMI - Senior Medical Animator/Illustrator
Michael D. Hickman, BA - Senior Technical Artist

Neuroscience Publications
Barrow Neurological Institute
St. Joseph's Hospital and Medical Center
Phoenix, Arizona, USA

714 illustrations

Thieme
New York • Stuttgart • Delhi • Rio de Janeiro

Library of Congress Cataloging-in-Publication Data is available with the publisher.

Thieme Publishers New York
333 Seventh Avenue, 18th Floor
New York, NY 10001, USA
www.thieme.com
+1 800 782 3488, customerservice@thieme.com

Illustrated by:
Peter M. Lawrence, MS, CMI - Senior Medical Illustrator
Kristen Larson Keil, MS, CMI - Manager/Senior Medical Illustrator
Danielle VanBrabant, MSMI, CMI - Senior Medical Animator/Illustrator
Michael D. Hickman, BA - Senior Technical Artist
Neuroscience Publications
Barrow Neurological Institute
St. Joseph's Hospital and Medical Center
Phoenix, Arizona, USA
No. of illustrations: [700+]

Cover design: © Thieme
On the Cover: Elevated cartography of the brain, as depicted in this volume, condenses a vast amount of anatomical information and preserves the brain's complexity while remaining understandable to a wide range of neurosurgeons. Eight such maps depict the cavernoma taxonomy and concepts. Each expresses the artistic collaboration and alchemy between the neurosurgeon-cartographer and the illustrators.
Cover image source: Cover art designed and illustrated by Peter M. Lawrence, MS, CMI.

Typesetting by TNQ Tech Private Limited, India

Printed in Germany by Beltz Printers 5 4 3 2

DOI: 10.1055/b000001256

ISBN: 978-1-68420-494-6

Also available as an e-book:
eISBN (PDF): 978-1-68420-495-3 eISBN (epub): 978-1-68420-494-6

In grateful remembrance of Lisa T. Hannegan, my clinical nurse practitioner for my first two decades in practice, for knowing, supporting, and elevating me during the most challenging years of my neurosurgical journey and for always reminding me that what happens at the bedside is as important as what happens under the operating microscope. Lisa imparted the wisdom of what came to be known as ***Hannegan's sign***: "When you have to stare at the clinical images for longer than 5 minutes trying to decide whether and how to operate, you probably should not." Her story is a reminder that time is precious, and the journey is richer when one finds an angel who helps along the way.
Lisa and Hannegan's sign reminded me to look for and listen to the guardian angels.

Michael T. Lawton

Contents

Videos

Foreword

In this fourth volume of surgical vascular entities, Dr. Michael Lawton tackles cavernomas. As in his previous three textbooks in this series of *Seven* pathologies, one is immediately fascinated with the quality of the illustrations and the easy-to-read and readily comprehensible prose. There is no similar publication in our neurosurgical literature that represents the surgical approach to brain cavernous malformations with such perspective and beauty. Michael has curated an impressive compendium of 65 surgical videos and 8 animations to accompany the text and illustrations.

This work begins with 10 tenets for the neurosurgical management of brain cavernous malformations. The first chapter describes a taxonomy that classifies cavernomas by their location and surface presentation into 7 types and 35 subtypes. The taxonomy established preferred surgical approaches to reach and resect targeted cavernomas safely. This framework uses natural corridors and vascular landmarks to navigate the subarachnoid space to lesions. The following chapters describe the brainstem and cerebral anatomy and dissection techniques in detail, with chapters on the triangle concept, arterial landmarks, hotspots of brain eloquence once thought to be noneloquent, recurrence, and patient selection. With Chapter 10 (Neurosurgical Cartography), Michael delves into his philosophical approach to his concept of the brain and our role as neurosurgeons in patient care. The next 7 chapters describe the 7 types and 35 subtypes of cavernomas and precisely how to approach them for resection. Finally, in Chapter 18 (Seven Cavernomas: Project Connectomunculus and the Mind), he comes full circle back to the future of neurosurgery's role in defining how the brain creates emotion, memory, neural plasticity, intelligence, and consciousness, noting that "These amazing facets of the mind make us human, and nothing is more important than understanding that."

I deeply admire Michael's commitment to the endless hours and meticulous attention to detail it took to compile this volume, the great deal of introspection and study that led him to discover what cavernomas have taught us, culminating in his taxonomy schema and vision into the future.

This volume belongs on the shelf of every vascular neurosurgeon, and the surgical lessons and the illumination contained in the taxonomy make it mandatory reading for anyone who practices our art.

It is a privilege to write the foreword to this volume, written by a former pupil who has fulfilled the goal of every dedicated teacher, which is to advance our specialty and to surpass the teacher. Michael Lawton has certainly achieved that!

Robert F. Spetzler, MD
JN Harbor Chairperson Emeritus, Department of Neurosurgery
Director Emeritus
Barrow Neurological Institute
St. Joseph's Hospital and Medical Center
Phoenix, Arizona, USA

Foreword

It was July 1994. I was starting my year as Robert Spetzler's Fellow at Barrow Neurological Institute in Phoenix, Arizona. No sooner had I arrived than I was told that a standout senior resident in the program was enamored with cerebrovascular surgery, intensely focused on learning all there was to learn from his iconic mentor, and he was fueled by a unique drive to excel. His name was Michael T. Lawton. The first time Mike and I scrubbed together, we discussed specifically how Spetzler might want us to carry out the cranio-orbito-zygomatic approach. Mike was full of inquisitive questions. Thirty years on, they never stopped.

Socrates stated: "The unexamined life is not worth living." I could paraphrase: "The unexamined craft is not worth practicing." Very few neurosurgeons have dissected and reported on the underpinnings of the craft of cerebrovascular microneurosurgery to the depth that Mike has. He is the embodiment of what becomes of a surgeon when he or she is blessed with or fosters a few key characteristics: curiosity, passion, ambition, courage, surgical skill, unquenched thirst for excellence, relentless self-assessment, an uncanny ability to analyze, then synthesize, then express thoughts and techniques to peers and students. Mike's major in college was engineering, and it shows very clearly in the constitution of the masterful surgeon he has become. His precise and analytical mind is evident throughout his writings. As he matured as a top-tier cerebrovascular neurosurgeon, he began to recognize a strong urge to describe, analyze, and classify every surgical lesion he tackled and every surgical move he made. He also discovered that the best way to learn was to teach. Thus began his remarkable "Seven Series" of books on aneurysms, AVMs, bypasses, and, now, this latest work of art, *Seven Cavernomas: Tenets and Techniques for Resection.*

This latest rendition of his thoughts and experience on the topic is illustrated in 18 chapters. Not surprisingly, Mike's obsession with order and structure compels him to start his book by developing a taxonomy to classify cavernoma locations into 7 categories that are further subcategorized into 35 locales. He goes on to describe the essence of subarachnoid dissection for each location and the "triangle" concept for the surgeon as the target is approached. In a Rhoton-esque manner, he allocates an "arterial address" to each cavernoma and further considers the useful concept—though debatable and in need of subtle analysis—of "safe entry zones." He goes on to discuss general techniques of cavernoma resection, the treachery of their blind spots in those deep dark holes, and the nebulous concept of "eloquence" and "eloquent noneloquence." He presents extensive outcome results from the combined Spetzler–Lawton surgical series and uses those results to propose a grading system for brainstem cavernomas that predicts surgical morbidity. In a touching segment, he pays posthumous tribute to Lisa Hannegan, his former nurse practitioner, who had long realized that not all things are measurable, verifiable, or even describable; "gut feelings" and that "je ne sais quoi" inner voice of an experienced surgeon still matter as much as if not more than all the grading systems, taxonomies, and predictive scales. If you have to study the scan of a patient with a brainstem cavernoma for more than 5 minutes, Lisa surmised, then perhaps there is no safe surgical approach to it.

By the time Chapter 10 comes along, it is very clear that if one were to choose a metaphor for the surgery of cavernomas, "cartography"—along with its rich history and visual appeal—is the perfect choice. Mike uses the metaphor to its full extent to demonstrate that the purpose of writing is a clear depiction of the complex rather than a complex depiction of the simple. The seven cavernoma locations are then each assigned a chapter, with links to superb surgical videos for each cavernoma location. It is most revealing and interesting, but not surprising, that only one chapter is dedicated to the cerebrum, even though it is by far the most voluminous portion of the brain. This conception is entirely appropriate, as Mike's analysis is commensurate with the surgical challenges and variables encountered rather than the prevalence of cavernomas at various locations. One can debate whether the "insula" should have been part of the cerebrum rather than lumped with the "putamen," but again, this book is written through a surgeon's lens, not an anatomist's.

The last chapter stands in clear contrast to the rest of the book. It is the only chapter that illustrates that our work as surgeons and thinkers is never done. Mike was clearly hoping to reach a definitive solution to the problem of reconciling "localization" and "connectomics." One can feel his intense need to have reached the neurosurgical equivalent of a "unified theory" for all surgical approaches to intra-axial lesions—what Mike named "connectomunculus." It was not meant to be, as our current understanding of the paths and interdependence of all those trillions of synaptic connections is highly rudimentary and does not allow proper synthesis—yet. In other words, the brain has first to understand itself fully before it can describe itself. Thus, Mike leaves an open door for future generations to persevere.

This book also demonstrates the sublime synergy that can be achieved when a brilliant surgeon collaborates with a superb medical illustrator. Peter Lawrence's artistry in every drawing is exquisite and almost stands by itself as a microneurosurgical storyline. The "Netterian" style of Kristen Larson Keil in depicting every brainstem syndrome and clinicopathological model is equally stunning and informative.

"The most powerful weapon on earth is the human soul on fire," said Ferdinand Foch. Passion without determination is but a dream or a state of mind; determination without passion is sterile or short-lived. It has been my distinct pleasure to watch the author's inquisitive, passionate, determined mind, which I first encountered in 1994, blossom into the making of a world authority on cerebrovascular neurosurgery. I have cherished our discussions and debates in private settings and conference halls. I have no doubt this latest fruit of his mind will entice legions of students to enter the field that Yaşargil heralded 60 years ago. If that is not a legacy, then I don't know what is.

Jacques J. Morcos, MD, FRCS(Eng), FRCS(Ed), FAANS
Chairman, Vivian L. Smith Department of Neurosurgery
Professor, McGovern Medical School at UTHealth Houston
John P. and Kathrine G. McGovern Distinguished Chair
Co-Director, UTHealth Houston Neurosciences
Director, Cerebrovascular and Skull Base Surgery
Houston, Texas, USA

Preface

The arachnoid membrane covers the brain like a sheet of ice on a frozen lake on a cold winter morning. Thickened areas are frosted to conceal the anatomy in fissures below, while thinned areas reveal arteries and veins, like looking through glass. The arachnoid is an overlooked structure supporting an organ so supple it would almost look like it had melted without it. Falling through ice into a frigid lake is a nightmarish danger, but dissecting into a pristine arachnoid is a neurosurgeon's dream. A nick with an up-facing no. 11 blade, then a few snips with microscissors break the ice and transport us into the otherworld of the subarachnoid space and its labyrinth of cisterns, sulci, and fissures. Cerebral prominences and protuberances are bathed in currents of cerebrospinal fluid, and it becomes clear that following these currents will lead the dissection to any point on the brain's surface. Deepening dissection slips past the blue delta of venous tributaries and into the pink arboretum of arterial branches. Intense illumination of the microscope and movements of instruments make the operative field twinkle with reflected light. The sparkle of arachnoid trabeculations spanning from one lobule to another catches the eye like holiday tinsel on a Christmas tree. Shimmering spider web-like filaments fill the cisterns, and with each arachnoid strand cut, the cortical walls retract, and spaces widen to turn narrow slots into majestic canyons. The brain bends and shifts as its connective tissue scaffold is progressively disassembled. Incising sylvian and carotid cisternal membranes frees the frontal lobe to unveil the optic nerves. The neurosurgeon dives through the optic-carotid triangle to reach Liliequist's membrane. Incising the ambient cisternal membranes frees the quadrangular lobule to descend with the pull of gravity and unveil the midbrain tegmentum. Potential spaces once dark and quiet now flood with light, color, and motion. The subarachnoid space transforms into a wonderland of glistening arteries, veins, cranial nerves, bony tubercles, and pia mater. The surreal view through the operating microscope is like peering into a forbidden world not meant for human eyes, like deep-water scuba diving, a Mount Everest ascent, or the video from an Apollo mission to the moon.

Seven Cavernomas is a book about cavernous malformations (CMs) in the brain, and in truth, it is just as much a book about the subarachnoid space. According to the Monro–Kellie doctrine, this space occupies approximately 10% of the intracranial volume, which is ample room to maneuver almost anywhere in the brain, be it superficial or deep. It can be navigated between layers of the pia mater with impunity, and the brain's pliability gives the neurosurgeon additional room to roam. Arguably, there is no better place to circumnavigate the brain than inside its fissures and folds. In contrast, brain tissue is certainly not ideal for brain surgery. Parenchymal transgression disrupts neural circuits and networks with costly neurological consequences for patients. Blood, the other liquid in the cranial compartment occupying another 10% of the intracranial volume, can be navigated endovascularly with wires and catheters. Still, we cannot see without radiology and intravenous contrast media, and actions are constrained by the arterial and venous walls, never truly touching the brain. The subarachnoid space is a microneurosurgical utopia and the stage for the *Seven Cavernomas* story.

Seven Cavernomas was conceived as a book about surgical approaches. CMs can occur in any area of the brain, and the therapeutic challenge is to resect them without neurological sequela. Meeting this challenge requires first selecting patients with symptomatic lesions presenting to an accessible pial surface and then selecting the surgical approaches that will expose them. Therefore, a comprehensive textbook about CMs can be organized and compiled into microsurgical approaches to a CM. *Seven Cavernomas* was intended to be an encyclopedia of every approach in the surgical armamentarium, celebrating subarachnoid corridors, anatomical details, and technical nuances. However, the writing process uncovered a more profound need. Amidst the almost daily requests from neurosurgeons worldwide seeking advice on whether and how best to operate on these lesions, it became clear that an encyclopedia of approaches was not as important as a framework for making these two critical patient selection and approach decisions. The original idea for *Seven Cavernomas* would have to wait as I pivoted to taxonomy, approach selection, the triangle concept, and grading systems for patient selection (▶ Table P.1). Abbreviations and their expansions are given in ▶ Table P.2, ▶ Table P.3, ▶ Table P.4, ▶ Table P.5, ▶ Table P.6, and ▶ Table P.7. In the end, I arrived at a framework and heuristics that would help neurosurgeons manage CMs with a common language, standardized selection criteria, and consistent approaches derived from clinical evidence from my experience and that of Robert Spetzler.

CMs have a fascinating neurosurgical history, and I landed in the middle of it as a resident at Barrow Neurological Institute in the 1990s. Not long before, neurosurgeons considered the brainstem a surgical backwoods where densely packed cranial nerve nuclei and ascending and descending tracts prevented operative transgression. Walter Dandy is credited with the first accurate diagnosis and successful removal of a brainstem CM in 1934. However, neurosurgeons considered surgical intervention in the brainstem too dangerous, and only a few cases were documented in the following decades. These lesions were misdiagnosed as "cryptic vascular malformations" after patients with intracerebral hemorrhages detected on CT scans would subsequently have negative angiograms. With the advent of MRI in the 1980s, CMs were characterized as pathological entities with pathognomonic findings, including a "popcorn" appearance, mixed signal intensities, and hemosiderin rings. CMs were more amenable to resection than arteriovenous malformations (AVMs) because they lacked arterial input and could be removed piecemeal. With these insights, a handful of brave vascular neurosurgeons advanced the idea that the brainstem was *not* inviolable territory and brainstem CMs were *not* inoperable.

Spetzler and colleagues published their first experience with 24 symptomatic brainstem cerebral CMs in 1991, selecting 16 patients for microsurgical treatment based on their neurological status, number of hemorrhages, and the lesion's proximity to the pial surface. All but one patient's neurological outcome improved postoperatively, leading to a surgical posture for symptomatic patients. My arrival in Phoenix as a resident coincided with this publication, and I experienced a wave of referrals from around the world to Barrow Neurological Institute. Other neurosurgeons, it seemed, believed that the brainstem was inviolable and brainstem surgery was impossible, so they referred their patients to someone brave enough to think that it was possible. That extensive referral network, combined with the prevalence of Hispanic patients in Phoenix, in whom CMs were common, fueled the discovery that the microsurgical resection of brainstem CMs was safe and even advisable for many patients. The convergence of case volume and a quintessential neurosurgeon like Robert Spetzler, who practiced high-level microsurgery and skull base surgery when other centers were moving toward endoscopic and endovascular techniques, shaped a new discipline within vascular neurosurgery. Brainstem CM surgery began with simple concepts like the two-point method to select the right approach to expose the lesion. This discipline adapted complex skull base surgical approaches developed for aneurysms and tumors to the simpler pathology of CMs. For example, the orbitozygomatic approach developed for high-riding basilar bifurcation aneurysms was ideal for midbrain brainstem CMs in the cerebral peduncle, interpeduncular fossa, and contralateral cerebral peduncle. Dr. Spetzler applied stereotactic navigation for submerged lesions, tractography for lesions near motor pathways, and lighted microinstruments that brought precision and light to deep, dark surgical corridors. Ultimately, our perception of the brainstem as an impenetrable monolith was transformed, and we appreciated it instead as a complex structure with zones that could be entered safely without causing neurological deficits in patients.

The cavernoma story, from early misdiagnosis and initial conservative management to the current state of its treatment, is a testament to open microsurgical technique, its application to a newly defined lesion, and its curative efficacy. With no endovascular or proven radiosurgical alternative, microsurgery occupies the dominant position in the therapeutic algorithm. CMs demonstrate that microsurgical skills are versatile, our surgical approaches can be refined, our repertoire can be expanded, and our techniques can become increasingly honed. This compelling story encompassed my training years, neurosurgical mentor, home institution, and current practice. Dr. Spetzler amassed an experience of over 400 brainstem CM resections, which I have surpassed, as part of an overall experience with over 1,300 brain CMs. Writing *Seven Cavernomas* and distilling this experience into teachable lessons felt like an imperative.

Seven Cavernomas is the fourth book in the "Seven Series" trilogy. By trilogy, I mean that this book was not supposed to be written. My first book, *Seven Aneurysms*, was imperative to preserve the endangered art of aneurysm surgery in the face of an endovascular revolution by simplifying and choreographing the microsurgical steps like a dance lesson for the seven most common aneurysms that account for three-quarters of all aneurysms. That book, with 224 pages, 90 illustrations, and 383 photographs, became a bestseller. *Seven AVMs* was my effort to make sense of surgery for AVMs. I had trained with the acknowledged AVM master at the mecca of AVM surgery but graduated feeling like I did not understand how to battle this enemy. This book presented a taxonomy for the spectrum of AVM pathology, conceptualized surgical steps, and developed specific battle plans for each subtype. This book, which Al Rhoton described in his foreword as *Seven Aneurysms'* "angry twin" because of its war metaphor, had 334 pages, 350 illustrations, and more than 700 photographs. My love of bypass surgery inspired *Seven Bypasses*. These operations are my favorite, embodying the importance of manual craftsmanship, the elegance of reconstructive surgery, and innovation without high technology. These operations are also the most challenging, requiring 1,000 perfect moves to complete successfully and doomed by only 1 imperfect move. *Seven Bypasses* aimed to elevate bypass surgery and turn "plumbing" into art by advancing intracranial-intracranial techniques, developing a taxonomy for bypasses, and introducing blueprints and codes for bypass designs with an architectural metaphor. *Seven Bypasses* had 698 pages, 1,519 illustrations, and more than 1,500 photographs. At this point, I promised my wife Suzanne that *Seven Bypasses* would be my last textbook, but my return to the hallowed halls of Barrow Neurological Institute, plus idle time during the COVID-19 pandemic, rekindled the energy to produce *Seven Cavernomas.*

Seven Cavernomas begins with 10 tenets of cavernoma surgery, starting with a comprehensive taxonomy meant to transform the spectrum of CM pathology into a system of 7 types and 35 subtypes. The endless variety of lesion sizes, shapes, and positions simplifies into superficial cerebral, deep cerebral (basal ganglia and thalamus), brainstem (midbrain, pons, and medulla), and cerebellar types. CMs are subtyped according to their surface presentation: anterior, lateral, posterior, medial, superior, etc. The combination of anatomical location (7 types) and surface presentation (35 subtypes) defines each CM analogous to the binomial nomenclature that classifies plants and animals zoologically by genus and species and yields a classification system with a finite number of recognizable subtypes, each with well-defined anatomy and a specific microsurgical plan (Chapter 1). Next, the seven subarachnoid corridors that comprise our neurosurgical highways are presented (Chapter 2). The "triangle concept" is introduced to precisely define surgical routes and accurately guide microdissection to the pathological targets, and a system of anatomical triangles is established for brainstem CM surgery, like what exists for cavernous sinus surgery (Chapter 3). Arteries cohabitating within the subarachnoid space are reimagined as arterial addresses and landmarks defining surgical routes and targets (Chapter 4). When the end of the road does not lead to the targeted pathology but to a buried cavernoma beneath a pial or ependymal surface, safe entry zones (SEZs) transgressing normal tissue are needed to reach the lesion (Chapter 5). If subarachnoid corridors are like lighted, well-signed highways, parenchymal corridors are like dark dirt roads, and trajectory, eloquence, and invisible triangles are factors to consider when resecting the CM (Chapter 6). In the cerebrum, parts of the brain that have long been considered by neurosurgeons to be noneloquent may actually be eloquent due to their involvement in large-scale networks. Thus, we must update our concept of cortical eloquence and our surgical strategies (Chapter 7). Residual or recurrent CMs require reoperation, and heuristics such as the right-angle method are presented to minimize this frustrating problem (Chapter 8). As with most surgeries, the secret to good outcomes is judicious patient selection, which is why a grading system for brainstem CMs was developed, validated, and incorporated into surgical decision-making (Chapter 9). Maps clarify and integrate information and concepts to plan and pilot the journey, and our artists share stunning maps for brainstem cavernoma surgery (Chapter 10).

In Section II, the neuroanatomy and resection techniques for the 7 cavernomas and 35 subtypes are covered in detail, traveling from superficial cerebral lesions (Chapter 11) to deep cerebral lesions (Chapters 12 and 13) and from brainstem lesions (Chapters 14–16) to cerebellar lesions (Chapter 17). Neural circuitry, bedside symptoms, signs and syndromes, craniotomy-surgical approach–triangle triads, and SEZs guide the approach to each cavernoma subtype. The artwork you are about to see, especially in this section, is superlative. Kristen Larson Keil brought neural circuitry to life in her illustrations of the neuroanatomy for each subtype and the clinical syndromes caused by CM hemorrhages, evoking Frank Netter's work correlating bedside neurological findings with the brain's complex wiring diagrams. Danielle VanBrabant generated three-dimensional computer models of the brain from high-resolution MRIs to capture and finesse the artist's pen, depicting the surface topology of the cerebrum and cerebellum. These models also revealed the connectomics of brain networks and their internal white matter connections (Chapter 18). Michael Hickman mastered surface renderings and textures to finish the models with vivid life-like colors, luster, and sheen that awakened this digital brain. Peter Lawrence created visual masterpieces showing the craniotomies, approach trajectories, anatomical triangles, SEZs, approach overviews, surgeon views, and arterial and cranial nerve anatomy. His illustrations distill countless photographs from my patients and led to my decision not to include intraoperative photographs as in the other Seven Series textbooks. This decision not only reduced the page count but also encouraged the inclusion of surgical videos. I have come to view videos as superior to still photographs because they capture the action, progression, movement, and technical nuance that sculpt the art of surgery. Technology and QR codes now make it easy to immerse oneself in videos on a mobile device, and I am pleased to transition to my first video textbook. I often wanted one of my Seven Series textbooks on my coffee table, but the esoteric content held little interest to lay people, and the photographs could be interpreted as too graphic and unsettling. *Seven Cavernomas* might just be the textbook worthy of the coffee table, exhibiting the astonishing beauty of the most magnificent organ in the body and the most powerful machine in our world, without any blood.

Finally, each Seven Series book has a metaphor. In *Seven Aneurysms*, the metaphor is ballet, with choreographed steps as aneurysm clipping progresses from subarachnoid dissection to proximal and distal control to aneurysm neck dissection to clip application. In *Seven AVMs*, AVM resection is like war, with types and subtypes that classify the AVM enemy. Battle plans are drawn for each AVM, and a stepwise campaign progresses from exposure to subarachnoid dissection to identification of the draining veins and feeding arteries to pial, parenchymal, and ependymal dissection, and, finally, to resection. In *Seven Bypasses*, the metaphor is architecture. Whether erecting a cathedral or performing a bypass, the arterial connections are envisioned, a bypass is designed on the basis of individualized anatomy, blueprints lay out the anastomotic sites and techniques, the anastomoses are constructed, and, finally, the bypass is brought to life with pulsations, flow, and reperfusion. You will notice that the metaphor for *Seven Cavernomas* is cartography. The subarachnoid space is the brain's open road for neurosurgeons, and this book is a collection of road trips through the cerebral terrain. Ralph Waldo Emerson is credited with the quote that joy is found not in reaching the destination but in taking the journey, and this quote aptly applies to cavernoma surgery. These capillary-fed malformations lack the hemodynamic fury of AVMs and the unnerving threat of intraoperative aneurysm rerupture. They are quickly and easily decompartmentalized, collapsed, and resected. Therefore, the thrill of cavernoma surgery comes not from reaching or removing the cavernoma but from the journey, that otherworldly passage down fissures and cisterns, past gyral undulations and twisting arteries, through triangles of cranial nerves and dural folds. This journey is the ultimate neurosurgical joyride, and nothing captures the thrill of a grand road trip like a map. We toss them into the glove compartment or program our navigation system before every trip. Maps show us routes, scenery, and distances through unfamiliar territory. They lead us to gas stations, restaurants, and rest stops. They alert us to accidents, road construction, hospitals, and hotels. Maps inform the trip and give confidence along the way that we will arrive safely without getting lost. They are valuable to those traveling to points unknown for the first time and to those who have been there countless times but are curious about a new route. Maps are the ticket to exploring the unknown.

Composing *Seven Cavernomas* has been like cartography for neurosurgical wanderlust. Our operations begin with craniotomies that access the intracranial wilderness like an on-ramp. Our microsurgical approaches set out along fissures and cisterns like highways. Intersecting cranial nerves and arteries form anatomical triangles that confirm our heading, like bridges crossing over rivers or tunnels bored through mountains. The faint hemosiderin stain on otherwise bright white brainstem pia alerts us like a signpost that the destination is near. Finally, the purple mulberry-like CM protruding through the pia is brought into view like an off-ramp, signaling the journey's end. The elements comprising cavernoma surgery can be bewildering but fit together like the elements of a road trip. The art and science of map-making is a way to crystallize the art and science of cavernoma surgery. As you read this book, I hope you enjoy the concepts, the ride, and the wind in your hair.

Michael T. Lawton, MD
President and CEO
Department of Neurosurgery Chair
Robert F. Spetzler Endowed
Neuroscience Chair
Chief of Neurovascular Surgery
Barrow Neurological Institute
St. Joseph's Hospital and Medical Center
Phoenix, Arizona, USA

Table P.1 Summary of taxonomy for cerebral CMs

Type	Subtype	Craniotomy	Approach	Triangle	Safe entry zone	Arterial target	Dissection code
Cerebral	Convexity	Convexity	TGyr, TSul	None		Cortical arteries (M4, A5, P4)	
	Medial	Bifrontal, biparieto-occipital	TGyr, TSul	None		ACA, PCA, ATA, TempPolA	
	Basal	Miscellaneous	TGyr, TSul	None		ACA, PCA,A1	
	Sylvian	Pterional	TSyl-TGyr, TSyl-TSul	None		M3	
Basal ganglia	Caudate	Bifrontal	cTCal-Vent	Caudate-thalamostriate		PcaA	
	Putaminal	Pterional	TSyl-AIns	None		M2	
	Pallidal	Orbitozygomatic	TSyl-SCIF	Supracarotid		A1, M1, mLSA, lLSA	
Thalamic	Anterior	Bifrontal	cTCal-iFor	Septocaudate		mPChA	
	Medial	Bifrontal	cTCal-cTChor; cTCal-iTChor	None		mPChA	
	Lateral	Pterional	TSyl-PIns	None		M2	
	Choroidal	Bifrontal	iTCal-Vent	None		mPChA	
	Pulvinar	Torcular	SCIT-Para	Infragalenic		mPChA	
	Geniculate	Torcular	cSCTT	Infragalenic		mPChA	
Midbrain	Interpeduncular	Orbitozygomatic	TSyl-IntPed; cTSyl-IntPed	Carotid-oculomotor	Interpeduncular	P1	M3-M2-M1-C6-AChA-PCoA-P1
	Peduncular	Orbitozygomatic	TSyl-Ped	Oculomotor-tentorial	Anterior mesencephalic	P2A, s1	M3-M2-M1-C6-AChA-PCoA-P2A
	Tegmental	Retrosigmoid	SCIT-Lat	Supra- and infratrochlear	Lateral mesencephalic sulcus	s3	s4-s3
	Quadrigeminal	Torcular	SCIT-Mid	Infragalenic	Intercollicular, supracollicular, infracollicular	mPChA, s4	s4-s3-P3-PreCenCblV-BVR-mPChA
	Periaqueductal	Bifrontal	TCal-TChor	None	None	None	CmaA-PcaA-ThaStrV-ICV-mPChA
Pontine	Basilar	Orbitozygomatic	Kaw; TSyl-Cav-Pon	Kawase/infratrigeminal, carotid-oculomotor	Supra-, infratrigeminal	BA, s1, a1	SPS-IPS-a2-a1-BA
	Peritrigeminal	Retrosigmoid	xRS-CPA	Supra- and infratrigeminal, glossopharyngeal-cochlear triangle	Supra-, infratrigeminal	s2	s4-s3-s2
	Middle peduncular	Retrosigmoid	xRS-MCP	Interlobular	Middle cerebellar peduncular/ lateral pontine	a3	a4-a3
	Inferior peduncular	Suboccipital	SOcc-TeVe	Subtonsillar	Area acustica	p4	p2-p3-p4
	Rhomboid	Suboccipital	SOcc-Vent	Vallecular	Median sulcus, suprafacial collicular, superior foveal	p3	L p3-R p3

(Continued)

Table P.1 (*Continued*) Summary of taxonomy for cerebral CMs

Type	Subtype	Craniotomy	Approach	Triangle	Safe entry zone	Arterial target	Dissection code
	Supraolivary	Far lateral	FL-PMS	Vagoaccessory (suprahypoglossal)	Pontomedullary sulcus	a2	V4-p3-p2-p1-a2
Medullary	Pyramidal	Far lateral	FL-PreMed	Junctional	Anterolateral sulcus	VBJ	V4-p1-ASA-VBJ
	Olivary	Far lateral	FL-Med	Vagoaccessory (supra- or hypoglossal-hypoglossal)	Olivary zone, posterolateral sulcus, lateral medullary zone	p2	V4-p3-p2
	Trigonal	Suboccipital	SOcc-Vent	Vallecular	Median sulcus, infrafacial collicular	p3	L p3-R p3
	Gracile	Suboccipital	SOcc-Magna	Vallecular	Posterior median sulcus	p3	L p3-R p3
	Cuneate	Suboccipital	SOcc-TeVe	Subtonsillar	Posterior intermediate sulcus	PSA	V4-p3-p2-PSA
Cerebellar	Suboccipital	Suboccipital	SOcc-Para	None		p5	
	Tentorial	Torcular	SCIT-Mid, SCIT-Para	None		s4	
	Petrosal	Retrosigmoid	xRS-CPA	Interlobular		a4	
	Vermian	Suboccipital	SOcc-Mid	None		s4, p5	
	Tonsillar	Suboccipital	SOcc-Magna	Vallecular		p5	
	Deep nuclear	Suboccipital	SOcc-TeVe, SOcc-SupraTons	Vallecular		p4	

Table P.2 Abbreviations for arteries

Abbreviation	Artery
ACA	Anterior cerebral
AChA	Anterior choroidal
ACoA	Anterior communicating
AICA	Anterior inferior cerebellar
AIFA	Anterior internal frontal
AngA	Angular
AntParA	Anterior parietal
AntSpA	Anterior spinal
AntThaP	Anterior thalamoperforators
Ao	Aorta
AscPharA	Ascending pharyngeal
ATA	Anterior temporal
ASA	Anterior spinal
BA	Basilar
CalcA	Calcarine
CaTr	Caudal trunk of superior cerebellar
CCA	Common carotid
CenA	Central
CirP	Circumflex perforators
CmaA	Callosomarginal
ECA	External carotid
FrPolA	Frontopolar
fSTA	Frontal branch of superficial temporal
HippoA	Hippocampal
ICA	Internal carotid
ILSA	Inferior lenticulostriate
IMA	Internal maxillary
InfParA	Inferior parietal
InfTr	Inferior trunk of middle cerebral
InsP	Insular perforators
IntHe	Intermediate hemispheric
iPChA	Inferior posterior choroidal
LatHe	Lateral hemispheric
LatTr	Lateral trunk of posterior inferior cerebellar
LingA	Lingual
lLSA	Lateral lenticulostriate
lPChA	Lateral posterior choroidal
LSA	Lenticulostriate
MCA	Middle cerebral
MedHe	Medial hemispheric
MedTr	Medial trunk of posterior inferior cerebellar
MidTempA	Middle temporal

(Continued)

Table P.2 *(Continued)* Abbreviations for arteries

Abbreviation	Artery
MidTr	Middle trunk of middle cerebral
MIFA	Middle internal frontal
mLSA	Medial lenticulostriate
MMA	Middle meningeal
mPChA	Medial posterior choroidal
OA	Occipital
OphA	Ophthalmic
OrbFrA	Orbitofrontal (ACA, MCA)
PAA	Posterior auricular
ParaCenA	Paracentral
ParOccA	Parieto-occipital
PCA	Posterior cerebral
PcaA	Pericallosal
PCoA	Posterior communicating
PedP	Peduncular perforators
Perf	Perforator
PICA	Posterior inferior cerebellar
PIFA	Posterior internal frontal
PoCenA	Postcentral
PosParA	Posterior parietal
PosTempA	Posterior temporal (MCA, PCA)
PosThaP	Posterior thalamoperforators
PreCenA	Precentral
PreCer	Precerebellar
PreFrA	Prefrontal
PSA	Posterior spinal
pSTA	Parietal branch of superficial temporal
RAH	Recurrent artery of Heubner
RoTr	Rostral trunk of superior cerebellar
SCA	Superior cerebellar
SclA	Subclavian
SHA	Superior hypophyseal
SplenA	Splenial
STA	Superficial temporal
SupParA	Superior parietal
SupThyrA	Superior thyroid
SupTr	Superior trunk of middle cerebral
TempOccA	Temporo-occipital
TempPolA	Temporopolar
ThaP	Thalamoperforators
ThGenP	Thalamogeniculate perforators
VA	Vertebral
VBJ	Vertebrobasilar junction
Ve	Vermian

Table P.3 Abbreviations for arterial segments

Abbreviation	Artery	Segment
C1	ICA	Cervical
C2	ICA	Petrous
C3	ICA	Lacerum
C4	ICA	Cavernous
C5	ICA	Clinoidal
C6	ICA	Ophthalmic
C7	ICA	Communicating
A1	ACA	Precommunicating or horizontal
A2	ACA	Postcommunicating or infracallosal
A3	ACA	Precallosal
A4	ACA	Supracallosal
A5	ACA	Postcallosal
M1	MCA	Sphenoidal
M2	MCA	Insular
M3	MCA	Opercular
M4	MCA	Cortical
P1	PCA	Precommunicating
P2	PCA	Postcommunicating
P2A	PCA	Crural
P2P	PCA	Ambient
P3	PCA	Quadrigeminal
P4	PCA	Calcarine
s1	SCA	Anterior pontomesencephalic
s2	SCA	Lateral pontomesencephalic
s3	SCA	Cerebellomesencephalic
s4	SCA	Cortical
a1	AICA	Anterior pontine
a2	AICA	Lateral pontine
a3	AICA	Flocculopeduncular
a4	AICA	Cortical
p1	PICA	Anterior medullary
p2	PICA	Lateral medullary
p3	PICA	Tonsillomedullary
p4	PICA	Telovelotonsillar
p5	PICA	Cortical
V1	VA	Preforaminal
V2	VA	Foraminal
V3	VA	Extradural
V4	VA	Intradural

Table P.4 Abbreviations for veins and venous sinuses

Abbreviation	Vein or sinus
AntHemV	Anterior hemispheric vein
AntCalcV	Anterior calcarine vein (internal occipital vein)
AntCaudV	Anterior caudate vein
AntFrV	Anterior frontal vein
AntParV	Anterior parietal vein
AntSepV	Anterior septal vein
AntTempV	Anterior temporal vein
AtrV	Atrial vein (medial, lateral)
BVR	Basal vein of Rosenthal
CaudV	Caudate vein (anterior, posterior)
CavS	Cavernous sinus
CenV	Central vein
ChorV	Choroidal vein (superior, inferior)
DeepSylV	Deep sylvian vein
FrPolV	Frontopolar vein
FrSylV	Frontosylvian vein
HippoV	Anterior hippocampal vein
ICV	Internal cerebral vein
IHemV	Inferior hemispheric vein
IJV	Internal jugular
IPetrV	Inferior petrosal vein
IPS	Inferior petrosal sinus
ISS	Inferior sagittal sinus
IVerV	Inferior vermian vein
Labbé	Vein of Labbé
LatAntMedV	Lateral anterior medullary vein
LatPonMesV	Lateral anterior pontomesencephalic vein
LatMedV	Lateral medullary vein
LatMesV	Lateral mesencephalic vein
MAMedV	Median anterior medullary vein
MAPonMesV	Median anterior pontomesencephalic vein
MAPosMedV	Median posterior medullary vein
MedFrV	Medial frontal vein (anterior, central, posterior)
MedParV	Medial parietal vein (anterior, posterior)
MedTempV	Medial temporal vein
MidFrV	Middle frontal vein
MidTempV	Middle temporal vein
OccBasV	Occipital basal vein
OccV	Occipital vein

(Continued)

Table P.4 (*Continued*) Abbreviations for veins and venous sinuses

Abbreviation	Vein or sinus
OlfV	Olfactory vein
OrbFrV	Orbitofrontal vein (anterior, posterior)
ParaCenV	Paracentral vein
PcaV	Pericallosal vein (anterior, posterior)
PedV	Peduncular vein
PosCalcV	Posterior calcarine vein
PosCenV	Postcentral vein
PosComV	Posterior communicating vein
PosFrV	Posterior frontal vein
PosParV	Posterior parietal vein
PosTempV	Posterior temporal vein
PreCenCblV	Precentral cerebellar vein
PreCenV	Precentral vein
ReOlvV	Retro-olivary vein
ReTonsV	Retrotonsillar vein
SepV	Septal vein (anterior, posterior)
SHemV	Superior hemispheric vein (anterior, posterior)
SigmS	Sigmoid sinus
SphBasS	Sphenobasal sinus
SphParS	Sphenoparietal sinus
SphPetS	Sphenopetrosal sinus
SplenV	Splenial vein
SPS	Superior petrosal sinus
SPV	Superior petrosal vein
SSS	Superior sagittal sinus
StrS	Straight sinus
STV	Superficial temporal
SupSylV	Superficial sylvian vein
SVerV	Superior vermian vein
TecV	Tectal vein
TempBasV	Temporal basal vein (anterior, middle, posterior)
TentS	Tentorial sinus
ThaStrV	Thalamostriate vein
TonsV	Tonsillar vein
Torc	Torcular
TrMedV	Transverse medullary vein
Trolard	Vein of Trolard
TrPonV	Transverse pontine vein
TrvS	Transverse sinus
UncV	Uncal vein
VCMedF	Vein of cerebellomedullary fissure
VCMesF	Vein of cerebellomesencephalic fissure
VCPonF	Vein of cerebellopontine fissure
VoG	Vein of Galen
VPonMedS	Vein of the pontomedullary sulcus
VPonMesS	Vein of the pontomesencephalic sulcus

Table P.5 Abbreviations for brain, gyri, nerves, cisterns, and miscellaneous

Type	Abbreviation	Name
Brain	ACP	Anterior clinoid process
	AVM	Arteriovenous malformation
	Cau	Caudate nucleus
	Cbl	Cerebellum
	CC	Corpus callosum
	CEN	Central executive network
	CenM	Centromedian (thalamus)
	CerMes	Cerebellomesencephalic
	CerPon	Cerebellopontine
	ChFis	Choroidal fissure
	Clau	Claustrum
	CP	Choroid plexus
	CPed	Cerebral peduncle
	CST	Corticospinal tract
	DAN	Dorsal attention network
	DMN	Default mode network
	EC	External capsule
	Floc	Flocculus
	FoM	Foramen of Monro
	GPe	Globus pallidus pars externa
	GPi	Globus pallidus pars interna
	IC	Internal capsule
	ICP	Inferior cerebellar peduncle
	INC	Interstitial nucleus of Cajal
	IPL	Inferior parietal lobule
	LD	Lateral dorsal nucleus
	Lent	Lentiform nucleus
	LGB	Lateral geniculate body
	LGN	Lateral geniculate nucleus
	LN	Limbic and paralimbic network
	LP	Lateral posterior nucleus
	MCP	Middle cerebellar peduncle
	MDl	Medial dorsal parvocellular
	MDm	Medial dorsal magnocellular
	MedVe	Medial vermian
	MGN	Medial geniculate nucleus
	MLF	Medial longitudinal fasciculus
	MoL	Membrane of Liliequist
	ParamedVe	Paramedian vermian
	PCP	Posterior clinoid process
	PetrFis	Petrosal fissure
	PMS	Pontomedullary sulcus
	PPRF	Paramedian pontine reticular formation
	PuA	Anterior pulvinar
	PuL	Lateral pulvinar

(Continued)

Table P.5 (*Continued*) Abbreviations for brain, gyri, nerves, cisterns, and miscellaneous

Type	Abbreviation	Name
	PuM	Medial pulvinar
	Put	Putamen
	riMLF	Rostral interstitial nucleus of medial longitudinal fasciculus
	RN	Red nucleus
	SCP	Superior cerebellar peduncle
	SMA	Supplementary motor area
	SMN	Sensorimotor network
	SN	Salience network
	SOF	Superior orbital fissure
	SPL	Superior parietal lobule
	STN	Subthalamic nucleus
	Tent	Tentorium
	Tha	Thalamus
	VA	Ventral anterior nucleus
	VAN	Ventral attention network
	Vent	Ventricle
	Vermohem	Vermohemispheric
	VI	Ventral intermediate nucleus
	VL	Ventral lateral nucleus
	VLa	Ventral lateral anterior subnucleus
	VLp	Ventral lateral posterior subnucleus
	VN	Visual network
	VPL	Ventral posterolateral nucleus
	VPM	Ventral posteromedial nucleus
Gyri	AOG	Anterior orbital
	IFG	Inferior frontal
	IOG	Inferior occipital
	ITG	Inferior temporal
	LOG	Lateral orbital
	MFG	Middle frontal
	MOG	Medial orbital
	MTG	Middle temporal
	OTG	Occipitotemporal
	POG	Posterior orbital
	SFG	Superior frontal
	SOG	Superior occipital
	STG	Superior temporal
Nerves	CN	Cranial nerve
	CN I, or I	Olfactory
	CN II, or II	Optic
	CN III, or III	Oculomotor
	CN IV, or IV	Trochlear
	CN V, or V	Trigeminal
	CN VI, or VI	Abducens
	CN VII, or VII	Facial
	CN VIII, or VIII	Vestibulocochlear

(Continued)

Table P.5 (*Continued*) Abbreviations for brain, gyri, nerves, cisterns, and miscellaneous

Type	Abbreviation	Name
	CN IX, or IX	Glossopharyngeal
	CN X, or X	Vagus
	CN XI, or XI	Spinal accessory
	CN XII, or XII	Hypoglossal
	GSPN	Greater superficial petrosal
	V2	Maxillary division of CN V
	V3	Mandibular division of CN V
Cisterns	AmbC	Ambient
	AntSpC	Anterior spinal
	CallC	Callosal
	CarC	Carotid
	CbMedC	Cerebellomedullary
	CbMesC	Cerebellomesencephalic
	CbPonC	Cerebellopontine
	ChiC	Chiasmatic
	CruC	Crural
	IpC	Interpeduncular
	LTC	Lamina terminalis
	MagnC	Cisterna magna
	MedC	Premedullary
	OlfC	Olfactory
	PonC	Prepontine
	PosSpC	Posterior spinal
	QuadC	Quadrigeminal
	SylC	Sylvian
Miscellaneous	A#B#C#	Age, bleeding, and compactness in Supplementary Grading Scale
	An	Aneurysm
	Ant	Anterior
	AUC	Area under the curve
	BiFr	Bifrontal
	BTO	Balloon test occlusion
	CM	Cavernous malformation
	Contra	Contralateral
	CSF	Cerebrospinal fluid
	CT	Computed tomography
	DDR	Distal dural ring
	Decuss	Decussation of the SCPs
	DVA	Developmental venous anomaly
	EAC	External auditory canal
	EC-IC	Extracranial-to-intracranial
	EEG	Electroencephalography
	Exo	Exophytic
	FLAIR	Fluid-attenuated inversion recovery
	fMRI	Functional magnetic resonance imaging
	GCT	Glossopharyngeal-cochlear triangle
	GOS	Glasgow Outcome Scale

(Continued)

Table P.5 (*Continued*) Abbreviations for brain, gyri, nerves, cisterns, and miscellaneous

Type	Abbreviation	Name
	HHT	Hypoglossal-hypoglossal triangle
	IAC	Internal auditory canal
	ICG	Indocyanine green
	IC-IC	Intracranial-to-intracranial
	IHT	Infrahypoglossal triangle
	Inf	Inferior
	INO	Internuclear ophthalmoplegia
	Ipsil	Ipsilateral
	IQR	Interquartile range
	L	Left
	Lat	Lateral
	Med	Medial
	MEP	Motor evoked potentials
	Mo	Month
	MRI	Magnetic resonance imaging
	mRS	Modified Rankin Scale
	N/A	Not applicable
	N/V	Nausea and vomiting
	NPV	Negative predictive value
	OR	Odds ratio
	OTT	Oculomotor-tentorial triangle
	OZ	Orbitozygomatic
	Para	Paramedian
	Pos	Posterior
	Postop	Postoperative
	PPV	Positive predictive value
	Preop	Preoperative
	Pt	Pterional
	R	Right
	RAG	Radial artery graft
	RCPM	Rectus capitis posterior major
	ROIs	Regions of interest
	RS	Retrosigmoid
	S#V#E#	Size, venous drainage, eloquence in Spetzler–Martin Grading Scale
	SAH	Subarachnoid hemorrhage
	SC	Supracerebellar
	SCM	Sternocleidomastoid muscle
	SD	Standard deviation
	SEZ	Safe entry zone
	SHT	Suprahypoglossal triangle
	SPECT	Single photon emission computed tomography
	SSEP	Somatosensory evoked potentials
	Sup	Superior
	Super	Superficial

Note: # indicates the grade.

Table P.6 Encyclopedia of approaches

Approach	Abbreviation	Name
Transgyral or transsulcal	TCbl	Transcerebellar
	TGyr	Transgyral
	TGyr-Fro	Frontal transgyral
	TGyr-Ins	Insular transgyral
	TGyr-Occ	Occipital transgyral
	TGyr-Par	Parietal transgyral
	TGyr-Tem	Temporal transgyral
	THem	Transhematoma
	TSul	Transsulcal
	TSul-Fro	Frontal transsulcal
	TSul-Ins	Insular transsulcal
	TSul-Occ	Occipital transsulcal
	TSul-Par	Parietal transsulcal
	TSul-Tem	Temporal transsulcal
Transsylvian	cTSyl-IntPed	Transsylvian-contralateral interpeduncular
	sFro-TLT	Subfrontal trans-lamina terminalis
	TSyl	Transsylvian
	TSyl-AIns	Transsylvian-anterior transinsular
	TSyl-Cav	Transsylvian-pretemporal-transcavernous
	TSyl-Cav-Pon	Transsylvian-transcavernous-transpontine
	TSyl-cPed	Transsylvian-contralateral transpeduncular
	TSyl-Fro	Transsylvian-transfrontal
	TSyl-IntPed	Transsylvian interpeduncular
	TSyl-LT	Transsylvian-subfrontal–trans-lamina terminalis
	TSyl-Ped	Transsylvian-transpeduncular
	TSyl-PIns	Transsylvian-posterior transinsular
	TSyl-SCIF	Transsylvian-supracarotid-infrafrontal
	TSyl-Tem	Transsylvian-transtemporal
	TSyl-TGyr	Transsylvian-transgyral
	TSyl-TSul	Transsylvian-transulcal
Interhemi-spheric	ATCal	Anterior transcallosal
	cAI	Contralateral anterior interhemispheric
	cAI-Falx	Contralateral anterior interhemispheric-transfalcine
	cATCal	Contralateral anterior transcallosal
	cPI	Contralateral posterior interhemispheric
	cPI-Falx	Contralateral posterior interhemispheric-transfalcine
	cPTCal	Contralateral posterior transcallosal
	cTCing	Contralateral transcingulate
	FarAI	Far anterior interhemispheric
	iAI	Ipsilateral anterior interhemispheric

(*Continued*)

Table P.6 (*Continued*) Encyclopedia of approaches

Approach	Abbreviation	Name
	iPI	Ipsilateral posterior interhemispheric
	iTCing	Ipsilateral transcingulate
	PTCal	Posterior transcallosal
	SFro	Subfrontal
	TCun	Transcuneal
Transventricular	cPTCal-Vent	Contralateral posterior transcallosal-transventricular
	cTCal-cTChor	Contralateral transcallosal–contralateral trans-choroidal fissure (subforniceal)
	cTCal-iFor	Contralateral transcallosal-ipsilateral transforaminal
	cTCal-iTChor	Contralateral transcallosal-ipsilateral transchoroidal fissure (supraforniceal)
	cTCal-Vent	Contralateral transcallosal-transventricular
	Fro-Sul-Vent	Frontal-transsulcal-transventricular
	iTCal-Vent	Ipsilateral transcallosal-transventricular
	PTCal-Vent	Posterior transcallosal-transventricular
	sFro-TLT	Subfrontal trans-lamina terminalis
	SPL-Atr	Superior parietal lobule-transatrial
	TCal-For	Transcallosal-transforaminal
	TCal-IF	Transcallosal-interforniceal
	TCal-SChor	Transcallosal–sub-choroidal fissure (subchoroidal)
	TCal-TChor	Transcallosal–trans-choroidal fissure (subforniceal)
	Tem-TChor	Transtemporal–trans-choroidal fissure
	Tem-Vent	Transtemporal-transventricular
	TLT	Subfrontal–trans-lamina terminalis
Transtentorial	cOTT	Contralateral occipital transtentorial
	cSCIT	Contralateral supracerebellar-infratentorial
	cSCTT	Contralateral supracerebellar-transtentorial
	iOTT	Ipsilateral occipital transtentorial
	iSCTT	Ipsilateral supracerebellar-transtentorial
	ITIT	Infratentorial-infratrochlear
	SCIT	Supracerebellar-infratentorial
	SCIT-IS	Supracerebellar-infratentorial inverted subchoroidal

(Continued)

Table P.6 (*Continued*) Encyclopedia of approaches

Approach	Abbreviation	Name
	SCIT-Lat	Lateral supracerebellar-infratentorial
	SCIT-Mid	Midline supracerebellar-infratentorial
	SCIT-Para	Paramedian supracerebellar-infratentorial
	SCST	Supracerebellar-supratrochlear
	SCTT	Supracerebellar-transtentorial
	ST	Subtemporal
	STIO	Supratentorial-infraoccipital
	STTT	Subtemporal-transtentorial
Transpetrous	Comb-SIT	Combined supra- and infratentorial
	Kaw	Kawase
	MidFos	Middle fossa approach
	RLab	Retrolabyrinthine
	RLab-Cru	Retrolabyrinthine-transcrural
	RLab-Sig	Retrolabyrinthine-transsigmoid
	RS-CPA	Retrosigmoid–trans-cerebellopontine angle
	TCliv-PonC	Transclival–trans-pontine cistern
	TCoc	Transcochlear
	TLab	Translabyrinthine
	xRS	Extended retrosigmoid
	xRS-CPA	Extended retrosigmoid–trans-cerebellopontine angle
	xRS-MCP	Extended retrosigmoid–trans-middle cerebellar peduncle
	xRS-Mea	Extended retrosigmoid-transmeatal
Transmagnum	FL	Far lateral
	FL-Med	Far lateral-transmedullary
	FL-PMS	Far lateral–trans-pontomedullary sulcus
	FL-PreMed	Far lateral–trans-premedullary cistern
	FL-xRS	Combined far lateral-retrosigmoid
	SOcc	Suboccipital
	SOcc-Magna	Suboccipital–trans-cisterna magna
	SOcc-Mid	Suboccipital-midline
	SOcc-Para	Suboccipital-paramedian
	SOcc-Supra-Tons	Suboccipital-supratonsillary
	SOcc-TeVe	Suboccipital-telovelar
	SOcc-Vent	Suboccipital-transventricular
	SOcc-Verm	Suboccipital-transvermian
	STons	Supratonsillar

Table P.7 Summary of cerebral gyri, sulci, and abbreviations of transgyral and transsulcal approaches

Lobe	Gyrus	Transgyral approach	Sulcus	Transsulcal approach
Frontal	Superior frontal gyrus	TGyr-SFG	Superior frontal sulcus	TSul-sfs
	Middle frontal gyrus	TGyr-MFG	Inferior frontal sulcus	TSul-ifs
	Inferior frontal gyrus	TGyr-IFG	Lateral sulcus, ascending ramus	TSul-las
	Precentral gyrus	TGyr-PRG	Lateral sulcus, anterior ramus	TSul-lat
	Pars opercularis	TGyr-IFGOp	Olfactory sulcus	TSul-ols
	Pars triangularis	TGyr-IFGTr	Orbital sulcus (lateral, medial, transverse)	TSul-ors
	Pars orbitalis	TGyr-IFGOr	Cingulate sulcus	TSul-cgs
	Gyrus rectus	TGyr-GR	Callosal sulcus	TSul-scc
	Orbital gyri (medial, lateral, anterior, posterior)	TGyr-MOrG, LOrG, AOrG, POrG	Precentral sulcus	TSul-pces
	Paracentral lobule	TGyr-PCL	Central sulcus	TSul-ces
	Cingulate gyrus	TGyr-CG	–	–
	Paraolfactory gyrus	TGyr-PaOG	–	–
	Subcallosal area/paraterminal gyrus	TGyr-SCA	–	–
Parietal	Postcentral gyrus	TGyr-POG	Postcentral sulcus	TSul-pcs
	Superior parietal lobule	TGyr-SPL	Intraparietal sulcus	TSul-ips
	Inferior parietal lobule	TGyr-IPL	Parieto-occipital sulcus	TSul-pos
	Supramarginal gyrus	TGyr-SMG	Lateral sulcus, posterior ramus	TSul-lpor
	Angular gyrus	TGyr-AG	Subparietal sulcus	TSul-sps
	Anterior paracentral gyrus	TGyr-APaG	–	–
	Posterior paracentral gyrus	TGyr-PPaG	–	–
	Precuneus	TGyr-PCun	–	–
Occipital	Superior occipital gyrus	TGyr-SOG	Calcarine sulcus	TSul-cas
	Middle occipital gyrus	TGyr-MOG	Lunate sulcus	TSul-ls
	Inferior occipital gyrus	TGyr-IOG	Intraoccipital sulcus	TSul-ios
	Cuneus	TGyr-Cun	Inferior occipital sulcus	TSul-ifos
	Lingual gyrus (medial occipitotem-poral)	TGyr-LG	Preoccipital incisura	TSul-poi
Temporal	Superior temporal gyrus	TGyr-STG	Superior temporal sulcus	TSul-sts
	Middle temporal gyrus	TGyr-MTG	Inferior temporal sulcus	TSul-its
	Inferior temporal gyrus	TGyr-ITG	Occipitotemporal sulcus	TSul-ots
	Fusiform gyrus (lateral occipitotem-poral)	TGyr-FG	Collateral sulcus	TSyl-cos
	Parahippocampal gyrus	TGyr-PHG	–	–
	Hippocampus, head	TGyr-HiH	–	–
	Hippocampus, body	TGyr-HiB	–	–
	Hippocampus, tail	TGyr-HiT	–	–
	Uncus (gyrus intralimbicus, uncinate gyrus, limbus Giacomini)	TGyr-Un	–	–
	Transverse temporal gyrus (Heschl's gyrus)	TGyr-TTG (anterior, posterior)	–	–
	Planum polare	TGyr-PPo	–	–
	Planum temporale	TGyr-PTe	–	–

Acknowledgments

Seven Cavernomas is the fourth book in the Seven Series of books, which began with *Seven Aneurysms*, followed by *Seven AVMs* and *Seven Bypasses* (Thieme). It is my most in-depth and complex book yet. *Seven Cavernomas* includes over 700+ exquisitely rendered illustrations and clinical images. Moreover, it incorporates 73 intraoperative videos and animations. This work was made possible with the support of Barrow Neurological Institute's talented and dedicated Neuroscience Publications team, for whom I am incredibly grateful. Samantha Soto, publishing specialist, tracked and coordinated all aspects of manuscript formatting, production, and submission. Cassie Todd, senior medical graphics specialist, tracked, coordinated, labeled, and formatted all images, with the help of Hannah Hunt, medical graphics specialist. Cassie also handled copyright and permissions for all images used in the book. Lynda Orescanin, managing editor, and Joseph Mills, editor, polished my prose and ensured consistency, clarity, and accuracy from chapter to chapter. Joseph also edited the video text. Marie Clarkson, medical video editor and multimedia specialist, and Julio Juarez-Alvarez, medical video editor and multimedia specialist, sifted through hours of intraoperative videos to select the pertinent sections to demonstrate each intended surgical nuance. They edited the recorded narrative and merged it with video footage into a cohesive story. Our multimedia team was led by Kristen Larson Keil, manager and senior medical illustrator, and included Peter M. Lawrence, senior medical illustrator, Danielle VanBrabant, senior medical animator/illustrator, and Michael D. Hickman, senior technical artist, with illustration support from Miranda Stano, medical illustrator. The team's artistic talent and depth of anatomical acumen are highlighted throughout the book. Peter M. Lawrence created the beautiful cover art, highlighting the brain cartography theme of the book.

I thank my family, especially my wife Suzanne, for their patience and ongoing support. Time to write and intrusion into family time are not insignificant, and I could not have finished without their understanding. I thank my colleagues here and elsewhere, including my current and former residents and fellows and those listed below for their contributions* to the series of articles, published in the *Journal of Neurosurgery*, that are the basis for this comprehensive compendium on cavernous malformations. Jim Rutka, Editor-in-Chief of the *Journal of Neurosurgery*, graciously agreed to publish these articles as the *Seven Cavernomas Collection*, and I am grateful to him and the editors for doing so.

Finally, I thank the team at Thieme Medical Publishers, including Karen Edmonson and Cathrin Weinstein, for their encouragement and assistance, without whom this book would not have been produced.

*Authors who contributed to the *Seven Cavernomas* articles published in the *Journal of Neurosurgery:*

Arnau Benet
Dimitri Benner
Joshua S. Catapano
Tyler S. Cole
Nicholas B. Dadario
Diego A. Devia
Adam T. Eberle
Roxanna M. Garcia
Christopher S. Graffeo
Benjamin K. Hendricks
Michael D. Hickman
Kate N. Jensen
Jubran H. Jubran
Katherine Karahalios
Anna R. Kimata
Stefan W. Koester
Mohamed A. Labib
Kristen Larson Keil
Peter M. Lawrence
Kevin L. Ma
Ramin A. Morshed
Taemin Oh
Redi Rahmani
Kunal P. Raygor
Emmajane G. Rhodenhiser
Kavelin Rumalla
Caleb Rutledge
Satvir Saggi
Lea Scherschinski
Mark Schornak
Nathan A. Shlobin
Robert F. Spetzler
Visish M. Srinivasan
Michael E. Sughrue
Ali Tayebi Meybodi
Danielle VanBrabant
Ethan A. Winkler

Section I

The Tenets

I

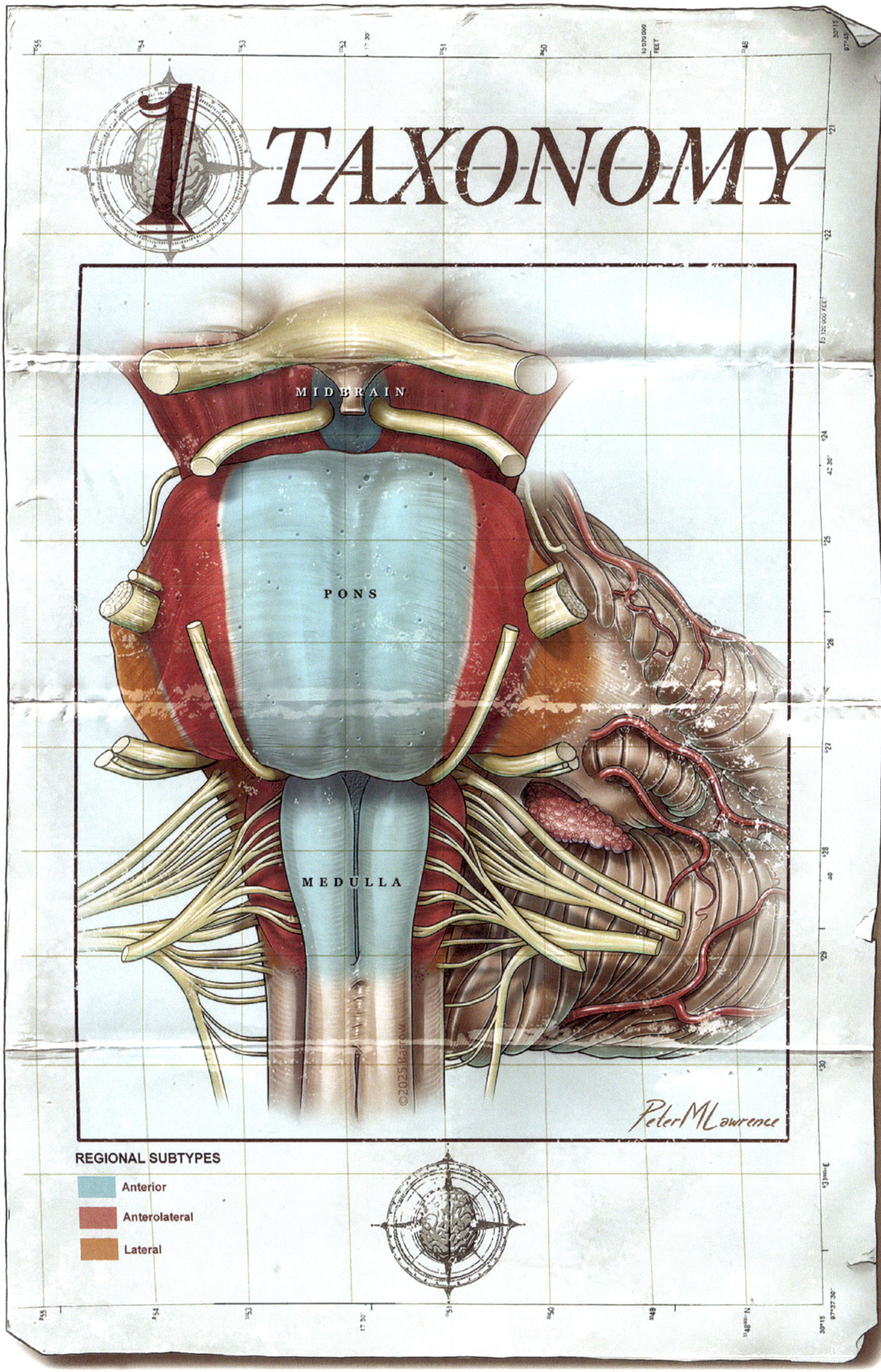

Reproduced with permission from Barrow Neurological Institute, Phoenix, AZ.

1 Taxonomy

Summary
Cavernous malformations are highly variable and seemingly random vascular anomalies that occur in every possible size, shape, and location in the central nervous system. This variability makes it difficult to envision the spectrum of disease caused by these lesions within a simplified framework. The creation of a taxonomy to organize cavernomas by neuroanatomical location and morphology brings order to an otherwise chaotic disease spectrum. The taxonomy defines seven cavernoma types and 35 subtypes and organizes them into a classification system that guides surgical strategy and patient management.

Keywords: brainstem, cavernous malformation, cerebellum, cerebrum, ependymal, hemorrhage, pial, resection, subtype, tenet

1.1 Classifying Surgical Pathology

Cavernomas occur in every imaginable size, shape, and location in the central nervous system, from cerebral convexity to conus medullaris. They range in size from submillimeter specks seen only on gradient echo sequences on magnetic resonance imaging (MRI) to the nearly holohemispheric 13 × 7-cm lesion I removed through a hemicraniotomy in a 12-year-old child. They can be shaped like freshly picked mulberries, intermixed with pockets of liquified or desiccated blood, or encapsulated in a thick rind. Cavernomas are far more variable than aneurysms, which occur regularly at specific branch points around the circle of Willis. Detailed knowledge of even just seven aneurysm types, and mastery of the basic surgical steps for treating them, empowers the neurosurgeon to manage more than three-quarters of all aneurysms seen in clinical practice. In contrast, cavernomas are seemingly random and endless in their distribution and morphology, making it difficult to encompass this spectrum of disease with a simplified framework.

Taxonomy is one method to bring order to an otherwise chaotic spectrum of disease. Taxonomy comes from the Greek word *taxis*, meaning arrangement or order, and *nomos*, meaning method or law, and is defined as the scientific classification of organisms and things. In zoology, for example, the study of animals' structure, physiology, embryology, habits, and habitats enables their classification into genera and species to make sense of the unlimited variety seen in the animal kingdom. The taxonomic binomial nomenclature uniquely defines the more than 1.5 million species of wildlife encountered in nature. Just as taxonomy classifies animals hierarchically into a system that enables biologists to identify animals in the wilderness, this cavernous malformation (CM) taxonomy classifies cavernomas hierarchically into a system that enables neurosurgeons to uniquely define the spectrum of pathology encountered in clinical practice (▶ Fig. 1.1). In short, taxonomy organizes a broad spectrum of pathology into a discrete number of entities that can be easily recognized to simplify and better understand the disease.

1.2 Informing Surgical Strategy

In addition to simplifying something complex, taxonomy enables scientists to find the information they need about a particular organism or thing. For example, a trip to Bali before starting my neurosurgical residency introduced me to the Komodo dragon. Tourists like me would ferry to the southeastern Indonesian island of Flores to observe these 70- to 90-kg (150- to 200-lb) beasts that grow to nearly 3 m (10 ft) in length and are capable of consuming livestock in several bites. These so-called dragons were first described by Europeans in 1910 as land crocodiles but are members of the monitor lizard family Varanidae (*Varanus komodoensis*), which also includes earless and Gray's monitors. Monitors are known as the most intelligent of lizards, forage for meat and fruits, and possess unidirectional pulmonary airflow. Just as taxonomy leads quickly to an understanding of the Komodo dragon in this example, it can also lead neurosurgeons to information needed to optimally manage patients with a particular CM in the brain.

Taxonomy has its greatest value when the differentiation of things leads to the differentiation of actions. Distinguishing one cavernoma type from another may be unimportant if the treatment for both is the same, but making such a distinction is crucial if their treatments are different. The classification of spinal arteriovenous malformations provides a dramatic example. The dural arteriovenous fistula (type 1) and the perimedullary arteriovenous fistula (type 4) can look similar on spinal angiography with arteriovenous shunting from a radicular artery to draining perimedullary veins. The fistulous site is located at the dural root sleeve in type 1 lesions and more distally at the pial surface in type 4 lesions. Surgical treatment of the former interrupts the fistula by coagulating and dividing the vein as it exits the fistula at the dura. In contrast, surgical treatment of the latter interrupts the fistula by clipping and dividing pathological branches from the anterior spinal artery on the ventral spinal cord. Misinterpretation of a type 4 fistula as a type 1 fistula might lead to the occlusion of an artery of Adamkiewicz as it enters the spinal subarachnoid space, with harmful neurological consequences and residual arteriovenous shunting. Conversely, misinterpretation of a type 1 fistula as a type 4 fistula might lead to the ineffectual remote occlusion of the draining vein from the fistula and residual arteriovenous shunting. In this example, successful treatment of the patient depends on the correct interpretation of the angiogram and classification of the arteriovenous pathology. Taxonomy for CMs has a similar potential to empower the management of this disease because the differentiation of cavernoma types and subtypes leads to different operations involving different craniotomies and surgical approaches. Therefore, a taxonomy for cavernomas has value because it informs surgical strategy.

1.3 Neuroanatomy

Like zoological taxonomy, neurosurgical taxonomy should be rooted scientifically in precise and reproducible facts, and in

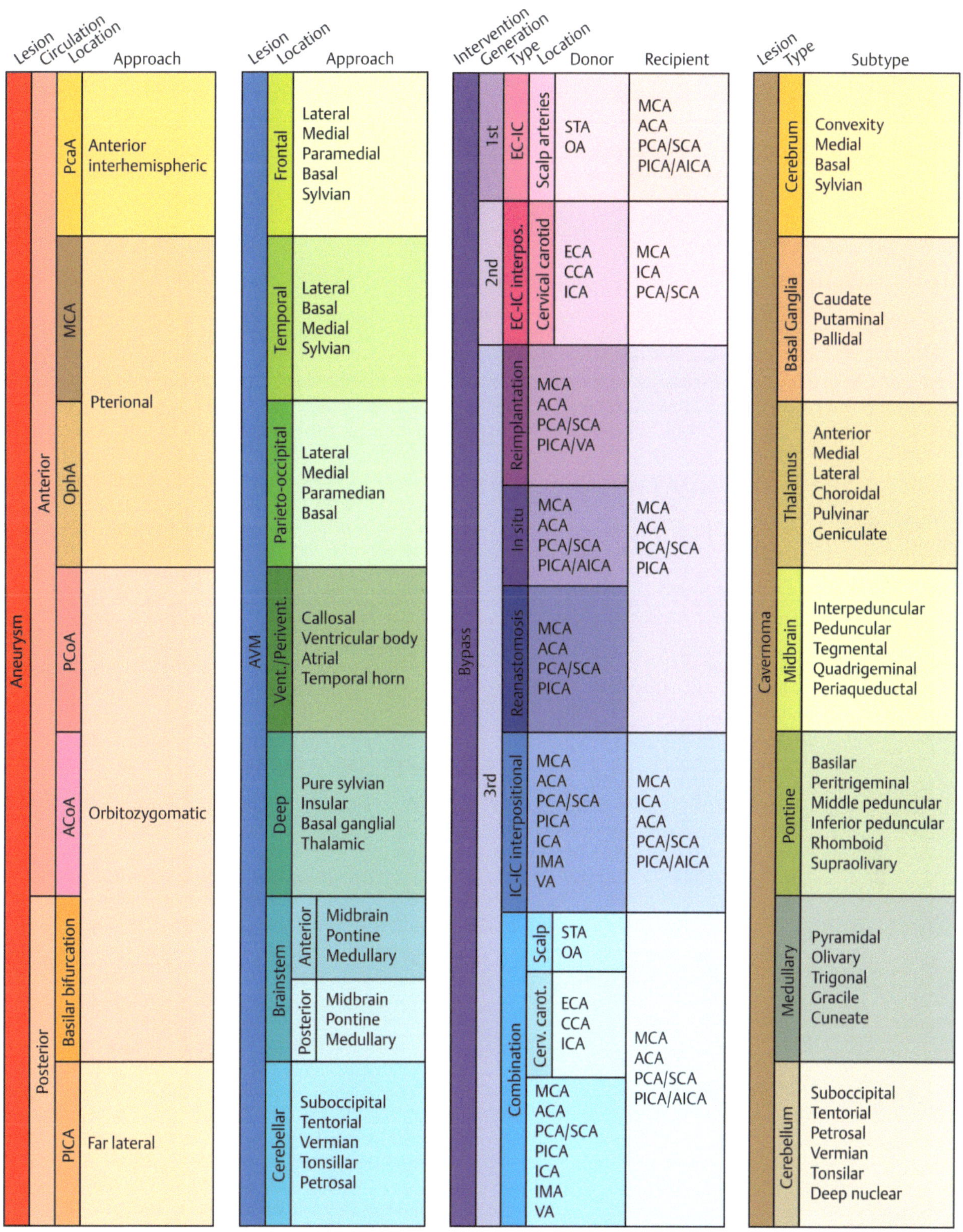

Fig. 1.1 The cavernous malformation taxonomy classifies cavernomas hierarchically into a system that enables neurosurgeons to uniquely define the spectrum of pathologies encountered in clinical practice. This taxonomy organizes a broad spectrum of pathologies into discrete entities that can be easily recognized to simplify and better understand the disease. Similar taxonomies have classified the spectrums of aneurysm and arteriovenous malformation pathologies, as well as the spectrum of bypass techniques. (Reproduced with permission from Barrow Neurological Institute, Phoenix, AZ.)

Table 1.1 Taxonomy of cavernoma types and subtypes

Type	Subtypes
Cerebrum	Convexity, medial, basal, and sylvian
Basal ganglia	Caudate, putaminal, and pallidal
Thalamus	Anterior, medial, lateral, choroidal, pulvinar, and geniculate
Midbrain	Interpeduncular, peduncular, tegmental, quadrigeminal, and periaqueductal
Pontine	Basilar, peritrigeminal, middle peduncular, inferior peduncular, rhomboid, and supraolivary
Medullary	Pyramidal, olivary, trigonal, gracile, and cuneate
Cerebellum	Suboccciptal, tentorial, petrosal, vermian, tonsillar, and deep nuclear

the case of cavernomas, that taxonomy should be based on neuroanatomy. The big idea in *Seven Cavernomas: Tenets and Techniques for Resection* is the introduction of a comprehensive taxonomy for all CMs encountered in the brain that is based on neuroanatomy, clearly defined, and applicable at the bedside. Like other taxonomies, the cavernoma taxonomy is a hierarchical system that characterizes a lesion's type and subtype (▶ Table 1.1). There are seven types according to lesion location in the brain: (1) cerebrum, (2) basal ganglia, (3) thalamus, (4) midbrain, (5) pons, (6) medulla, and (7) cerebellum. Cavernomas in the gyri, sulci, and subcortical white matter of the superficial cerebrum are the most common in clinical practice because this territory comprises 85% of the brain's volume. Deep cerebral cavernomas reside in the basal ganglia and thalami, which together make up the central core of the brain and serve as the brain's information gateway, relaying and modulating signals from the periphery to the cortex. The brainstem occupies only roughly 5% of the brain's overall territory, but brainstem cavernomas account for three of the seven cavernoma types because their central location and depth make surgical strategy nuanced and complex. The seventh type comprises cavernomas in the cerebellum, the so-called little brain. The borders and boundaries of the seven types satisfy our conditions of clarity and applicability for a meaningful taxonomy.

Cavernoma types are defined by general brain regions, and subtypes are defined by the surface within that region where the lesion presents (▶ Fig. 1.2, ▶ Fig. 1.3). Surface presentation is a fundamental concept in surgical strategy because it guides approach selection and minimizes brain transgression. Lesions presenting at (superficial) or protruding through (exophytic) the pial or ependymal surfaces are accessed with minimal violation of normal tissue and resected with an inherently lower risk of neurological injury. In contrast, lesions presenting beneath the pial and ependymal surfaces (deep) are accessed only by violation of normal tissue, which raises the risks. Each cavernoma type has multiple pial or ependymal surfaces that define the subtypes. The cerebral hemispheres have four surfaces—convexity, medial, basal, and sylvian surfaces—throughout the frontal, parietal, occipital, and temporal lobes. The brainstem has anterior, anterolateral, lateral, posterolateral, and posterior surfaces, giving five or six subtypes for each type. The cerebellum has six subtypes, of which five are based on surfaces: suboccipital, tentorial, petrosal, vermian, and tonsillar. The thalamus and basal ganglia have limited or no communication with subarachnoid surfaces, and subtyping for these deep cerebral types is based on buried surfaces and nuclear anatomy. Similarly, the sixth cerebellar subtype is based on the deep anatomy of the dentate, emboliform, globose, and fastigial nuclei rather than surface presentation.

The comprehensive taxonomy for all CMs contains 7 types, 3 to 6 subtypes within each type, and 35 subtypes overall. The neuroanatomy of the 35 subtypes follows in Section II of the book, each defined with prominent surface landmarks that can be identified radiographically and microsurgically. The borders and boundaries of the 35 subtypes also satisfy our conditions of clarity and applicability for a meaningful taxonomy. From the cartographer's perspective, taxonomy partitions the brain into types like countries on the map and into subtypes like states within each country. Collectively, taxonomy systematically classifies every conceivable cavernoma, just as nationality and state or province of residence help classify every citizen's home.

1.4 Neuroradiology

The MRI appearance of cavernomas makes them easy to diagnose. Their popcorn-like morphology, mixed signal intensities, hemosiderin ring, and associated developmental venous anomalies are pathognomonic. Immediately after the diagnosis is established, thoughts turn to the surgical plan. The exquisite anatomical and pathological details of MRI make neuroradiology essential to surgical strategizing. These plans are needed first to calculate the surgical risk, which hangs in the balance with natural history risk to arrive at a therapeutic recommendation. Heuristics like the two-point method were devised to select the surgical approach (▶ Fig. 1.4). This method places the first point at the center of the lesion, and the second point is where the lesion comes to a pial or an ependymal surface. The line connecting these two points defines the lesion's axis. Extending this line outward to the cranium suggests an operative corridor that might lead inward to the lesion. The lesion's axis is compared with operative trajectories from the menu of surgical options, and the best match is selected. The two-point method is a crude guide at best. It relies on simple geometries on single MRI slices to draw the lesion axis, rough approximations of surgical axes, and inclusion by the neurosurgeon of appropriate approaches from the operative menu.

Taxonomy offers a completely different approach. Instead of jumping immediately to the surgical plan, the cavernoma is classified on the basis of the pathoanatomical MRI appearance. The lesion's type and subtype then indicate the best

Brain CM Subtypes

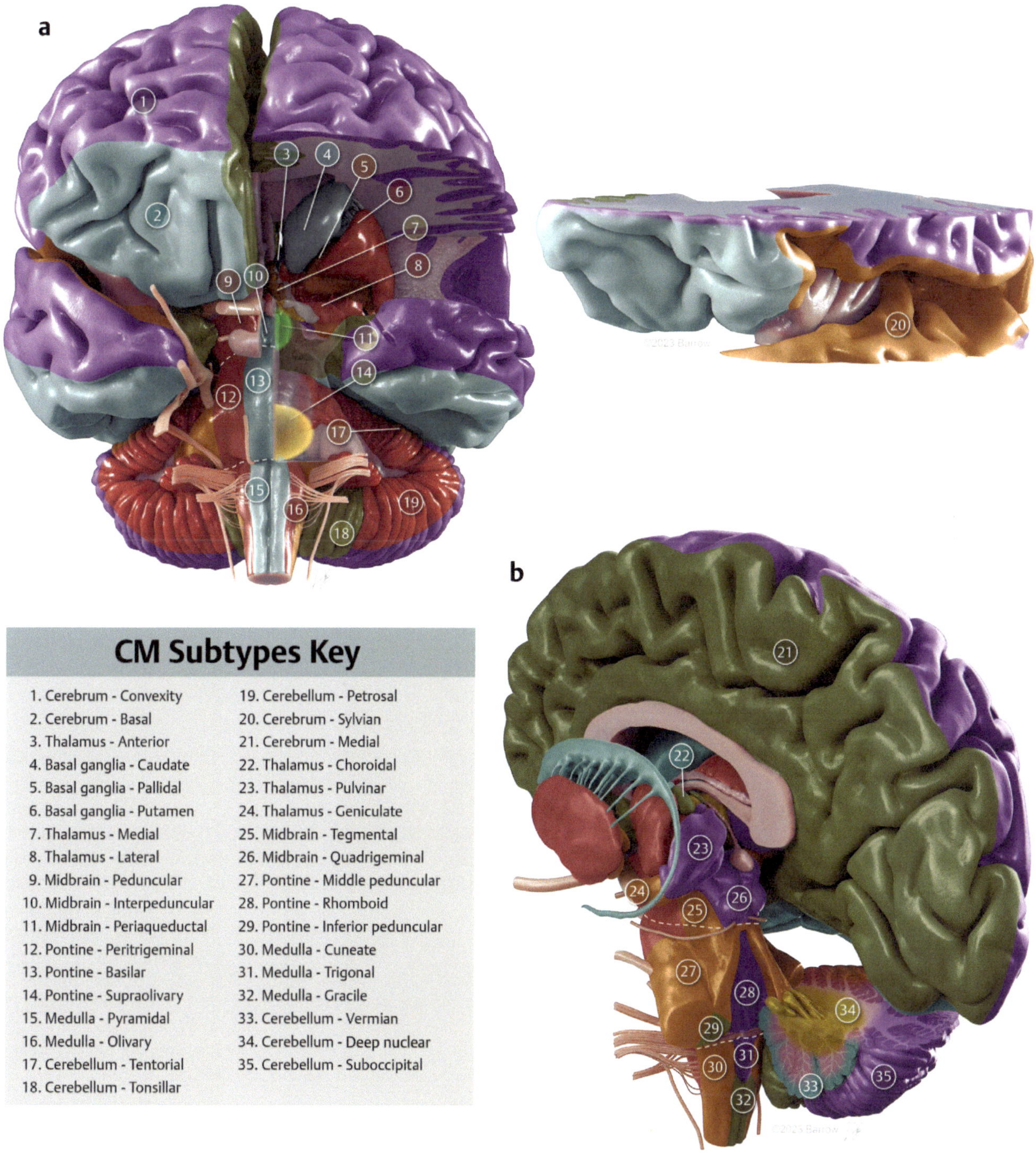

Fig. 1.2 Comprehensive taxonomy for seven cavernoma types and 35 subtypes. **(a)** The cerebrum, brainstem, and cerebellum are shown from an anterior view. An axial section of the left frontal, parietal, and temporal lobes is removed at the level of the sylvian fissure and insula to show some of the basal ganglia and thalamic subtypes. **(b)** The right cerebrum and cerebellum, left basal ganglia and thalamus, and brainstem are shown from a posterior oblique view. Cavernoma types and subtypes are numbered in the subtype key (*inset*). (Reproduced with permission from Barrow Neurological Institute, Phoenix, AZ.)

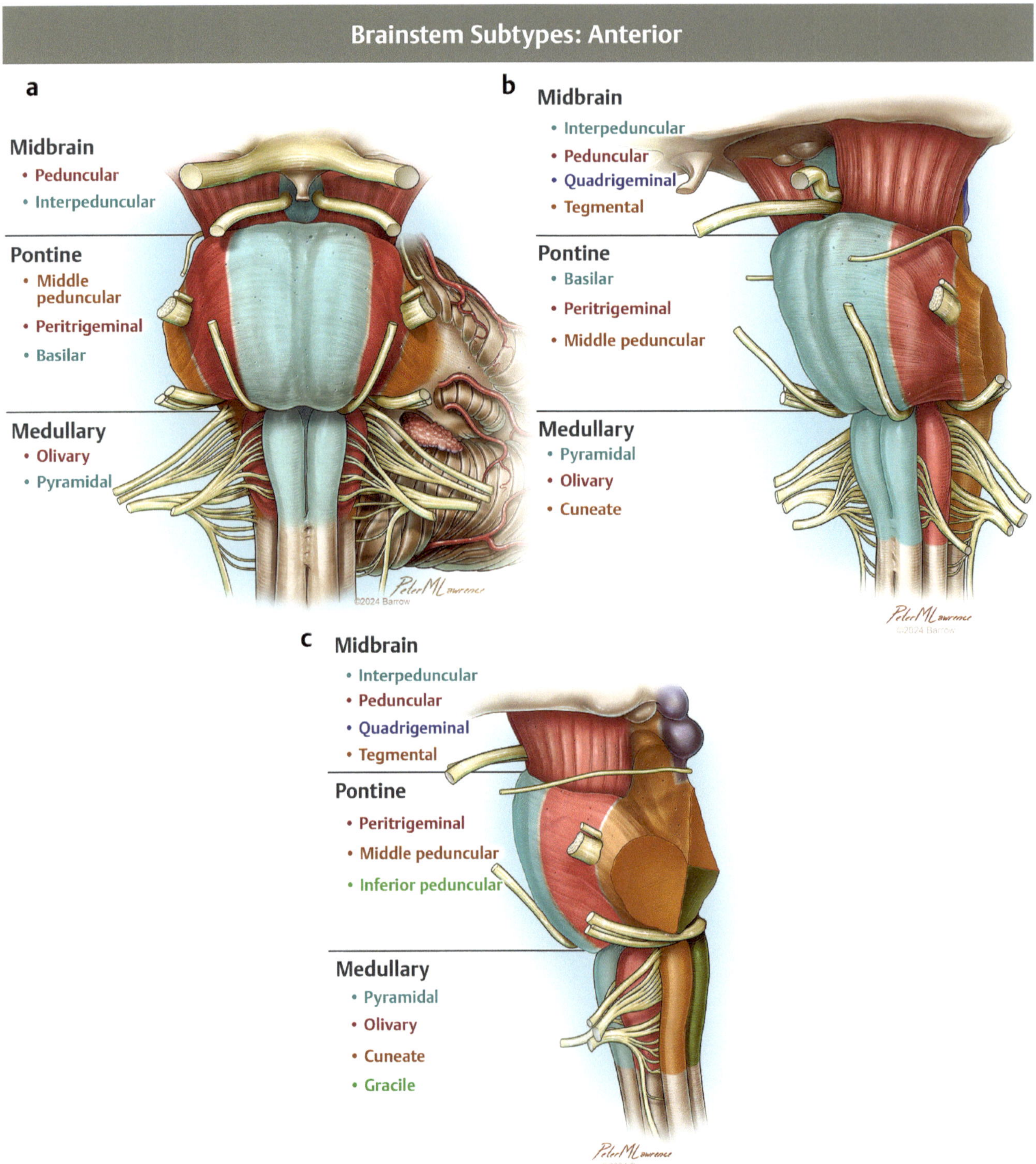

Fig. 1.3 The taxonomy for brainstem types and subtypes is shown in various perspectives: **(a)** anterior, **(b)** anterolateral, **(c)** lateral,

(Continued)

craniotomy and surgical approach based on surgical experience and clinical evidence (▶ Table 1.2). The recommendations tabulated for the various cavernomas in the taxonomy were derived from the combinations of Dr. Robert Spetzler's and my surgical experiences, as well as in others' works, described in this textbook and the *7 Cavernomas* series of articles published in the *Journal of Neurosurgery*. Accurate analysis and taxonomic interpretation of a patient's lesion on MRI is the first step that initiates a cascade of suggestions and decisions. Therefore, neuroradiological imaging is critical in translating pathoanatomy into an individualized classification that clarifies the course of management.

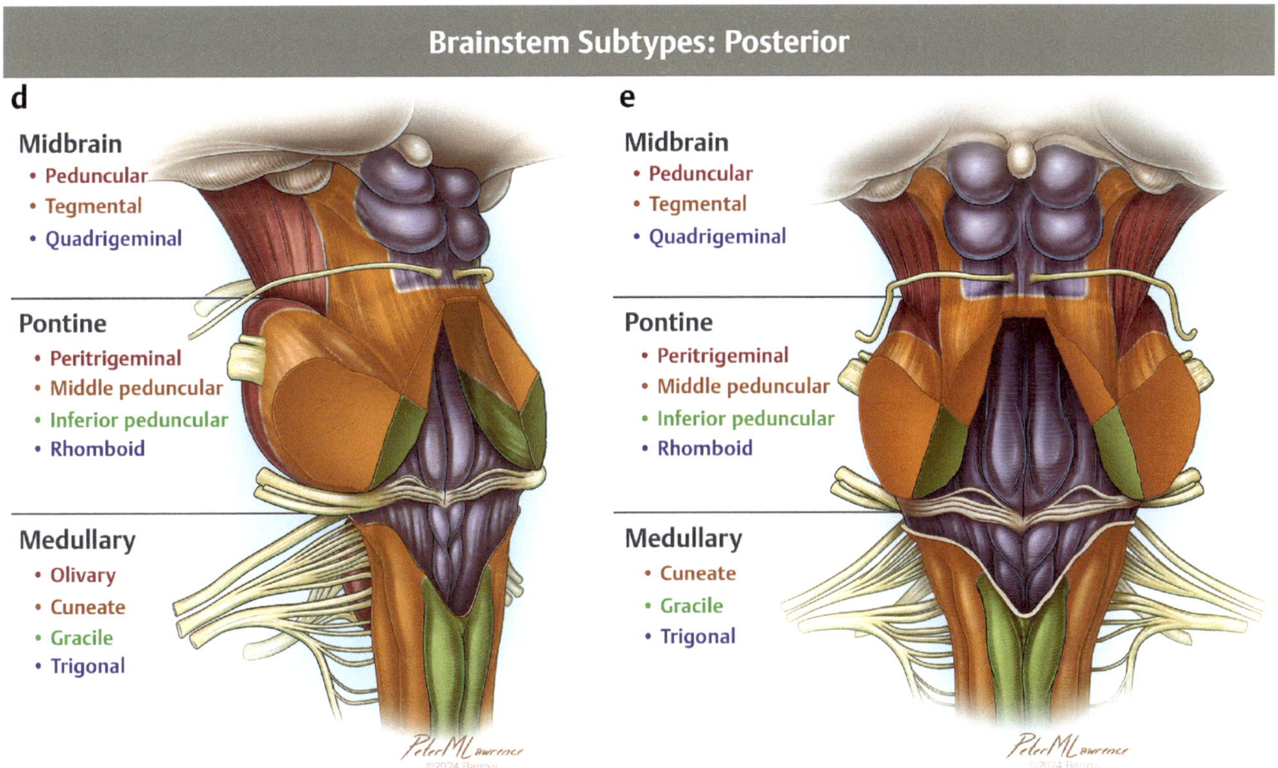

Fig. 1.3 *(Continued)* **(d)** posterolateral, and **(e)** posterior. (Reproduced with permission from Barrow Neurological Institute, Phoenix, AZ.)

1.5 Neurology

Findings from a neurological examination can localize and classify the cavernoma even before the brain MRI is ordered. Neurosurgery has always been the subspecialty of neurology focused on disorders and diseases requiring surgical treatment. This surgical focus encourages the incorporation of sophisticated equipment, advanced imaging, innovative devices, and high technology, often de-emphasizing fundamental skills like bedside examination. However, neurological findings are remarkably accurate at localizing lesions, especially in areas densely packed with tracts, cranial nerves, and their nuclei. In his remarks at the opening of the new building of the Boston Medical Library in 1901, Sir William Osler said, "Listen to your patient, he is telling you the diagnosis." Nowhere is this truer than in the patient with a brainstem cavernoma. For example, diplopia and the presence of an isolated abducens nerve palsy are clues that the patient has a supraolivary pontine CM. In addition, the presence of a preoperative deficit resulting from cavernoma hemorrhage may influence the approach selection. A patient with abducens nerve palsy without contralateral hemiparesis or hemiplegia (i.e., without Millard–Gubler syndrome) may be a better candidate for a far lateral craniotomy and trans-pontomedullary sulcus approach than an extended retrosigmoid craniotomy and transmiddle cerebellar peduncle approach because the former avoids transgressing a laterally displaced corticospinal tract. Therefore, taxonomy may boost the value of bedside acumen in neurosurgical practice. The examination findings of our patients are often minimized or overlooked in fast-paced clinical rounds and operative routines. However, they may lead to the classification of the cavernoma long before reviewing the MRIs or confirming the subtype suggested by the images.

Osler was described as one of the greatest diagnosticians ever to wield a stethoscope. The list of signs, symptoms, and diseases that bear his name is long, including Osler's sign (artificially elevated systolic blood pressure readings due to calcified atherosclerotic arteries), Osler's nodes (raised tender nodules on the pulps of fingertips and toes in the setting of subacute bacterial endocarditis), and Osler-Weber-Rendu disease (hereditary hemorrhagic telangiectasia with arteriovenous malformations in brain, lung, and liver), to name a few. Like Osler wielding the stethoscope, skilled neurologists wielding the reflex hammer, flashlight, and pin can localize a stroke from the findings on a neurological examination. Weber's, Wallenberg's, and Dejerine's syndromes arose from the constellation of symptoms and signs resulting from strokes in ascending and descending tracts, decussations, and cranial nerve nuclei. Knowledge of these classic stroke syndromes and the ability to diagnose them on the basis of subtle bedside clues is empowering. The examination becomes a puzzle of localization and a valuable tool, challenging and reinvigorating our understanding of underlying neural circuitry.

Stroke syndromes might have been abandoned in the MRI era, but cavernoma taxonomy could revive their use (▶ Table 1.3). Midbrain CMs cause Claude's, Weber's, Nothnagel's, and

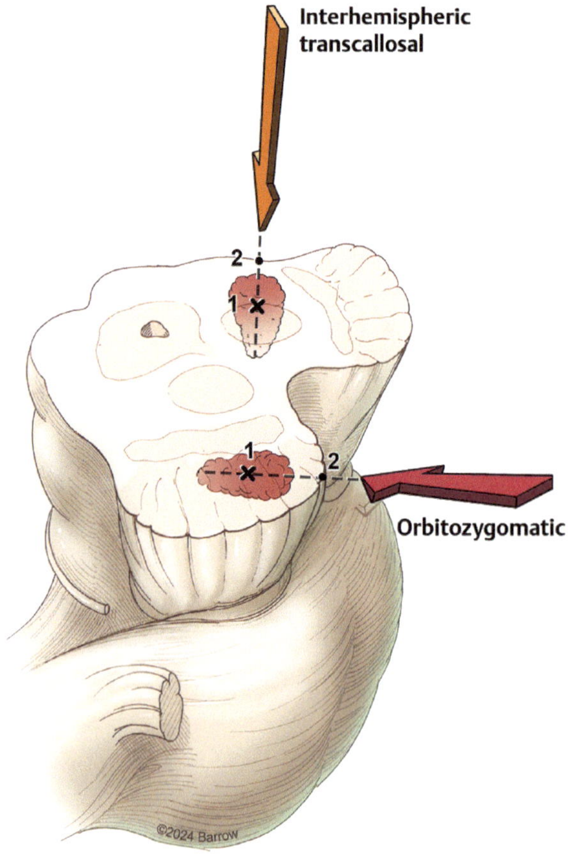

Fig. 1.4 Two-point method to determine the gross surgical approach to avoid the disturbance of eloquent brain parenchyma. The surgeon determines the center of the longest axis of the cavernoma and marks the center (x) as point 1; point 2 is then placed where the lesion comes to a pial or ependymal surface or nearest the least eloquent entry point closest to the surface of the brainstem. The line connecting these two points defines the lesion's axis. Extension of this line outward to the cranium suggests an operative corridor that leads toward the cavernoma (*orange and red arrows*). The cavernoma's axis is compared with the operative trajectories from the menu of surgical options considering the cavernoma's taxonomy and anatomical triangles, and the best match is selected. (Reproduced with permission from Barrow Neurological Institute, Phoenix, AZ.)

Parinaud's syndromes with interpeduncular, peduncular, quadrigeminal, and periaqueductal lesions, respectively. Pontine CMs cause locked-in, Marie–Foix, Millard–Gubler, and Foville's syndromes with basilar, middle peduncular, rhomboid, and supraolivary lesions, respectively. Medullary CMs cause Dejerine's and Wallenberg's syndromes with pyramidal, olivary, and cuneate CMs. In addition, novel syndromes can be defined by lesional hemorrhage by a particular subtype. For example, a new lemniscal syndrome can be described for tegmental midbrain CMs characterized by contralateral hemisensory loss of vibration and fine touch sensations, contralateral loss of pain and temperature sensations, contralateral facial hemisensory loss, and contralateral hearing impairment and tinnitus. CMs here affect the medial lemniscus, trigeminal lemniscus, lateral lemniscus, and spinothalamic tracts, where they ascend to the thalamus. Similarly, a novel trigonal medullary syndrome can be characterized by dysphagia or dysphonia, nausea, vomiting, and tongue weakness associated with CMs in the medullary floor of the fourth ventricle. A stroke cannot cause this syndrome because the vascular territory of the medullary perforators precludes it, and consequently, this syndrome has not been reported previously.

Bleeding from a CM is like a stroke, affecting a discrete area of the brain or brainstem to cause focal deficits, but is often more focal. A stroke's effect is determined not only by the location of the arterial blockage but also by the downstream ischemia in the blocked vascular territory. In contrast, a cavernoma's effect is determined only by the location of the lesion. For example, Wallenberg's or lateral medullary syndromes are caused by a posterior inferior cerebellar artery occlusion and infarction involving the entire lateral medulla, including the inferior cerebellar peduncle, spinal trigeminal nucleus and tract, vestibular nuclei, dorsal motor nucleus of cranial nerve X, solitary nucleus, and nucleus ambiguus. Olivary CMs reside in the anterolateral portion of the medulla, and cuneate CMs reside in the posterolateral portion of the medulla. Together, olivary and cuneate CMs produce the classic Wallenberg syndrome; individually, each produces either the anterior or posterior signs and symptoms of Wallenberg's syndrome, respectively. Therefore, cavernoma syndromes have greater specificity than stroke syndromes, and the definition and redefinition of cavernoma syndromes associated with the subtypes are presented throughout the book to increase our neurosurgical acumen and empower us as diagnosticians.

1.6 Neurosurgery

Taxonomy is most valuable while designing and executing surgical strategies in the operating room. Neuroanatomy organizes and simplifies the spectrum of pathology, neuroradiology translates individual cavernomas into one of the 35 subtypes, and neurological findings confirm the classification. These steps ultimately lead to a specific surgical plan that includes craniotomy, approach, anatomical triangle, safe entry zone, arterial address, and arterial dissection codes. In short, taxonomy integrates neuroanatomy, neuroradiology, and neurology to inform neurosurgical intervention.

The goals of cavernoma surgery are twofold: first, curative resection of the pathology and, second, no surgical morbidity. Prevention of future hemorrhage and protection from its harmful effects cannot be accomplished without complete resection, which is easier for cavernomas than for other pathologies in vascular and skull base surgery, like brain arteriovenous malformations, petroclival meningiomas, and acoustic neuromas. Cavernomas are not fed by arteries and can be confronted without significant bleeding. They can be entered, decompartmentalized, and resected piecemeal, unlike arteriovenous malformations. The resection technique is basic and similar for all subtypes, and the discussion of the resection technique is limited to a single chapter in this book. The second goal is not as easy to achieve. Surgical morbidity can result from many situations. The journey from craniotomy to subarachnoid corridor to triangle to target can be long and deep, with pitfalls and traps along the way.

Table 1.2 Comprehensive taxonomy for all cavernoma types and subtypes and their associated craniotomies, approaches, and anatomical triangles

Type, subtype	Craniotomy	Approach	Triangle
Cerebral			
Convexity	Convexity	TGyr, TSul	None
Medial	Bifrontal, biparieto-occipital	TGyr, TSul	None
Basal	Various	TGyr, TSul	None
Sylvian	Pterional	TSyl-TGyr, TSyl-TSul	None
Basal ganglia			
Caudate	Bifrontal	cTCal-Vent	Caudate-thalamostriate
Putaminal	Pterional	TSyl-AIns	None
Pallidal	Orbitozygomatic	TSyl-SCIF	Supracarotid
Thalamic			
Anterior	Bifrontal	cTCal-iFor	Septocaudate
Medial	Bifrontal	cTCal-cTChor, cTCal-iTChor	None
Lateral	Pterional	TSyl-PIns	None
Choroidal	Bifrontal	iTCal-Vent	None
Pulvinar	Torcular	SCIT-Para	Infragalenic
Geniculate	Torcular	cSCTT	Infragalenic
Midbrain			
Interpeduncular	Orbitozygomatic	TSyl-IntPed, cTSyl-IntPed	Carotid-oculomotor
Peduncular	Orbitozygomatic	TSyl-Ped	Oculomotor-tentorial
Tegmental	Retrosigmoid	SCIT-Lat	Supra- and infratrochlear
Quadrigeminal	Torcular	SCIT-Mid	Infragalenic
Periaqueductal	Bifrontal	TCal-TChor	None
Pontine			
Basilar	Orbitozygomatic	Kaw, TSyl-Cav-Pon	Kawase/infratrigeminal, carotid-oculomotor
Peritrigeminal	Retrosigmoid	xRS-CPA	Supra- and infratrigeminal, GCT
Middle peduncular	Retrosigmoid	xRS-MCP	Interlobular
Inferior peduncular	Suboccipital	SOcc-TeVe	Subtonsillar
Rhomboid	Suboccipital	SOcc-Vent	Vallecular
Supraolivary	Far lateral	FL-PMS	Vagoaccessory (suprahypoglossal)
Medullary			
Pyramidal	Far lateral	FL-PreMed	Junctional
Olivary	Far lateral	FL-Med	Vagoaccessory (supra- or hypoglossal-hypoglossal)
Trigonal	Suboccipital	SOcc-Vent	Vallecular
Gracile	Suboccipital	SOcc-Magna	Vallecular
Cuneate	Suboccipital	SOcc-TeVe	Subtonsillar
Cerebellum			
Suboccciptal	Suboccipital	SOcc-Para	None
Tentorial	Torcular	SCIT-Mid, SCIT-Para	None
Petrosal	Retrosigmoid	xRS-CPA	Interlobular
Vermian	Suboccipital	SOcc-Mid	None
Tonsillar	Suboccipital	SOcc-Magna	Vallecular
Deep nuclear	Suboccipital	SOcc-TeVe, SOcc-SupraTons	Vallecular

Table 1.3 Summary of brainstem taxonomy and associated neurological syndromes

Type, subtype	Syndrome
Midbrain	
Interpeduncular	Claude; Benedikt
Peduncular	Weber
Tegmental	Lemniscal syndrome
Quadrigeminal	Parinaud
Periaqueductal	Nothnagel; Claude
Pontine	
Basilar	Medial pontine; locked in
Peritrigeminal	Peritrigeminal pontine syndrome
Middle cerebellar peduncular	Marie–Foix (lateral pontine)
Supraolivary	Millard–Gubler; Foville
Rhomboid	INO; reverse INO; one-and-a-half; eight-and-a-half (facial colliculus syndrome)
Inferior cerebellar peduncular	Acute vestibular syndrome
Medulla	
Pyramidal	Dejerine
Olivary	Anterior Wallenberg
Trigonal	Trigonal medullary syndrome
Gracile	Leg numbness
Cuneate	Posterior Wallenberg

Normal tissue overlying the cavernoma might need to be transgressed to reach the lesion because the adherent capsule might not separate from the adjacent eloquent brain, and the mobilization of normal tissue might be needed to visualize hidden portions of the cavernoma within the working corridor. Achieving zero morbidity during the various phases of the operation demands meticulous dissection technique and skill. It also demands forethought and insight before entering the operating room to orchestrate a proverbial surgical strike.

The surgeon's surgical strike takes the most direct pathway from the skin to the cavernoma, opens a wide corridor to the target, exposes critical neurovascular structures, exposes pathology throughout the resection, and optimizes the chances of a cure. In the words of Al Rhoton, "a well-designed surgical strike should be accurate, simple, and safe." During beautiful surgery, strategic preoperative planning is probably more important and harder to see than meticulous operative technique. Surprisingly, the strategic aspects of cavernoma surgery are easier to teach in the pages of a book than the technical aspects. Taxonomy attempts to codify surgical strategy to choose the best approaches, guide the execution, and optimize intraoperative performance to improve patient outcomes. It might be fair to say that cavernoma surgery is the ultimate game of surgical strategy because the design and execution of the strategy have a greater effect on the results than the surgeon's resection of the pathology. That said, CM taxonomy organizes the many surgical strategies and approaches into a coherent and applicable framework.

1.7 Seven Cavernomas Framework

With 7 types and 35 subtypes in the taxonomy for cavernomas, the 7 cavernomas framework may seem complex and impractical. However, the subtypes are intuitive and easy to remember. The interconnections between taxonomy, neuroanatomy, neuroradiology, neurology, and neurosurgery are shown in ▶ Table 1.2, which is a Rosetta stone of sorts that decodes the seven cavernomas framework and summarizes the topics covered in this book. Armed with the correct subtype for the patient's cavernoma, a surgeon can consult this table, which guides surgical planning and execution. Anatomical classification leads to a unique set of recommendations for each of the 35 subtypes in the taxonomy.

We are advancing rapidly toward a future where artificial intelligence on computers and smartphones will guide these steps. I worry that we will be beholden to our workstations, feeding MRIs into a black box and waiting for the algorithm to deliver the subtype and surgical directive. Neurosurgeons would be reduced to nonthinking technicians, much like drivers who rely on dashboard navigation to prompt the next turn or exit. I prefer a future where neurosurgeons embrace the metacognitive challenges of cavernoma surgery and apply their knowledge of neuroanatomy and heuristics like taxonomy and grading systems to practice the art of neurosurgery. The more we engage in the analysis and strategy for every patient, the more adept we become at achieving our goal of safe and curative surgery. Real drivers study their road maps, design their routes, and anticipate key turns. They know their travel times, fuel needs, and arrival times. These drivers actively orienteer their way to their destination, in contrast with those who passively follow their technology for directions. The cartography metaphor is meant to encourage the learning and application of the seven cavernomas framework in pursuit of elegant and safe neurosurgery. It is also meant to encourage neurosurgeons to take the high road of thinking and strategizing their way through the subarachnoid space rather than the low road of just following directions.

2 SUBARACHNOID DISSECTION

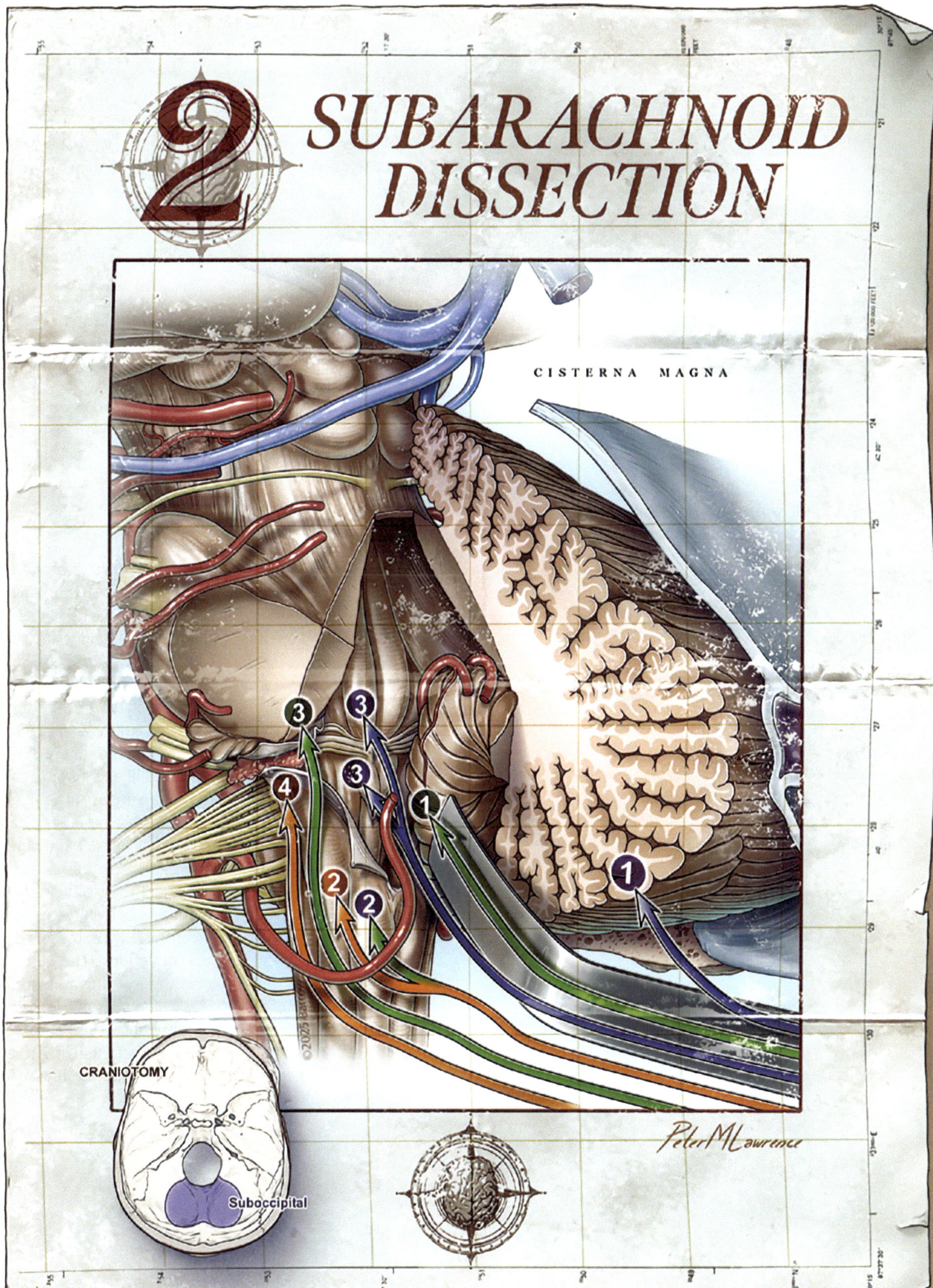

Reproduced with permission from Barrow Neurological Institute, Phoenix, AZ.

2 Subarachnoid Dissection

2

Summary
The subarachnoid space provides a passageway through the brain to navigate to cavernoma targets. Meticulous dissection of the subarachnoid membrane opens corridors beneath the cerebral convexity into the subarachnoid space through which the central depths of the brain and brainstem are reached using tissue-sparing techniques. Seven subarachnoid corridors are defined, comprising the cerebral sulci, sylvian fissure, interhemispheric fissure, ventricular system, tentorial fissure, cerebellopontine cistern, and cisterna magna. Any cavernoma target can be resected with minimal or no tissue transgression or neurological sequela using this subarachnoid-centered technique. Surgical nuances, such as gravity retraction, cerebrospinal fluid release, brain shifting, and dynamic retraction, are designed to help navigate these spaces. Patient positioning is the key to aligning the trajectory to a cavernoma target and opening the surgical corridor in a way that allows a deep dive into the recesses and ventricles without fixed retraction or brain transgression. These strategic moves, combined with expert dissection, make difficult surgery easier and dangerous surgery safer.

Keywords: approach, cavernoma, cavernous malformation, cerebrum, fissure, gravity retraction, gyrus, resection, sulcus, taxonomy

2.1 Seven Surgical Corridors

The subarachnoid space is the secret to cavernoma surgery because, with meticulous dissection that preserves the protective pia, it is a passageway that takes you anywhere you want to go. From the sulci beneath the cerebral convexity to the basal cisterns around the central core and brainstem, subarachnoid spaces are the roads traveled to reach target cavernomas with microsurgical dissection. *Seven Cavernomas: Tenets and Techniques for Resection* was initially conceived as a textbook about tissue-sparing approaches through subarachnoid spaces. Seven refers to seven subarachnoid corridors, including the cerebral sulci, sylvian fissure, interhemispheric fissure, ventricular system, tentorial fissure, cerebellopontine cistern, and cisterna magna. Each chapter would compile various approaches through a corridor to produce an encyclopedia of approaches. The cavernous malformation (CM) was almost incidental, and the big idea was that any cavernoma target could be removed with minimal or no tissue transgression or neurological sequela with this subarachnoid-centered technique. However, *Seven Cavernomas* evolved into something different and more valuable: Taxonomy became the big idea, and the titular seven refers to the cavernoma types. This chapter examines the seven surgical corridors to engage with the original *Seven Cavernomas* theme.

2.2 Cerebral Sulci

The nearly 40 gyri and over 20 sulci in each hemisphere form a vast network of sulcal corridors, leading to the superficial cerebral subtypes and their approaches (▸ Table 2.1, ▸ Table 2.2). Dissection into a sulcus exposes an enormous amount of cortical surface area inaccessible on the convexity of the cerebrum alone. When parenchymal entry is required to access a cavernoma beneath the cortical surface, sulcal dissection drops the entry below the convexity surface to minimize brain transgression (▸ Fig. 2.1). The typical sulcus is closed off by a thick arachnoid membrane spanning adjacent gyri at the brain's convexity and by arachnoid trabeculations pulling together gyrus

Table 2.1 Summary of cerebral gyri, sulci, and abbreviations of transgyral and transsulcal approaches

Lobe	Gyrus	Transgyral approach	Sulcus	Transsulcal approach
Frontal	Superior frontal	TGyr-SFG	Superior frontal sulcus	TSul-sfs
	Middle frontal	TGyr-MFG	Inferior frontal sulcus	TSul-ifs
	Inferior frontal	TGyr-IFG	Lateral sulcus, ascending ramus	TSul-las
	Precentral	TGyr-PRG	Lateral sulcus, anterior ramus	TSul-lat
	Pars opercularis	TGyr-IFGOp	Olfactory sulcus	TSul-ols
	Pars triangularis	TGyr-IFGTr	Orbital sulcus (lateral, medial, transverse)	TSul-ors
	Pars orbitalis	TGyr-IFGOr	Cingulate sulcus	TSul-cgs
	Gyrus rectus	TGyr-GR	Callosal sulcus	TSul-scc
	Orbital (medial, lateral, anterior, posterior)	TGyr-MOrG, LOrG, AOrG, POrG	Precentral sulcus	TSul-pces
	Paracentral lobule	TGyr-PCL	Central sulcus	TSul-ces
	Cingulate	TGyr-CG	–	–
	Paraolfactory	TGyr-PaOG	–	–
	Subcallosal area, paraterminal	TGyr-SCA	–	–

(Continued)

Table 2.1 (*Continued*) Summary of cerebral gyri, sulci, and abbreviations of transgyral and transsulcal approaches

Lobe	Gyrus	Transgyral approach	Sulcus	Transsulcal approach
Parietal	Postcentral	TGyr-POG	Postcentral sulcus	TSul-pcs
	Superior parietal lobule	TGyr-SPL	Intraparietal sulcus	TSul-ips
	Inferior parietal lobule	TGyr-IPL	Parieto-occipital sulcus	TSul-pos
	Supramarginal	TGyr-SMG	Lateral sulcus, posterior ramus	TSul-lpor
	Angular	TGyr-AG	Subparietal sulcus	TSul-sps
	Anterior paracentral	TGyr-APaG	–	–
	Posterior paracentral	TGyr-PPaG	–	–
	Precuneus	TGyr-PCun	–	–
Occipital	Superior occipital	TGyr-SOG	Calcarine sulcus	TSul-cas
	Middle occipital	TGyr-MOG	Lunate sulcus	TSul-ls
	Inferior occipital	TGyr-IOG	Intraoccipital sulcus	TSul-ios
	Cuneus	TGyr-Cun	Inferior occipital sulcus	TSul-ifos
	Lingual (medial occipitotemporal)	TGyr-LG	Preoccipital incisura	TSul-poi
Temporal	Superior temporal	TGyr-STG	Superior temporal sulcus	TSul-sts
	Middle temporal	TGyr-MTG	Inferior temporal sulcus	TSul-its
	Inferior temporal	TGyr-ITG	Occipitotemporal sulcus	TSul-ots
	Fusiform gyrus (lateral occipitotemporal)	TGyr-FG	Collateral sulcus	TSyl-cos
	Parahippocampal gyrus	TGyr-PHG	–	–
	Hippocampus, head	TGyr-HiH	–	–
	Hippocampus, body	TGyr-HiB	–	–
	Hippocampus, tail	TGyr-HiT	–	–
	Uncus (gyrus intralimbicus, uncinate gyrus, limbus Giacomini)	TGyr-Un	–	–
	Transverse temporal (Heschl's gyrus)	TGyr-TTG (anterior, posterior)	–	–
	Planum polare	TGyr-PPo	–	–
	Planum temporale	TGyr-PTe	–	–

Table 2.2 Subarachnoid dissection approaches through the cerebral gyri and sulci

Approach	Abbreviation	Dissection level[a]
Frontal transgyral	TGyr-Fro	1
Frontal transsulcal	TSul-Fro	1
Temporal transgyral	TGyr-Tem	1
Temporal transsulcal	TSul-Tem	1
Parietal transgyral	TGyr-Par	1
Parietal transsulcal	TSul-Par	1
Occipital transgyral	TGyr-Occ	1
Occipital transsulcal	TSul-Occ	1
Insular transgyral	TGyr-Ins	2
Insular transsulcal	TSul-Ins	2
Transhematoma	THem	1

[a]Depth of dissection from superficial (level 1) to deep (level 4).

walls within the sulcus. Sharp transsulcal dissection penetrates the sulcus and disconnects the pia-to-pia connections without breaching the pia. The arachnoid membrane covering the sulcus is incised, and overlying veins are mobilized to one side. Cortical arteries traverse the sulcus and naturally separate the pial planes, which reduces the dissection to simply following the artery lying in the sulcus. An artery emerging from the sulcus of interest is followed in the retrograde direction into the sulcus, just as when splitting the sylvian fissure. The artery separates the pia from the opposing gyri, producing a natural separation plane in the center of the field. Centrifugal dissection away from the artery leads to pial adhesions, which are placed on traction and cut sharply to widen and deepen the dissection. The guiding artery may not lead directly to the cavernoma but establishes a separation plane that can be shifted to reach the lesion. An artery is a blessing when initiating transsulcal dissection because it facilitates the split, but it can become a curse during resection of the lesion because the passage of instruments into and out of the sulcus can injure the artery or its tiny branches. Venules lining the sulcus are less important but more delicate and may bleed, especially with the dynamic retraction needed to stretch the arachnoid bands for sharp dissection. Dissection is extended vertically to the bottom of the sulcus and radially outward to widen the mouth of the sulcus to shape the corridor into a cone rather than a cylinder.

The basic maneuvers of subarachnoid dissection include cutting with microscissors, spreading with bipolar forceps,

Subarachnoid Dissection: Sulci

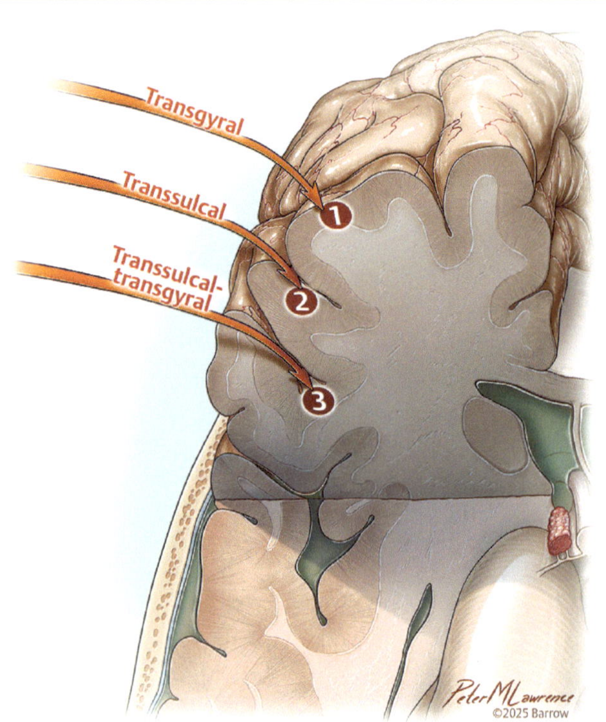

Fig. 2.1 Transgyral, transsulcal, and transsulcal-transgyral approaches. Transgyral approaches (level 1 dissection) are selected for superficial cerebral cavernomas on or near the convexity and do not require subarachnoid dissection to open a sulcus as a surgical corridor. Transgyral approaches access surface lesions or proceed through parenchymal tissue to access lesions below the surface. Transsulcal approaches (level 2) are selected for superficial cerebral cavernomas that lie below the convexity and near a sulcus whose dissection would open a surgical corridor to the target. Transsulcal approaches access lesions presenting to a sulcal surface and require little or no parenchymal transgression. Transsulcal-transgyral approaches (level 3) are selected for cerebral cavernomas that extend beyond the depths of a sulcus into deep white matter. Transsulcal-transgyral approaches require subarachnoid dissection to open the sulcus and parenchymal dissection to reach the lesion. (Reproduced with permission from Barrow Neurological Institute, Phoenix, AZ.)

and probing with a slightly curved dissector (Rhoton no. 6). Microscissors are used to open arachnoid membranes and cisterns sharply, whereas spreading and probing release internal arachnoid webs and identify resistant bands that require cutting. The arachnoid cuts cleanly when placed under tension by traction with the suction. Closed microscissor blades are used to dissect bluntly, and open microscissor blades can lift the arachnoid away from underlying arteries and veins before cutting it, which turns the microscissors into a dissecting instrument to set up cuts. The gentle opening force of bipolar forceps can be applied to tissues to spread and open dissection planes. Bipolar forceps are aligned parallel to arteries and pial surfaces to direct the opening forces perpendicular to these surfaces. Bipolar forceps aligned perpendicular to the arteries will not distribute the instrument's opening force to the opposing gyri, and its tips might dig into the brain.

Blunt dissection with a Rhoton no. 6 dissector is like an extension of one's index finger, feeling the tissue planes, pushing on arteries and nerves, and developing lines of dissection. Interfaces between arteries and lobules are loosened with blunt dissection, transitioning to sharp dissection when blunt dissection reaches its limits. The art of subarachnoid dissection is reducible to these basic maneuvers with three simple instruments. The rhythm of subarachnoid dissection is a cycle from blunt to sharp to spreading dissection and back around again.

Dynamic retraction is essential to opening narrow sulcal corridors. It is the suction tip and hand holding it that act as a roving retractor while also drying the field. The surgeon applies countertraction at the point of dissection with the suction tip and gentle retraction pressure to the brain with its shaft. The bullet-tipped no. 7 microsuction tip is smooth and atraumatic. Suction strength is regulated by rolling the thumb forward to cover the keyhole fenestration for more suction or backward to uncover the fenestration for less suction. The thumb rests in a middle position to partially cover the hole, with a constant whistling noise confirming an uncovered fenestration and preventing the aspiration of adjacent structures. The tip's malleable shaft is straightened to apply retraction pressure to the brain and curved gently to the hand.

Properly adjusted suction naturally compliments the dissecting instrument. These instruments lie directly opposite one another at the depth of the field, with the microsuction tip providing microretraction for each maneuver of the dissecting instrument. Unlike a fixed retractor blade, the tip adjusts constantly to the dissection. Lateral pressure with the suction tip provides countertraction when cutting tissue and retracts tissues to visualize the dissection plane. The suction tip can be directed to cross to the side of the dissecting instrument to apply traction or help with visualization. A dynamic suction hand all but eliminates the need for a fixed retractor.

The suction shaft also functions as a dynamic brain retractor. Laying the shaft against the brain gently pulls the brain back and opens the corridor like a funnel. The position of the tip is unaffected by this lateral hand movement. Like suction tip retraction, shaft retraction is also dynamic and ever adapting to the changing course of the dissection. Dissecting instruments in the dominant hand also function as brain retractors. The shaft of microscissors or bipolar forceps can lay gently against their side of the surgical corridor and open the other side of the funnel.

Transsulcal dissection is the systematic disassembly of the arachnoid scaffold holding the gyri together to liberate the tissue, enable it to move, and expand the sulcal corridor. There is a fine line between deconstructing subarachnoid structures and violating the protective pia mater. The soft and defenseless brain depends on the pia for protection, and subpial transgressions can transform the gentle push and pull of dynamic retraction into traumatic blows and contusions. Delicate microdissection transforms the potential spaces in the sulcal landscape into innumerable surgical corridors that reveal the targeted superficial cerebral cavernomas.

2.3 Sylvian Fissure

The sylvian fissure, or lateral sulcus, is the most important of the seven corridors because it provides a direct highway from the cortical surface to the cranium's geographic center, with four levels of dissection along the way (▸ Table 2.3). Superficially, the sylvian fissure provides access to cerebral cavernomas in the sylvian cortex (frontal, parietal, and temporal) in and around the operculum (level 1). At the depth below the operculum, the sylvian fissure provides access to the insular cortex and the basal ganglial (putamen) and thalamic (lateral) subtypes that reside in the central core (level 2). At the next depth, the sylvian fissure gives access to the carotid cistern, circle of Willis, and subtypes in the basal frontal and medial temporal cortex and pallidal basal ganglia (level 3). At the deepest level, beyond the membrane of Liliequist, the sylvian fissure provides access to brainstem cavernomas in the interpeduncular fossa for interpeduncular and peduncular midbrain and even certain basilar pontine subtypes (level 4). The range and depth of transsylvian approaches make the sylvian fissure the crucial gateway to the subarachnoid network (▸ Fig. 2.2).

This versatility makes splitting the sylvian fissure an essential technical skill. The superficial sylvian veins are the guardians of the sylvian fissure, and dissection beyond the veins is the first step in splitting the fissure (▸ Fig. 2.3a). These superficial veins are mobilized to the temporal side of the fissure because they course inferiorly and bridge to the sphenoparietal sinus under the sphenoid ridge. Dissection along the temporal side of the veins would cross their outflow connections, whereas dissection along the frontal side preserves these connections. The arachnoid is incised along the superficial sylvian vein from distal to proximal (▸ Fig. 2.3b, c), coagulating and cutting venous tributaries from the frontal lobe to gradually detach the vein from the frontal lobe and mobilize it temporally. Some patients have a single vein; others have an inviting sheet of arachnoid between frontal and temporal lobes with no veins; and others have a complex of veins coursing along the lips of the sylvian fissure. A single sylvian vein can be preserved by rolling it away from the frontal lobe. Sometimes, the plane between multiple sylvian veins may be the best pathway into the fissure. Occasionally, an unmovable vein may need to be divided, which is tolerable when it connects with other venous systems, namely the anterior system that drains into the sphenoparietal sinus, the posterior system that drains into the lateral temporal veins and vein of Labbé, or the superior system that drains into the vein of Trolard and the superior sagittal sinus (SSS).

As dissection along the superficial sylvian vein reaches the temporal pole, the cortical arachnoid descends into the sphenoidal arachnoid. From the surgeon's perspective, the sphenoidal arachnoid is vertically oriented, and the cortical arachnoid is horizontally oriented. The sphenoidal arachnoid should be opened before initiating deep sylvian dissection because it connects the frontal and temporal lobes and resists deep spreading dissection. Superficial sylvian veins lie beneath the sphenoidal arachnoid membrane or can penetrate it en route to the sphenoparietal sinus.

After mobilizing the superficial veins temporally and opening the lateral sylvian arachnoid membrane (▸ Fig. 2.3d), a cortical M4 branch of the middle cerebral artery (MCA) is identified as it emerges from the fissure. Arteries naturally separate the frontal and temporal lobes and define the dissection plane. The M3 segment is followed into the depths of the fissure to further the separation plane. Deep sylvian dissection along M3 arteries helps the neurosurgeon align the microscope at a steep, downward angle, almost looking back toward the surgeon. Cutting the arachnoid bands between the frontal and temporal lobes disconnects the lobes (▸ Fig. 2.3e). The working area around an M3 artery is circumferentially widened like a funnel instead of a cylinder to avoid constricted holes. Similar separation planes around adjacent arteries are developed and interconnected to reach level 1 target CMs.

Opercular M3 segments lead to arterial bifurcations and larger M2 insular segments. Larger arteries widely separate the frontal and temporal lobes to make dissection easier as it deepens. Spreading dissection along insular M2 trunks parts the lobes from the inside out, following a wide plane of separation deep in the sylvian fissure toward narrow and more adherent areas superficially. Yaşargil analogized this process to splitting an orange, where the radial force directed outward from the center easily divides the wedges. The sylvian fissure is often the most adherent superficially near the pterion, where the frontal and temporal lobes meet with few arteries in between to separate the lobes. Lobules can interdigitate, adding a rolling contour to this plane of contact. Spreading inside-out dissection is the best method for opening these difficult planes. When tissues still do not separate, an artery might be found under the sphenoidal arachnoid in the proximal fissure to reestablish the separation plane.

Table 2.3 Subarachnoid dissection approaches through the sylvian fissure

Approach	Abbreviation	Dissection level[a]
Transsylvian	TSyl	1
Transsylvian transfrontal	TSyl-Fro	1
Transsylvian transtemporal	TSyl-Tem	1
Transsylvian-anterior transinsular	TSyl-AIns	2
Transsylvian-posterior transinsular	TSyl-PIns	2
Supracarotid infrafrontal (transperforate)	TSyl-SCIF	3
Subfrontal trans-lamina terminalis	sFro-TLT	3
Transsylvian interpeduncular	TSyl-IPed	4
Transsylvian transpeduncular	TSyl-Ped	4
Transsylvian-contralateral interpeduncular	cTSyl-IntPed	4
Pretemporal transcavernous	TSyl-Cav	4
Transcavernous transpontine	TSyl-Cav-Pon	4

[a]Depth of dissection from superficial (level 1) to deep (level 4).

Subarachnoid Dissection: Sylvian Fissure

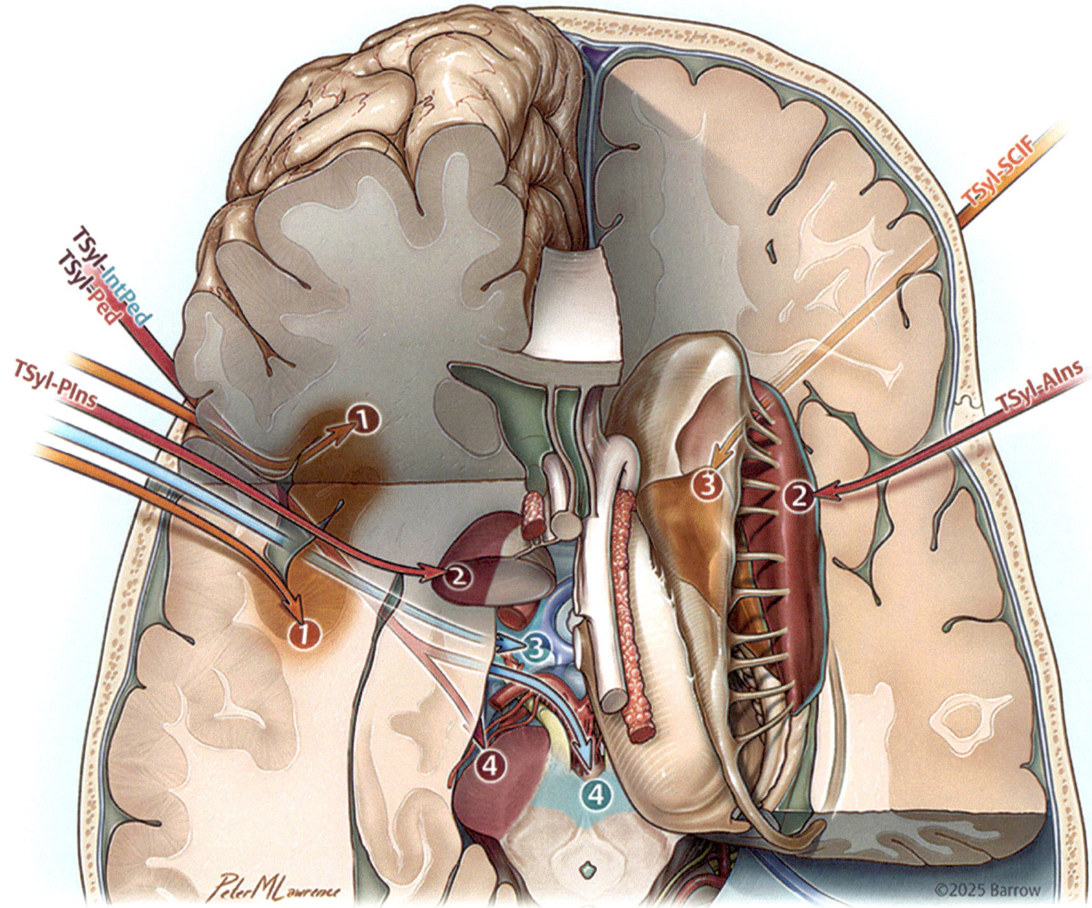

Fig. 2.2 Transsylvian approaches. Superficially, the sylvian fissure provides access to cerebral cavernomas in the sylvian cortex (frontal, parietal, and temporal) in and around the operculum (level 1). At the depth below the operculum, the sylvian fissure provides access to the insular cortex and the basal ganglial (putamen) and thalamic (lateral) subtypes that reside in the central core (level 2; TSyl-AIns and TSyl-PIns approaches). At the next depth, the sylvian fissure gives access to the carotid cistern, circle of Willis, and subtypes in the basal frontal and medial temporal cortex and pallidal basal ganglia (level 3; TSyl-Fro, TSyl-Tem, and TSyl-SCIF approaches). At the deepest level, beyond the membrane of Liliequist, the sylvian fissure provides access to brainstem cavernomas in the interpeduncular fossa for interpeduncular and peduncular midbrain and certain basilar pontine subtypes (level 4; TSyl-IntPed, TSyl-Ped, TSyl-Cav, and TSyl-Cav-Pon approaches). The range and depth of transsylvian approaches make the sylvian fissure the crucial gateway to the subarachnoid network. Numbered circles represent the four depths of dissection from superficial to deep. (Reproduced with permission from Barrow Neurological Institute, Phoenix, AZ.)

Once inside the sylvian cistern, the insula (limen insulae, short and long gyri) is exposed (▸ Fig. 2.3f) and level 2 targets in the basal ganglia and thalamus can be reached with transinsular approaches. For level 3 targets in the carotid cistern, the challenge shifts from separating lobes to unscrambling arteries. Inferior, middle, and superior divisions of the M2 segment of the MCA, anterior temporal artery, lenticulostriate arteries, and other branch arteries are untangled to complete the fissure split. Arteries supply only one lobe, coursing temporally or frontally but not both. Consequently, arteries in the sylvian cistern are moved to one side or the other. A temporal artery that adheres to the frontal lobe before looping back to the temporal lobe will bridge the fissure and might be compromised if this anatomy is not appreciated. Branch arteries that are traced from origin to destination will be correctly interpreted and mobilized. Bridging arteries with confusing anatomy require more dissection and another review of the anatomy.

Unlike arteries, which supply one lobe, veins can branch into both lobes and frequently bridge the sylvian fissure. Deep sylvian veins are encountered at the bottom of the fissure dissection over or under the M1 segment, and their caliber is inversely related to that of the superficial sylvian veins. The thick arachnoid between the carotid and sylvian cisterns is the final tether between the frontal and temporal

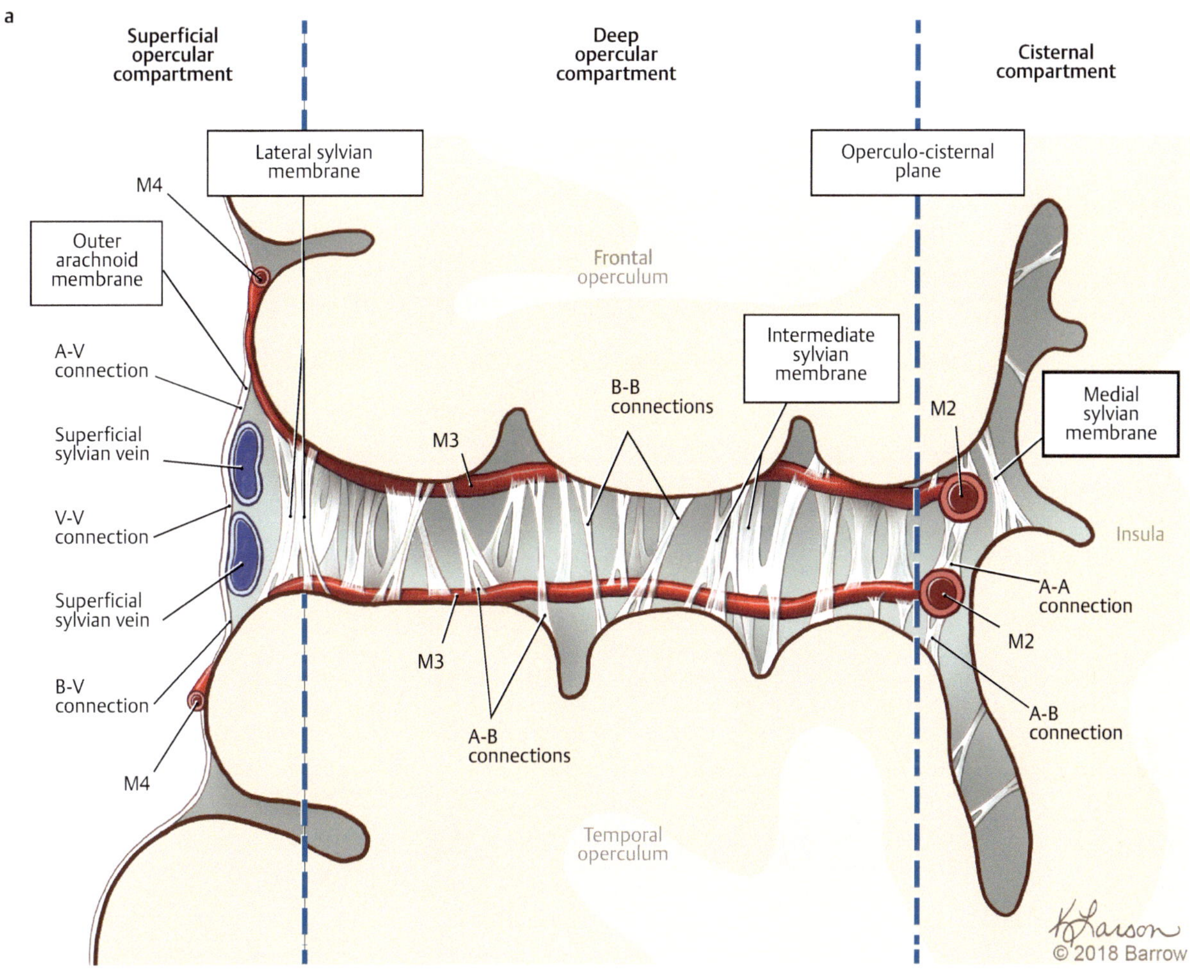

Fig. 2.3 Splitting the sylvian fissure. **(a)** Sylvian fissure anatomy is shown in coronal cross-section between the frontal and temporal opercula and the insular cortex. The sylvian fissure is covered by an outer arachnoid membrane, below which lie the superficial sylvian veins, and below them, the lateral sylvian membrane. The opercular surfaces of the fissure are joined by arachnoid trabeculae that form brain to brain (B-B) connections, between arteries and brain (A-B connections), and between brain and veins (B-V connections). In addition, arachnoid trabeculae join arteries and veins with artery to artery (A-A) connections, artery to vein (A-V) connections, and vein to vein (V-V) connections. A medial sylvian membrane lies at the depths of the operculum at the level of the operculo-cisternal plane. The M2 segments of the MCA reside in the cisternal compartment, M3 segments in the deep opercular compartment, and M4 segments in the superficial opercular compartment and on the cortical surface.

(Continued)

lobes (▶ Fig. 2.3g). Once this tether is cut, the sylvian fissure split is complete (▶ Fig. 2.3h), and the MCA candelabra can be followed through its four segments to the supraclinoid internal carotid artery.

Splitting the sylvian fissure distally to proximally, as described above, is easier than splitting it proximally to distally. Distal-to-proximal dissection proceeds sequentially to deep arterial trunks. Inside-out dissection is effective, brain retraction is unnecessary, and the cerebrospinal fluid (CSF) remains in the sylvian cistern to separate the lobes. In contrast, proximal-to-distal dissection follows the M1 segment of the MCA and may require frontal lobe retraction and early CSF release that collapses the cistern. Proximal-to-distal dissection gains proximal control during approaches to MCA aneurysms, whereas control is not an issue in cavernoma surgery.

Additional dissection beyond the carotid cistern leads to level 4 brainstem CM targets. The carotid-oculomotor triangle is entered, and the posterior communicating artery (PCoA) and anterior choroidal artery are mobilized medially. The PCoA is followed from its origin on the internal carotid artery to the junction between P1 (precommunicating) and P2 (postcommunicating) on the posterior cerebral artery (PCA). The P1 segment is followed proximally to Liliequist's membrane, the dense arachnoid sheet that extends from the dorsum sellae to the mammillary bodies and between the oculomotor nerves, separating the chiasmatic and interpeduncular cisterns. An incision

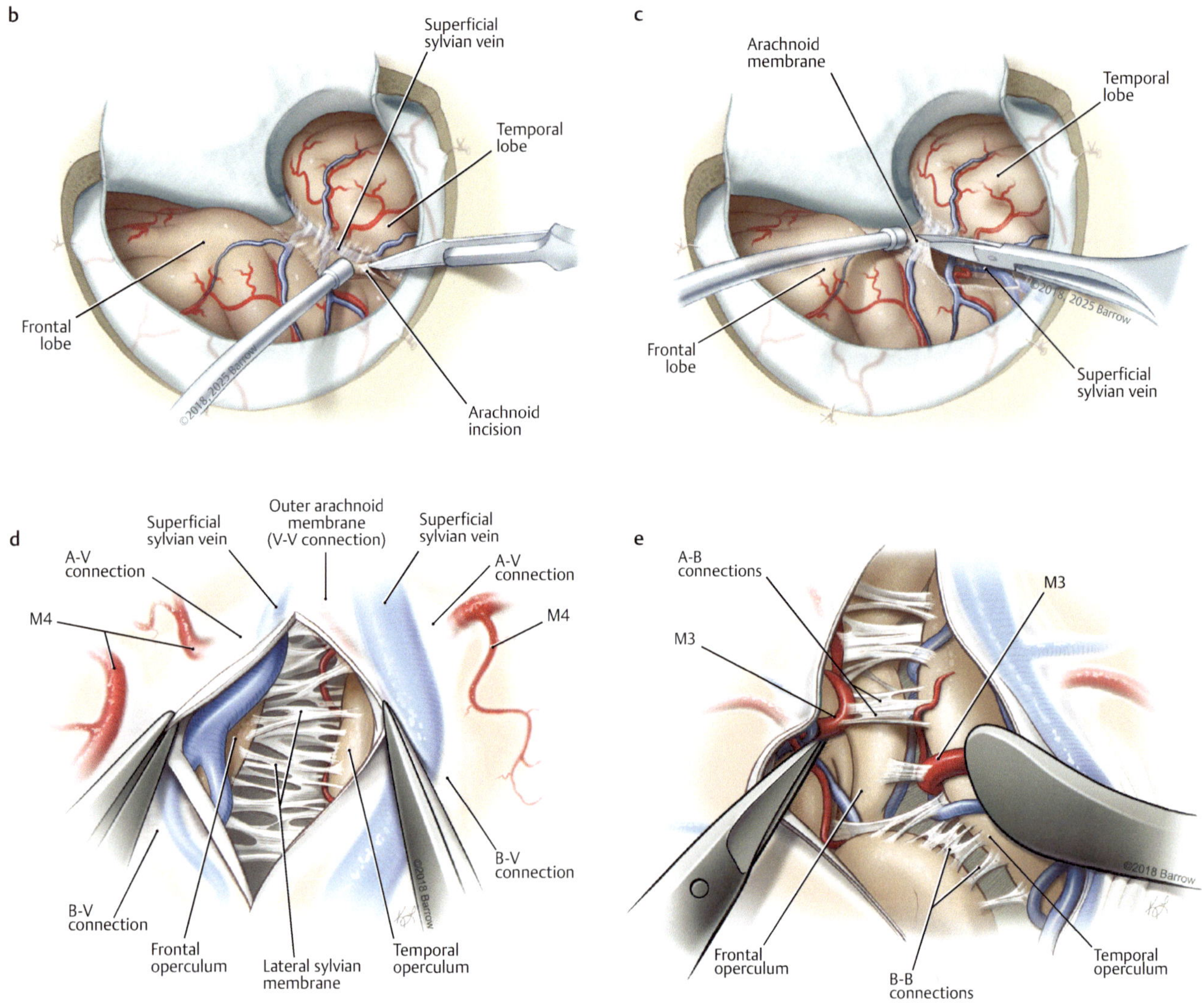

Fig. 2.3 *(Continued)* **(b)** The sylvian split begins with an arachnoid incision along the frontal side of the superficial sylvian veins. **(c)** These veins are mobilized to the temporal side of the fissure to preserve their distal connection to the sphenoparietal sinus. **(d)** The lateral sylvian membrane is opened to enter the operculum. **(e)** A cortical M4 branch emerging from the fissure is followed proximally to its opercular M3 segment to define the separation plane, and the arachnoid trabeculae connecting the brain, arteries, and veins are cut to widen the operculum.

(Continued)

behind the posterior clinoid process and medial to the oculomotor nerve opens Liliequist's membrane and extends posteriorly to the undersurface of the P1 segment, where it pierces the membrane (▶ Fig. 2.3i). The undersurface of the P1 segment is followed medially to the s1 (anterior pontomesencephalic) segment of the superior cerebellar artery (SCA) and basilar trunk to avoid the thalamoperforating arteries on the upper surface. The s1 segment lies below the oculomotor nerve and is crossed carefully with the incision in Liliequist's membrane. Dissection of the anterior choroidal artery's cisternal segment releases the medial attachments of the temporal lobe and enters the crural cistern, where the P2 and s2 (lateral pontomesencephalic) segments are visualized through the tentorial incisura.

The PCoA and its anterior thalamoperforating arteries are moved superiorly to open the medial corridor. A small PCoA that tethers the P1 segment or compromises the view can be cauterized and divided if its anterior thalamoperforating arteries can be preserved; however, when the PCoA has fetal anatomy, it cannot be sacrificed. The transsylvian-pretemporal corridor through the middle cranial fossa descends to the midbrain (peduncular and interpeduncular) and pontine (basilar) CM targets. Dissection across the basilar apex to the contralateral SCA and PCA opens a contralateral interpeduncular corridor to cavernomas in the lateral wall of the interpeduncular fossa. The contralateral SCA lies in the line of sight through the carotid-oculomotor triangle, and the

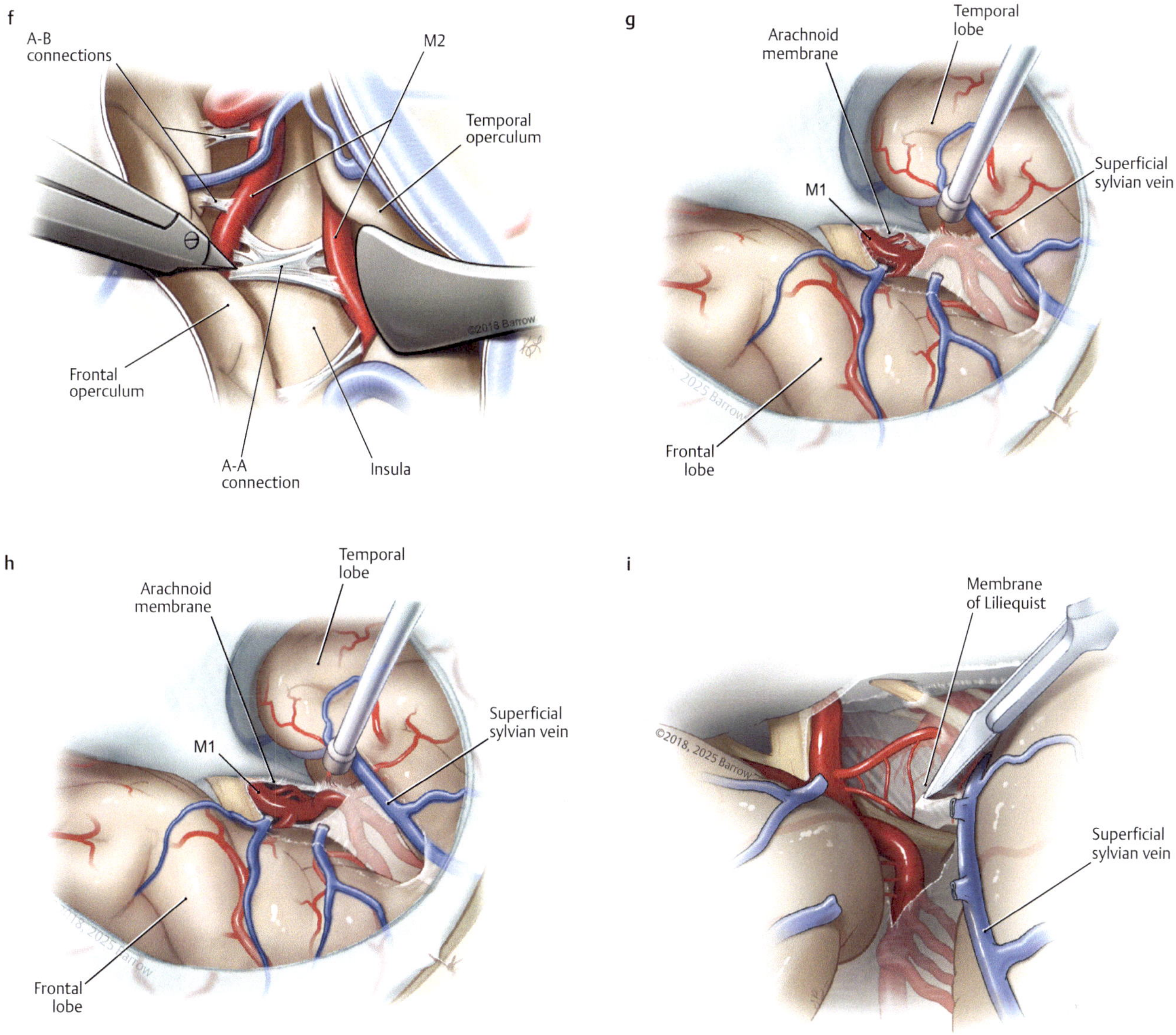

Fig. 2.3 *(Continued)* **(f)** Deepening dissection along M3 segments lead to M2 segments at the level of the operculo-cisternal plane and insula. **(g)** Thick arachnoid between the sylvian and carotid cisterns is encountered along the M1 segment of the MCA and is the final tether between the frontal and temporal lobes. **(h)** Incising these deep cisternal layers completes the sylvian split and joins the carotid and sylvian cisterns. **(i)** Dissection along the anterior choroidal artery leads to the crural cistern and releases the deepest arachnoid connections joining the frontal and temporal lobes, and dissection along PCoA and oculomotor nerve incises Liliequist's membrane to communicate with the interpeduncular cistern. Roman numerals denote CNs. (Reproduced with permission from Barrow Neurological Institute, Phoenix, AZ.)

contralateral oculomotor nerve is an orienting landmark that differentiates the SCA (below the nerve) from the PCA (above the nerve). The identification of the five major arteries (basilar trunk, bilateral PCAs, and bilateral SCAs) gives the neurosurgeon vascular control and anatomic orientation. This contralateral interpeduncular approach typically reaches over the shoulder of the opposite P1 segment of the PCA. Additional exposure and depth can be added to this level 4 transsylvian dissection with a posterior clinoidectomy, transcavernous dissection, and anterior petrosectomy (Kawase approach) as indicated, just as with complex basilar apex aneurysms.

2.4 Interhemispheric Fissure

The interhemispheric, or longitudinal, fissure is the brain's longest fissure and the corridor to medial cerebral cavernomas on the medial hemispheric surface. Scarce bridging veins from the convexity to the SSS in its anterior and posterior thirds make the interhemispheric fissure amenable to gravity-assisted subarachnoid dissection. Interhemispheric dissection relies on head position, with the sagittal midline oriented horizontally to allow gravity to pull on the dependent hemisphere and widen the fissure naturally, whereas transsulcal and transsylvian dissections rely on dynamic retraction (▸ Fig. 2.4; ▸ Table 2.4).

Subarachnoid Dissection: Interhemispheric and Transventricular

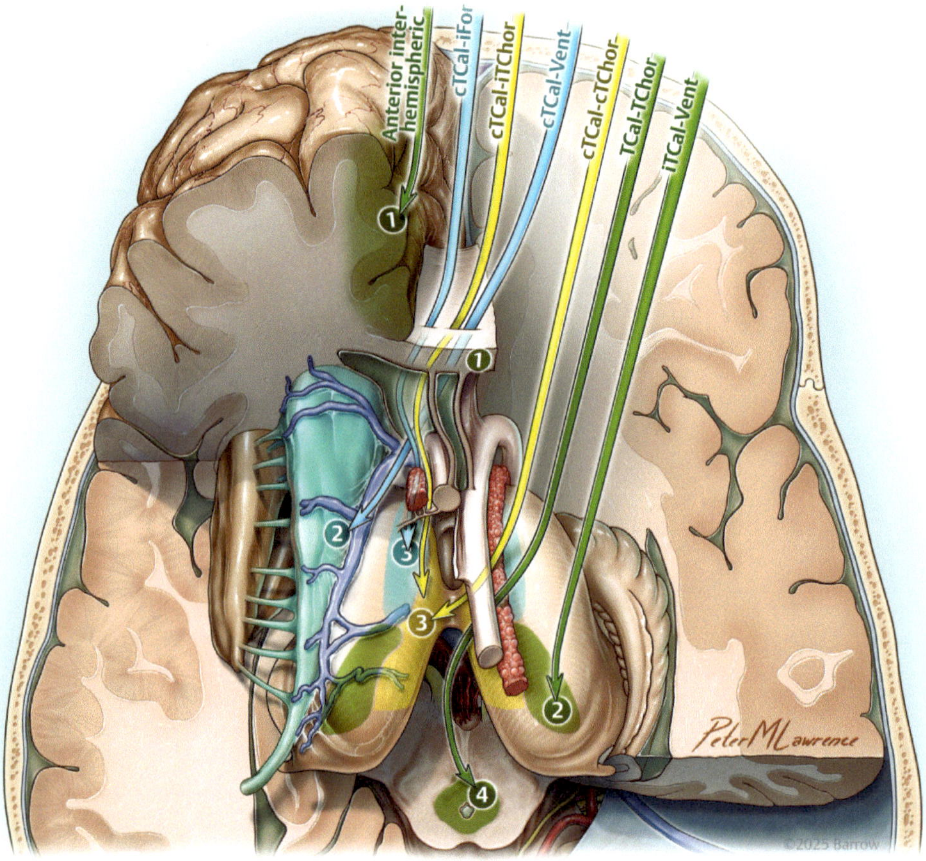

Fig. 2.4 Interhemispheric approaches. The interhemispheric, or longitudinal, fissure is the brain's longest fissure and the corridor to medial cerebral cavernomas on the medial hemispheric surface. The anterior interhemispheric approach accesses medial frontal cavernomas and the posterior interhemispheric approach accesses medial parieto-occipital cavernomas. These approaches also expose cavernomas in the corpus callosum (level 1). Transcallosal approaches access cavernomas in the basal ganglia (caudate subtype) and thalamus (choroidal subtype) that present to an ependymal surface (level 2; cTCal-Vent and iTCal-Vent approaches, respectively). Transforaminal and transchoroidal approaches deepen into the third ventricle to access thalamic lesions (anterior and medial subtypes, respectively; level 3; cTCal-iFor, cTCal-cTChor, and cTCal-iTChor approaches). Transchoroidal approaches can extend through the floor of the third ventricle to reach periaqueductal midbrain subtypes (level 4; TCal-TChor approach). Like the transsylvian corridor, which also has four levels, the interhemispheric-transventricular corridor has range and depth that make it the essential route to distant midline and paramedian cavernoma targets. (Reproduced with permission from Barrow Neurological Institute, Phoenix, AZ.)

The anterior interhemispheric approach is centered just in front of the coronal suture, with a bifrontal craniotomy placed two-thirds in front and one-third behind the coronal suture, crossing the SSS. Dural reflection to the opposite side with taut tacking sutures facilitates access to a subdural plane down the falx from the SSS to the inferior sagittal sinus (ISS). This approach is obstructed only by arachnoid granulations and adhesions along the paramedian space, which are easily released. The interhemispheric fissure is entered between the bridging veins. Veins that fuse with the parasagittal dura before reaching the midline can be preserved by splitting the dural flap and creating a dural sleeve over the vein. This parafalcine dissection exposes the superior frontal gyrus and the anterior part of the cingulate sulcus.

Subdural dissection transitions to subarachnoid dissection beneath the free edge of the falx at the roof of the callosal cistern. This cistern is entered in the midline along an ascending branch of the callosomarginal artery (CmaA) or one of the internal frontal arteries. The cortical surfaces of the medial frontal lobes can be adherent, and the technique for opening the interhemispheric fissure is the same as that for splitting the sylvian fissure. A peripheral artery is followed in the retrograde direction toward deeper and larger trunks using a combination of sharp and spreading

Table 2.4 Subarachnoid dissection approaches through the interhemispheric fissure

Approach	Abbreviation	Dissection level[a]
Far anterior interhemispheric	FarAI	1
Ipsilateral anterior interhemispheric	iAI	1
Contralateral anterior interhemispheric	cAI	1
Contralateral anterior interhemispheric-transfalcine	cAI-Falx	1
Ipsilateral transcingulate	iTCing	1
Contralateral transcingulate	cTCing	1
Anterior transcallosal	ATCal	2
Contralateral anterior transcallosal	cATCal	2
Ipsilateral posterior interhemispheric	iPI	1
Contralateral posterior interhemispheric	cPI	1
Contralateral posterior interhemispheric-transfalcine	cPI-Falx	1
Transcuneal	TCun	1
Posterior transcallosal	PTCal	2
Contralateral posterior transcallosal	cPTCal	2
Subfrontal	SFro	1

[a]Depth of dissection from superficial (level 1) to deep (level 4).

dissection. Gravity places the arachnoid bands in traction and facilitates the split. However, the corpus callosal cistern is uniformly narrow and does not widen with deepening dissection like the sylvian cistern. In addition, the caliber of the anterior cerebral artery branches does not enlarge in the way that the MCA branches enlarge to separate the sylvian surfaces of the frontal and temporal lobes. The pericallosal artery (PcaA) can hide beneath the inferior edge of the cingulate gyrus, but the pure white color of the corpus callosum signals the arrival at the PcaA's depth. The laterality of the PcaA and CmaA may be unclear when encountered unpaired, but the direction of its branches indicates the side with which that artery is associated.

Once the corpus callosum has been reached, the PcaA is followed anteriorly and posteriorly to open the interhemispheric fissure from the inside out. The fissure is opened from the depth of the PcaA upward to the depth of the CmaA and upward still to the falx's free edge. Dissection progresses distally or proximally along the arteries depending on the location of the cavernoma. Medial lesions located superficially in the ipsilateral hemisphere are easily accessed through the superior frontal and cingulate gyri (anterior interhemispheric-transgyral approach). Medial lesions located deeper in the ipsilateral hemisphere may require an approach through a superior frontal or cingulate sulcus (anterior interhemispheric-transsulcal approach). The crossing trajectory of a contralateral approach may optimize the lateral reach to deeper lesions in the frontal white matter, with variations that include the contralateral anterior interhemispheric, contralateral transcingulate, and contralateral transfalcine approaches.

The posterior interhemispheric approach is centered around the parieto-occipital fissure. With the patient positioned laterally, the head turned nose down about 60 degrees toward the floor, and the neck slightly flexed, the occipital lobe falls away from the falx with gravity retraction. The neurosurgeon faces the field from behind the patient, with the posterior third of the SSS oriented horizontally and the interhemispheric fissure widened naturally. A lumbar drain or ventriculostomy is unnecessary when CSF drainage from the quadrigeminal cistern is performed quickly as the first step after the dural opening to relax the brain. I prefer a semicircular scalp incision exposing the anterior margin of the surgical corridor, crossing the midline, and curving inferiorly along the SSS. A biparietal or bioccipital craniotomy is performed, which places most of the craniotomy on the approach side but crosses the SSS and exposes some of the opposite side. The dura is opened in a semicircular flap based along the SSS and tacked up medially. Releasing the arachnoid adhesions between the dura and the paramedian hemisphere opens the interhemispheric fissure. Bridging lateral veins course anteriorly, and the interhemispheric fissure is entered from behind them. Dissection deepens down the medial hemisphere to the falcotentorial junction and posterior incisural space, where the callosal and quadrigeminal cisterns are drained of CSF. This maneuver slackens the brain, further drops the occipital lobe, and widens the surgical corridor. The falx leads to the bottom of the fissure without subarachnoid dissection, and deep cisterns can be entered quickly.

Medial parietal and occipital cavernomas are accessed along this ipsilateral surface in the precuneus, cuneus, and lingual gyrus (posterior interhemispheric-transgyral approach). Deeper parietal and occipital cavernomas may require transsulcal dissection in the parieto-occipital, subparietal, or calcarine sulci (posterior interhemispheric-transsulcal approach). The crossing trajectory of a contralateral approach may optimize lateral reach to deeper lesions in the parietal or occipital white matter, and these CMs are accessed through a transfalcine window made between the SSS, ISS, and straight sinus (contralateral posterior interhemispheric-transfalcine approach). Contralateral arteries and veins may adhere to the falx out of view, and these incisions are performed layer by layer with traction on the falx away from the lesion. The subarachnoid dissection crosses through the falx into the opposite interhemispheric fissure to expose the lesion. With circumferential dissection, the CM mobilizes into the interhemispheric fissure with gravity, the lateral margin is easier to visualize, and the falx holds the ipsilateral hemisphere in position. This approach improves visualization of the margin that is most difficult to see.

2.5 Ventricular System

Although not strictly a subarachnoid corridor, the ventricular system is another versatile pathway to deep cavernomas extending from the corpus callosum to the brainstem. Although fissures and sulci are potential spaces that must be opened, ventricles are natural spaces that are interconnected and easily entered (▸ Table 2.5). Two key maneuvers, callosotomy and dissection of the choroidal fissure, define four levels of transventricular dissection (▸ Fig. 2.4). First, callosotomy accesses cavernomas in the corpus callosum and roof of the lateral ventricles (level 1). Transcallosal approaches access cavernomas in the basal ganglia (caudate subtype) and thalamus (choroidal subtype) that present to an ependymal surface (level 2). Transforaminal and transchoroidal approaches deepen into the third ventricle to access thalamic lesions (anterior and medial subtypes, respectively; level 3). Transchoroidal approaches can extend through the floor of the third ventricle to reach periaqueductal midbrain subtypes (level 4). Like the transsylvian corridor, which also has four levels, the transventricular corridor has range and depth that make it the essential route to distant midline targets.

The rostrum, genu, body, and splenium form the largest part of the ventricular wall. CMs in the corpus callosum may reside in any of these parts and are accessed through the interhemispheric fissure. Transcallosal approaches traverse the body of the corpus callosum in two variations: ipsilateral (iTCal-Vent) and contralateral (cTCal-Vent), relative to the cavernoma. Ipsilateral approaches enter the corpus callosum off the midline toward the lesion, which is on the downward or dependent side with gravity retraction. This entry keeps the septum pellucidum and fornix at the top of the corridor and comes down on the superior aspect of the thalamus for choroidal CMs. Contralateral approaches traverse the corpus callosum across the midline underneath the PcaA on the opposite side. Gravity retraction of the dependent hemisphere facilitates this crossing trajectory, and passage underneath the PcaA ensures entry into the opposite ventricle. This trajectory brings the ventricle's lateral wall into view for targeted cavernomas in the head and body of the caudate nucleus. The contralateral transcallosal approach also aligns with anterior thalamic subtypes that appear within the foramen of Monro (FoM) from this crossing perspective (cTCal-iFor).

The choroidal fissure is a narrow cleft between the fornix and the thalamus, where the choroid plexus attaches to the ventricular body, atrium, and temporal horn. The choroidal fissure extends in a C-shaped arc from the FoM, around the thalamic surfaces, to the inferior choroidal point behind the head of the hippocampus. The tela choroidea, the clear membrane from which the choroid plexus arises, attaches to neural structures via small ridges called teniae, including the tenia thalami, tenia fornicis, and tenia fimbriae. The body portion of the choroidal fissure opens into the velum interpositum and the roof of the third ventricle. The roof of the third ventricle comprises four layers: the fornix, two membranes of the tela choroidea, and a layer of blood vessels between the tela (medial posterior choroidal artery and internal cerebral vein [ICV]). The velum interpositum is the space between the two layers of tela in the roof of the third ventricle. The veins of the lateral ventricle and frontal horn are the thalamostriate, caudate, and septal veins, and they converge on the ICV in the velum interpositum just behind the FoM.

Transchoroidal approaches disassemble this complex anatomy to enlarge the FoM posteriorly and unroof the anterior third ventricle. Choroidal fissure dissection sweeps the ventricular body's choroid plexus laterally, incises the tela choroidea between the choroid plexus laterally and fornix medially (tenia fornicis), and traces the thalamostriate vein (ThaStrV) through the FoM into its convergence with the ICV. The anteromedial aspect of the ThaStrV–ICV junction is followed posteriorly and may require interruption of the anterior septal vein, which is tolerable when the ThaStrV and ICV are preserved. Posterior dissection between the paired ICVs extends the opening into the roof of the third ventricle as far back as the posterior commissure, if needed, where the crus of fornix courses laterally around the thalamus. Fissure dissection doubles or triples the caliber of the FoM for a panoramic view into the third ventricle. Some neurosurgeons prefer transchoroidal dissection through the tenia thalami, lateral to the choroid plexus, to place

Table 2.5 Subarachnoid dissection approaches through the ventricles

Approach	Abbreviation	Dissection level[a]
Ipsilateral transcallosal-transventricular	iTCal-Vent	2
Contralateral transcallosal-transventricular	cTCal-Vent	2
Transcallosal-transforaminal	TCal-For	3
Transcallosal-interforniceal	TCal-IF	3
Contralateral transcallosal-contralateral transchoroidal fissure (subforniceal)	cTCal-cTChor	3
Contralateral transcallosal-ipsilateral transchoroidal fissure (supraforniceal)	cTCal-iTChor	3
Transcallosal–sub-choroidal fissure (subchoroidal)	TCal-SChor	3
Posterior transcallosal-transventricular	PTCal-Vent	2
Contralateral posterior transcallosal-transventricular	cPTCal-Vent	2
Transtemporal-transventricular	Tem-Vent	3
Transtemporal-transchoroidal fissure	Tem-TChor	3
Superior parietal lobule-transatrial	SPL-Atr	2
Subfrontal trans-lamina terminalis	sFro-TLT	3

[a]Depth of dissection from superficial (level 1) to deep (level 4).

this tuft of the choroid as a protective barrier between the dissection plane and the fornix. However, this trajectory lands between the ThaStrV and the ICV, which allows the ThaStrV to tether the fornix to the thalamus and close the choroidal fissure. Thin cottonoids can be placed as a protective buffer on the fornix when dissecting through the tenia fornicis.

The fornix is a delicate structure critical to short-term memory and composed of hippocampomammillary tract fibers that arise as fimbria on the ventricular surface of the hippocampal formation in the temporal horn. They form the crus of the fornix, which courses posteriorly, wraps around the pulvinar of the thalamus, and joins the opposite crus in the body of the lateral ventricle to become the body of the fornix. The fornix continues along the superomedial thalami in the medial wall of the lateral ventricular body, splits anteriorly into two columns, and then dives into the anterior margin of FoM to end in the mammillary bodies. Two variations of transchoroidal approaches have evolved to manage the fornix safely, both using a contralateral transcallosal approach, with one coursing under and the other over the fornix. The contralateral transcallosal-contralateral transchoroidal (cTCal-cTChor) approach accesses small or low-lying medial thalamic (level 3) and periaqueductal midbrain (level 4) CMs. The slight crossing trajectory passes safely under the fornix without needing much retraction on the fornix. However, medial thalamic CMs that are large or high lying require dissection more laterally, with lifting retraction of the fornix. A contralateral transcallosal-ipsilateral transchoroidal (cTCal-iTChor) approach crosses above the fornix at the level of the corpus callosum to spare the fornix this harmful retraction. The cTCal-cTChor approach travels under the fornix and elevates it, whereas the cTCal-iTChor approach travels over the fornix and drops it, removing it from harm's way. The midline is crossed with the transcallosal incision, and choroidal fissure dissection allows the fornix to fall away and reach unimpeded into the superolateral corner.

2.6 Tentorial Fissure

The tentorium cerebelli, the tent of the cerebellum, lies between the inferior surface of the temporal and occipital lobes and the superior surface of the cerebellum, partitioning the brain into the supra- and infratentorial compartments and giving passage to the midbrain through its incisura. The tentorium cerebelli is anchored to the petrous bones bilaterally, bears the weight of the cerebrum, and shields the posterior fossa contents. The tentorial fissure is the space occupied by the tentorium cerebelli and rivals the longitudinal and sylvian fissures as one of the great surgical corridors. The subarachnoid spaces and cisterns around the tentorium lead directly to deep targets in the basal surfaces, thalamus, and brainstem (▶ Fig. 2.5). This corridor has only two levels of dissection depth to reach cavernomas in the basal surfaces of the occipital and temporal lobes and the tentorial surface of the cerebellum (level 1) and tegmental and quadrigeminal midbrain as well as pulvinar and geniculate thalamic cavernomas (level 2). However, there are three variations of approach into the tentorium: infratentorial, supratentorial, and transtentorial. In addition, the tentorium's semicircular shape produces three variations of trajectory: posterior midline, paramedian, and lateral. Thus, there are eight distinct approaches to traverse the tentorial fissure (▶ Table 2.6).

The tentorium's ability to separate the cerebrum from the cerebellum and bear its weight makes the supracerebellar-infratentorial (SCIT) corridor, widened by gravity retraction, one of the most spectacular of the seven corridors. With the patient in the sitting position and extensive CSF drainage from the cisterna magna, the cerebellum sags to open the infratentorial space, opens inward to the quadrigeminal and ambient cisterns, offers panoramic exposures, and, in the process, improves operative indices like blood loss, operative duration, and patient outcomes. Fixed retractors are unnecessary, operative corridors remain unencumbered, and natural subarachnoid planes open to deep targets. The tentorium has a semicircular shape with a complex roofline that creates a peaked attic in the midline for navigation to cavernoma subtypes in the vermian cerebellar and quadrigeminal midbrain (via a midline SCIT [SCIT-Mid] approach). The roofline descends off the midline, but the posterior incisura still allows access to lesions in the pulvinar of the thalamus through the paramedian SCIT (SCIT-Para) approach. The SCIT-Para approach is also ideal for tentorial cerebellar subtypes more superficially. Laterally, the tentorium flattens at its insertion to the petrous ridge. The infratentorial space widens by gravity retraction on the cerebellum and easily reaches cavernomas in the ambient cistern and tegmental midbrain as well as superficial tentorial cerebellar cavernomas.

Gravity-assisted SCIT approaches are performed with the patient in the sitting position. The operating table is maximally flexed to position the patient's back vertically, with the head flexed forward to flatten the angle of the tentorium. The SCIT-Mid and SCIT-Para approaches are performed through a midline linear incision, torcular craniotomy, and dural flap based superiorly on the transverse sinus and tented with sutures to elevate the sinuses. The lateral SCIT (SCIT-Lat) approach is performed through a linear or lazy-S incision midway between the inion and the mastoid bone, with the craniotomy extending laterally to the transverse–sigmoid junction, superiorly above the transverse sinus, and inferiorly above the foramen magnum. The dura is opened in a flap superiorly along the transverse sinus and tented with sutures to elevate the sinus. The sitting position can be awkward for the neurosurgeon, holding the hands high to reach the surgical field. A rolling chair with raised armrests can support the elbows, whereas the end of the operating table can support the hands at shoulder level. The hands remain relaxed and stabilized in this position. The sitting position also requires preoperative patient screening for a patent foramen ovale with preoperative echocardiography and a bubble test. Patients with a patent foramen ovale, a steep tentorial angle, advanced age, or thin, adherent dura might be better positioned prone with the neck flexed for the SCIT-Mid or SCIT-Para approach or laterally for the SCIT-Lat approach. Air embolism is a major concern with craniotomies that cross major venous sinuses and have a risk of dural tears.

Early CSF release from the cisterna magna and the deep cisterns relaxes the cerebellum and obviates the need for a lumbar drain. The cerebellum is untethered by releasing arachnoid adhesions bridging from the posterior edge of the superior cerebellum to the outer edge of the tentorium. Bridging veins to the tentorium may need to be divided to open the corridor to the free edge of the tentorium or can be mobilized by releasing incisions

Subarachnoid Dissection: Tentorial Fissure

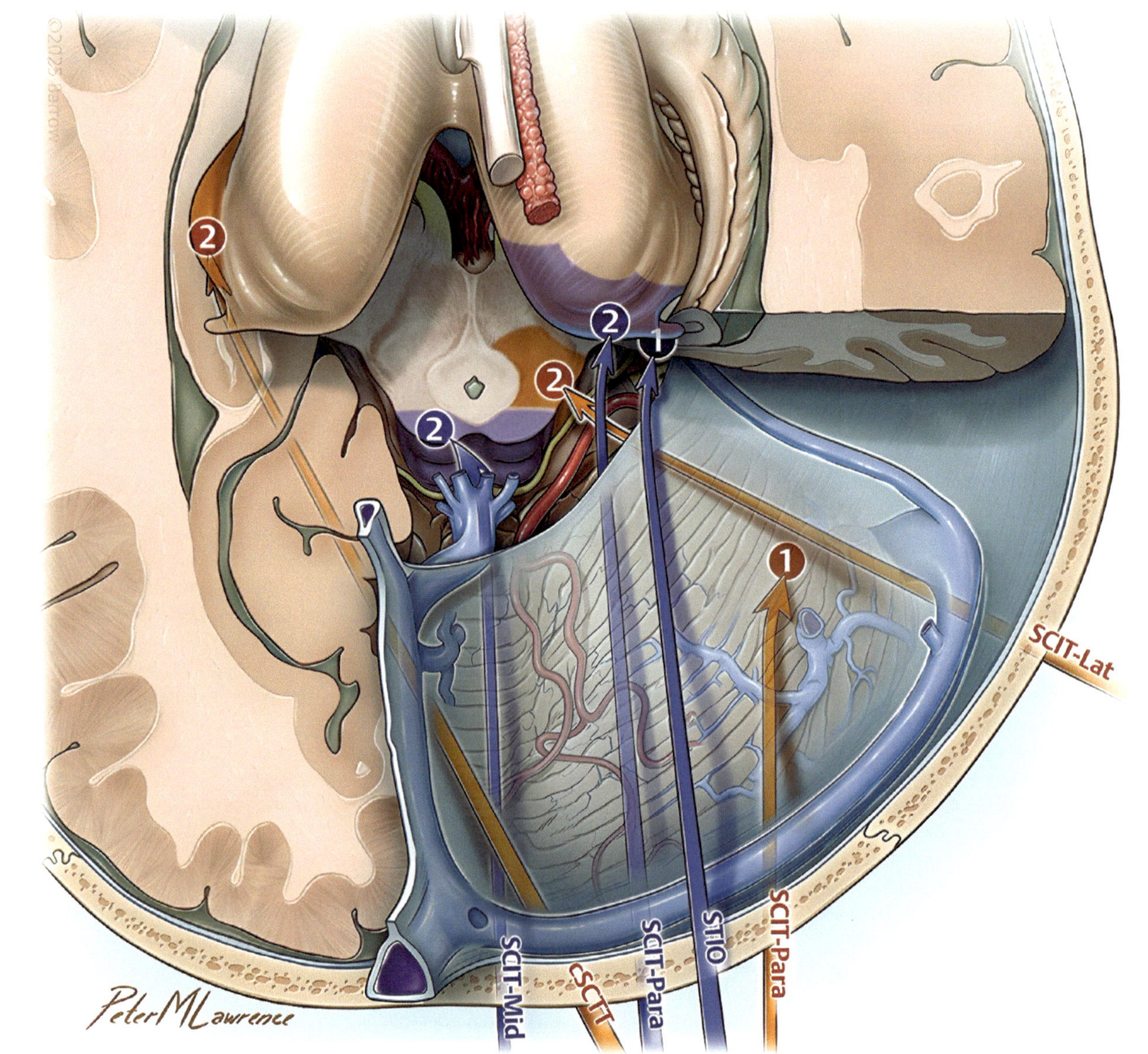

Fig. 2.5 Transtentorial approaches. The tentorial fissure is the space occupied by the tentorium cerebelli and rivals the longitudinal and sylvian fissures as one of the great surgical corridors. The subarachnoid spaces and cisterns around the tentorium lead directly to deep targets in the cerebrum's basal surfaces, thalamus, and brainstem. This corridor has only two levels of dissection depth to reach cavernomas in the basal surfaces of the occipital and temporal lobes and the tentorial surface of the cerebellum (level 1), and tegmental and quadrigeminal midbrain as well as pulvinar and geniculate thalamic cavernomas (level 2). However, there are three variations of approach into the tentorium: infratentorial (SCIT), supratentorial (STIO), and transtentorial (SCTT). In addition, the tentorium's semicircular shape produces three variations of trajectory: posterior midline (SCIT-Mid), paramedian (SCIT-Para), and lateral (SCIT-Lat). Thus, there are at least eight distinct approaches to traverse the tentorial fissure. (Reproduced with permission from Barrow Neurological Institute, Phoenix, AZ.)

Table 2.6 Subarachnoid dissection approaches through the tentorial fissure

Approach	Abbreviation	Dissection level[a]
Supracerebellar-infratentorial (midline)	SCIT-Mid	2
Supracerebellar-infratentorial (paramedian)	SCIT-Para	2
Supracerebellar-infratentorial (lateral)	SCIT-Lat	2
Supracerebellar-infratentorial (contralateral)	cSCIT	2
Supracerebellar-transtentorial (ipsilateral)	iSCTT	2
Supracerebellar-transtentorial (contralateral)	cSCTT	2
Supracerebellar-supratrochlear	SCST	2
Infratentorial-infratrochlear	ITIT	2
Supratentorial-infraoccipital	STIO	1
Subtemporal	ST	1
Subtemporal-transtentorial	STTT	2
Occipital transtentorial (ipsilateral)	iOTT	2
Occipital transtentorial (contralateral)	cOTT	2
Supracerebellar-infratentorial inverted subchoroidal	SCIT-IS	2

[a]Depth of dissection from superficial (level 1) to deep (level 4).

in the tentorium. With the SCIT-Mid and SCIT-Lat approaches, the arachnoid of the posterior incisural space is incised to drain the quadrigeminal cistern and expose the posterior midbrain. Orienting landmarks include the pineal gland, superior and inferior colliculi, the Galenic venous complex, loops of the P3 (quadrigeminal) segment of the PCA, and medial posterior choroidal artery coursing over the superior colliculus. With the SCIT-Lat approach, the arachnoid of the middle incisural space is incised to drain the ambient cistern. The orienting anatomy consists of the rostral and caudal trunks of the SCA (a2 lateral pontomesencephalic and a3 cerebellomesencephalic segments) and trochlear nerve as it originates beneath the inferior colliculus, ascends in the cerebellomesencephalic fissure, and parallels the free edge of the tentorium. The lateral mesencephalic vein courses in the sulcus that separates the cerebral peduncle anteriorly from the superior cerebellar peduncle and tegmentum posteriorly. The surface anatomy of the midbrain tegmentum includes the brachium of the inferior colliculus, lemniscal trigone, interpeduncular sulcus between the superior cerebellar peduncle and the middle cerebellar peduncle (MCP), and the rostral portion of the MCP.

Like the infratentorial approaches through the tentorial fissure, the supratentorial approaches exploit this expansive anatomic corridor but not gravity retraction, being on the tentorium's upside. The supratentorial-infraoccipital (STIO) approach accesses basal occipital and posteromedial temporal cavernomas, and the subtemporal approach accesses basal temporal cavernomas. The STIO approach (▸ Fig. 2.6) fans out along the basal occipital lobe between the straight and superior petrosal sinuses. The patient is positioned in the lateral or park bench position with the head rotated until the patient's head is nearly facing the floor, with the head gently flexed to account for the rise of the tentorium. An L- or U-shaped incision is made with the vertical portion paralleling the SSS and curving laterally over the parietal region. A torcular craniotomy is elevated in two pieces with an occipital flap raised first to allow stripping of the SSS, transverse sinus, and torcular Herophili under direct visualization. A second, L-shaped flap extends the exposure across these venous sinuses. The dura is opened in a curvilinear fashion from the SSS to the transverse sinus and then bisected with an incision down to the corner of the torcular Herophili, thereby releasing the occipital pole and opening the inferomedial infraoccipital corridor. Under microscopic visualization, infraoccipital dissection is extended downward into the quadrigeminal cistern for rapid CSF release, brain relaxation, and wider subarachnoid dissection. Important anatomic landmarks in the quadrigeminal and ambient cisterns include the tentorial incisura, PCA branches, and veins draining to the basal veins of Rosenthal.

The popular subtemporal approach uses a temporal craniotomy with the patient positioned supine, the head rotated 90 degrees (midline horizontal), and the neck flexed laterally to drop the vertex downward toward the floor, allowing the temporal lobe to fall away from the middle fossa floor. The inferior extent of the craniotomy is flattened to remove the lip of the temporal squamosal bone and widen exposure to the floor. Subtemporal dissection exposes cavernomas along the basal temporal surface. Release of tentorial adhesions and arachnoid granulations frees the temporal lobe, and CSF drainage from carotid and ambient cisterns slackens the brain. This approach typically requires fixed retraction for lesions located more medially.

The transtentorial approaches are the third variation of approaches through the tentorial fissure. They begin on one side of the tentorium and cross to the other through a tentoriotomy incision and include the contralateral supracerebellar-transtentorial (cSCTT), occipital-transtentorial (OTT), and subtemporal-transtentorial approaches. The cSCTT approach was introduced as a modification of the SCIT-Mid approach, adding a horizontal incision in the tentorial incisura to obtain better superolateral exposure of the thalamus and extend forward into the ambient cistern. The relaxing incision widens the posterior incisural space to follow the basal vein of Rosenthal around the midbrain, bringing the inferior pulvinar surface and the geniculate nuclei of the thalamus into view. This anterolateral divergence ipsilateral to the cavernoma moves the neurosurgeon to the opposite side at the level of the craniotomy, making this a contralateral approach with a trajectory crossing the midline. Geniculate thalamic cavernomas can be exposed and entered from below with excellent visualization of the anterior, superior, and lateral margins of the lesion, which are difficult to appreciate from an ipsilateral perspective. The cSCTT extends the inferolateral exposure of the thalamus in the ambient cistern and reaches upward into the thalamus to the level of the posterior limb of the internal capsule, which would be unsafe from any other trajectory.

The occipital-transtentorial approach combines a posterior interhemispheric dissection with a tentorial incision that parallels the straight sinus to open the posterior incisural space and travel infratentorially into the quadrigeminal cistern and cerebellomesencephalic fissure. Infratentorial approaches seldom reach this low into the cerebellomesencephalic fissure without significant retraction or resection of the tissue in the quadrangular lobule. The occipital-transtentorial approach provides a direct line of sight below the quadrigeminal plate to the level of the trochlear nerve root exit zone. Target lesions include low-lying quadrigeminal midbrain and vermian cerebellar cavernomas presenting to the cisternal side of the posterolateral midbrain or central lobule. The targeted CM is located on the upside of the surgical corridor and the occipital lobe on the downside, with gravity creating a generous working corridor.

Finally, the subtemporal-transtentorial approach extends the subtemporal exposure with an incision in the tentorium behind the entrance of the trochlear nerve into its dural sleeve, bringing the lateral midbrain into view to access tegmental midbrain and upper peritrigeminal pontine cavernomas. This approach is also used for posteriorly projecting basilar aneurysms and superficial temporal artery-SCA bypasses. The trajectory of the transtentorial approach descends infratentorially and lessens the retraction on the temporal lobe. cSCTT, occipital-transtentorial, and subtemporal-transtentorial approaches modify the standard SCIT, posterior interhemispheric, and subtemporal approaches described above and add a tentoriotomy incision for a more favorable trajectory and additional reach.

2.7 Cerebellopontine Cistern

Rhoton created the concept of triplets to describe the posterior fossa structures. The brainstem comprises three parts (midbrain, pons, and medulla); three cerebellar peduncles connect the brainstem and cerebellum (superior, middle, and inferior); and three fissures divide the brainstem and the cerebellum (cerebellomesencephalic, cerebellopontine, and cerebellomedullary). The cerebellum has three surfaces (tentorial, petrosal, and suboccipital), and three arteries supply the brainstem and the cerebellum (SCA, anterior inferior cerebellar artery [AICA], and posterior inferior cerebellar artery [PICA]). There are three neurovascular complexes with one of the three brainstem parts, one of the three cerebellar surfaces, one of the three peduncles, one of the three major fissures, and one of the three cerebellar arteries. In addition, each neurovascular complex contains a group of cranial nerves (CNs): the upper complex includes the oculomotor, trochlear, and trigeminal nerves; the middle complex includes the abducens, facial, and vestibulocochlear nerves; and the lower complex includes the glossopharyngeal, vagus, accessory, and hypoglossal nerves. Dissection into the cerebellopontine cistern encounters parts of all three neurovascular complexes but dives squarely into the middle neurovascular complex with the AICA, pons, MCP, cerebellopontine fissure, petrosal surface, and CNs VI, VII, and VIII. In keeping with Rhoton's triplets, dissection in this cistern has three depths: superficially to the petrosal cerebellar surface for petrosal cavernomas (level 1), through the petrosal fissure and into the MCP for middle peduncular cavernomas in the lateral pons (level 2), and deep past CNs V, VII, VIII, IX, X, and XI to reach targeted peritrigeminal cavernomas in the anterolateral pons (level 3; ▶ Table 2.7).

The extended retrosigmoid craniotomy is used for trans-cerebellopontine cistern approaches (▶ Fig. 2.6). Skeletonizing the sigmoid sinus from the transverse–sigmoid sinus junction to the jugular bulb widens the access corridor ventrally. In addition, mobilizing the sigmoid sinus anteriorly with tension on the dural flap allows for a range of trajectories anteriorly along the petrous face or posteriorly through

Table 2.7 Approaches through the cerebellopontine cistern

Approach	Abbreviation	Dissection level[a]
Retrosigmoid–transcerebellopontine angle	RS-CPA	1
Extended retrosigmoid–trans-cerebellopontine angle	xRS-CPA	2, 3
Extended retrosigmoid–trans-middle cerebellar peduncle	xRS-MCP	2
Extended retrosigmoid-transmeatal	xRS-Mea	3
Retrolabyrinthine	RLab	3
Translabyrinthine	TLab	3
Transcochlear	TCoc	3
Combined supra- and infratentorial	Comb-SIT	3
Middle fossa	MidFos	3
Anterior transpetrous (Kawase)	Kaw	3
Retrolabyrinthine-transcrural	RLab-Cru	3
Retrolabyrinthine-transsigmoid	RLab-Sig	3
Transclival–trans-pontine cistern	TCliv-PonC	3

[a]Depth of dissection from superficial (level 1) to deep (level 4).

Subarachnoid Dissection: Cerebellopontine Cistern

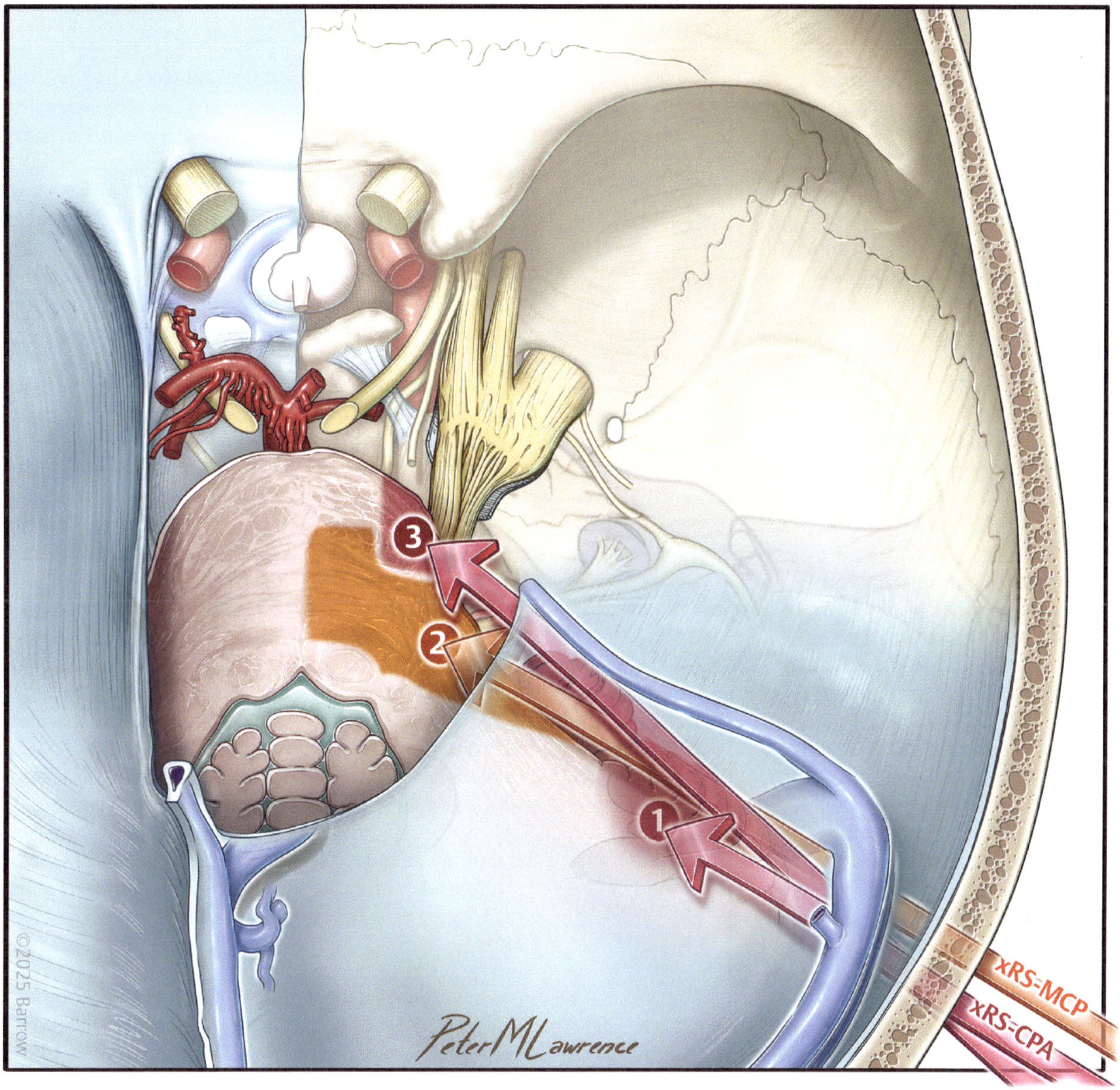

Fig. 2.6 Trans-cerebellopontine cistern approaches. Dissection in the cerebellopontine cistern has three depths: superficially to the petrosal cerebellar surface for petrosal cavernomas (level 1; xRS-CPA); through the petrosal fissure and into the MCP for middle peduncular cavernomas in the lateral pons (level 2; xRS-MCP); and deep past CNs V, VII, VIII, IX, X, and XI to reach targeted peritrigeminal cavernomas in the anterolateral pons (level 3; xRS-CPA). The xRS or RS approach is used for most of these cavernomas, but transpetrous approaches may occasionally be needed (retrolabyrinthine [RLab]; translabyrinthine [TLab]; transcochlear [TCoc]; combined supra- and infratentorial [Comb-SIT]; middle fossa [MidFos]; and anterior transpetrous/Kawase [Kaw]). (Reproduced with permission from Barrow Neurological Institute, Phoenix, AZ.)

the MCP. Skeletonization of the sigmoid sinus down to the jugular bulb provides inferior exposure to aim the surgical trajectory superiorly for pontine lesions extending into the midbrain. Following craniotomy and dural opening, the immediate release of the CSF from the lateral cerebellomedullary cistern relaxes the cerebellum. Widely opening the cerebellopontine cistern reveals the lower CN complex (CNs IX, X, XI, and XII), middle CN complex (CNs VI, VII, and VIII), and part of the upper CN complex (CNs IV and V).

Level 1 dissection leads to the cerebellar lobules that overhang into the cerebellopontine cistern and compose the petrosal surface. Petrosal cerebellar cavernomas are easily accessed and resected with minimal dissection. Level 2 dissection requires the opening of the petrosal (horizontal) fissure along the ventrolateral cerebellum between the superior and inferior semilunar lobules to reveal the MCP. Sharp arachnoid dissection widely splits the petrosal fissure, proceeding from posterolateral to anteromedial. The AICA arises at the pontine level, courses under CN VI and along CNs VII and VIII to reach the surface of the MCP, where it dives into the petrosal fissure before it emerges laterally at the cerebellopontine angle to supply the petrosal surface. Opening the petrosal fissure allows the surgeon to follow the AICA in reverse, akin to a classic sylvian split where a4 (cortical) branches take the place of M4 branches in guiding dissection, and the semilunar lobules are separated instead of the frontal and temporal lobes. The interlobular triangle is opened as the corridor to the MCP, which provides the corridor's insula-like floor. Splitting the petrosal fissure exposes the MCP safe entry zone for the trans-MCP approach. A lateral entry site on the MCP, near the intersection of superior and inferior semilunar lobules, is identified, and neuronavigation guides entry point optimization. For most lesions, a trajectory aligned with the long axis of a brainstem CM is preferred. After the selection of an ideal entry point, the pial surface is cauterized and opened sharply, after which gentle bimanual spreading dissection with lighted bipolar forceps and a long, microscopic suction tip is used to produce a narrow corridor to the lesion. This corridor gives access to the lateral pons and can extend deeper into the central pons.

Level 3 dissection travels directly through the cerebellopontine cistern to the CNs, opening their intervening dissection triangles (supra- and infratrigeminal and glossopharyngeal-cochlear triangles). Dissection through the triangles and deep to these nerve bundles leads to targeted peritrigeminal pontine cavernomas. These lesions do not necessarily require splitting the petrosal fissure to reach them, but this step mobilizes the overhanging cerebellar lobules to improve exposure and maneuverability in the cistern.

2.8 Cisterna Magna

The cisterna magna is the last of the seven corridors, providing access to the inferior cerebellum, medulla, and posterior pons (▶ Table 2.8). As the cerebellopontine cistern leads into the middle neurovascular complex, the cisterna magna leads into the lower neurovascular complex that includes the PICA, medulla, inferior cerebellar peduncle, cerebellomedullary fissure, suboccipital surface, and CNs IX, X, XI, and XII. This territory has four levels of dissection (▶ Fig. 2.7). Level 1, superficial dissection through the cisterna magna, exposes the cerebellar cortex and targeted cavernomas located inferiorly within the suboccipital, vermian, and tonsillar regions. Level 2, dissection through the cisterna magna, exposes the posterior medulla outside the fourth ventricle to reach gracile and cuneate medullary cavernoma subtypes. Level 3, deep dissection, extends into the fourth ventricle to expose targeted trigonal and rhomboid cavernomas that surface in the ventricular floor and the inferior peduncular cavernomas in the lateral recess. Level 4 is the deepest dissection level and extends into the cerebellomedullary fissure, where the PICA encircles the medulla and passes between the lower CNs.

Levels 1 to 3 are accessed through a standard suboccipital craniotomy with the patient positioned prone and the neck flexed to tuck the chin two fingerbreadths from the manubrium to open the occipital-cervical angle. Soft-tissue dissection consists of a midline linear scalp incision, a Y-shaped incision in the cervical fascia to create three leaflets for closure, and a T-shaped incision in the muscle to mobilize the paraspinal muscles inferolaterally. A suboccipital craniotomy and C1 laminectomy are performed, and rongeurs are used to nip the lateral bone of the foramen magnum to expose the region. A Y-shaped dural opening reveals the funnel of thickened arachnoid encircling the medulla and inferior cerebellum. The arachnoid of the cisterna magna is preserved to keep blood out of the subarachnoid space until the microscope is placed in the surgical field. An incision through this arachnoid layer provides access to the cisterna magna, where the trabeculated arachnoid webs between the medulla and the cisternal wall are released. At this point, level 1 targeted cerebellar cavernomas can be removed through the suboccipital, vermian, and tonsillar surfaces. Level 2 targeted deep nuclear cerebellar cavernomas lie beneath the cerebellar surface. They are accessed through either a telovelar approach, described below, or a supratonsillar approach, which is a transsulcal approach through the tonsillobiventral fissure to the region lateral of the dentate nucleus. The posterior medulla is reached by opening the cerebellomedullary fissure, which transmits the p3 (tonsillomedullary) segment of the PICA. The caudal loops of the PICA are identified at or under the inferior

Table 2.8 Subarachnoid dissection approaches through the cisterna magna

Approach	Abbreviation	Dissection level[a]
Suboccipital	SOcc	1
Suboccipital-transvermian	SOcc-Verm	2
Supratonsillar	STons	2
Suboccipital-transventricular	SOcc-Vent	3
Suboccipital-telovelar	SOcc-TeVe	3
Far lateral-transmedullary	FL-Med	4
Far lateral-transpontomedullary sulcus	FL-PMS	4
Combined far lateral-extended retrosigmoid	FL-xRS	4

[a]Depth of dissection from superficial (level 1) to deep (level 4).

Subarachnoid Dissection: Cisterna Magna

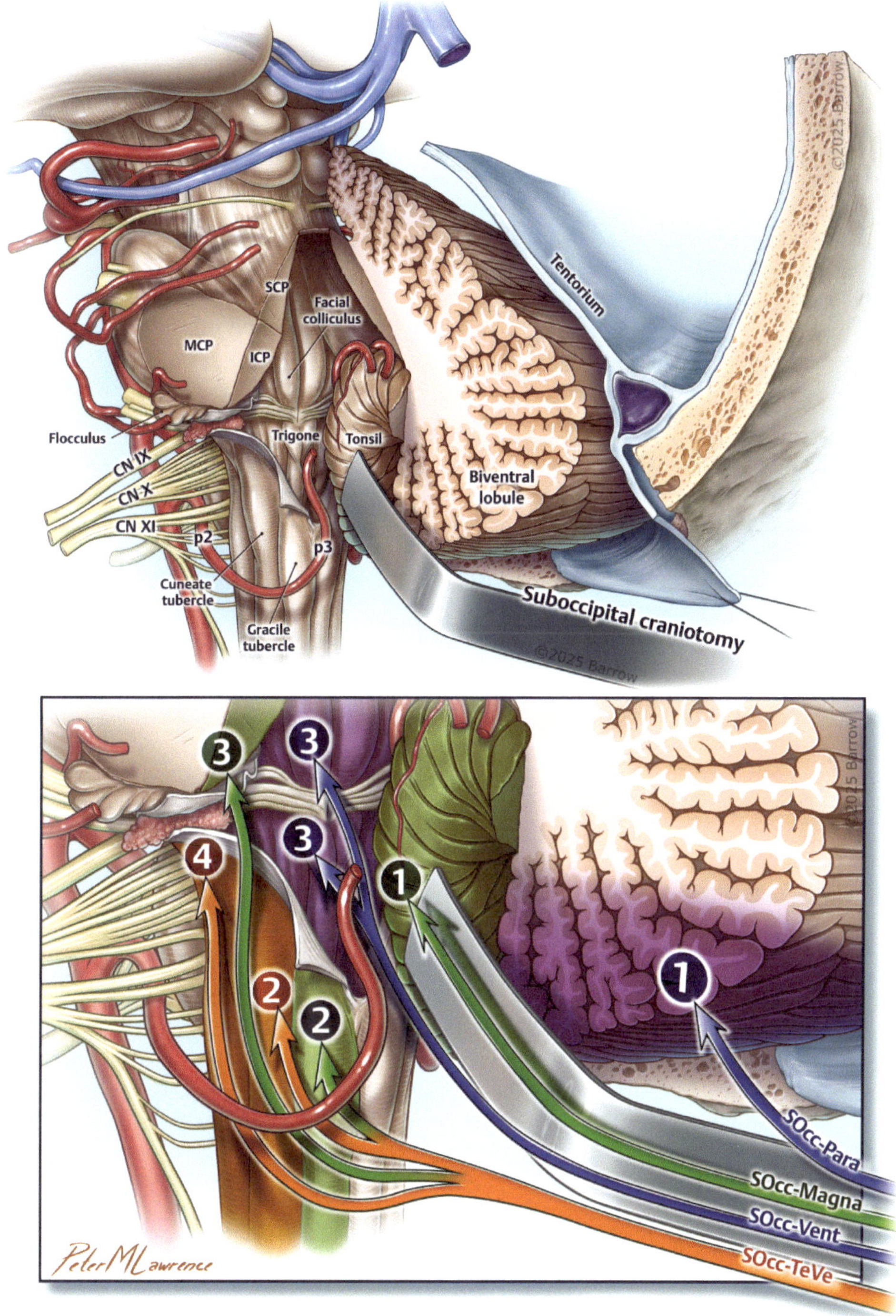

Fig. 2.7 Trans-cisterna magna approaches. The cisterna magna has four levels of dissection (*inset*). Level 1, superficial dissection through the cisterna magna, exposes the cerebellar cortex and targeted cavernomas located inferiorly within the suboccipital, vermian, and tonsillar regions (SOcc-Magna, SOcc-Verm, and SOcc-Para approaches). Level 2, dissection through the cisterna magna, exposes the posterior medulla, outside the fourth ventricle, to reach gracile and cuneate medullary cavernoma subtypes (SOcc-Magna approach). Level 3, deep dissection, extends into the fourth ventricle to expose targeted trigonal and rhomboid cavernomas that surface in the ventricular floor, as well as inferior peduncular cavernomas in the lateral recess (SOcc-Vent and SOcc-TeVe approaches). Level 4 is the deepest dissection level and extends into the cerebellomedullary fissure, where the PICA encircles the medulla and passes between the lower CNs. These deeper dissection routes require use of far lateral approaches (FL-Med and FL-PMS). (Reproduced with permission from Barrow Neurological Institute, Phoenix, AZ.)

aspect of the tonsils, and dissection along the caudal loop opens this fissure, liberates the tonsils, and enables their mobilization. These level 2 targeted extraventricular medullary cavernomas, as well as high cervical spinal cord cavernomas, are removed through this posterior brainstem surface.

Level 3 intraventricular targets require additional superior dissection. The tonsils hang from the inferomedial cerebellum and block the ventricular entrance. With their lateral mobilization, the potential space of the vallecula opens to reveal the choroid plexus in the foramen of Magendie. Cautery is used to shrink the bulky choroid plexus. Progressive widening of the vallecular triangle exposes the inferior medullar velum. The triangle-shaped velum attaches to the lateral margin of the ventricle and is an expendable arachnoid membrane. It is detached along the tela choroidea, the clear membrane from which the choroid plexus arises. This detachment of the velum along the tela choroidea defines the telovelar approach and unroofs the fourth ventricle. Although necessary for targets in the lateral recess, bilateral telovelar dissection is equally valuable for midline targets in the ventricular floor because it widens and deepens the exposure. With progressive detachment of the velum, the tonsils separate further, and the vallecular triangle widens. These maneuvers are helpful for trigonal medullary cavernomas and necessary for rhomboid pontine cavernomas, where the full extent of upward dissection and tonsillar separation is needed. Unilateral telovelar dissection out to the foramen of Luschka with the opening of the subtonsillar triangle exposes inferior peduncular cavernomas in the lateral recess. Thorough dissection and fixed upward retraction on the tonsil reveal the choroid plexus exiting the foramen of Luschka into the lateral cerebellomedullary cistern on top of the glossopharyngeal nerve.

The far lateral craniotomy enables level 4 anterolateral dissection through the cisterna magna and into the lateral cerebellomedullary cistern. The V4 (intradural) segment of the vertebral artery (VA) is identified as it pierces the dura under the dentate ligament; this ligament is then divided. The dentate ligament is a pure white fibrous sheet that attaches to the lateral margin of the spinal cord between the dorsal and ventral rootlets along the length of the spinal cord. It inserts on the dura at the level of the foramen magnum above the VA's dural penetration and fans out inferiorly over the VA. Cutting the dentate ligament at its dural insertion allows access to the VA anteriorly and detaches the upper cervical spinal cord to widen the surgical corridor. A lattice of accessory nerve rootlets crosses the VA obliquely; the C1 rootlets join the undersurface of the VA at its dural ring, and the posterior spinal arteries course to the spinal cord at this location. Liberating the caudal loop of the PICA from the inferior tonsil allows tonsillar retraction. The smooth, distinct surfaces of the medulla and anterior tonsil are easily separated, and the cerebellomedullary fissure widens to expose the proximal p3 tonsillomedullary segment of the PICA. This p3 segment is followed in the retrograde direction as it encircles the medulla and leads to the olive and p2 lateral medullary segment. The CNs arrange themselves in two layers: (1) a retro-olivary layer that extends from the retro-olivary sulcus to the jugular foramen and contains the roots of CNs IX, X, and XI and (2) a preolivary layer that extends from the preolivary sulcus to the hypoglossal foramen and contains the hypoglossal roots. Triangles through these two layers of nerve roots are opened to reach the PICA–VA confluence and lateral brainstem, specifically the vagoaccessory triangle and its internal subdivision, the suprahypoglossal, infrahypoglossal, and sometimes the hypoglossal-hypoglossal triangles. The vagoaccessory triangle is traversed to reach targeted olivary cavernomas in the medulla and supraolivary cavernomas in the underbelly of the pons. Dissection anterior to the vagoaccessory triangle into the premedullary cistern and vertebrobasilar junctional triangle exposes targeted pyramidal medullary cavernomas.

2.9 Conclusion

Subarachnoid corridors are often narrow or potential spaces that cannot be opened easily. Meticulous dissection is required, but our aptitude is greatly increased by tricks and tweaks such as gravity retraction, CSF release, brain shift, and dynamic retraction. The patient is positioned to align with the surgical corridor for a comfortable look into the brain; gravity is invoked whenever possible to open natural planes. Dural structures like the falx and tentorium are used to hold the brain, which would otherwise shift and close the plane. Deep dissections into recesses and ventricles without fixed retraction or brain transgression are what make cavernoma surgery elegant and dramatic. Strategic moves combined with expert dissection make difficult surgery easier and dangerous surgery safer. Delicate dissection and strategic maneuvers in these seven corridors make almost any cavernoma target reachable for dissection. Arachnoid sheets, bands, and trabeculae that maintain the brain's natural structure require thorough disassembly before neurosurgeons can develop and navigate naturally occurring extraparenchymal tissue planes as surgical corridors.

3 TRIANGLES

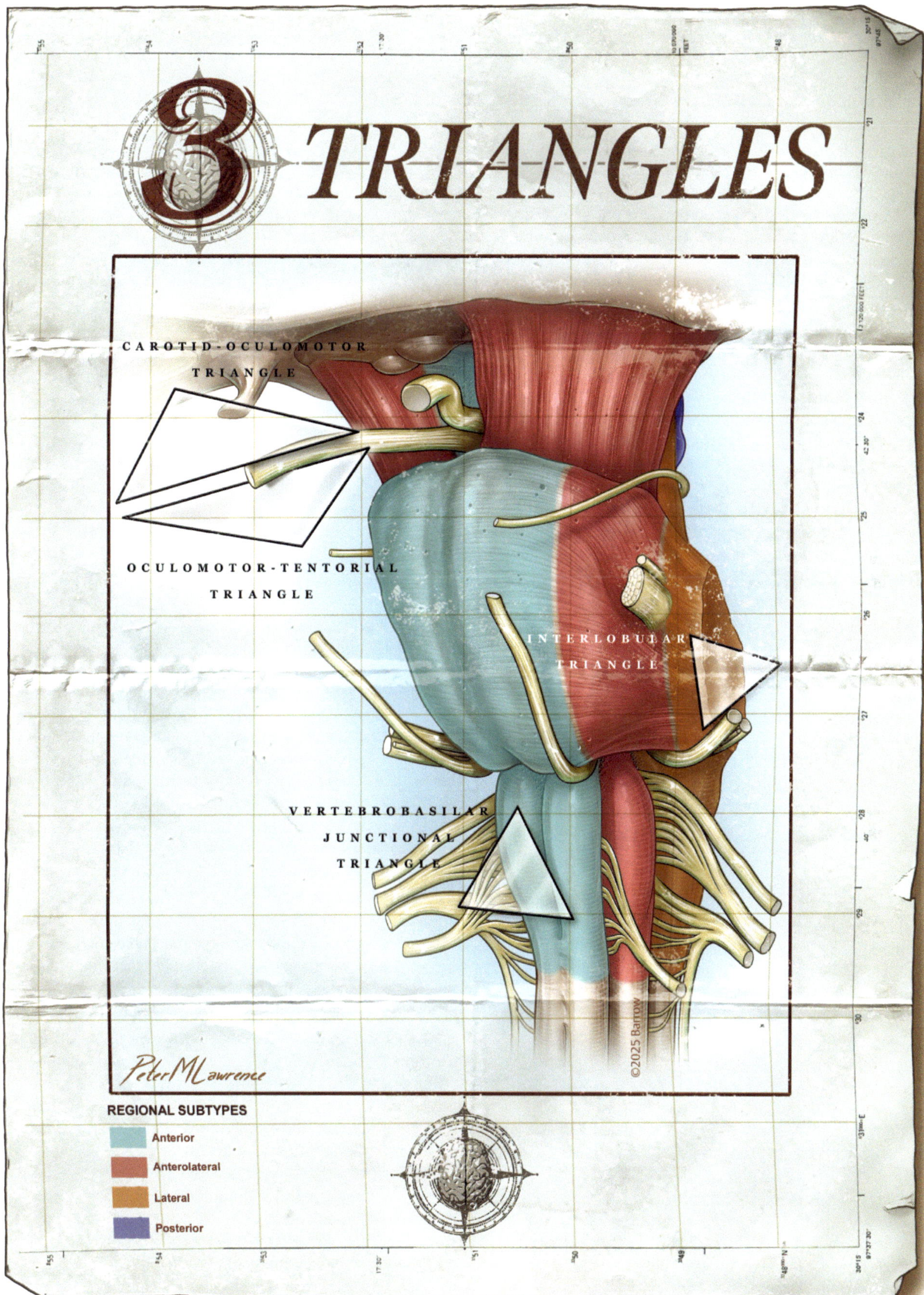

Reproduced with permission from Barrow Neurological Institute, Phoenix, AZ.

3 Triangle Concept

Summary
Anatomical triangles are defined by intersecting neurovascular structures. These triangles fine-tune surgical routes to pathological targets such as aneurysms and cavernous malformations (CMs). Although the craniotomy and approach typically delineate dissection pathways, they may fail to define the precise dissection route. The addition of the appropriate anatomical triangle combined with the craniotomy and approach expedites the mapping of the exact pathway to the target CM and reduces errors and uncertainty. One can think of the combination of craniotomy, approach, and triangle as analogous to the sights on a rifle that facilitate taking perfect aim. The triangle concept increases specificity beyond the craniotomy and approach to guide accurate dissection to the target. A system of 14 primary triangles complementary to the taxonomy refines dissection routes to brainstem target CMs and clarifies the approach through arachnoid corridors to reach specific brainstem CM subtypes. Most cerebral and cerebellar CMs have no associated triangles because they occur superficially on hemispheric surfaces. The triangle concept, along with a detailed knowledge of surface anatomy and safe entry zones, is a reliable and precise anatomical navigation tool to guide dissection to targeted CM lesions.

Keywords: approach, arachnoid membrane, artery, brainstem, cavernous malformation, dissection, fissure, safe entry zone, sulcus

3.1 The Triangle Concept

Geometric concepts have value in planning and executing microneurosurgical strategies. For example, the box concept for brain arteriovenous malformations (AVMs) applies an orthogonal structure to a complex tangle of vessels. It simplifies the nidus into six sides, defined anatomically as medial, lateral, anterior, posterior, deep, and superficial, and structurally as pial, parenchymal, and ependymal. Each side of the box can be characterized by relationships between feeding arteries, draining veins, cortical landmarks, and eloquence that categorize the AVM into hot and cold sides based on the presence or absence of these key features. With the box concept, the dissection strategy leads surgeons to confront the hot sides early to dearterialize the AVM and the eloquent sides after the nidus has quieted. The box concept paces the dissection by progressing from the top (pial) to the four sides (parenchymal) to the bottom (ependymal) of the box.

The triangle concept for cavernous malformations (CMs) is analogous to the box concept for brain AVMs. CMs do not need conceptualization of resection steps like AVMs because their removal is much simpler. Instead, CMs require greater precision in the dissection pathway to reach the pathological target. Although the craniotomy and approach describe this pathway, these descriptors may fail to define the exact dissection route. With the addition of a triangle, the combination of the craniotomy, approach, and triangle maps the exact pathway to the target CM and reduces errors and uncertainty.

The sights of a rifle are a helpful analogy. The rear sight on the back of the gun barrel and the front sight at the end of the barrel allow the shooter to align the two sights between the shooter's eye and the target to aim the rifle. Without the second sight, the shot is unlikely to be accurate. Microsurgically, the craniotomy is analogous to the rear sight, the approach is the line of sight down the gun barrel, and the triangle is the front sight. Without the triangle, the trajectory of the approach is unlikely to be accurate. The addition of the triangle better defines the pathway taken through the craniotomy and refines our conceptualization of the surgical approach. The triangle concept adds this second sight, or extra specificity, to the surgical strategy, which then guides dissection through subarachnoid corridors, enhances microsurgical execution, and could improve patient outcomes.

The triangle concept informs the dissection approach better than the craniotomy alone. There are three times as many CM subtypes as there are craniotomies for the treatment of brainstem CMs, and the large windows of these craniotomies often accommodate multiple approaches. Therefore, the craniotomy strategy is inferior to the triangle concept for choosing surgical approaches to reach the target lesion. The triangle concept increases specificity beyond the craniotomy and guides accurate dissection to the target CM. Triangles are defined by discrete anatomical borders within the subarachnoid space that can be identified despite hemorrhage, distortion of the brainstem surface anatomy from hematoma or edema, or inaccuracies in the intraoperative navigation system. Modern neurosurgical operating room technology continues to advance, and frameless stereotactic navigation is the standard of care for microsurgical resection of CMs. However, head movement, brain shift, and inherent inaccuracies make stereotactic navigation less reliable than triangle landmarks. A system of triangles, combined with a detailed knowledge of surface anatomy and safe entry zones, is an accurate and dependable navigation tool that guides dissection to the target lesions.

3.2 A System of Anatomical Triangles

Intersecting neurovascular structures define anatomical triangles that deepen our anatomical knowledge, define surgical routes to pathological targets, and guide neurosurgeons during dissection steps. Triangles are particularly useful in vascular neurosurgery because most dissection is within the subarachnoid space that contains these neurovascular structures. As a proponent of this triangle concept, I have introduced or tried to popularize the use of several new triangles in vascular neurosurgery, including the vagoaccessory, suprahypoglossal, hypoglossal-hypoglossal, and infrahypoglossal triangles to guide dissection to posterior inferior cerebellar artery (PICA) aneurysms through the network of the overlying glossopharyngeal, vagus, accessory, and hypoglossal nerves. These triangles clarify the borders of the operative corridors and the depth of dissection through the nerves. The A1-A1 precommunicating triangle (formed by the precommunicating segment of the anterior cerebral artery [ACA]) and the A1-A2 junctional triangle (formed by the precommunicating and postcommunicating segments of the ACA) were introduced to guide dissection to anterior communicating artery (ACoA) aneurysms through the complex of five parent and seven branch arteries at the anterior circle of Willis. The precommunicating triangle exposes ACoA aneurysms that project anteriorly and inferiorly. The precommunicating triangle allows the surgeon to exert proximal control. In contrast, the junctional triangle leads to the region behind the ACoA complex for dissection of the branch arteries, visualization of the posterior clip blade during application, and perforator preservation with superiorly and posteriorly projecting ACoA aneurysms. The oculomotor-tentorial triangle (OTT) was introduced to guide dissection in and around the crural and ambient cisterns to a variety of pathologies like posterior cerebral artery (PCA) aneurysms, brainstem CMs, and dural arteriovenous fistulas. The OTT is an essential workspace for posterior circulation bypasses, providing a pretemporal alternative to traditional subtemporal routes.

Collections or systems of anatomical triangles have proven helpful for specific surgical subspecialties, notably skull base surgery. Although the intersection of cranial nerves, arteries, and venous sinuses makes the cavernous sinus anatomy among the most complex in the human body, a triangle system of landmarks has made skull base surgery in this workspace navigable and safer. Anterior clinoidectomy and dissection of the clinoidal (Dolenc) triangle provide access to the proximal and distal dural rings and the clinoidal segment of the internal carotid artery (ICA). The dissection of the oculomotor (Hakuba) triangle allows access to the oculomotor nerve, the intracavernous segment of the abducens nerve, and the cavernous ICA. Dissection of the infratrochlear (Parkinson) triangle opens the center of the cavernous sinus to access the cavernous ICA, meningohypophyseal trunk, and abducens nerve. Eight other cavernous sinus triangles, including the (1) supratrochlear, (2) anterolateral, (3) anteromedial, (4) posteromedial (Kawase), (5) posterolateral (Glasscock), (6) lateral, (7) inferomedial, and (8) inferolateral, form a collage of dissection routes that informs the skull base surgeon's selection of the approach and route to specific target pathologies (▸ Fig. 3.1; ▸ Video 3.1, ▸ Video 3.2, ▸ Video 3.3).

A similar system of anatomical triangles would be advantageous for targeted brainstem CMs located at the geographic center of the cranium, which are reached at the end of long surgical corridors described by the craniotomy and approach (▸ Table 3.1). For example, a pterional craniotomy may be used with a transsylvian approach to describe the route to a basilar artery bifurcation aneurysm and differentiate it from a temporal craniotomy and subtemporal approach to this lesion. Although the combination of craniotomy and approach is more descriptive than the craniotomy alone, deep dissection routes used with brainstem CMs require the additional specificity of the triangle concept. In this example, transsylvian dissection of a basilar bifurcation aneurysm ultimately leads into the carotid-oculomotor triangle; however, the transsylvian dissection of an anterior midbrain CM requires a choice between the carotid-oculomotor triangle for interpeduncular lesions and the OTT for peduncular lesions. The anatomical triangle adds specificity to the description of the approach and further guides the neurosurgeon during the final dissection to reach the lesion.

Fourteen triangles are defined, with additional secondary triangles subdividing some primary triangles (▸ Fig. 3.2). Five triangles are well established and described, including the carotid-oculomotor, oculomotor-tentorial, Kawase, vagoaccessory, and glossopharyngeal-cochlear triangles. These triangles were developed and popularized for other lesions, like aneurysms and tumors, and are applied here to brainstem CMs. Four other triangles define known routes that have been used intuitively but not named formally as triangles, like the vallecular triangle associated with a suboccipital transventricular approach, the supra- and infratrigeminal triangles associated with an extended retrosigmoid–trans-cerebellopontine cistern approach, and the subtonsillar triangle associated with the telovelar approach. The naming of these triangles helps formalize this system for brainstem CMs and provides standardization in the literature and our discourse.

Five other triangles are newly defined: (1) infragalenic, (2) supracerebellar-supratrochlear, (3) supracerebellar-infratrochlear, (4) interlobular, and (5) vertebrobasilar junctional. These additions to the system emphasize the anatomical details of particular routes or the technical nuances of the exposures. For example, the interlobular triangle is a potential space underneath the superior and inferior semilunar lobules that becomes apparent only after dissecting the course of the anterior inferior cerebellar artery (AICA), splitting the petrosal fissure, and separating these apposed surfaces of the cerebellum. The pairing of the interlobular triangle with the middle peduncular pontine subtype of CM emphasizes that these dissection steps are necessary for safe lateral entry into the middle cerebellar peduncle (MCP) to resect this target lesion. Similarly, the infragalenic triangle emphasizes the importance of preserving the trunks of the deep venous system, especially the basal vein of Rosenthal (BVR) and precentral cerebellar vein, by resecting targeted quadrigeminal brainstem CMs beneath them. In addition, the infragalenic triangle can be widened laterally with a transtentorial incision and dissection along the BVR into the ambient cistern to access CMs in the thalamus that surface at the lateral geniculate nucleus (geniculate subtype of thalamic CM). This triangle emphasizes that anatomy can be used as a dissection guide in deep corridors without a panoramic field of view, and triangles introduced for brainstem CMs might have applications to CMs and other lesions outside of the brainstem.

3.3 Midbrain Triangles

Six triangles represent wayfinding landmarks within the midbrain: (1) the carotid-oculomotor triangle, (2) the OTT, (3) the lemniscal (Reil's) trigone triangle, (4) the supratrochlear triangle, (5) infratrochlear triangle, and (6) the infragalenic triangle. Each triangle leads the approach to deeper corridors that have limited visibility at the lesion. Thus, they help guide dissection to targeted CMs.

3

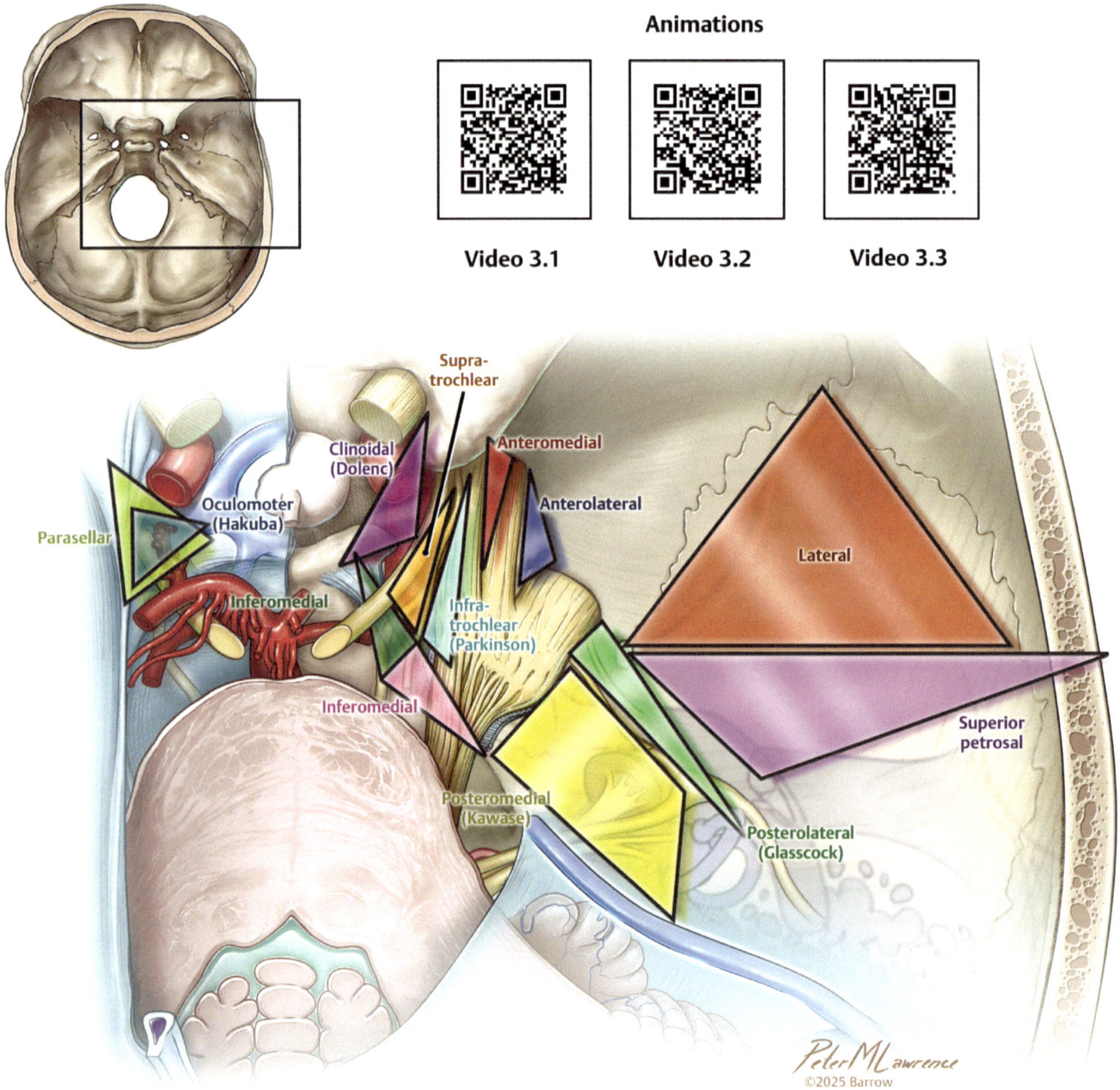

Fig. 3.1 Illustration of the three divisions of the triangles within the middle cranial fossa: the medial fossa and cavernous sinus, lateral fossa, and paraclival triangles. Six of the seven medial fossa and cavernous sinus region triangles are shown: parasellar, clinoidal, oculomotor, supratrochlear, infratrochlear, and anteromedial. Five of the six lateral fossa triangles are shown: anterolateral, posteromedial, posterolateral, lateral, and superior petrosal. Two of the three paraclival triangles are shown: inferomedial and inferolateral. *Inset* shows craniotomy (animations, ▶ Video 3.1, Midbrain triangles, ▶ Video 3.2, Pontine triangles, ▶ Video 3.3 Medullary triangles, QR codes). (Reproduced with permission from Barrow Neurological Institute, Phoenix, AZ.)

Table 3.1 Summary of brainstem cavernous malformations subtypes, approaches, and triangles

Type	Subtype	Craniotomy	Approach	Triangle
Midbrain	Interpeduncular	Orbitozygomatic-pterional	TSyl-IntPed	Carotid-oculomotor
	Peduncular	Orbitozygomatic-pterional	TSyl-Ped	Oculomotor-tentorial
	Tegmental	Retrosigmoid	SCIT-Para	Supracerebellar-supratrochlear, supracerebellar-infratrochlear
	Quadrigeminal	Torcular	SCIT-Mid	Infragalenic
	Periaqueductal	Bifrontal	TCal-TChor	None
Pontine	Basilar	Orbitozygomatic-pterional	Kaw, TSyl-Cav-Pon	Kawase, carotid-oculomotor
	Peritrigeminal	Extended retrosigmoid	xRS-CPA	Supratrigeminal, infratrigeminal, glossopharyngeal-cochlear
	Middle peduncular	Extended retrosigmoid	xRS-MCP	Interlobular
	Inferior peduncular	Suboccipital	SOcc-TeVe	Subtonsillar
	Rhomboid	Suboccipital	SOcc-Vent	Vallecular
	Supraolivary	Far lateral	FL-PMS	Vagoaccessory (SHT)
Medullary	Pyramidal	Far lateral	FL-Med	Junctional
	Olivary	Far lateral	FL-Med	Vagoaccessory (SHT), vagoaccessory (HHT)
	Trigonal	Suboccipital	SOcc-Vent	Vallecular
	Gracile	Suboccipital	SOcc-Magna	Vallecular
	Cuneate	Suboccipital	SOcc-TeVe	Subtonsillar

3.3.1 Carotid-Oculomotor Triangle

The carotid-oculomotor triangle is bordered by the supraclinoid ICA segment medially, a line from the anterior clinoid process to the porus oculomotorius anterolaterally, and a line from the ICA bifurcation to the location where the oculomotor nerve intersects the tentorium posterolaterally (▶ Fig. 3.3; ▶ Table 3.2). The carotid-oculomotor triangle is a critical window for approach to the basilar quadrifurcation, upper basilar trunk, the P1 (precommunicating) and P2A (crural) segments of the PCA, and s1 (anterior pontomesencephalic) segment of the superior cerebellar artery (SCA). Anterior thalamoperforators from the posterior communicating artery (PCoA) ascend out of the triangle, and the anterior choroidal artery (AChA) sweeps medially. This triangle can be widened with an anterior clinoidectomy, liberation of the oculomotor nerve from its dural sheath, and mobilization of the nerve laterally. The triangle can be widened posteriorly with a posterior clinoidectomy and mobilization of the ICA medially. The carotid-oculomotor triangle has been used for approaches to the basilar artery but had remained unnamed until reported as the carotid-oculomotor window by Youssef and colleagues in 2004. The carotid-oculomotor triangle differs from the oculomotor or medial triangle. The oculomotor or medial triangle is bordered by the anterior petroclinoid, posterior petroclinoid, and interclinoid dural folds.

3.3.2 Oculomotor-Tentorial Triangle

The OTT is defined by the cisternal segment of the oculomotor nerve medially, the medial edge of the tentorium laterally, and the cerebral peduncle posteriorly (▶ Fig. 3.3). It is a potential space opened with posterolateral mobilization of the temporal pole. This triangle contains the P2A segment of the PCA, the s2 (lateral pontomesencephalic) segment of the SCA, and the peduncular, circumflex, and thalamogeniculate perforators; it provides access to the ventrolateral pontomesencephalic region and cerebral peduncle. This triangle provides access to aneurysms originating from these segments and is useful for posterior circulation bypasses and dural arteriovenous fistulas along the anterior incisural space. The OTT was first described in 2019 by Lawton and colleagues.

3.3.3 Supracerebellar-Supratrochlear and Supracerebellar-Infratrochlear Triangles

Supra- and infratrochlear (i.e., Parkinson's) triangles are best known as part of the system of cavernous sinus triangles, each providing entrance into the cavernous sinus through its lateral wall (▶ Fig. 3.1, ▶ Fig. 3.4). However, supra- and infratrochlear triangles also exist within the paramedian and lateral supracerebellar-infratentorial (SCIT) corridors (▶ Fig. 3.3, ▶ Fig. 3.4). The trochlear nerve originates beneath the inferior colliculus, courses through the cerebellomesencephalic fissure, continues through the middle incisural space, and enters the undersurface of the tentorium's free edge at the crus of the cerebral peduncle. The nerve becomes sheathed in an arachnoid sleeve in the lateral arachnoid of the ambient cistern. The supracerebellar-supratrochlear triangle is bordered by the lateral border of the tectum medially, tentorium superiorly, and trochlear nerve inferiorly. The supratrochlear triangle is the widest in the posterior incisural space where the tentorium slopes steeply up to the falcotentorial junction and is the narrowest in the middle incisural space where the trochlear nerve ascends into its dural sleeve.

3

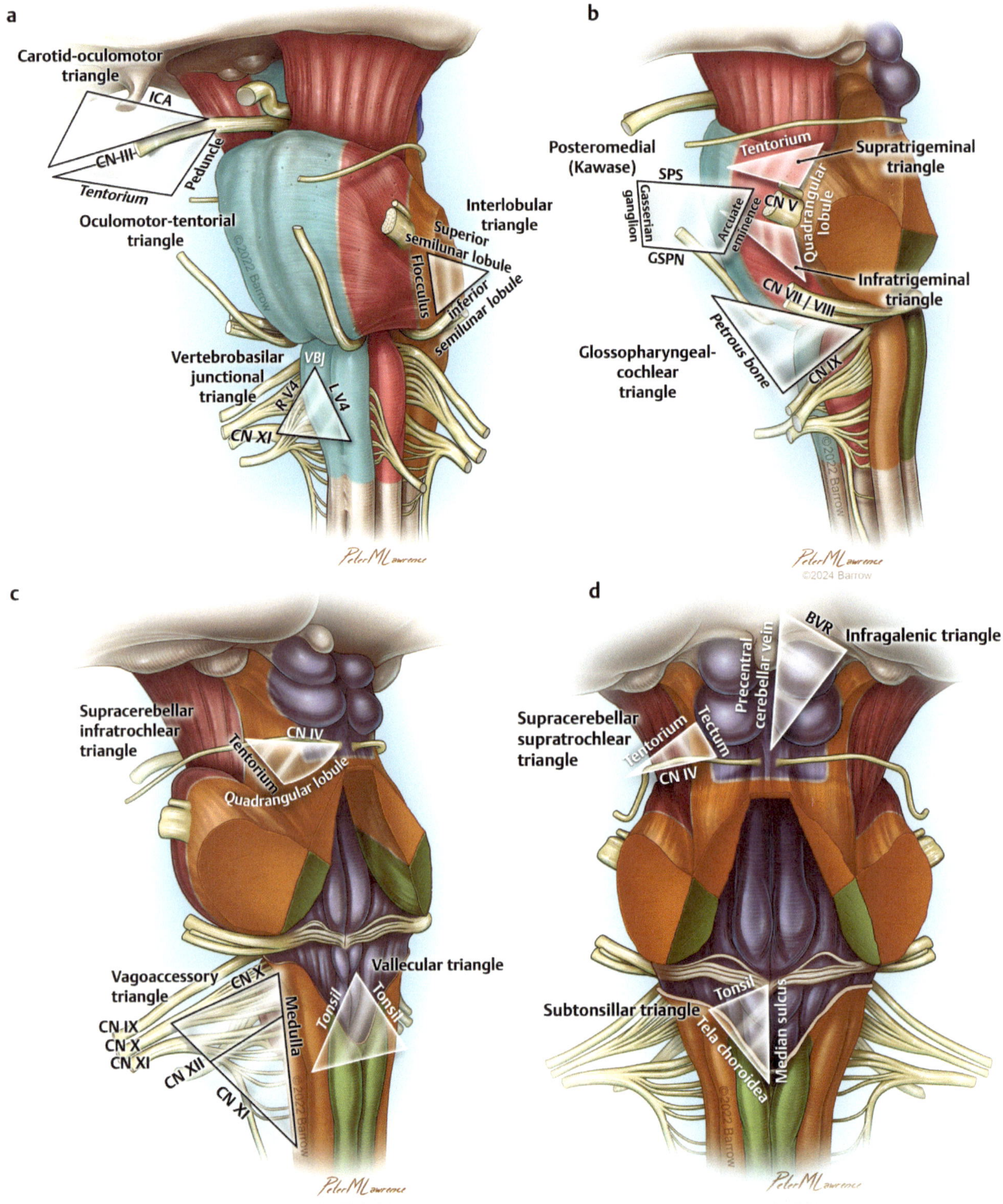

Fig. 3.2 The system of 14 anatomical triangles defining dissection routes to brainstem CMs is depicted in **(a)** anterolateral, **(b)** lateral, **(c)** posterolateral, and **(d)** posterior views. These illustrations show brainstem and cranial nerve anatomy only; other defining vascular, dural, or skull base borders are labeled on the triangles. Anterior subtypes comprise interpeduncular, basilar, and pyramidal (*teal*); anterolateral subtypes are peduncular, peritrigeminal, and olivary (*red*); lateral subtypes are tegmental, middle peduncular, and cuneate (*orange*); posterolateral subtypes are inferior peduncular and gracile (*green*); and posterior subtypes are quadrigeminal, rhomboid, and trigonal (*purple*); periaqueductal and supraolivary subtypes are not shown. (Reproduced with permission from Barrow Neurological Institute, Phoenix, AZ.)

Anterior Midbrain Triangles

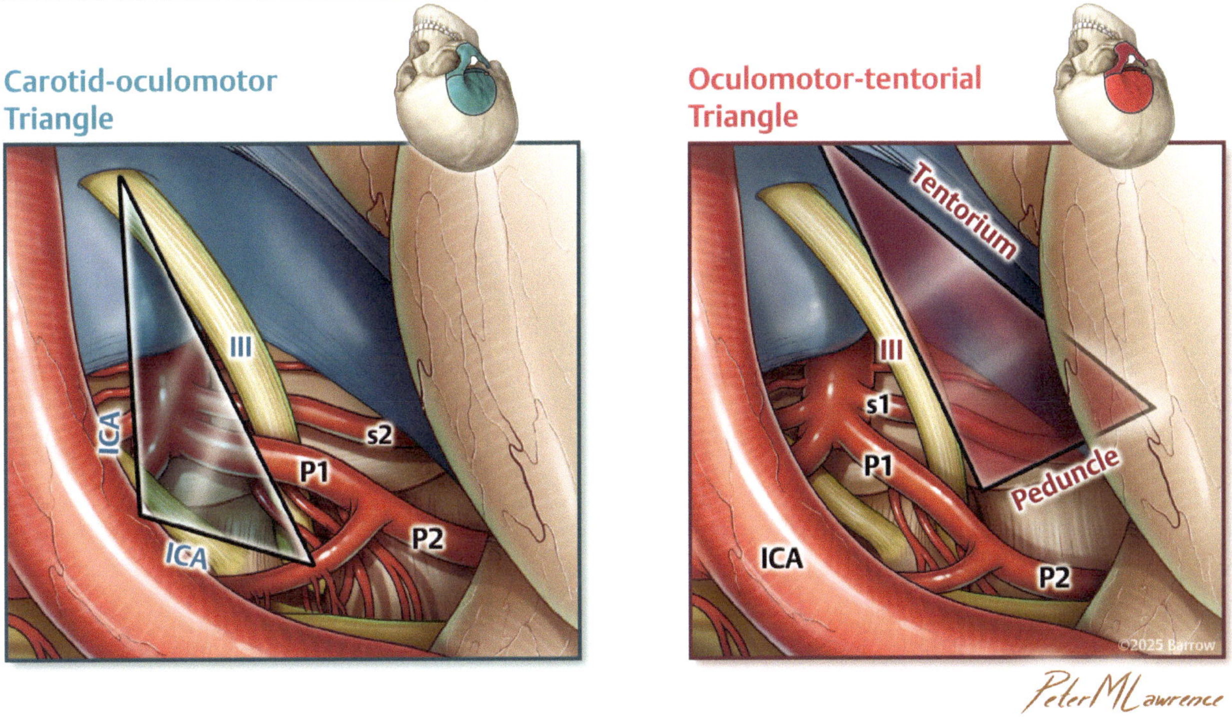

Fig. 3.3 Illustration depicting anterior midbrain triangles. The carotid-oculomotor triangle (*teal*) guides dissection to interpeduncular CMs, and the oculomotor-tentorial triangle (*red*) guides dissection to peduncular CMs. *Insets* show craniotomies. Roman numerals denote cranial nerves. (Reproduced with permission from Barrow Neurological Institute, Phoenix, AZ.)

Table 3.2 Anatomical triangles for accessing midbrain CMs

Triangle	Orientation	Borders	Contents and significance	Safe entry zone
Carotid-oculomotor	Medial	Supraclinoid ICA segment	Basilar quadrifurcation P1, P2A, s1	Interpeduncular
	Posterolateral	Line from the CN III–tentorial intersection to ICA bifurcation		
	Anterolateral	Line from the ACP to porus oculomotorius		
Oculomotor-tentorial	Medial	Cisternal CN III segment	P2A, s1, s2 Perforators: peduncular, circumflex, thalamogeniculate	Anterior mesencephalic
	Lateral	Medial edge of the tentorium		
	Posterior	Ventrolateral cerebral peduncle		
Supracerebellar-supratrochlear	Medial	Lateral border of the tectum	Widest in posterior incisural space Best access with SCIT-Para	Lateral mesencephalic sulcus
	Superior	Tentorium CN IV		
	Inferior	CN IV		
Supracerebellar-infratrochlear	Anterosuperior	Free edge of the tentorium	Widest in middle incisural space Best access with SCIT-Lat	Lateral mesencephalic sulcus
	Posterosuperior	CN IV		
	Inferior	Quadrangular lobule		
Infragalenic	Medial	Precentral cerebellar vein	Medial quadrigeminal cistern Pineal region and tectal plate P3, s3, s4, mPChA, vein of Galen	Intercollicular Supracollicular Infracollicular
	Superolateral	Basal vein of Rosenthal		
	Inferior	Quadrangular lobule		

3

Posterior Midbrain Triangles

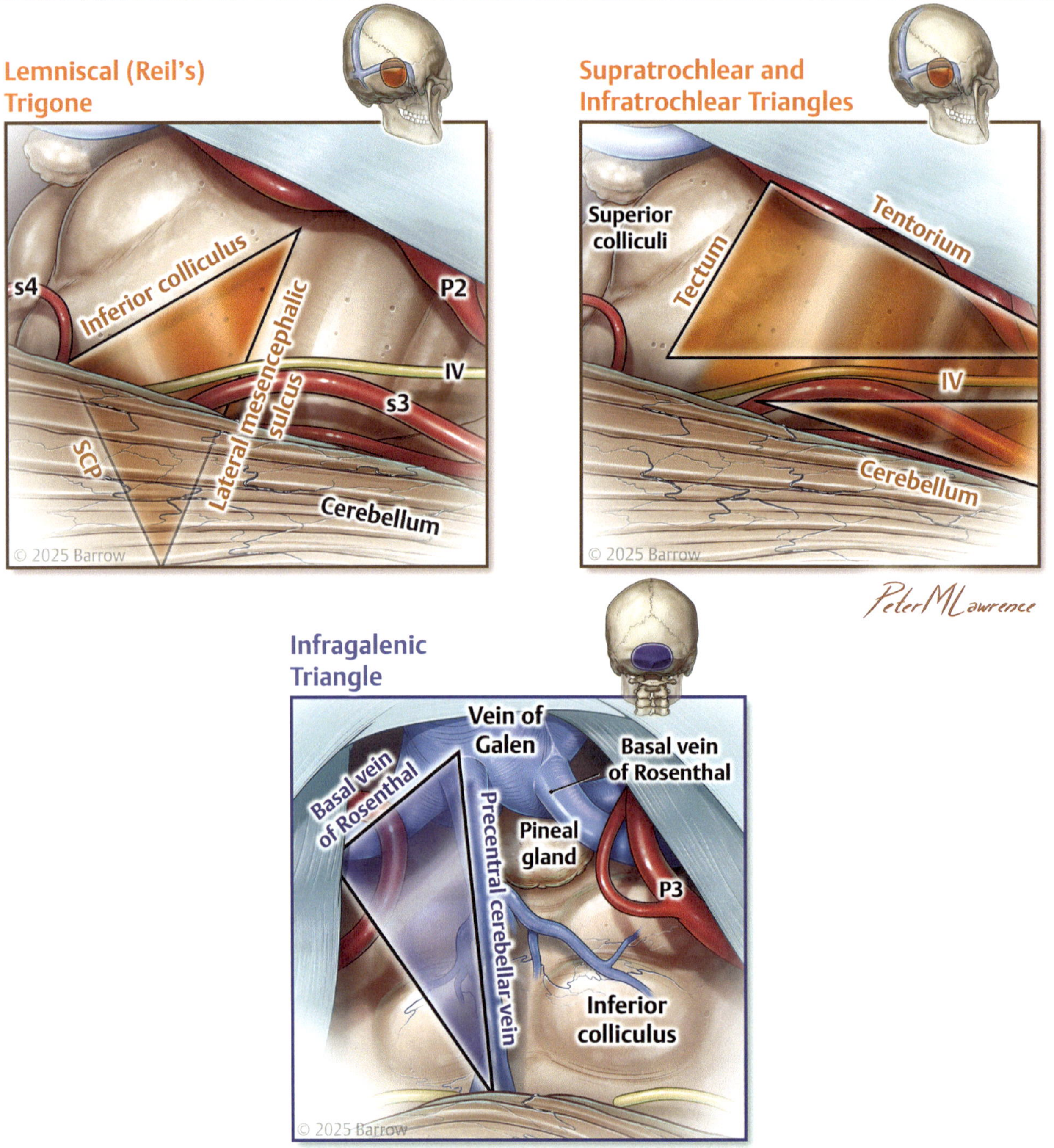

Fig. 3.4 Illustration depicting posterior midbrain triangles. The supracerebellar-supratrochlear and supracerebellar-infratrochlear triangles (*orange*) to tegmental CMs, and infragalenic triangle (*purple*) to quadrigeminal CMs. Note that Reil's trigone is a prominent triangular landmark on the midbrain tegmentum and spans both the supracerebellar-supratrochlear and supracerebellar-infratrochlear triangles. *Insets* show craniotomies. Roman numerals denote cranial nerves. (Reproduced with permission from Barrow Neurological Institute, Phoenix, AZ.)

The supracerebellar-infratrochlear triangle is bordered by the trochlear nerve posterosuperiorly, the free edge of tentorium anterosuperiorly, and the quadrangular lobule inferiorly. With an SCIT approach, gravity retraction of the cerebellum due to the sitting position and release of CSF from the cisterna magna lower the inferior border of the triangle and widen the triangle. The infratrochlear triangle is widest in the middle incisural space and narrowest posteriorly, where the quadrangular lobule rises to join the superior vermis and central lobule. Therefore, the supratrochlear triangle is more accessible with a paramedian SCIT approach, whereas the infratrochlear triangle is more accessible with a lateral SCIT approach. The supratrochlear triangle allows access to the quadrigeminal cistern, posterior tegmentum, P2 P (ambient) and P3 (quadrigeminal) segments of the PCA, and the midbrain above the BVR. The infratrochlear triangle provides access to the ambient cistern, cerebellomesencephalic fissure, anterior tegmentum, s3 segments of the SCA, circumflex perforators, and lateral mesencephalic vein. Supratrochlear access can be created in the middle incisural space by mobilizing the trochlear nerve inferiorly and making a transtentorial incision. Supracerebellar supra- and infratrochlear triangles are introduced here but were suggested by Sanai and colleagues in our differentiation of gravity-dependent variation of the lateral approaches over the cerebellum.

3.3.4 Infragalenic Triangle

The infragalenic triangle is bordered by the midline precentral cerebellar vein, the BVR superolaterally, and the quadrangular lobule of the cerebellum inferiorly (▶ Fig. 3.4). This triangular space extends laterally to the lateral border of the tectum, where the trochlear nerve emerges, and the supratrochlear triangle begins. The infragalenic triangle exposes the medial quadrigeminal cistern, the superior and inferior colliculi on one side, the pineal gland, distal s3 and s4 (cortical) segments of the SCA, loops of the P3 segment of the PCA, medial posterior choroidal artery, and the vein of Galen and its tributaries. Sagging of the cerebellum with the sitting position and gravity retraction lowers the inferior border of the triangle and widens the triangle. This working space has been used with approaches to the pineal region but has not previously been defined as an infragalenic triangle.

3.4 Pontine Triangles

Five pontine triangles and three pontomedullary triangles represent wayfinding landmarks within the pons. The pontine triangles include (1) the Kawase (posteromedial) triangle (quadrangle), (2) the glossopharyngeal-cochlear triangle, (3) the supratrigeminal triangle, (4) the infratrigeminal triangle, and (5) the interlobular triangle. The pontomedullary triangles include (1) the vallecular triangle, (2) the subtonsillar triangle, and (3) the vagoaccessory triangle. Each triangle leads the approach to deeper corridors that have limited visibility at the lesion. Thus, they help guide dissection to targeted CMs.

3.4.1 Posteromedial (Kawase) Triangle

The posteromedial triangle is also referred to as the Kawase triangle, the rhomboid space, and the Kawase–Shiobara triangle (▶ Fig. 3.1, ▶ Fig. 3.5). This triangle was first described in 1977 by Kanzaki and colleagues and later in 1985 by Kawase and colleagues. The triangle was defined as an anatomical triangle by Dolenc in 1989 and Day and colleagues in 1994. The borders of this space are the greater superficial petrosal nerve laterally, the arcuate eminence posteriorly, the superior petrosal sinus medially, and the gasserian ganglion anteriorly (▶ Table 3.3). The anterior petrous bone fills this space, with the cochlea lying at the posterolateral edge of the Kawase quadrangle. Anticipation of the cochlea within the posteromedial triangle is crucial to preserve hearing function. Drilling the temporal bone within this region exposes the petrous segment of the ICA, anterolateral pons, vertebrobasilar junction, a1 (anterior pontine) segment of the AICA, and petroclival region via a subtemporal trajectory.

3.4.2 Glossopharyngeal-Cochlear Triangle

The glossopharyngeal-cochlear triangle is defined laterally by the dural entry points of the glossopharyngeal and cochlear nerves into the jugular foramen and internal auditory meatus, respectively, and medially by their brainstem entry zone, which are anatomically adjacent to each other (▶ Fig. 3.5). The ascending course of the vestibulocochlear nerve (cranial nerve VIII) relative to the lower cranial nerves creates this small triangle of access to the cerebellopontine and cerebellomedullary cisterns and inferomedial pons lateral to the abducens nerve. The cisternal segments of cranial nerve VIII and the AICA, PICA, the distal V4 (intradural) segment of the vertebral artery (VA), and the basilar artery are exposed through this triangle. This triangle was first described as the acousticofacial-glossopharyngeal triangle in 2010 by Surek and colleagues. It was later characterized in detail and renamed the glossopharyngeal-cochlear triangle by Zhao and colleagues and Baranoski and colleagues. This workspace is used to access tumors in the posterior fossa. However, its importance for clipping high-riding PICA aneurysms led to further anatomical definition and the renaming of this triangle.

3.4.3 Supra- and Infratrigeminal Triangles

The dissection through the cerebellopontine cistern leads to cranial nerves in the three neurovascular complexes of the posterior fossa: the trigeminal nerve in the upper complex; the facial and vestibulocochlear nerves in the middle complex; and the glossopharyngeal, vagus, and accessory nerves in the lower complex. These nerve complexes define three triangular dissection routes to target CMs in this region (▶ Fig. 3.5): (1) the supratrigeminal triangle, superior to the trigeminal nerve and inferior to the tentorium and trochlear nerve; (2) the infratrigeminal triangle, inferior to the trigeminal nerve and superior to the vestibular nerve; and (3) the glossopharyngeal-cochlear

Pontine Triangles

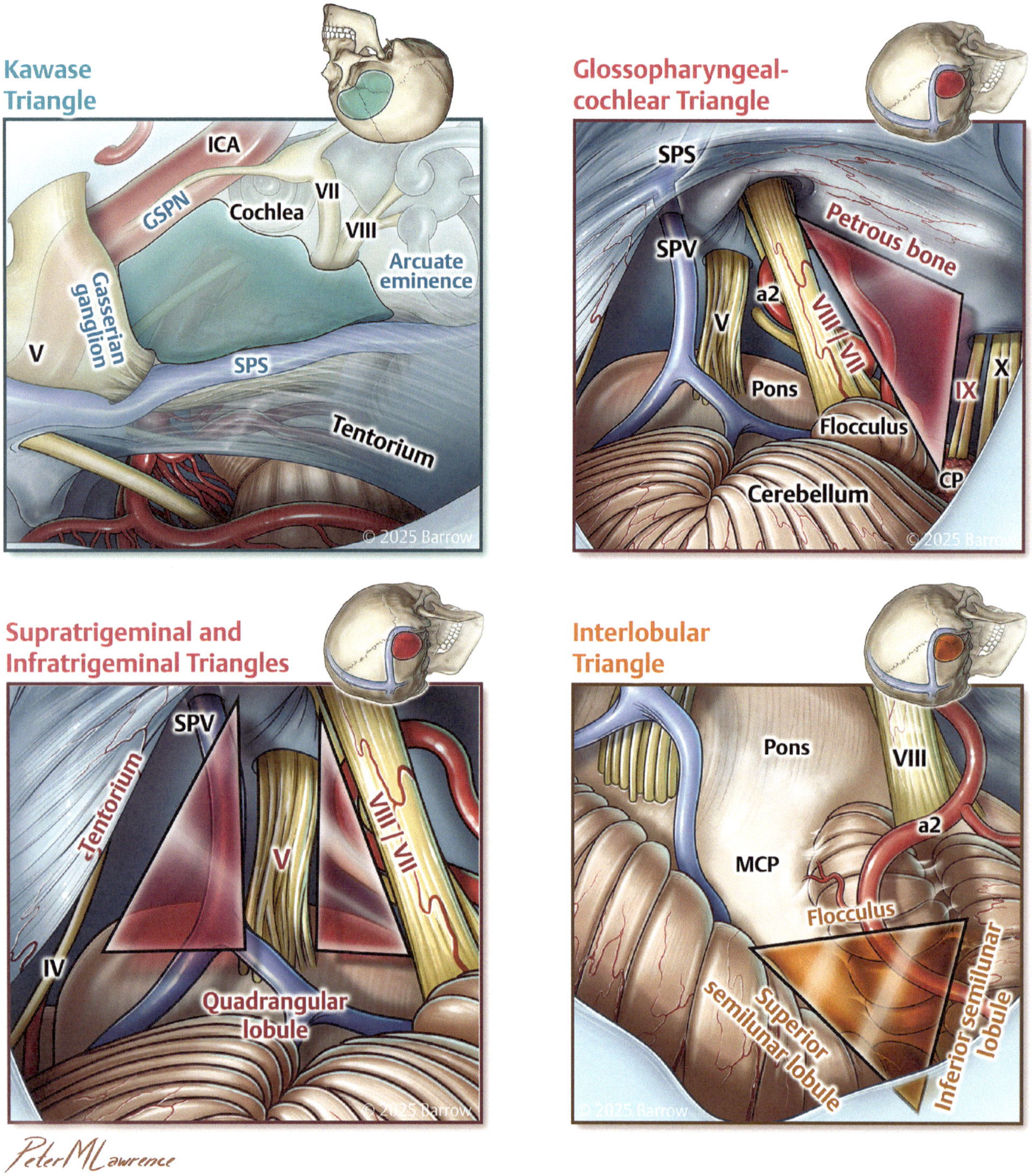

Fig. 3.5 Illustration depicting pontine triangles. The Kawase triangle (*teal quadrangle*) is a quadrangle that guides dissection to basilar CMs. The *teal* region also indicates the area of bone removal for the anterior transpetrous approach. The glossopharyngeal-cochlear triangle (*red*) guides dissection to inferior peritrigeminal CMs, supra- and infratrigeminal triangles (*red*) to superior and middle peritrigeminal CMs, respectively, and interlobular triangle (*orange*) to middle peduncular CMs. *Insets* show craniotomies. Roman numerals denote cranial nerves. (Reproduced with permission from Barrow Neurological Institute, Phoenix, AZ.)

Table 3.3 Anatomical triangles for accessing pontine CMs

Triangle	Orientation	Borders	Contents and significance	Safe entry zone
Posteromedial (Kawase)	Medial	Superior petrosal sinus	Anterior petrous bone Cochlea at the posterolateral edge, anterolateral pons Petrous ICA segment, vertebrobasilar junction	None
	Lateral	Greater superficial petrosal nerve		
	Posterior	Arcuate eminence		
	Anterior	Gasserian ganglion, V3		
Supratrigeminal	Medial	Quadrangular lobule	Meckel's cave, superior petrosal sinus, petrosal (Dandy's) vein Cerebellomesencephalic fissure, anterolateral pons, cerebral peduncular crus s3	Supratrigeminal
	Superior	Tentorium		
	Inferior	Upper edge of CN V		
Infratrigeminal	Superior	Lower edge of CN V	Porus trigeminus, porus acusticus Largest corridor to the anterior pons	Infratrigeminal
	Posterior	Quadrangular lobule		
	Inferior	Superior vestibular nerve		
	Anterior	Petrous bone		
Glossopharyngeal-cochlear	Superior	Acousticofacial complex	High-riding PICA aneurysms Distal V4, AICA, PICA	Pontomedullary sulcus
	Lateral	Petrous bone		
	Inferior	CN IX		
Interlobular	Medial	Flocculus	a3	Middle cerebellar peduncle Lateral pontine
	Superior	Inferior margin of the superior semilunar lobule		
	Inferior	Superior margin of the inferior semilunar lobule		

triangle, inferior to the cochlear nerve and superior to the glossopharyngeal nerve. The supratrigeminal triangle is defined by the upper edge of the trigeminal nerve inferiorly, the tentorium superiorly, and the quadrangular lobule medially. The porus trigeminus (Meckel's cave) and the superior petrosal sinus lie at the lateral corner of the triangle, and the petrosal vein (i.e., Dandy's vein) and its tributaries lie in front of the triangle. The motor root of the trigeminal nerve sits on the superior surface of the trigeminal nerve. The supratrigeminal triangle exposes the mouth of the cerebellomesencephalic fissure, the anterolateral pons, the crus of the cerebral peduncle, and the s3 (cerebellomesencephalic) segment of the SCA.

The infratrigeminal triangle is actually a quadrangle defined by the lower edge of the trigeminal nerve superiorly, the superior vestibular nerve inferiorly, the petrous bone anteriorly, and the quadrangular lobule of the cerebellum posteriorly. The porus trigeminus and porus acusticus lie at the anterior border of this space. The infratrigeminal triangle provides the largest corridor and best exposure to the anterolateral pontine surface. The low position of the vestibulocochlear nerve and the high position of the trigeminal nerve within the triangle contribute to this exceptional exposure.

3.4.4 Interlobular Triangle

The interlobular triangle is in the cerebellopontine angle, defined by the inferior margin of the superior semilunar lobule, the superior margin of the inferior semilunar lobule, and the flocculus medially (▶ Fig. 3.5). These lobular margins appose each other in the petrosal (horizontal) fissure and form the cerebellopontine angle. The interlobular triangle is a potential space opened by splitting the petrosal fissure. The a3 (flocculopeduncular) segment of the AICA and its branches course into this space and define the petrosal fissure. The MCP lies at the bottom of the petrosal fissure within the interlobular triangle. The wide opening of the interlobular triangle reveals the distal or lateral extent of the MCP, where it is safest to enter. At the triangle's medial border, the flocculus can be mobilized inferiorly, superiorly, or medially to expose the proximal peduncle. Although petrosal fissure access to the distal MCP is well known, the introduction of an interlobular triangle emphasizes this hidden entry zone and the technique for access.

3.4.5 Pontomedullary Triangles

Three additional triangles are used to access pontine CMs: the vallecular triangle for the rhomboid pontine subtype, the subtonsillar triangle for the inferior peduncular pontine subtype, and the vagoaccessory triangle for the supraolivary pontine subtype (▶ Fig. 3.6). These triangles are described below as medullary triangles because they are located at the level of the medulla but serve as portals to reach upward into the pons.

3.5 Medullary Triangles

Four triangles represent wayfinding landmarks within the medulla: (1) the vertebrobasilar junction triangle, (2) the

3

Pontomedullary Triangles

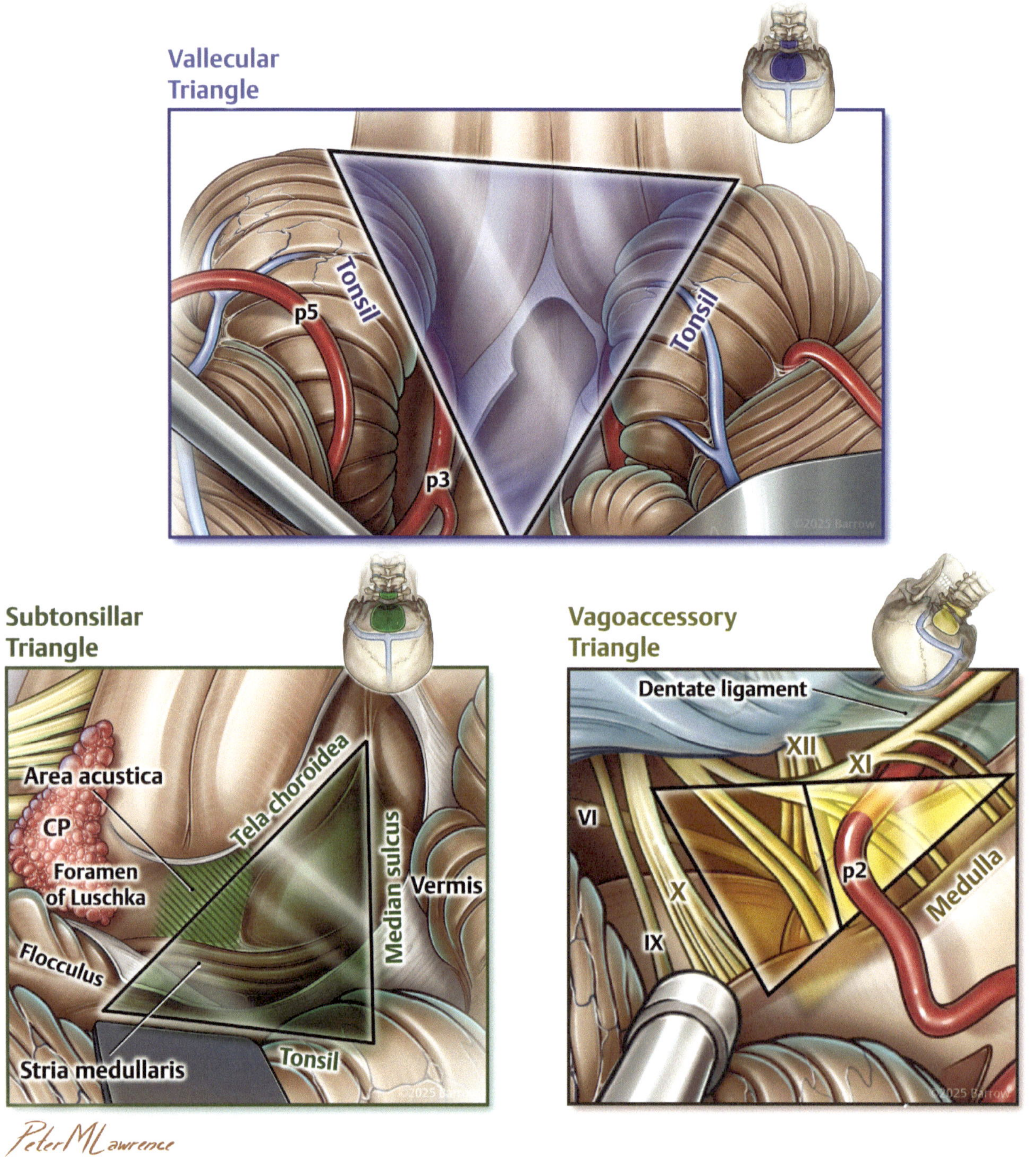

Fig. 3.6 Illustration depicting pontomedullary triangles. Pontomedullary triangles are located at the level of the medulla but serve as portals to reach upward into pontine territories. The vallecular triangle (*purple*) guides dissection to rhomboid pontine CMs. The subtonsillar triangle (*green*) guides dissection to inferior peduncular pontine CMs, and the vagoaccessory triangle (*yellow*) guides dissection to supraolivary pontine CMs. *Insets* show craniotomies. Roman numerals denote cranial nerves. (Reproduced with permission from Barrow Neurological Institute, Phoenix, AZ.)

subtonsillar triangle, (3) the vagoaccessory triangle, and (4) the triangles of the median eminence, which include the vallecular triangle, the vagal trigone, and the hypoglossal trigone. Each triangle leads the approach to deeper corridors that have limited visibility at the lesion. Thus, they help guide dissection to targeted CMs.

3.5.1 Vertebrobasilar Junctional Triangle

The junctional triangle is described as the space between the ipsilateral V4 segment of the VA, the contralateral V4 segment, and the spinal accessory nerve (▸ Fig. 3.7; ▸ Table 3.4). The triangle is named after the vertebrobasilar junction, which lies at the superior apex of the triangle. This triangle lies in front of the vagoaccessory triangle. Medially mobilizing the spinal accessory nerve with the medulla and dissecting anterior to it maximizes the anteromedial view along the clivus. This triangle is opened with an aggressive condylectomy and the vantage of the far lateral approach, with the head positioned so that the clivus is perpendicular to the floor and the viewing axis is down the barrel of the ipsilateral V4 segment. The triangular space opens only with the division of the dentate ligaments, dissection into the premedullary cistern, and some posteromedial mobilization of the medulla and upper spinal cord. The PICA is outside the triangle, but bilateral anterior spinal arteries are within it. This surgical trajectory brings the clivus and arterial anatomy into view but is tangential to the anterior medullary surface. The anterolateral sulcus may be visible, but the anterior median fissure and median anterior medullary vein are not. Hypoglossal rootlets originate from within this triangle and are easily identified laterally in the cerebellomedullary cistern and traced back to the anterolateral sulcus. The transverse medullary vein can also be traced medially toward the median anterior medullary vein.

3.5.2 Subtonsillar Triangle

The subtonsillar triangle is formed by the midline, the insertion of the tela choroidea of the fourth ventricle inferolaterally, and the medial border of the tonsil superolaterally (▸ Fig. 3.7). The lateral apex of the triangle is the intersection of the tela choroidea and the retracted tonsil, which makes the height of the triangle variable and dependent on the extent of telovelar dissection. Appropriate dissection should extend laterally to the lateral recess of the fourth ventricle, giving full height to the triangle. The combination of dividing the tela choroidea's insertion and mobilizing the tonsil provides access to the cerebellomedullary cistern and a working space that is subtonsillar. These ovoid structures on the inferomedial aspect of the cerebellar hemispheres attach to the cerebellum superolaterally through the tonsillar peduncles. The tonsils are otherwise free, which allows them to be mobilized with or without fixed retraction to open the subtonsillar triangle. Dissection into the vallecular triangle mobilizes both tonsils, whereas dissection into the subtonsillar triangle mobilizes only one. Distal p3 tonsillomedullary and proximal p4 (telovelotonsillar) segments of the PICA on the involved side are exposed, and a view into the foramen of Luschka is opened.

3.5.3 Vagoaccessory Triangle

The vagoaccessory triangle is bordered by the vagus nerve superiorly, the spinal accessory nerve laterally, and the medulla medially (▸ Fig. 3.7). Rodriguez-Hernandez and colleagues described this triangle in 2011 as the main corridor to the ventromedial compartment of the posterior fossa through the far lateral approach for clipping of proximal PICA or V4 aneurysms. The medullary rootlets of the accessory nerve traverse this triangle and must be protected when dissecting through this triangle. The rootlets of the hypoglossal nerve subdivide the vagoaccessory triangle into the suprahypoglossal, hypoglossal-hypoglossal, and infrahypoglossal triangles. The suprahypoglossal triangle occupies the superior aspect of the vagoaccessory triangle, bordered by the hypoglossal nerve inferiorly, the spinal accessory nerve laterally, the vagus nerve superiorly, and the medulla medially. This quadrangular space leads to PICA aneurysms within the anterior medullary zone, anterior to the hypoglossal nerve rootlets, and to the inferior olivary nucleus, pontomedullary sulcus, and pontine underbelly.

The hypoglossal-hypoglossal triangle, defined by Tayebi Meybodi and colleagues in 2019, lies between the highest hypoglossal nerve rootlets superiorly, the lowest hypoglossal nerve rootlets inferiorly, and the medulla medially. The origination of the PICA from the V4 segment of the VA is most common in this triangle, making it a vital route for clipping PICA aneurysms. The infrahypoglossal triangle occupies the inferior aspect of the vagoaccessory triangle, bordered by the spinal accessory nerve laterally, the hypoglossal nerve superiorly, and the medulla medially. The infrahypoglossal triangle leads to targeted PICA aneurysms associated with PICAs that originate early from the parent V4 segment of the VA within the lateral medullary zone. This triangle is the location where proximal control of the VA can be established by cutting the superior insertion of the dentate ligament.

3.5.4 Cerebellar Vallecular Triangle

The cerebellar vallecular triangle is the space between the tonsils bilaterally and the uvula of the inferior vermis superiorly (▸ Fig. 3.7). The medial tonsillar surfaces are normally apposed and close to the vallecula. Midline dissection separates them. The uvula forms the lower margin of the vermis and the upper limit of the vallecular triangle. The tonsils extend as low as the foramen magnum and conceal the fourth ventricle, obex, and gracile and cuneate nuclei. Lysis of arachnoid adhesions, slight lateral tonsillar retraction, incision of the inferior medullary velum, and exposure through the vallecular triangle allow the neurosurgeon to reach above the stria medullaris to the upper rhomboid fossa in the pons. The caudal loops and distal p3 (tonsillomedullary) segments of the PICA course along the medial borders of the tonsils and are mobilized laterally out of the triangle. The choroid plexus is often located at the superior apex of the triangle. Although the potential space of the vallecula is well known, the introduction of a vallecular

3

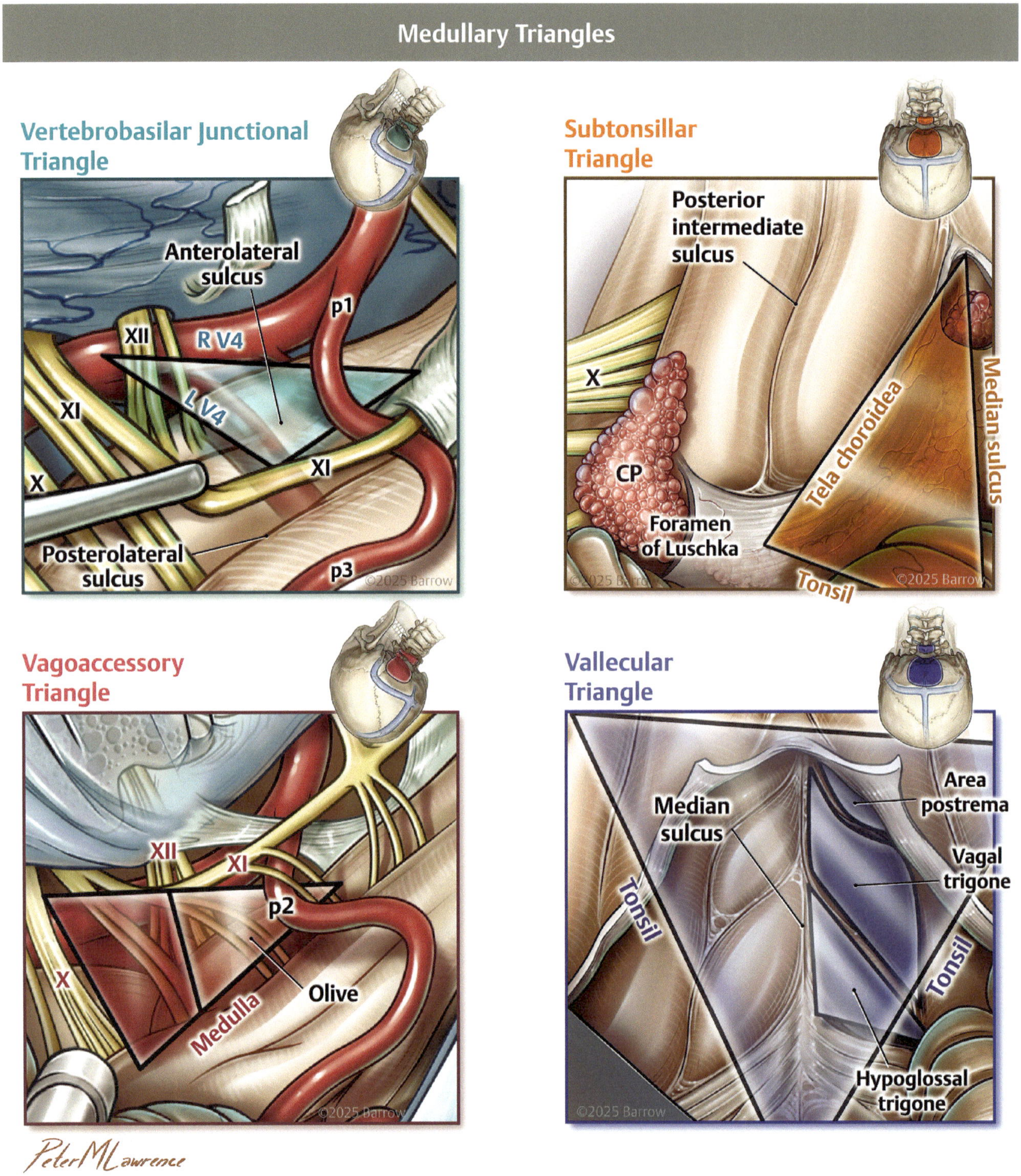

Fig. 3.7 Illustration depicting medullary triangles. The vertebrobasilar junctional triangle (*teal*) guides dissection to pyramidal CMs. The subtonsillar triangle (*orange*) guides dissection to cuneate CMs, the vagoaccessory triangle (*red*) to olivary CMs, and the vallecular triangle (*purple*) to trigonal and gracile CMs. Note that the trigones forming the calamus scriptorius on the fourth ventricular floor are prominent triangular landmarks in the median eminence of the medulla seen through the vallecular triangle. *Insets* show craniotomies. Roman numerals denote cranial nerves. (Reproduced with permission from Barrow Neurological Institute, Phoenix, AZ.)

Table 3.4 Anatomical triangles for accessing medullary CMs

Triangle	Orientation	Borders	Contents and significance	Safe entry zone
Vertebrobasilar junction	Superior	Vertebrobasilar junction	Dentate ligament division, dissection into premedullary cistern AntSpA transverse medullary vein CN XII rootlets	Anterolateral sulcus
	Inferior	CN XI		
	Medial	Contralateral V4		
	Lateral	Ipsilateral V4		
Vagoaccessory (SHT)	Medial	Medulla	V4, p1, p2 Inferior olivary nucleus, pontomedullary sulcus, pontine underbelly	Pontomedullary sulcus Posterolateral retro-olivary sulcus Olivary Lateral medullary zone
	Superior	CN X		
	Lateral	CN XI		
	Inferior	CN XII		
Vagoaccessory (HHT)	Medial	Medulla	V4, p1, p2	Posterolateral retro-olivary sulcus
	Superior	Highest CN XII rootlets		
	Inferior	Lowest CN XII rootlets		
Vagoaccessory (IHT)	Medial	Medulla	V4, p1, p2 Proximal control of VA by cutting dentate ligament	Lateral medullary zone
	Superior	CN XII		
	Inferior	CN XI		
Vallecular	Superior	Uvula of the inferior vermis	Fourth ventricle, obex, rhomboid fossa Gracile and cuneate nuclei p3	Median sulcus Infrafacial collicular sulcus
	Lateral (two-sided)	Medial surface of the cerebellar tonsils		
	Inferior	Line between the inferior extent of the cerebellar tonsils		
Subtonsillar	Medial	Midline	Lateral recess of the fourth ventricle, cerebellomedullary cistern, foramen of Luschka p3, p4	Area acustica Posterior intermediate sulcus
	Superolateral	Medial border of the tonsil		
	Inferolateral	Tela choroidea of the fourth ventricle		

triangle emphasizes this hidden entry zone and the technique needed to access it.

3.6 Thalamic and Basal Ganglial Triangles

Three triangles represent wayfinding landmarks within the thalamus and basal ganglia: (1) the supracarotid-infrafrontal triangle, (2) the caudate-thalamostriate triangle, and (3) the septocaudate triangle. Each triangle leads the approach to deeper corridors that have limited visibility at the lesion. Thus, they help guide dissection to targeted CMs.

3.6.1 Supracarotid-Infrafrontal Triangle

Basal ganglia CMs in the globus pallidus that present inferiorly near the anterior perforated substance are exposed through the supracarotid-infrafrontal triangle (▶ Fig. 3.8). This triangle is formed by the initial portions of the A1 segment medially and the M1 (sphenoidal) segment laterally as they originate from the carotid terminus. The base of this triangle is the anterior perforated substance superiorly. Superficial pallidal CMs are directly accessed through the anterior perforated substance. In contrast, superiorly located lesions require parenchymal transgression through the posterior part of the medial orbital gyrus and lateral olfactory stria to climb up into the substantia innominata. The supracarotid triangle contains lenticulostriate perforators that originate from the A1 (medial lenticulostriate arteries) and M1 (lateral lenticulostriate arteries) segments and perforators from the terminal ICA and AChA. The recurrent artery of Heubner originates from the A2 segment just distal to the ACoA and courses through the supracarotid triangle parallel to its base, in contrast to other perforators that run perpendicular to its base. This dense collection of perforators in the supracarotid triangle supplies the caudate nucleus, globus pallidus, putamen, internal capsule, and anterior thalamus and is the critical obstacle with the approach. Cavernoma resection is performed between and deep to these crisscrossing perforators.

3.6.2 Caudate-Thalamostriate Triangle

The anterior caudate vein overlies and identifies the caudate head. The thalamostriate vein runs between the thalamus and caudate nucleus atop the stria terminalis. This vein identifies the inferior border of the caudate subtype of basal ganglia CMs and the lateral border of the choroidal thalamic subtype. The caudate-thalamostriate triangle is a geometric construct defining the inferior border of the caudate nucleus, with the contralateral transcallosal-transventricular (cTCal-Vent) approach used to reach across the body of the lateral ventricle to the lesion (▶ Fig. 3.8).

3.6.3 Septocaudate Triangle

The thalamus and basal ganglia are deep nuclei embedded in the cerebral parenchyma with limited surface anatomy that

3

Thalamic & Basal Ganglia Triangles

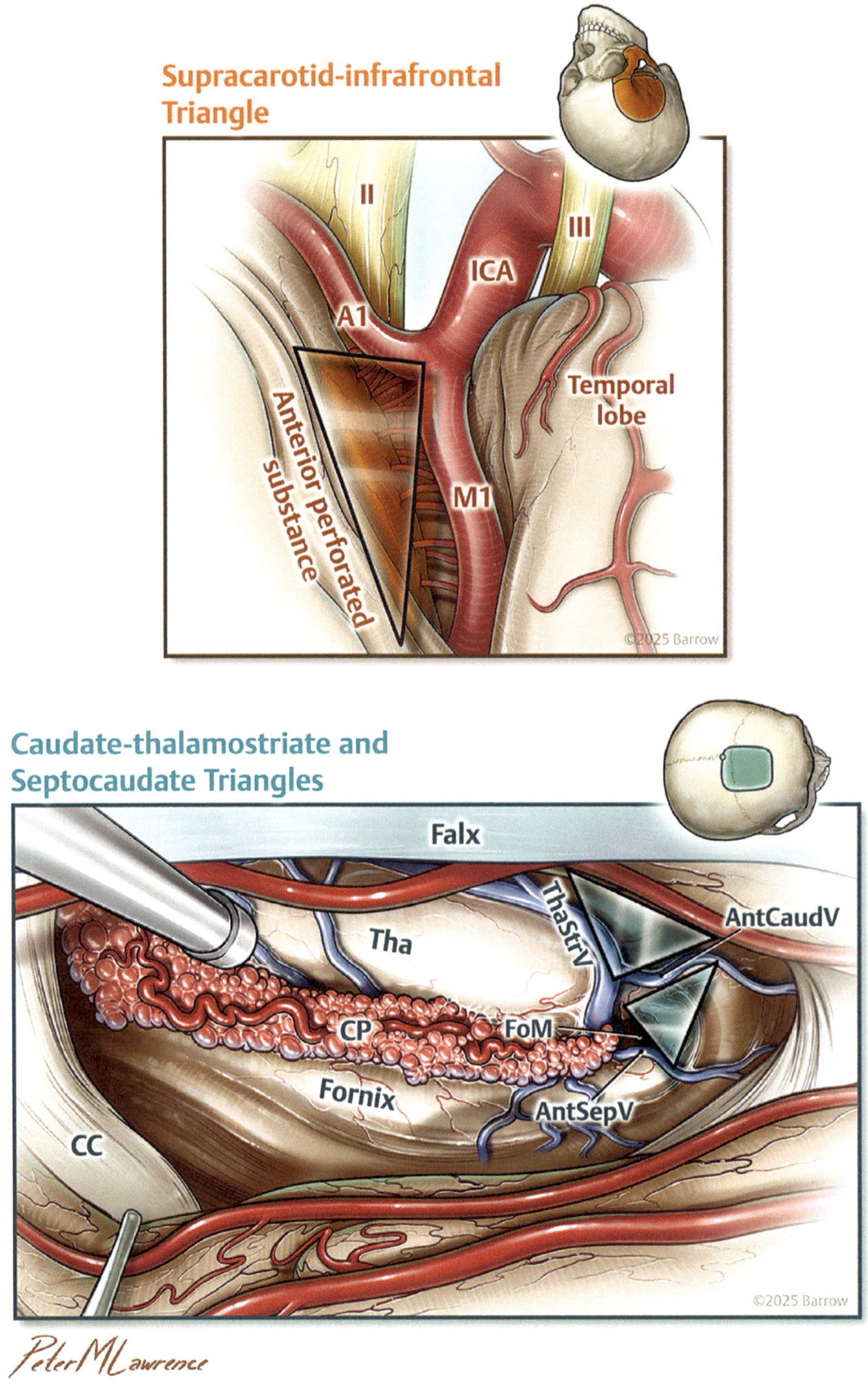

Fig. 3.8 Illustration depicting thalamic and basal ganglia triangles. The supracarotid-infrafrontal triangle (*orange*) guides dissection to pallidal CMs, working through anterior perforated substance and between lenticulostriate arteries to reach CMs located inferiorly in the globus pallidus. The caudate-thalamostriate triangle (*teal, upper triangle*) guides dissection to caudate CMs through a cTCal-Vent approach. The septocaudate triangle (*teal, lower triangle*) guides dissection to caudate CMs in the head of the caudate nucleus and anterior thalamic CMs through the foramen of Monro. *Insets* show craniotomies. Roman numerals denote cranial nerves. (Reproduced with permission from Barrow Neurological Institute, Phoenix, AZ.)

presents to the subarachnoid spaces or ependyma. Consequently, the thalamus and basal ganglia have a few relevant triangles. One such triangle is the septocaudate triangle, which is defined by the ependymal veins in the body of the lateral ventricle (▸ Fig. 3.8). The venous angle is formed by the confluence of the thalamostriate vein posterolaterally, caudate vein anterolaterally, and septal vein anteromedially. The triangle between the septal and anterior caudate veins is the septocaudate triangle. The foramen of Monro lies at the apex of this triangle, and the descending column of the fornix courses along the base of the triangle. Targeted CMs in the anterior thalamus reside laterally and inferiorly to the foramen of Monro. They are reached with a contralateral transcallosal-ipsilateral transforaminal (cTCal-iFor) approach to the anterior thalamic tubercle at the posterior edge of the foramen. Caudate subtypes in the head of the caudate nucleus are also reached through this septocaudate triangle.

3.6.4 Infragalenic Triangle

The infragalenic triangle (▸ Fig. 3.2, ▸ Fig. 3.3, ▸ Fig. 3.4) was previously described for accessing quadrigeminal midbrain CMs (see section 3.3.4). It is also used for navigation to pulvinar and geniculate thalamic CMs. The triangular space formed by the confluence of the precentral cerebellar vein, BVR, and the vein of Galen is entered to reach thalamic CM subtypes, requiring a steep upward climb to reach the pulvinar (paramedian supracerebellar-infratentorial [SCIT-Para] approach) and a lateral transtentorial climb to reach the geniculate nuclei (contralateral supracerebellar-transtentorial [cSCTT] approach). Excursions over the shoulder of the BVR, rather than under its axilla, may be needed to reach the lateral pulvinar. The BVR descends laterally, which makes the over-the-shoulder route routine to reach geniculate CMs. The P3 segment of the PCA courses supratentorially and vanishes behind the tentorium, as does the medial occipital vein. A loop of P3 can stand between the neurosurgeon and the infragalenic triangle, but dissection can proceed through the loop. The prominent medial occipital vein can be misinterpreted as the BVR but is differentiated by its supratentorial crossing of the tentorial incisura.

3.7 Cerebral and Cerebellar Triangles

Cerebral and most cerebellar CMs have no associated triangles because they are superficial on hemispheric surfaces without the intersecting vessels and nerves seen with deeper lesions. However, two previously described triangles are relevant for cerebellar CMs around or adjacent to the cerebellar tonsils and petrosal CMs: the vallecular triangle and the interlobular triangle.

3.7.1 Vallecular Triangle

Tonsillar, inferior vermian, and deep nuclear cerebellar CMs are targeted through the vallecular triangle, separating the tonsils in the midline and opening the vallecula to access the medial tonsil and inferior vermis. The vallecular triangle leads into the fissures around the superior tonsil that provide access to the deep nuclei with a telovelar approach for medial CMs in the fastigial, globose, and emboliform nuclei or a supratonsillar approach for lateral CMs in the dentate nuclei (▸ Fig. 3.6). The suboccipital-telovelar approach (SOcc-TeVe) progresses from the medial side of the tonsil, through the inferior medullary velum toward the lateral recess of the fourth ventricle, and over the superomedial tonsillar surface between the uvula and the tonsil. The suboccipital-supratonsillar approach (SOcc-SupraTons) progresses through the tonsillobiventral fissure, over the superolateral tonsillar surface, and into the deep white matter adjacent to the dentate nucleus.

3.7.2 Interlobular Triangle

Petrosal cerebellar CMs are located on the petrosal cerebellar surface, where exposure is often limited in the cerebellopontine cistern and increased by opening the interlobular triangle described above for middle peduncular pontine CMs. The interlobular triangle (▸ Fig. 3.5) between the superior and inferior semilunar lobules opens after the petrosal fissure is split along the a3 AICA segment to access petrosal cerebellar CMs along this surface. The interlobular triangle exposes floccular CMs and the MCP at its depth, and petrosal cerebellar CMs are superficial to the MCP in these lobules.

3.8 Clinical Evidence

The anatomical triangle through which a brainstem CM was resected microsurgically was determined for patients treated who had brain magnetic resonance imaging and intraoperative photographs or videos available for review during a 23-year period from 1997 through 2020. Of 183 patients who met the inclusion criteria, 50 (27%) had midbrain lesions, 102 (56%) had pontine lesions, and 31 (17%) had medullary lesions. The craniotomies used to resect these brainstem CMs included the extended retrosigmoid (66 [36%]), midline suboccipital (46 [25%]), far lateral (30 [16%]), pterional orbitozygomatic (17 [9%]), torcular (8 [4%]), and lateral suboccipital retrosigmoid (8 [4%]) approaches. The anatomical triangles through which brainstem CMs were most frequently resected were the interlobular (37 [20%]), vallecular (32 [17.5%]), vagoaccessory (30 [16%]), supracerebellar-infratrochlear (16 [9%]), subtonsillar (14 [8%]), oculomotor-tentorial (11 [6%]), infragalenic (8 [4%]), and supracerebellar-supratrochlear (8 [4%]) triangles. New and infrequently used triangles included the vertebrobasilar junctional (1 [0.5%]), supratrigeminal (3 [2%]), and infratrigeminal (5 [3%]) triangles. The 16 brainstem subtypes of CMs were exposed through 6 craniotomies, and the approach was redirected to the CM by 1 of the 14 triangles paired with the CM subtype (▸ Fig. 3.9, ▸ Fig. 3.10, ▸ Fig. 3.11). The 6 craniotomies lacked the specificity to guide the dissection to the brainstem CM, but the 14 anatomical triangles associated with the CM subtypes added this anatomical specificity to guide the dissection accurately to the brainstem CM (▸ Fig. 3.12).

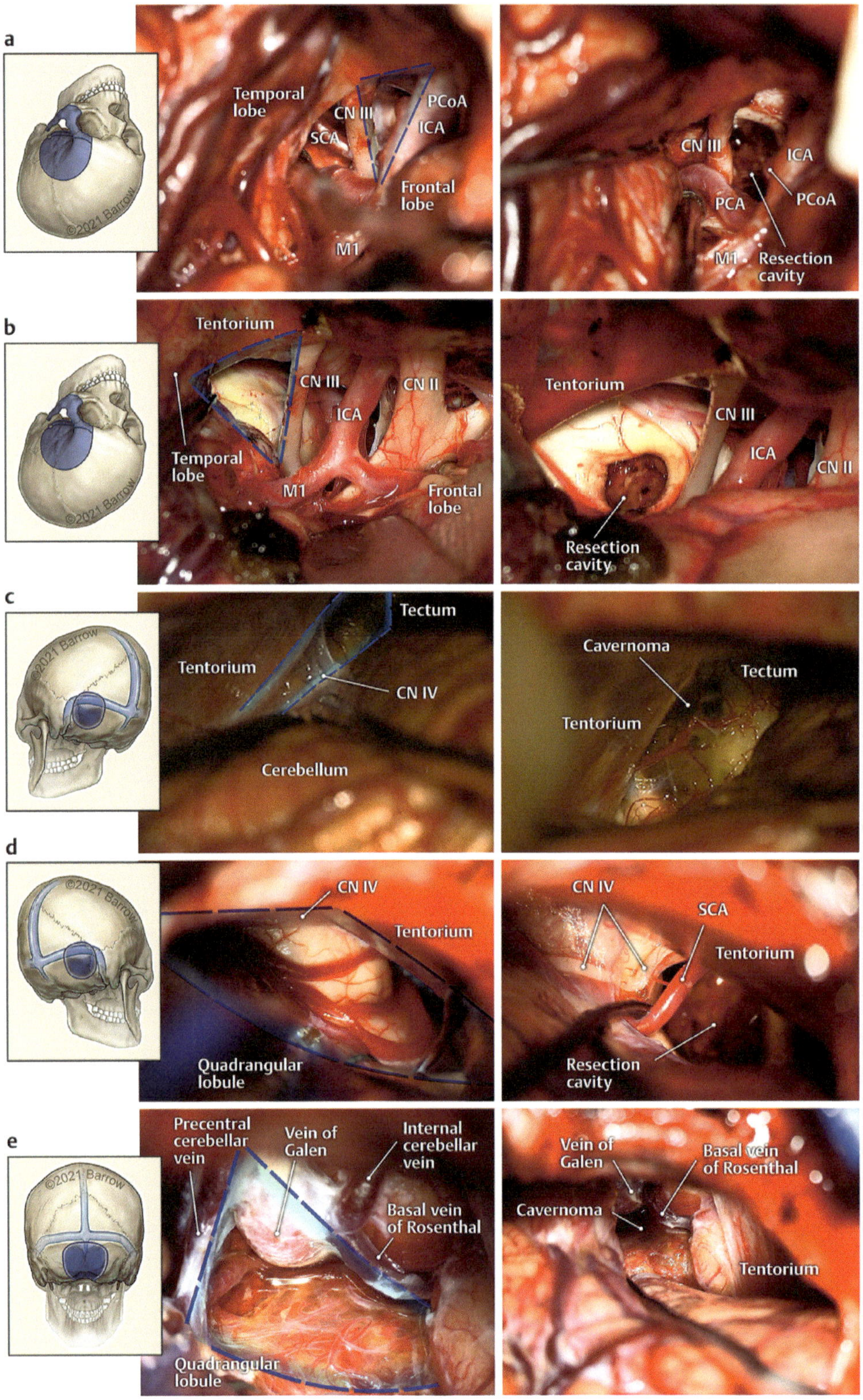

Fig. 3.9 Surgical views of midbrain anatomical triangles (*outlined* in left panels). **(a)** This interpeduncular midbrain CM was resected through the carotid-oculomotor triangle using a left orbitozygomatic-pterional craniotomy and transsylvian approach. **(b)** This left peduncular midbrain CM was resected through the oculomotor-tentorial triangle using a left orbitozygomatic-pterional craniotomy and transsylvian approach. **(c)** This left tegmental midbrain CM was resected through the supracerebellar-supratrochlear triangle using a left extended retrosigmoid craniotomy and supracerebellar-infratentorial approach (sitting position). **(d)** This right tegmental midbrain CM was resected through the supracerebellar-infratrochlear triangle using a right extended retrosigmoid craniotomy and supracerebellar-infratentorial approach (sitting position). **(e)** This quadrigeminal midbrain CM was resected through the infragalenic triangle using a torcular craniotomy and midline supracerebellar-infratentorial approach (sitting position). *Insets* show craniotomies. (Surgical images are reproduced with permission from Benner D, Hendricks BK, Benet A, et al. A system of anatomical triangles defining dissection routes to brainstem cavernous malformations: definitions and application to a cohort of 183 patients. J Neurosurg. 2022;138(3):768–784. Insets are reproduced with permission from Barrow Neurological Institute, Phoenix, AZ.)

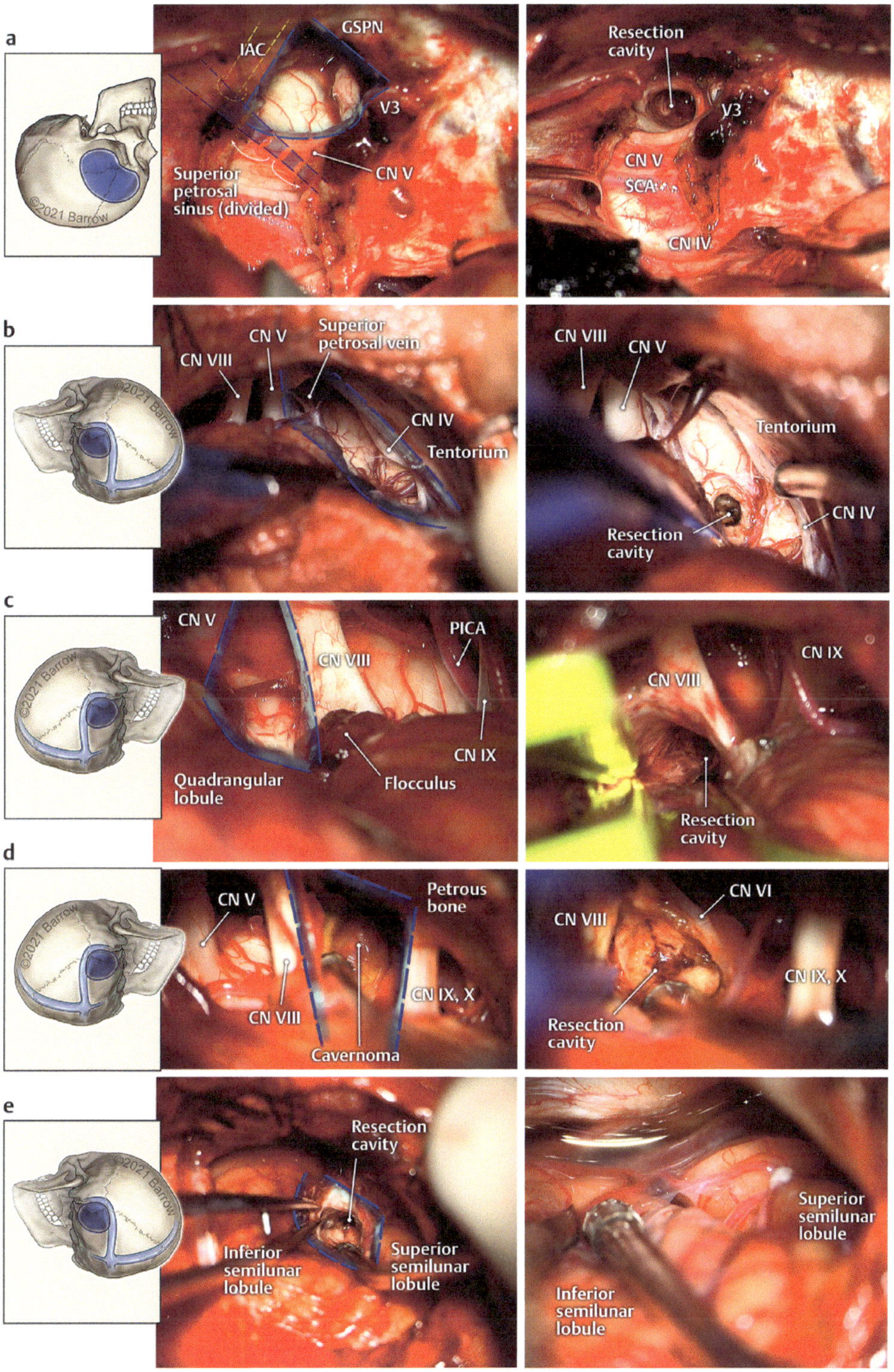

Fig. 3.10 Surgical views of pontine anatomical triangles (*outlined* in left panels). **(a)** This basilar pontine CM was resected through the Kawase *triangle* (quadrangle) using a pterional craniotomy and anterior transpetrosal (Kawase) approach. The Kawase triangle was visible only after dividing the tentorium, transecting the superior petrosal sinus (ghosted in *blue*), and entering the extradural space that had been drilled previously. **(b)** This left peritrigeminal pontine CM was resected through the supratrigeminal triangle using a left extended retrosigmoid craniotomy and trans-cerebellopontine angle approach. **(c)** This right peritrigeminal pontine CM was resected through the infratrigeminal triangle using a right extended retrosigmoid craniotomy and trans-cerebellopontine angle approach. **(d)** This right peritrigeminal pontine CM was resected through the glossopharyngeal-cochlear triangle using a right extended retrosigmoid craniotomy and trans-cerebellopontine angle approach. **(e)** This left middle peduncular pontine CM was resected through the interlobular triangle using a left extended retrosigmoid craniotomy and trans-middle cerebellar peduncle approach. *Insets* show craniotomies. (Surgical images are reproduced with permission from Benner D, Hendricks BK, Benet A, et al. A system of anatomical triangles defining dissection routes to brainstem cavernous malformations: definitions and application to a cohort of 183 patients. J Neurosurg 2022;138(3): 768–784. Insets are reproduced with permission from Barrow Neurological Institute, Phoenix, AZ.)

3

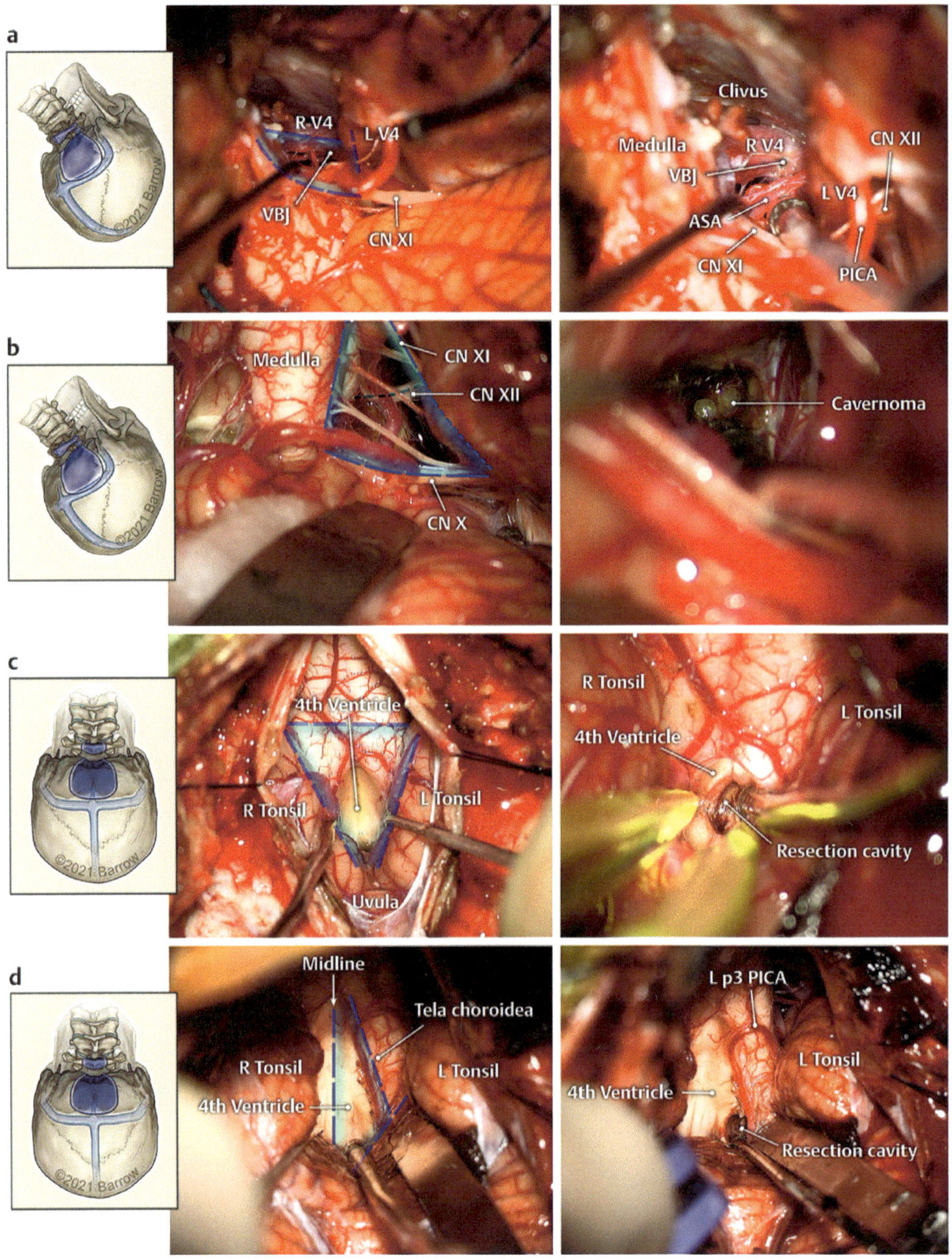

Fig. 3.11 Surgical views of medullary anatomical triangles (*outlined* in the left panels). **(a)** This left pyramidal medullary CM was resected through the vertebrobasilar junctional triangle using a left far lateral craniotomy and transpremedullary cistern approach. **(b)** This left olivary medullary CM was resected through the vago-accessory triangle using a left far lateral craniotomy and transcerebellomedullary cistern approach. **(c)** This trigonal medullary CM was resected through the vallecular triangle using a midline suboccipital craniotomy and transventricular approach. **(d)** This left inferior peduncular pontine CM was resected through the subtonsillar triangle using a midline suboccipital craniotomy and left telovelar approach. *Insets* show craniotomies. (Surgical images are reproduced with permission from Benner D, Hendricks BK, Benet A, et al. A system of anatomical triangles defining dissection routes to brainstem cavernous malformations: definitions and application to a cohort of 183 patients. J Neurosurg 2022;138(3):768–784. Insets are reproduced with permission from Barrow Neurological Institute, Phoenix, AZ.)

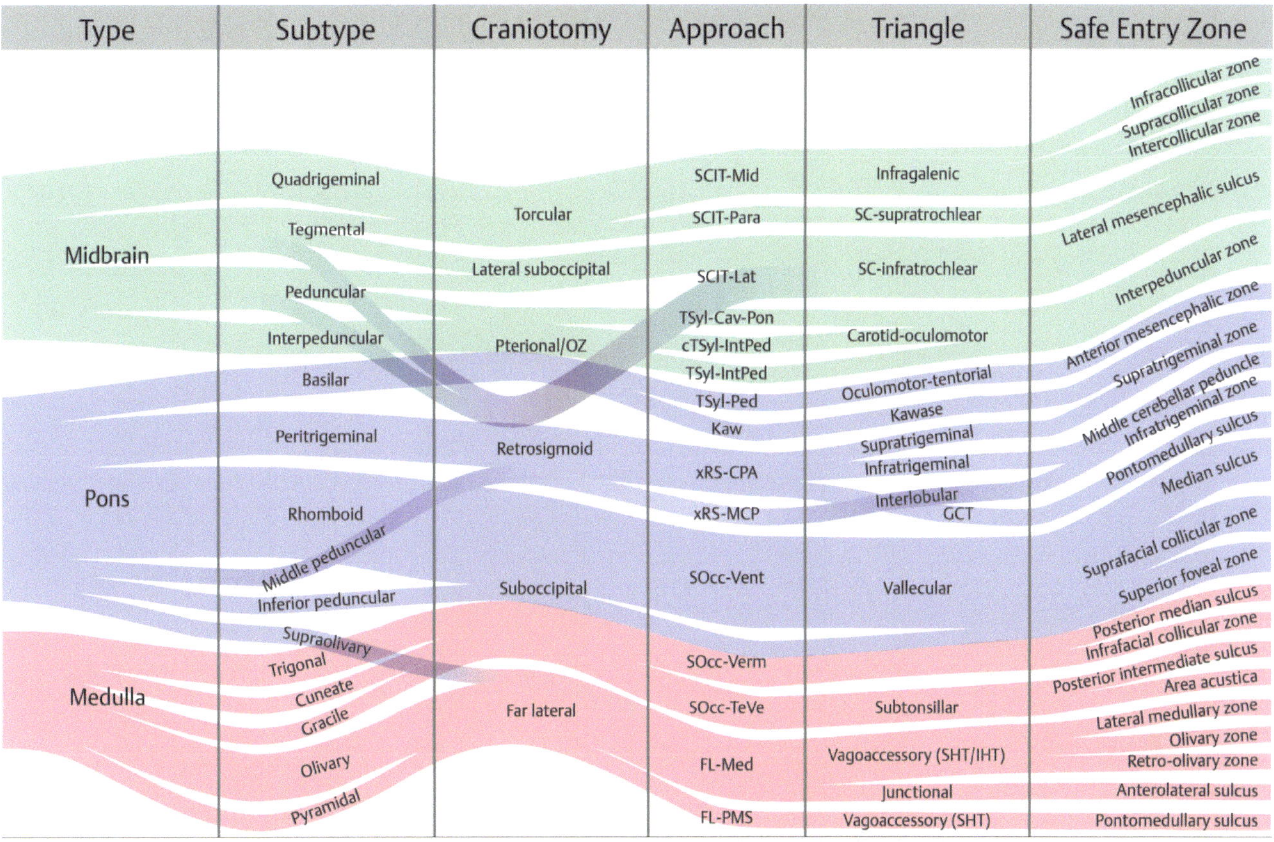

Fig. 3.12 Sankey diagram showing the flow from brainstem CM type and subtype to craniotomy, dissection approach, and anatomical triangle through which the target lesion was resected. The safe entry zone exposed within the anatomical triangle is also shown. Midbrain subtypes are shown in *green*, pontine subtypes in *purple*, and medullary subtypes in *pink*. The bandwidths are proportional to the number of patients in each group. Periaqueductal midbrain CMs are resected transventricularly without an associated anatomical triangle, and these patients were excluded. Once through the craniotomy, the approach to the CM was redirected by the anatomical triangle paired with the specific CM subtype. (Reproduced with permission from Benner D, Hendricks BK, Benet A, et al. A system of anatomical triangles defining dissection routes to brainstem cavernous malformations: definitions and application to a cohort of 183 patients. J Neurosurg 2022;138(3):768–784.)

3.9 Conclusion

Anatomical triangles defined by intersecting neurovascular structures define surgical routes to pathological targets and guide neurosurgeons during dissection steps. Collections or systems of anatomical triangles have been integrated into skull base surgery to help navigate complex regions like the cavernous sinus. A system of brainstem CM triangles, including nine newly defined triangles, guides dissection to these lesions. The use of an anatomical triangle better defines the pathway taken through the craniotomy to the lesion and refines the conceptualization of surgical approaches (▶ Fig. 3.13, ▶ Fig. 3.14, ▶ Fig. 3.15). The triangle concept and the brainstem CM triangle system increase the precision of dissection through subarachnoid corridors, enhance microsurgical execution, and potentially improve patient outcomes.

The triangle concept was developed to complement the taxonomy for brainstem CMs. However, the 16 brainstem subtypes in the taxonomy do not pair 1-to-1 with the 14 triangles. Different brainstem CM subtypes were sometimes approached through different trajectories within the same triangle. For example, rhomboid and trigonal brainstem CMs were approached through the vallecular triangle, and inferior peduncular and cuneate brainstem CMs were approached through the subtonsillar triangle. Conversely, one subtype can be accessed through multiple triangles, as with tegmental midbrain and peritrigeminal pontine brainstem CMs. Tegmental lesions can be removed above or below the trochlear nerve through the supra- or infratrochlear triangles, whereas the long length of the peritrigeminal territory opens three triangles of exposure: the supratrigeminal, infratrigeminal, and glossopharyngeal-cochlear triangles. Some triangles introduced here may have limited use, as with the vertebrobasilar junctional triangle, which was used for one pyramidal lesion. Nonetheless, the triangle concept combines craniotomy, approach, and triangle with each brainstem CM subtype to inform surgical planning and microsurgical dissection. The system of triangles assembled here is the first of its kind for brainstem CMs. By adopting the new names and new triangles proposed, others can join this effort to standardize the description and reporting of approaches and techniques applied to the microsurgical management of brainstem CMs.

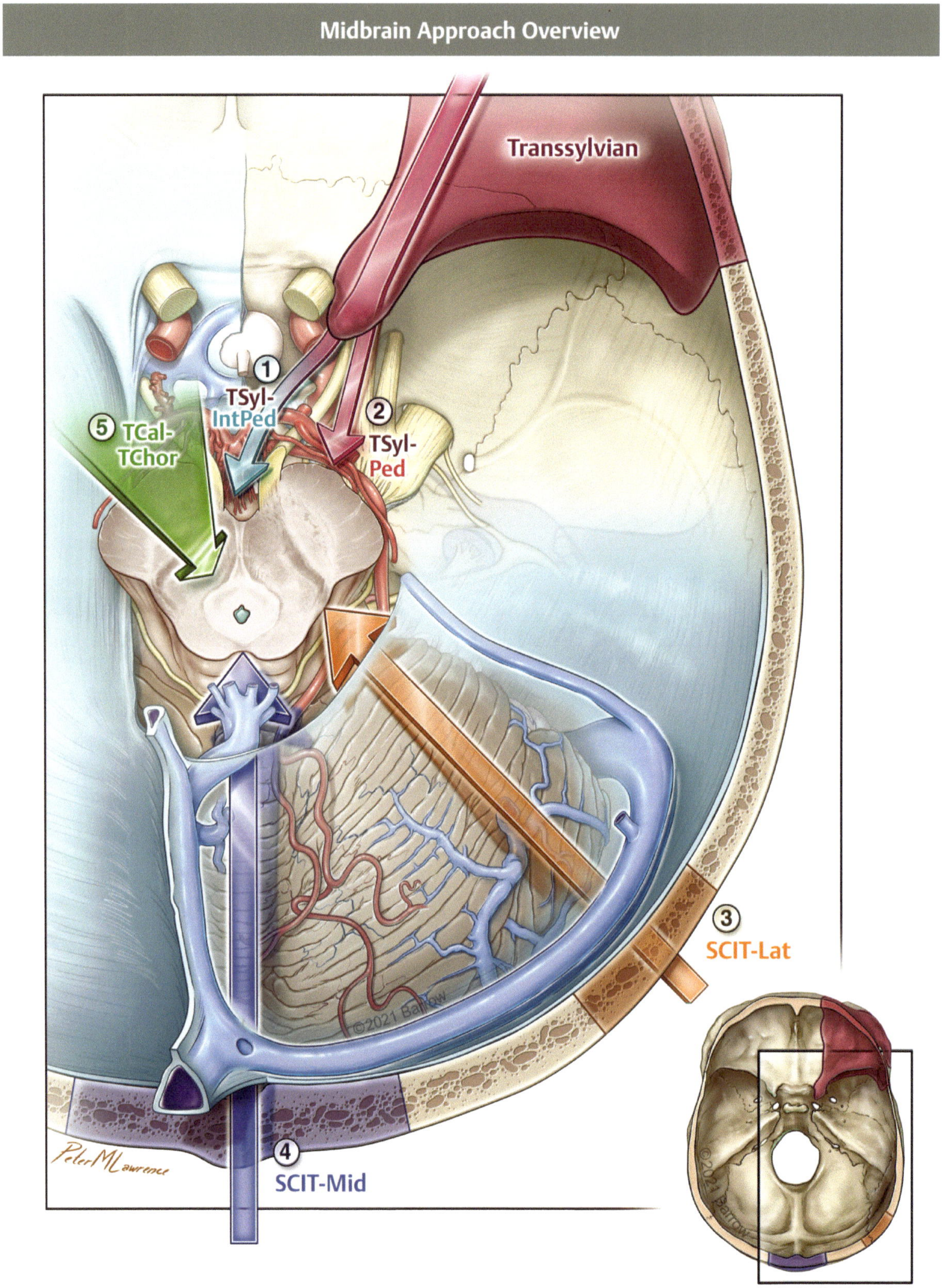

Fig. 3.13 Summary of five midbrain surgical approaches. *Inset* shows craniotomy. (Reproduced with permission from Barrow Neurological Institute, Phoenix, AZ.)

Pontine Approach Overview

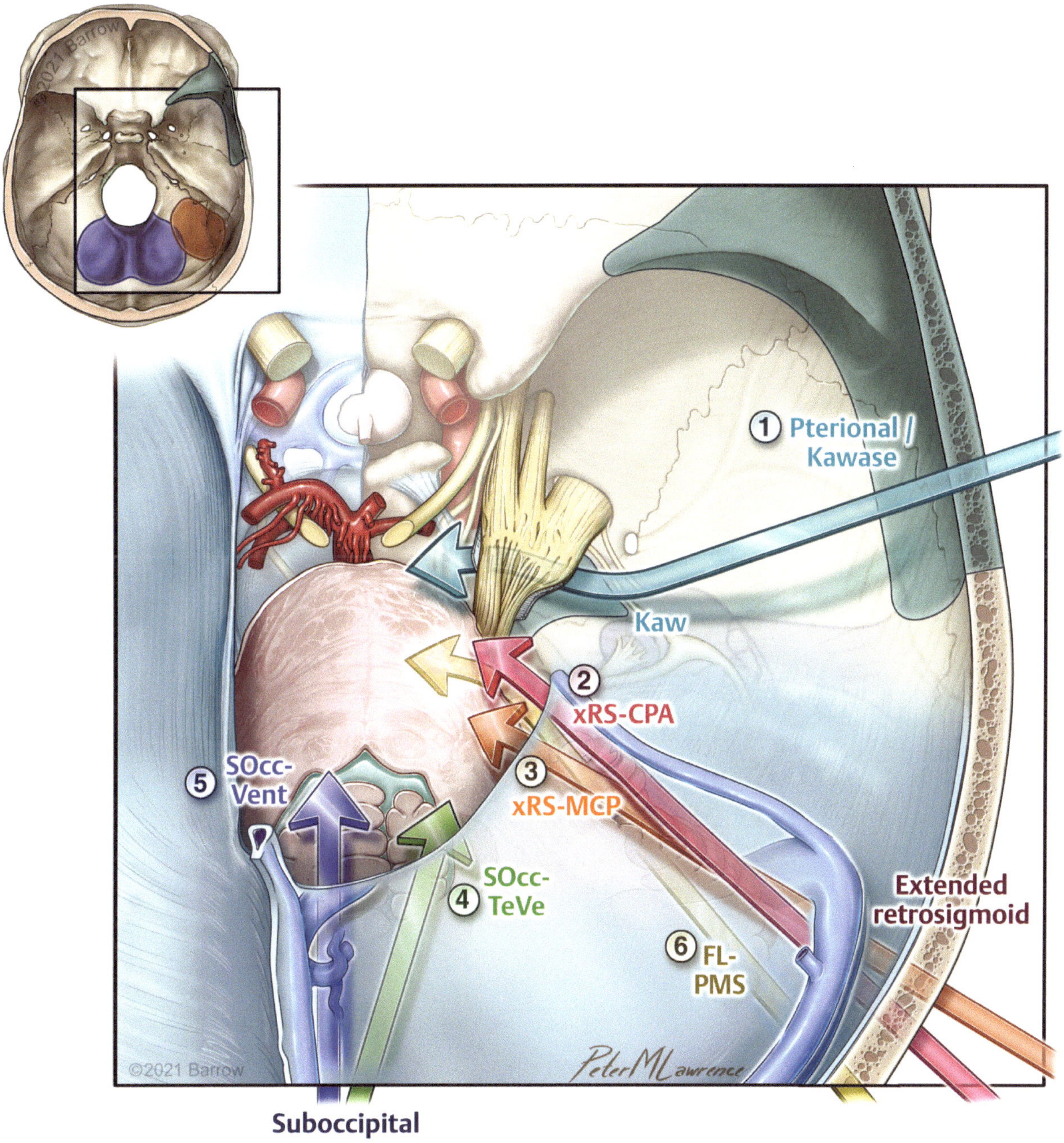

Fig. 3.14 Summary of six pontine surgical approaches. Two translabyrinthine approaches are not shown because they are no longer used for these CM subtypes. *Inset* shows craniotomy. (Reproduced with permission from Barrow Neurological Institute, Phoenix, AZ.)

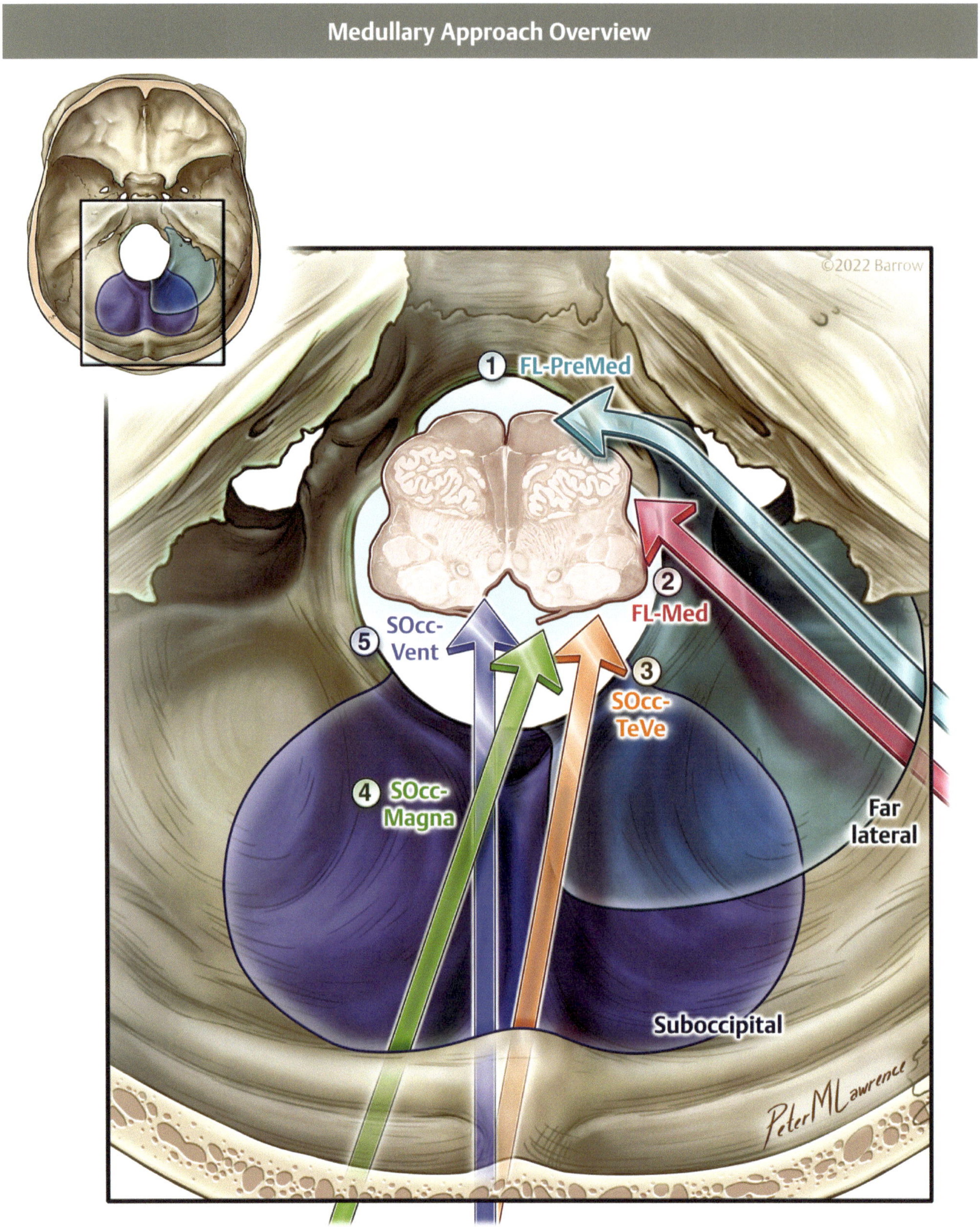

Fig. 3.15 Summary of five medullary surgical approaches. (Reproduced with permission from Barrow Neurological Institute, Phoenix, AZ.)

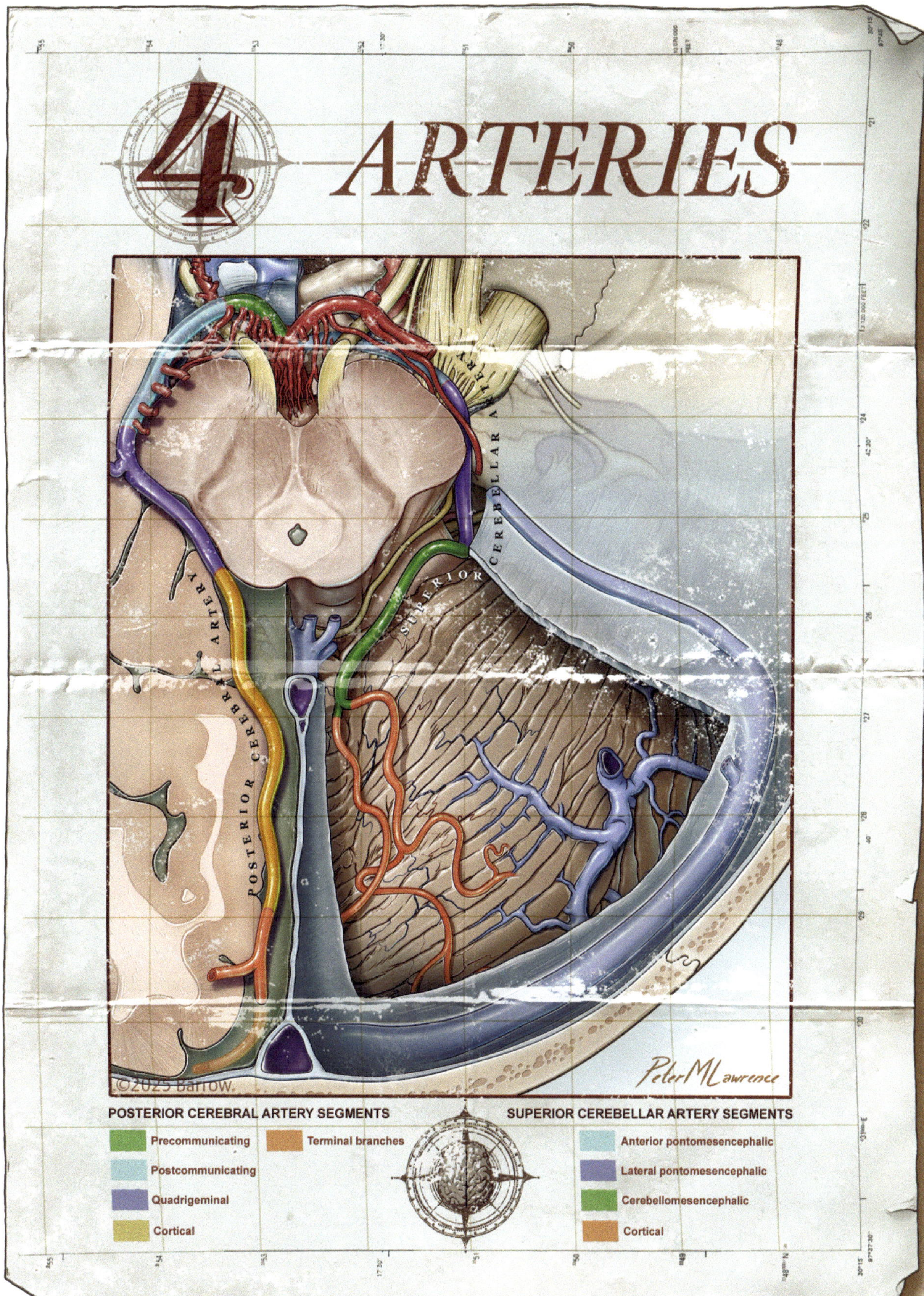

Reproduced with permission from Barrow Neurological Institute, Phoenix, AZ.

4 Arterial Landmarks

Summary
Within the subarachnoid space, navigation to target cavernous malformations (CMs) is easier with the help of arteries that separate adherent pial surfaces of cisterns and sulci. An artery emerging from a fissure is an invitation to enter its separation plane. The arterial tree splits and diverges in the direction of blood flow and converges in the reverse direction of dissection. This arterial tree is like a network of arterial trails leading inward to the circle of Willis and vertebrobasilar circulation. The neurosurgeon needs only to dissect alongside arteries to widen corridors and reach key target lesions. Thus, arteries are landmarks that define our trails and direct us to our resection targets. Each brainstem CM subtype has a unique arterial segment associated with its surface presentation, and this *arterial address* serves as a dissection guide. Arterial segment alphanumerics are easy shorthand and act as arterial addresses for CMs that can develop throughout the brain, as described in the taxonomy. Like rivers and streams in the wilderness, these arterial landmarks deserve a place on our neurosurgical map to guide our dissection routes.

Keywords: address, arterial segment, brainstem, cistern, dissection guide, fissure, network, plane, subarachnoid space, sulci

4.1 Rivers of the Brain

Arteries are the main occupants of the subarachnoid space. Because subarachnoid spaces and corridors are the secrets to cavernoma surgery, as discussed in Chapter 2, working with the arteries to navigate the network is an essential component of that secret to success. Arteries separate adherent pial surfaces as they course in the center of cisterns and sulci, helping open these spaces. An artery emerging from a fissure is a gift and an invitation to enter a naturally occurring separation plane. The arterial tree bifurcates and diverges in the anterograde direction of blood flow, but it converges and enlarges in the reverse, retrograde direction of dissection. Branches turn into stems and then into trunks with deepening dissection, and separation planes widen progressively into cisterns. This confluence of the arterial tree is like a network of arterial trails leading inward to the circle of Willis and vertebrobasilar circulation, reminiscent of creeks and streams in nature guiding the route to rivers and waterfalls. Wilderness trails often follow waterways for the same reason: flowing water finds the most direct route and often has already cleared the way. Just as the astute hiker proceeds alongside the stream to arrive at a destination, the neurosurgeon needs only to dissect alongside arteries to widen corridors and reach key targets. The artery is followed in parallel when it aligns with the corridor, and when an artery intersects the corridor, it orients and informs like a bridge on a map. Thus, arteries are landmarks that define our trails and direct us to crossroads. One artery may guide the first leg of the journey, and another artery may guide the next leg, each connecting to arrive at the target.

An insight struck me while tabulating the taxonomy for brainstem cavernous malformations (CMs), with their associated craniotomies, approaches, and triangles: each subtype also has a unique arterial segment associated with its surface presentation, and this *arterial address* serves as another dissection guide, just like the triangle concept (▸ Table 4.1). Rhoton and colleagues partitioned the arterial tree into building blocks or segments defined by arterial branches or adjacent anatomy (▸ Table 4.2). For example, the supraclinoid internal carotid artery (ICA) is partitioned into C6 (ophthalmic) and C7 (communicating) segments by the posterior communicating artery (PCoA). The bend in the middle cerebral artery (MCA) around the limen insula partitions the M1 (sphenoidal) segment proximally from the M2 (insular) segment distally. Segmental alphanumerics are easy shorthand and act as arterial addresses for many of the cavernomas dispersed throughout the brain and described in the taxonomy. Just like rivers and streams in the wilderness, these arterial landmarks deserve a place on our neurosurgical map to guide our dissection routes.

4.2 Middle Cerebral Arteries

The MCA courses from the carotid terminus to the cerebral convexity; it has four segments, makes three right-angle turns,

Table 4.1 Superficial and deep cerebral and cerebellar CM taxonomy of types and subtypes and their associated craniotomies, approaches, anatomic triangles, and arterial segments

Type	Subtype	Craniotomy	Approach	Triangle	Arterial target
Cerebral	Convexity	Convexity	Transgyral, transsulcal		M4
	Medial	Bifrontal, biparieto-occipital	Transgyral, transsulcal		A2, A3, A4, A5, P4
	Basal	Pterional, temporal, torcular	Transgyral, transsulcal		A1, HippoA, PosTempA
	Sylvian	Pterional	Transgyral, transsulcal		M3
Basal ganglia	Caudate	Bifrontal	cTCal-Vent	Anterior caudate-thalamostriate	ThaStrV
	Putaminal	Pterional	TSyl-AIns		M2
	Pallidal	Orbitozygomatic	TSyl-SCIF	Supracarotid	A1, M1

(Continued)

Table 4.1 *(Continued)* Superficial and deep cerebral and cerebellar CM taxonomy of types and subtypes and their associated craniotomies, approaches, anatomic triangles, and arterial segments

Type	Subtype	Craniotomy	Approach	Triangle	Arterial target
Thalamic	Anterior	Bifrontal	cTCal-iFor	Septocaudate triangle	SepV
	Medial	Bifrontal	cTCal-cTChor		
	Lateral	Pterional	TSyl-PIns		M2
	Choroidal	Bifrontal	iTCal-Vent		mPChA
	Pulvinar	Torcular	SCIT-Para; (SPL-Atr; cPTCal-Vent)	Infragalenic	P3, mPChA
	Geniculate	Torcular	cSCTT	Infragalenic	P3, mPChA
Cerebellar	Suboccipital	Suboccipital	SOcc-Para, SOcc-Mid		p5
	Tentorial	Torcular	SCIT-Para, SCIT-Mid		s4
	Petrosal	Extended retrosigmoid	xRS-CPA	Interlobular	a4
	Vermian	Suboccipital	SOcc-Mid		s4, p5
	Tonsillar	Suboccipital	SOcc-Magna		p5
	Deep nuclear	Suboccipital	SOcc-SupraTons, SOcc-TeVe		p4

Table 4.2 Brainstem CM taxonomy of types and subtypes and their associated craniotomies, approaches, anatomic triangles, SEZs, and arterial segments

Type	Subtype	Craniotomy	Approach	Triangle	Safe entry zone	Arterial target
Midbrain	Interpeduncular	Orbitozygomatic	TSyl-IntPed; cTSyl-IntPed	Carotid-oculomotor	Interpeduncular	P1
	Peduncular	Orbitozygomatic	TSyl-Ped	Oculomotor-tentorial	Anterior mesencephalic sulcus	P2A
	Tegmental	Retrosigmoid	SCIT-Lat	Supratrochlear and infratrochlear	Lateral mesencephalic sulcus	s3
	Quadrigeminal	Torcular	SCIT-Mid	Infragalenic	Intercollicular; supracollicular; infracollicular	mPChA
	Periaqueductal	Bifrontal	TCal-TChor	None	None	None
Pontine	Basilar	Orbitozygomatic	Kaw; TSyl-Cav-Pon	Kawase/infratrigeminal; carotid-oculomotor	Supratrigeminal; infratrigeminal	BA, s1
	Peritrigeminal	Retrosigmoid	xRS-CPA	Supratrigeminal and infratrigeminal, GCT	Supratrigeminal; infratrigeminal	s2
	Middle peduncular	Retrosigmoid	xRS-MCP	Interlobular	Middle cerebellar peduncle/lateral pontine	a3
	Inferior peduncular	Suboccipital	SOcc-TeVe	Subtonsillar	Area acustica	p4
	Rhomboid	Suboccipital	SOcc-Vent	Vallecular	Median sulcus; suprafacial collicular; superior foveal	p3
	Supraolivary	Far lateral	FL-PMS	Vagoaccessory (suprahypoglossal)	Pontomedullary sulcus	a2
Medullary	Pyramidal	Far lateral	FL-PreMed	Junctional	Anterolateral sulcus	V4, VBJ, p1
	Olivary	Far lateral	FL-Med	Vagoaccessory (supra- or hypoglossal-hypoglossal)	Olivary zone; posterolateral sulcus; lateral medullary zone	p2
	Trigonal	Suboccipital	SOcc-Vent	Vallecular	Median sulcus; infrafacial collicular	p3
	Gracile	Suboccipital	SOcc-Magna	Vallecular	Posterior median sulcus	p3
	Cuneate	Suboccipital	SOcc-TeVe	Subtonsillar	Posterior intermediate sulcus	PSA

alternates twice from horizontal to vertical, and branches into a candelabra of insular, opercular, and cortical arteries (▶ Fig. 4.1). The M1 (sphenoidal) segment begins at the terminal bifurcation of the ICA and ends at the genu in the artery as it courses over the limen insula. The M1 segment is the arterial landmark for globus pallidus CMs that present at the lateral two-thirds of the anterior perforated substance surface. Passage through the supracarotid triangle circumvents lateral lenticulostriate arteries (LSAs) originating from the superior surface of the M1 segment, entering anterior perforated substance, and ascending to basal ganglia structures including the caudate nucleus, putamen, globus pallidus, and superior half of the internal capsule.

The M2 (insular) segment begins at the genu, runs in the insular cleft, and terminates at the circular sulcus of the insula, where the arteries make their next right-angle turn. The MCA bifurcates into superior and inferior trunks, with the bifurcation located on the M1 segment if it is proximal to the genu at the limen insula, on the M2 segment if it is distal to the genu, or at the M1–M2 junction if it is at the genu. MCA trifurcations and quadrifurcations result in additional middle trunks. Trunks branch into stem arteries that course through the insular cleft, with the insular cortex beneath this arterial candelabra. M2 segments are the alphanumeric address for putaminal basal ganglial CMs deep to the short gyri and lateral thalamic CMs deep to the long gyri.

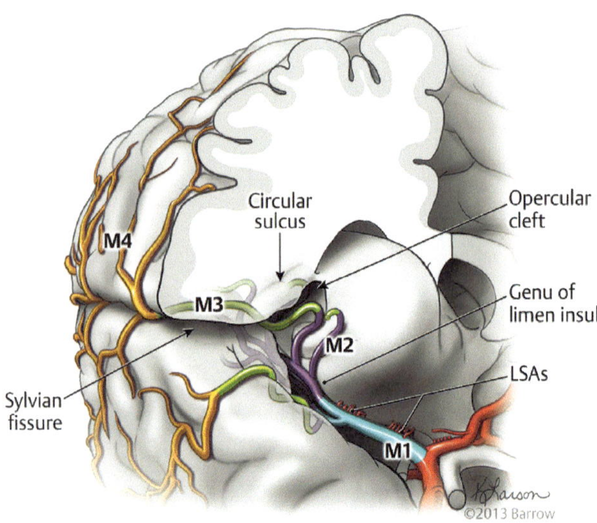

Fig. 4.1 MCA segments, as seen from a right anterior oblique view with the frontal lobe transected. The MCA courses from the carotid terminus to the cerebral convexity; it has four segments, makes three right-angle turns, alternates twice from horizontal to vertical, and branches into a candelabra of M2 insular, M3 opercular, and M4 cortical arteries. The M1 segment is the arterial landmark for globus pallidus CMs. M2 segments are the alphanumeric address for putaminal basal ganglial CMs deep to the short gyri and lateral thalamic CMs deep to the long gyri. M3 segments in the operculum overlie sylvian CMs (frontal, parietal, and temporal). Convexity cerebral CMs, especially those in a sulcus, are associated with a cortical M4 branch. (Reproduced with permission from Barrow Neurological Institute, Phoenix, AZ.)

The MCA transitions from M2 segments along insular surfaces with a right-angle genu to M3 (opercular) segments along opercular surfaces. M3 segments leave the insular surface, run in the opercular cleft, and terminate at the cortical surface of the sylvian fissure. Retrograde dissection from M4 (cortical) arteries on the convexity to M3 segments in the operculum exposes sylvian CMs (frontal, parietal, and temporal). Periarterial dissection along several of these exiting arteries creates nodes of separation in an area where frontotemporal adhesions can be tight, and progressively connecting these dissection nodes opens the operculum. The M3 segments are 2 to 3 cm long, and dissection into the insular cleft opens into the superolateral extension of the sylvian cistern.

The M4 segment consists of branches supplying the lateral convexity from their emergence from the sylvian fissure to their final territory. Convexity cerebral CMs, especially those in a sulcus, are associated with a cortical branch of the MCA and have M4 as their alphanumeric address. Several named cortical branches around the sylvian fissure are helpful with sylvian subtypes: four frontal cortical arteries climb from the fissure (orbitofrontal artery [OrbFrA], prefrontal artery, precentral artery, and central artery); four temporal arteries drop from the fissure (middle temporal, posterior temporal, temporo-occipital, and angular arteries), and two parietal arteries exit the distal fissure (anterior and posterior parietal arteries). The OrbFrA is the most anteroinferior branch and helps guide entrance into the sylvian fissure nearest the pars orbitalis. The prefrontal artery is associated with CMs in the eloquent pars triangularis and pars opercularis in the dominant hemisphere. M4 segments on the temporal lobe are collectively called superior temporal arteries. They lead to targeted CMs in the superior and middle temporal gyri. The temporopolar artery and the anterior temporal artery are branches that arise from the inferior surface of the M1 segment proximal to the MCA bifurcation; these branches are landmarks that lead to targeted medial temporal CMs.

4.3 Anterior Cerebral Arteries

The anterior cerebral artery (ACA) is the arterial landmark for basal and medial frontal CMs as well as those in the globus pallidus (▶ Fig. 4.2). The A1 (precommunicating) segment begins at the terminal bifurcation of the ICA and ends at the anterior communicating artery (ACoA). This A1 segment forms the medial boundary of the supracarotid triangle through which pallidal cavernomas are accessed. Medial LSAs originate from the superior surface of the A1 segment and ascend to the anterior perforated substance, subfrontal area, hypothalamus, anterior commissure, septum pellucidum, and paraolfactory structures. These medial LSAs are carefully avoided during pallidal CM resection, as is the recurrent artery of Heubner, which is considered the medial-most LSA, defining the inner border of the collection of perforators along A1 medial LSA and M1 lateral LSA segments. As its name implies, the recurrent artery of Heubner travels back along the A1 segment after originating from the lateral wall of the proximal A2 (postcommunicating) segment just distal to the ACoA, almost as a lateral continuation of the ACoA.

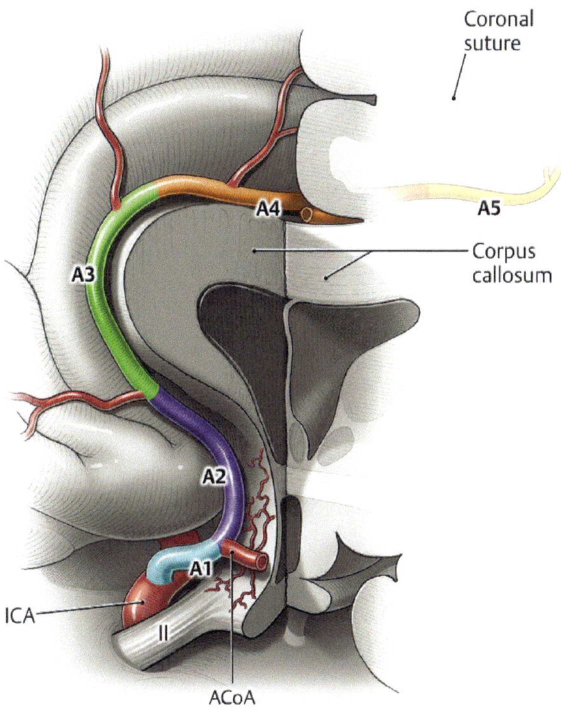

Fig. 4.2 ACA segments, as seen from a left medial view of the right hemisphere. The ACA is the arterial landmark for basal and medial frontal CMs as well as those in the globus pallidus. The A1 segment forms the medial boundary of the supracarotid triangle through which pallidal cavernomas are accessed. Ten cortical branches radiate from the ACA as it courses around the corpus callosum. The first two terminal A5 cortical arteries (OrbFrA and FrPolA) overlie targeted basal CMs in the frontal lobe. The next six branches (CmaA, AIFA, MIFA, PIFA, paracentral artery, and PcaA) overlie medial CMs in the frontal lobe. The last two (superior and inferior parietal arteries) branches overlie targeted medial CMs in the parietal lobe. Roman numeral denotes CN. (Reproduced with permission from Barrow Neurological Institute, Phoenix, AZ.)

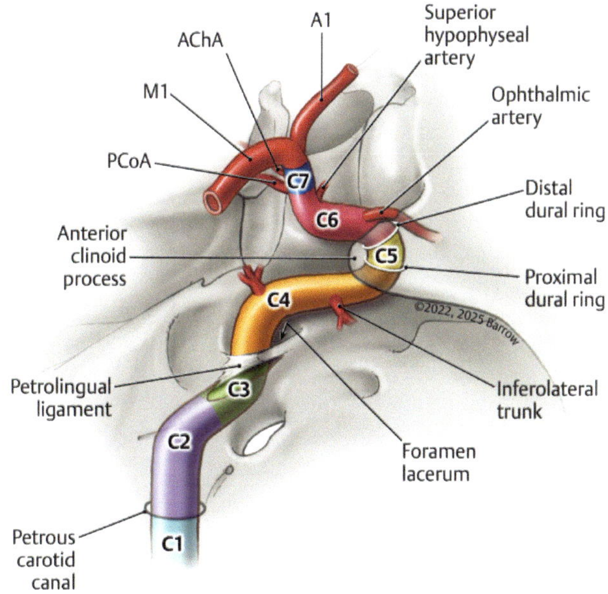

Fig. 4.3 ICA segments, as seen from the right lateral view. Only the last two segments (C6 and C7) reside in the subarachnoid space, and while neither one has an associated cavernoma subtype, they are relevant to cavernoma dissection. The PCoA is a trail from the supratentorial to infratentorial compartments through Liliequist's membrane. The AChA is a trail to the crural cistern and anterior incisural space. AChA and oculomotor nerve dissection releases the medial temporal lobe to expose the P2A (crural) segment of the PCA and s2 (lateral pontomesencephalic) segment of the SCA to reach interpeduncular and peduncular midbrain CMs as well as some basilar pontine CMs. (Reproduced with permission from Barrow Neurological Institute, Phoenix, AZ.)

The A2 segment begins at the ACoA and follows the rostrum of the corpus callosum. The A3 (precallosal) segment curves around the anterior corpus callosum and follows the genu until the artery assumes a posterior course. The A4 (supracallosal) and A5 (postcallosal) segments continue over the anterior and posterior halves, respectively, of the body of the corpus callosum, with the vertical plane of coronal suture dividing them. This segmental anatomy at the deep margin of the medial hemisphere is not useful as a localizing landmark. However, the OrbFrA and frontopolar artery (FrPolA) offer guidance to reach basal frontal CMs. The OrbFrA is the first cortical ACA branch, arising from the anterolateral surface of the A2 segment approximately 5 mm distal to the ACoA and coursing perpendicularly over the gyrus rectus and olfactory tract. The FrPolA is the second cortical ACA branch, originating from the A2 segment approximately 14 mm from the ACoA and coursing anteriorly in interhemispheric fissure to the ventromedial frontal lobes.

Ten cortical branches radiate from the ACA as it courses around the corpus callosum: the (1) OrbFrA, (2) FrPolA, (3) callosomarginal artery (CmaA), (4) anterior internal frontal artery, (5) middle internal frontal artery, (6) posterior internal frontal artery, (7) paracentral artery, (8) pericallosal artery, (9) superior parietal artery, and (10) inferior parietal artery. The first two terminal A5 cortical arteries overlie targeted basal CMs in the frontal lobe. The next six branches overlie medial CMs in the frontal lobe, and the last two overlie targeted medial CMs in the parietal lobe. The specific identities of vertically ascending A5 segments may not be apparent during interhemispheric dissection. Nonetheless, the horizontally traversing CmaA and pericallosal artery are recognizable on either side of the cingulate gyrus in the corpus callosum cistern. The anterior internal frontal artery originates from the A2 segment adjacent to the rostrum, the middle internal frontal artery originates from the A3 segment adjacent to the genu or from the CmaA, and the posterior internal frontal artery originates from the A4 segment adjacent to the body of the corpus callosum.

4.4 Internal Carotid Artery

Branches from the carotid artery are like roads to Rome: the carotid artery lies at the center of the cerebral circulation, and many arterial landmarks connect to or leave from it (▶ Fig. 4.3). The ICA may not be an address for many cavernoma subtypes, but the ICA pathways are critical stepping stones to many targeted CM subtypes. Simple classifications like Rhoton's describe four ICA segments: C1 (cervical), C2 (petrous), C3 (cavernous), and C4 (supraclinoid). A contemporary classification by van Loveren and colleagues defines seven segments using the surrounding anatomy and the compartments through which the ICA travels, also numbered in the direction of antegrade blood flow: C1 (cervical), C2 (petrous), C3 (lacerum), C4 (cavernous), C5 (clinoidal), C6 (ophthalmic), and C7 (communicating). Only the last two segments reside in the subarachnoid space and are relevant to cavernoma dissection.

The C6 segment courses from the distal dural ring to the PCoA and has two named branches: (1) the ophthalmic artery, arising from the superior surface of the ICA just beyond the distal dural ring and running anteriorly under the optic nerve to enter the optic canal and the orbit, and (2) the superior hypophyseal artery, arising from the medial surface of the ICA, also beyond the distal dural ring, but more posterior to the ophthalmic artery origin. The C7 segment runs from the PCoA to the ICA terminus. The PCoA arises from the posterior carotid wall. It courses posteriorly and medially along the superior surface of the oculomotor nerve and intersects the posterior cerebral artery (PCA) to mark the end of the P1 (precommunicating) segment and the beginning of the P2 (postcommunicating) segment. Therefore, the PCoA is a trail from the supratentorial to infratentorial compartments. Anterior thalamoperforating arteries or premammillary arteries originate from the superior surface of the PCoA along its course and ascend to the hypothalamus, anterior thalamus, internal capsule, and optic chiasm and tract. They can obscure the critical view through the carotid-oculomotor triangle. The division of the PCoA allows it to ascend into the interpeduncular fossa with its anterior thalamoperforating arteries and open the corridor to targeted interpeduncular midbrain CMs. However, the fetal PCA is a critical variant in as many as 20% of patients; in these patients, the fetal PCA must be preserved because the P1 segment remains hypoplastic or atretic, and compromising the fetal PCA can result in occipital lobe infarction.

The anterior choroidal artery (AChA) arises from the posterior wall of the communicating segment of the ICA. This segment is usually a single artery, but it can be two arteries. Its initial cisternal segment runs posteromedially behind the ICA, following the contour of the medial uncus through the crural cistern and supplying the optic tract, lateral thalamus, and internal capsule (genu and posterior limb). The cisternal segment ends at the plexal point where the AChA pierces the tela choroidea of the temporal horn of the lateral ventricle. The plexal segment runs from the temporal horn to the atrium and has diminishing surgical significance. The cisternal segment is a vital artery because its compromise causes deficits (hemiplegia, hemianesthesia, and hemianopsia) out of proportion to its small size. Additionally, the dissection of this cisternal segment liberates the uncus from the frontal lobe and midbrain to widen the carotid-oculomotor and oculomotor-tentorial triangles for deep dissection. Thorough AChA dissection into the crural cistern releases the medial temporal lobe and oculomotor nerve. It opens the anterior incisural space and exposes the P2A (crural) segment of the PCA and s2 (lateral pontomesencephalic) segment of the superior cerebellar artery (SCA) segments to reach targeted CMs in the anterior midbrain and pons.

4.5 Posterior Cerebral Arteries

The basilar artery terminates in a quadrifurcation from which two PCAs and two SCAs originate (▶ Fig. 4.4). The P1 segment of the PCA begins at the basilar bifurcation and ends at the

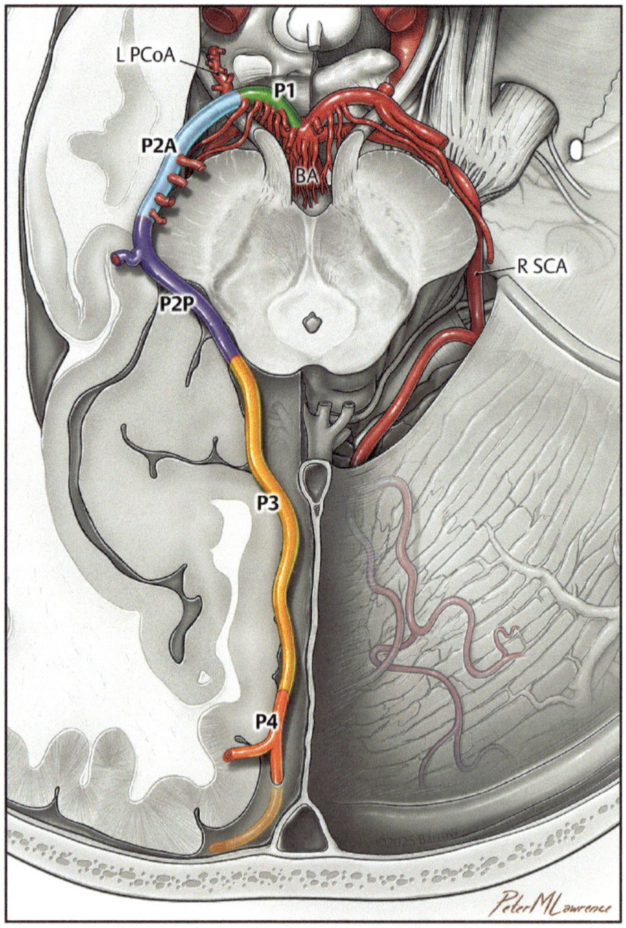

Fig. 4.4 PCA segments, as seen from above with the midbrain and occipital lobes cross-sectioned. The P1 segment is the arterial address for interpeduncular midbrain CMs between the cerebral peduncles and oculomotor nerves, with access above the basilar bifurcation and between the posterior thalamoperforating arteries that originate from the P1 segments. The P2A is the arterial address for peduncular midbrain CMs, with access through the oculomotor-tentorial triangle lateral to CN III, inferior to the P2A, and superior to the s2 segment of the SCA. P3 segments are exposed during SCIT and SCTT approaches to targeted quadrigeminal midbrain, pulvinar thalamic, and geniculate thalamic CMs. Rather than serving as an address, they are often landmarks that must be passed en route to deeper targets. The P4 segment provides landmarks to medial parietal and occipital CMs. The P4 divides into the CalcA as it enters the calcarine fissure and fans out over the lingula, inferior cuneus, and occipital pole and into the ParOccA as it enters the parieto-occipital fissure and supplies the cuneus and precuneus. The splenial artery arises proximally from the ParOccA and guides dissection to the posterior corpus callosum CMs. Not shown is the mPChA, whose circuitous course through crural, ambient, and quadrigeminal cisterns to reach the choroid plexus in the roof of the third ventricle and the floor of lateral ventricles makes the mPChA an arterial address for quadrigeminal midbrain and five (geniculate, pulvinar, choroidal, medial, and anterior thalamic) of the six thalamic subtypes. (Reproduced with permission from Barrow Neurological Institute, Phoenix, AZ.)

junction with the PCoA. This segment is typically larger in caliber than the PCoA but may be smaller in patients with fetal anatomy. The P1 segment is the arterial address for CMs that arise in the interpeduncular midbrain between the cerebral peduncles and oculomotor nerves. This access corridor runs above the basilar bifurcation and between the posterior thalamoperforating arteries that originate from the P1 segments. Most posterior thalamoperforating arteries arise from the middle third of the P1 segment as individual branches or branching trunks that can be bilateral and symmetric, bilateral and asymmetric, or unilateral with bilateral territories (artery of Percheron). Posterior thalamoperforating arteries are vital because they supply the anterior and part of the posterior thalamus, hypothalamus, subthalamus, medial midbrain, substantia nigra, red nucleus, oculomotor and trochlear nuclei, oculomotor nerve, reticular formation, and posterior internal capsule. Thalamoperforating artery compromise can cause sensory disturbances, weakness, memory deficits, autonomic imbalance, diplopia, alterations of consciousness, and endocrine disturbances.

The P2 segment begins at the junction with the PCoA and ends lateral to the posterior margin of the midbrain. The P2 segment is divided into anterior and posterior halves, with the P2A segment coursing around the cerebral peduncle to its lateral edge through the crural cistern and the P2P (ambient) segment coursing around the lateral midbrain through the ambient cistern. P2A is the arterial address for CMs that develop in the peduncular midbrain. This access corridor runs through the oculomotor-tentorial triangle lateral to cranial nerve (CN) III, inferior to the P2A, and superior to the s2 segment of the SCA. Peduncular and thalamogeniculate perforators arise from the P2 segments but ascend superiorly away from this access corridor. Long and short circumflex perforators originate from the P1 and P2 segments of the PCA and course parallel and medial to the PCA and away from this access corridor.

The P3 (quadrigeminal) segment begins lateral to the posterior margin of the midbrain, climbs over the free edge of the tentorium, courses through the quadrigeminal cistern, and ends at the anterior limit of the calcarine fissure. The PCA typically branches along this segment into its major terminal arteries, the calcarine artery (CalcA), and the parieto-occipital artery (ParOccA). P3 segments are exposed during supracerebellar-infratentorial approaches to targeted quadrigeminal midbrain, pulvinar thalamic, and geniculate thalamic CMs. Rather than serving as an address, they are often landmarks that must be passed en route to deeper targets. Contralateral supracerebellar-transtentorial approaches proceed through the tentorium and into the ambient cistern; in some cases, they proceed laterally to this P3 loop and over the tentorial edge.

The P4 (calcarine) segment begins at the anterior limit of the calcarine fissure and ends at the cortical surface of the occipital lobe. After dividing into the CalcA and ParOccA along its P3 segment, these trunks climb from the posterior margin of the midbrain, over the free edge of the tentorium, through the quadrigeminal cistern, and into the anterior limit of the calcarine fissure. The CalcA becomes the P4 segment after it enters the calcarine fissure and courses to the cortical surface of the occipital lobe, fanning out over the lingula, the inferior cuneus, and the occipital pole. The ParOccA runs in the parieto-occipital fissure and supplies the cuneus and precuneus. These sizable trunks provide landmarks to locate medial parietal and occipital CMs. The splenial artery arises proximally from the ParOccA and guides dissection to the posterior corpus callosum.

The PCA also supplies the medial and basal surfaces of the temporal lobe with hippocampal and posterior temporal arteries originating from the P2 segment. The hippocampal artery is the first PCA cortical branch, arising in the crural or ambient cistern and supplying the uncus, anterior parahippocampal gyrus, hippocampus, and dentate gyrus. The posterior temporal artery can arise as a common trunk that branches into anterior, middle, and posterior branches or as individual anterior, middle, and posterior branches. Collectively, the hippocampal and posterior temporal arteries are called inferior temporal arteries. They serve as arterial landmarks to target basal temporal and basal occipital CMs as they course over the tentorial incisura in the subtemporal plane.

One final PCA branch of importance is the medial posterior choroidal artery (mPChA), which arises from the PCA along its distal P1 or proximal P2 segment on its medial wall. The mPChA encircles the midbrain, paralleling the PCA trunk before curling forward at the superior colliculus and ascending over the pineal gland to reach the roof of the third ventricle. There, it enters the velum interpositum, courses between the thalami, and arrives at the foramen of Monro adjacent to the choroidal fissure. It makes a hairpin turn to enter the lateral ventricles and course posteriorly in the lateral ventricular floor. This course of the mPChA on angiography has been characterized as the *3-sign* from the curvature in the artery as it drapes over the superior colliculus and pineal gland. The course of the mPChA has two complete reversals of direction, one gradually around the pineal region posteriorly and the other sharply through the foramen of Monro anteriorly. This circuitous course through crural, ambient, and quadrigeminal cisterns to reach the choroid plexus in the roof of the third ventricle and the floor of lateral ventricles makes the mPChA an arterial address for quadrigeminal midbrain and five (geniculate, pulvinar, choroidal, medial, and anterior thalamic) of the six thalamic subtypes.

4.6 Superior Cerebellar Artery

The SCA is partitioned into four segments: s1 (anterior pontomesencephalic), s2 (lateral pontomesencephalic), s3 (cerebellomesencephalic), and s4 (cortical) segments (▸ Fig. 4.5). The s1 segment begins at the SCA origin, courses underneath CN III, and ends at the anterolateral brainstem, medial to the tentorial edge. The distal s1 segment is another arterial address for targeted CMs in the peduncular midbrain, forming the inferior border of the access corridor. The superior border of this access corridor is the P2A segment described above. The s1 segment also runs in or near the pontomesencephalic sulcus and, therefore, lies superior to high-riding basilar pontine CMs in the overbelly of the pons. However, the basilar artery is the primary arterial address for CMs in the basilar pons.

The s2 segment begins at the anterolateral brainstem, dips caudally to the trigeminal root, and terminates at the entrance to the cerebellomesencephalic fissure. Therefore, the low-lying s2 segment is a landmark for targeted peritrigeminal pontine CMs in the upper pons and supratrigeminal triangle. The s3 segment courses posteriorly within the cerebellomesencephalic

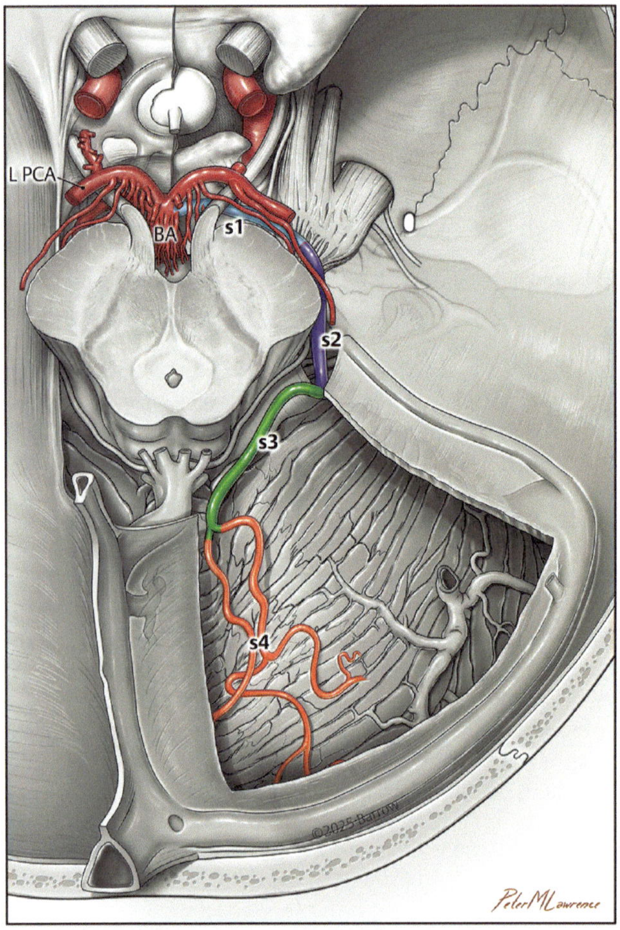

Fig. 4.5 SCA segments, as seen from above in an axial cross-section through the midbrain. The distal s1 segment is another arterial address for targeted peduncular midbrain CMs, forming the inferior border of the access corridor. The s1 segment also runs in or near the pontomesencephalic sulcus and, therefore, is a superior address for high-riding basilar pontine CMs in the overbelly of the pons. The s2 segment is a landmark for targeted peritrigeminal pontine CMs in the upper pons and supratrigeminal triangle. The s3 segment is the dominant landmark in the ambient cistern and the arterial address of targeted tegmental midbrain CMs and low-lying quadrigeminal midbrain CMs. The rostral trunk of s4 is the arterial address for vermian cerebellar CMs and the caudal trunk is the arterial addresses for tentorial cerebellar CMs. (Reproduced with permission from Barrow Neurological Institute, Phoenix, AZ.)

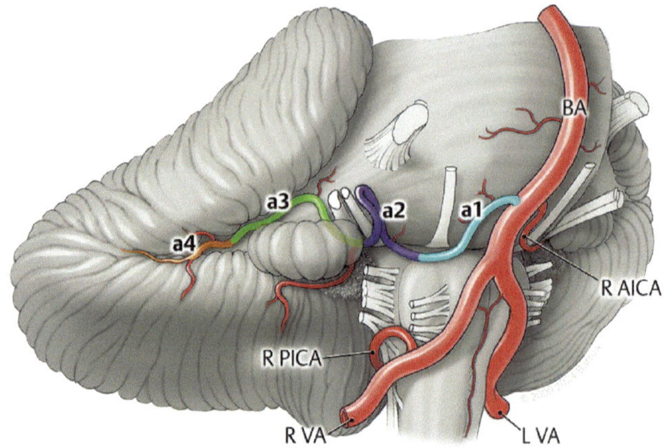

Fig. 4.6 AICA segments, as seen from a right anterior oblique view. Low-lying basilar pontine CMs are exposed through a Kawase or anterior transpetrous approach, which visualizes these lesions in the corner formed by the basilar artery and a1. The a2 segment parallels the pontomedullary sulcus between the superior olive and the pontine underbelly, making the a2 segment the landmark for supraolivary pontine CMs. The a3 segment courses through the petrosal fissure, making it the principal arterial landmark for splitting this fissure and accessing the entry zone for middle peduncular pontine CMs. Cortical a4 segments distal to the cerebellopontine fissure are the arterial address for petrosal cerebellar CMs. (Reproduced with permission from Barrow Neurological Institute, Phoenix, AZ.)

fissure, following the trochlear nerve. The SCA usually bifurcates into rostral and caudal trunks within this segment, but it can duplicate at its origin from the basilar artery or bifurcate within s1 or s2 proximal segments. The s3 segment is the dominant landmark in the ambient cistern; it is the arterial address of targeted tegmental midbrain CMs and low-lying quadrigeminal midbrain CMs.

The s4 segments begin as distal s3 branches exit the cerebellomesencephalic fissure and supply the cerebellum's tentorial surface. The rostral trunk supplies the superior vermis and the caudal trunk supplies the tentorial surface, making them arterial addresses for vermian and tentorial cerebellar CMs, respectively.

4.7 Anterior Inferior Cerebellar Artery

The anterior inferior cerebellar artery (AICA) is partitioned into four segments: a1 (anterior pontine), a2 (lateral pontine), a3 (flocculopeduncular), and a4 (cortical) segments (▶ Fig. 4.6). The a1 segment begins at the AICA's origin from the basilar trunk. It ends at the transolivary line, drawn through the long axis of the inferior olive extended upward on the pons. This segment courses below CN VI as it ascends to Dorello's canal. Low-lying basilar pontine CMs are exposed through a Kawase or anterior transpetrous approach, which visualizes these lesions in the corner formed by the basilar artery and a1.

The a2 segment begins at the anterolateral margin of the pons (transolivary line). It passes through the cerebellopontine angle alongside CNs VII and VIII, the internal auditory meatus, the lateral recess, and the choroid plexus protruding from the foramen of Luschka. The labyrinthine artery, recurrent perforating arteries, and subarcuate artery arise from this segment. The a2 segment parallels the pontomedullary sulcus, where the superior olive and the pontine underbelly intersect. Supraolivary pontine CMs can present at this sulcus, making the a2 segment the landmark for this subtype.

The a3 segment begins as the artery passes the flocculus and middle cerebellar peduncle. It enters the petrosal fissure, courses between superior and inferior semilunar lobules, and ends as it exits the petrosal fissure at the cerebellopontine angle. It commonly bifurcates near CNs VII and VIII into rostral and caudal trunks, with the former supplying the middle cerebellar peduncle and superior lip of the cerebellopontine fissure, and the latter supplying the inferior lip of the cerebellopontine fissure, flocculus, and choroid plexus. The course of this a3 segment through the petrosal fissure makes it the principal arterial landmark for splitting this fissure and accessing the entry zone for middle peduncular pontine CMs.

Cortical a4 segments supply the petrosal surface distal to the cerebellopontine fissure. They are the arterial address for petrosal cerebellar CMs.

4.8 Posterior Inferior Cerebellar Artery

The posterior inferior cerebellar artery (PICA) is the significant arterial landmark for medullary and pontine cavernomas because it guides dissection around the medulla and into the fourth ventricle (▶ Fig. 4.7). The PICA has five arterial segments defined by its relationship to lower CNs as it winds around the medulla and posterior surface of the cerebellum: p1 (anterior medullary), p2 (lateral medullary), p3 (tonsillomedullary), p4 (telovelotonsillar), and p5 (cortical) segments. The p1 segment begins at the PICA's origin, lies anterior to the medulla, and extends past the hypoglossal rootlets at the medial edge of the inferior olive. The distal V4 (intradural) segments of the vertebral arteries (VAs) plus the vertebrobasilar junction (VBJ) can be used as the arterial address for pyramidal medullary CMs, and the p1 segment may course near this confluence and provide guidance.

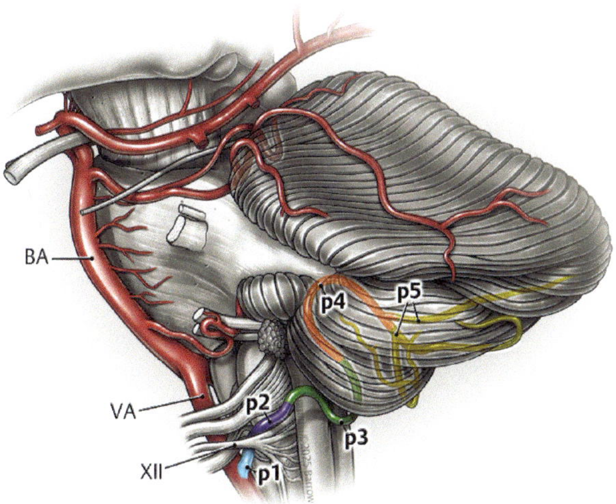

Fig. 4.7 PICA segments, as seen from a right lateral view. The distal V4 (intradural) segments of the vertebral arteries plus the vertebrobasilar junction are the arterial address for pyramidal medullary CMs, and the p1 segment offer arterial guidance to this confluence. The course of p2 over the olive makes it the natural landmark for targeted olivary medullary CMs. The p3 segment is an arterial landmark for gracile and trigonal medullary CMs and rhomboid pontine CMs. The additional dissection needed to expose the p4 segment makes it the landmark for inferior peduncular pontine CMs on the pontine side of the lateral recess and foramen of Luschka. In addition, p4 leads to entry zones medial to or superior to the tonsil for supratonsillar access to deep nuclear CMs in the cerebellum, specifically adjacent to the dentate nucleus. The p5 segments are used as arterial landmarks for superficial suboccipital, vermian, and tonsillar cerebellar CMs. The PSA (not shown) is an arterial landmark for cuneate medullary CMs. Roman numeral denotes CN. (Reproduced with permission from Barrow Neurological Institute, Phoenix, AZ.)

The p2 segment extends from the olive to the rootlets of CNs IX, X, and XI at the lateral edge of the olive. The course of p2 over the olive makes it the natural landmark for targeted olivary medullary CMs. The p3 segment begins where the PICA passes under or between the rootlets of the CN IX–X–XI triad, descends to the inferior pole of the cerebellar tonsil, reverses course in the caudal or infratonsillar loop, and ascends along the medial tonsil to its midpoint. The p3 caudal loop is positioned ideally to open the cerebellomedullary fissures, separate the tonsils from the medulla, widen the vallecular triangle, and enter the fourth ventricle. Therefore, the p3 segment is an arterial landmark for targeted gracile and trigonal medullary and rhomboid pontine CMs.

The p4 segment begins at the midpoint of the PICA's ascent along the medial tonsil, continues toward the roof of the fourth ventricle, turns around again to form a cranial or supratonsillar loop, and courses downward and posteriorly to the tonsillobiventral fissure. This segment derives its name from its branches to the choroid plexus of the fourth ventricle (tela choroidea) and its association with the roof of the fourth ventricle (inferior medullary velum). The additional dissection needed to expose the p4 segment makes it the landmark for inferior peduncular pontine lesions on the pontine side of the lateral recess and foramen of Luschka. In addition, p4 leads to entry zones medial or superior to the tonsil for access to deep nuclear CMs in the cerebellum.

The p5 segments begin as the PICA emerges from the tonsillobiventral fissure where the tonsil, vermis, and biventral lobule of the cerebellar hemisphere meet. These p5 segments consist of numerous trunks and branches, with a medial trunk supplying the vermian surface and a lateral trunk supplying tonsillar and hemispheric surfaces. The p5 segments are used as arterial landmarks for superficial suboccipital, vermian, and tonsillar cerebellar CMs, as well as with the supratonsillar approach to deep nuclear cerebellar CMs.

As mentioned above, the VBJ is an arterial address for CMs that develop in the pyramids of the medulla. The V4 segment begins as it pierces the dura behind the occipital condyle. The V4 segment passes over the dorsal and ventral roots of the first cervical nerve and crosses anteriorly to the dentate ligament and spinal portion of the accessory nerve. It courses from the lower lateral to the upper anterior surface of the medulla, giving off perforators along the way. It passes across the pyramid, joins the contralateral VA at or near the pontomedullary sulcus, and forms the VBJ and basilar trunk below targeted pyramidal CMs. The anterior spinal artery is the last branch proximal to the VBJ. It joins the contralateral artery to form a single midline anterior spinal artery that descends through the foramen magnum on the ventral surface of the medulla and spinal cord in or near the anterior median fissure. This important artery is another landmark and must be carefully protected during cavernoma resection because it supplies the pyramids and their decussation, medial lemniscus, and hypoglossal nuclei and nerves.

The posterior spinal artery (PSA) is the first intracranial branch of the VA. However, it sometimes arises extradurally and travels with the VA through the dural ring into the subarachnoid space. The PSA courses medially behind the dentate ligament and divides into ascending and descending branches that supply dorsal columns and portions of the dorsal cervical spinal cord. The PSA is an arterial landmark for CMs that arise in the cuneate nucleus in the medulla.

4.9 Arterial Dissection Codes

Segmental alphanumerics serve as specific arterial addresses that can empower the dissection of cavernomas, akin to delivering mail to residential addresses in the postal system (▶ Table 4.2). The arterial segments can be viewed as defining landmarks in surgical corridors that identify target lesions, with or without surface presentation. In a cohort of 128 patients with brainstem CMs, preoperative MRIs for subtyping, and intraoperative photographs or videos, segmental arterial targets were associated with lesions in 117 (91%) patients

Table 4.3 Brainstem CM subtypes and the presence of the arterial segments and veins associated with each subtype within the surgical field, based on analysis of intraoperative images

				Brainstem CMs, *n* (%)			
Type	**Subtype**	**Arterial target**	**Venous target**	**All**	**Artery observed**	**Vein observed**	**Dissection code**[a]
All				128	117/128 (91)	96/128 (75)	
Midbrain	Interpeduncular	P1	Anterior pontomesencephalic vein	1 (0.78)	1/1 (100)	1/1 (100)	M3-M2-M1-C6-AChA-PCoA-P1
	Peduncular	P2A	Peduncular vein	8 (6.3)	8/8 (100)	7/8 (88)	M3-M2-M1-C6-AChA-PCoA-P2A
	Tegmental	s3	Lateral mesencephalic vein	12 (9.4)	11/12 (92)	7/12 (58)	s4-s3
	Quadrigeminal	mPChA	Internal cerebral vein	8 (6.3)	8/8 (100)	6/8 (75)	s4-s3-P3-PreCenCblV-BVR-mPChA
	Periaqueductal	None	None	0	0	0	CmaA-PcaA-ThaStrV-ICV-mPChA
Pontine	Basilar	BA	Anterior pontomesencephalic vein	3 (2.3)	1/3 (33)	2/3 (67)	SPS-IPS-a2-a1-BA
	Peritrigeminal	s2	Superior petrosal vein	11 (8.6)	10/11 (91)	10/11 (91)	s4-s3-s2
	Middle peduncular	a3	Vein of the middle cerebellar peduncle	28 (21.9)	24/28 (86)	21/28 (75)	a4-a3
	Inferior peduncular	p4	Vein of the inferior cerebellar peduncle	6 (4.7)	5/6 (83)	4/6 (67)	p2-p3-p4
	Rhomboid	p3	Vein of the cerebellomedullary fissure	14 (11.0)	13/14 (93)	10/14 (71)	L p3-R p3
	Supraolivary	a2	Vein of the pontomedullary sulcus	13 (10.1)	13/13 (100)	12/13 (92)	V4-p3-p2-p1-a2
Medullary	Pyramidal	VBJ	Lateral anterior medullary vein	0	0	0	V4-p1-ASA-VBJ
	Olivary	p2	Retro-olivary vein	14 (10.9)	14/14 (100)	9/14 (64)	V4-p3-p2
	Trigonal	p3	Median posterior medullary vein/vein of the inferior cerebellar peduncle	4 (3.1)	4/4 (100)	3/4 (75)	L p3-R p3
	Gracile	p3	Median posterior medullary vein/vein of the inferior cerebellar peduncle	2 (1.6)	2/2 (100)	2/2 (100)	L p3-R p3
	Cuneate	PSA	Median posterior medullary vein	4 (3.1)	3/4 (75)	2/4 (50)	V4-p3-p2-PSA

[a]The dissection code is the sequence of arterial segments (in some cases, veins of the ventricles or deep venous system) followed through the subarachnoid corridor to reach the target lesion.

(▶ Table 4.3). Thus, arterial targets complement the Seven Cavernomas taxonomy and have excellent reliability. Centering dissection on an artery might seem to risk injury or bleeding, but arteries are rugged, elastic, and manipulable.

In addition to their utility in specifying the target of dissection, arterial segments can be followed through the subarachnoid spaces to reach the arterial target, creating a *dissection code* for each brainstem CM subtype to guide methodical, stepwise microsurgery (▶ Table 4.3; ▶ Fig. 4.8, ▶ Fig. 4.9, ▶ Fig. 4.10, ▶ Fig. 4.11, ▶ Fig. 4.12). A dissection sequence along contiguous arterial segments can lead to the target, creating an alphanumeric code for dissection steps that functions like cairns or blazes along a trail. For example, peduncular midbrain lesions associated with the P2A segment of the PCA are accessed with an orbitozygomatic craniotomy, transsylvian approach, and passage through the oculomotor-tentorial triangle. This dissection traces arteries through the sylvian fissure and carotid, crural, and interpeduncular cisterns to finally reach the lesion, giving it the following dissection code: M3-M2-M1-C6-AChA-PCoA-P2A. The specific arterial address of the target is the last alphanumeric in the code. In this example, the code provides wayfinding to the lesion from beginning to end; in other cases, the code may describe only one segment of the trail. For example, with middle peduncular pontine lesions, the AICA provides guidance into the petrosal fissure to reach the middle cerebellar peduncle (a4–a3). However, the remainder of the trans-middle cerebellar peduncle dissection is through parenchyma and, therefore, without arterial guidance to the target CM.

Venous anatomy is less reliable as a wayfinding instrument than arterial anatomy (75 vs. 91% association with brainstem CM subtypes). Some veins are highly reliable, such as the veins of the galenic complex, but smaller veins may be hypoplastic, absent, or in unusual locations. Consequently, veins are not included in the Seven Cavernomas framework. However,

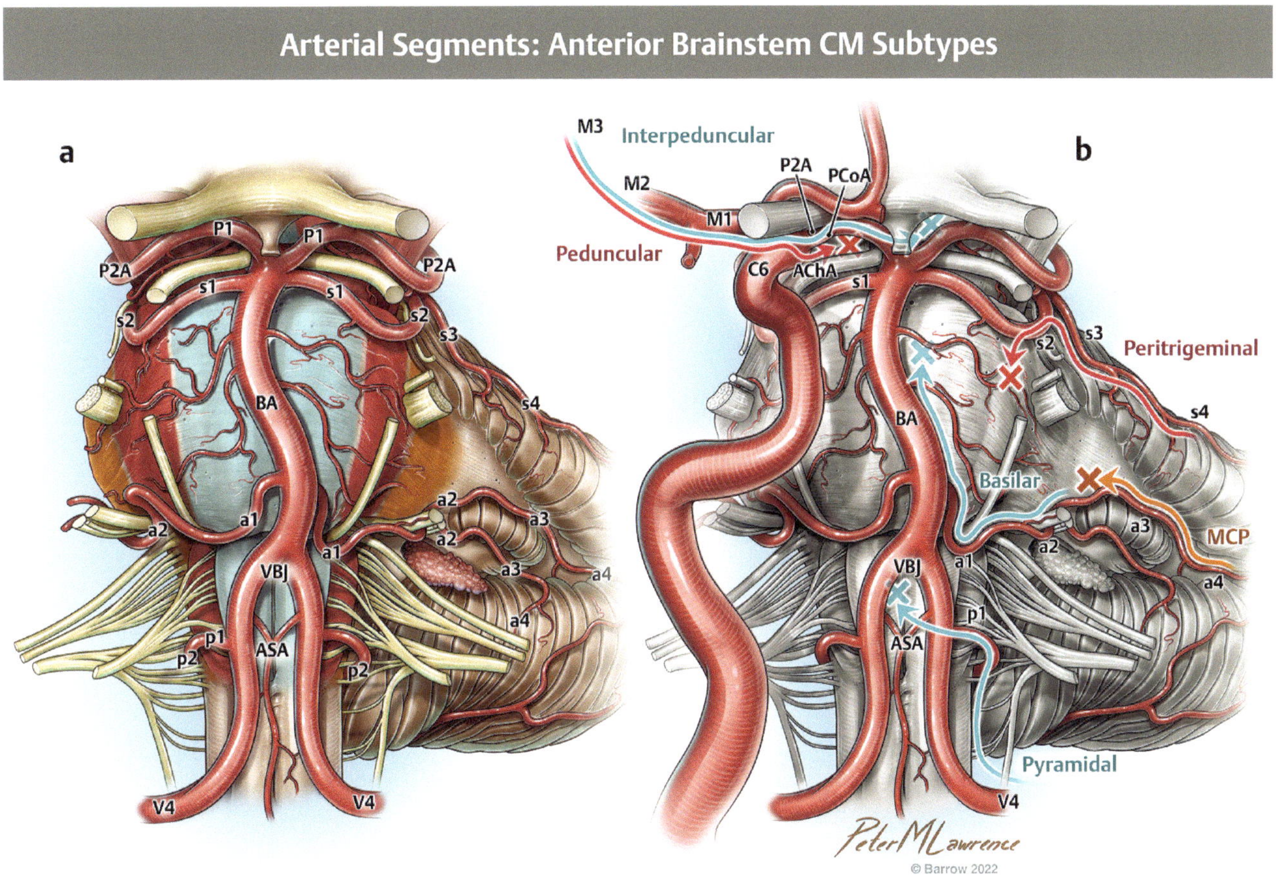

Fig. 4.8 Arterial segments associated with specific brainstem CM subtypes. **(a)** Anterior view of the brainstem shows the surface locations of anterior (*teal*), anterolateral (*red*), and lateral (*orange*) CM subtypes. Anterior subtypes comprise interpeduncular, basilar, and pyramidal (*teal*); anterolateral subtypes are peduncular, peritrigeminal, and olivary (*red*); and lateral subtypes are tegmental, middle peduncular, and cuneate (*orange*). **(b)** Dissection routes to six specific CM subtypes that follow arterial waypoints are depicted with *arrows* that match the colors of the brainstem's anatomic surfaces (shown in **a**). The target CM is depicted with a matching colored *X*. (Reproduced with permission from Barrow Neurological Institute, Phoenix, AZ.)

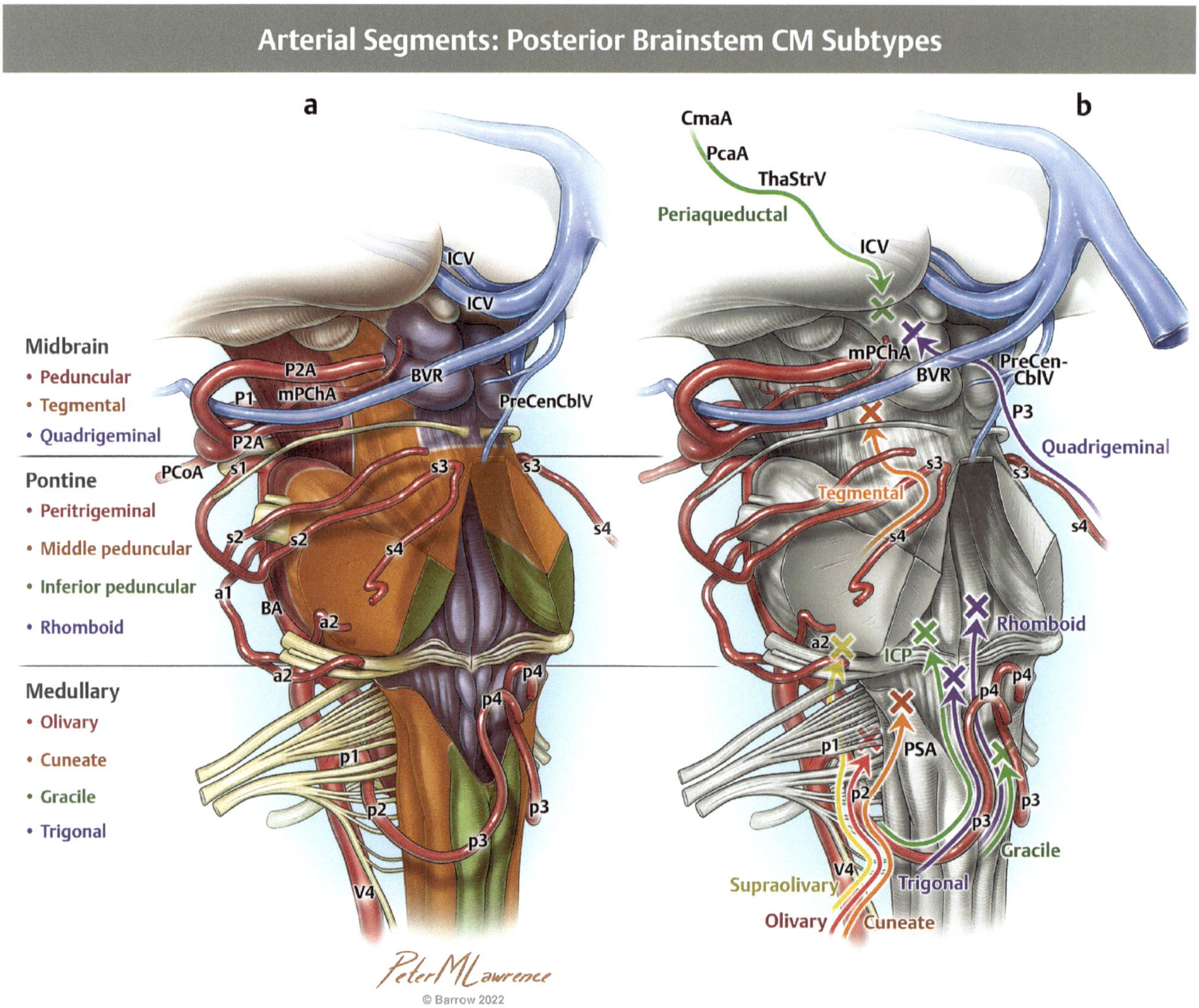

Fig. 4.9 Arterial segments associated with specific brainstem CM subtypes. **(a)** Posterolateral views of the brainstem surface locations show posterior (*purple*), posterolateral (*green*), lateral (*orange*), and anterolateral (*red*) CM subtypes. Posterior subtypes are quadrigeminal, rhomboid, and trigonal (*purple*); posterolateral subtypes are inferior peduncular and gracile (*green*); lateral subtypes are tegmental, middle peduncular, and cuneate (*orange*); anterolateral subtypes comprise peduncular, peritrigeminal, and olivary (*red*; also in ▶ Fig. 4.8), and periaqueductal and supraolivary subtypes are not shown. **(b)** Dissection routes to 10 specific brainstem CM subtypes that follow vascular waypoints are depicted with *arrows* that match the colors of the brainstem's anatomic surface (shown in **a**). The target CM is depicted with a matching colored *X*. Periaqueductal (*green*) and supraolivary (*yellow*) subtypes are shown. (Reproduced with permission from Barrow Neurological Institute, Phoenix, AZ.)

recognizing the potential value of a venous malformation or developmental venous anomaly is important because it is intimately associated with the target CM and provides localizing clues to the CM through the subarachnoid system and parenchyma. These pathognomonic veins are typically distinct from other veins, larger in caliber, and identifiable preoperatively on contrast-enhanced imaging. Their role in guiding dissection ultimately depends on the conformation of the lesion, the developmental venous anomaly itself, and the approach, mandating an individualized surgical plan.

Midbrain Artery Paths

Interpeduncular

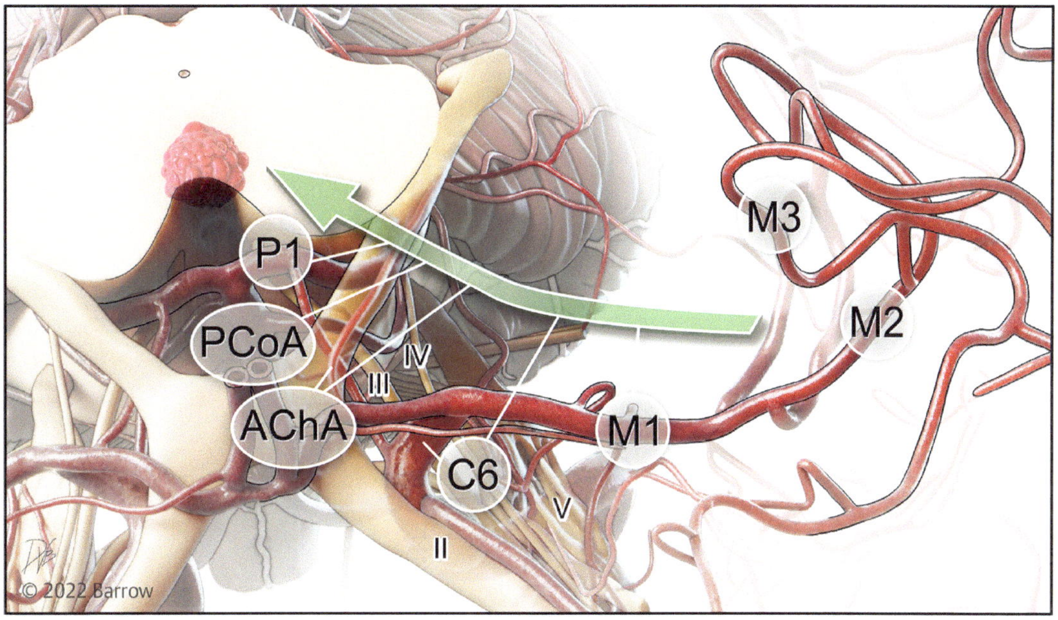

Peduncular

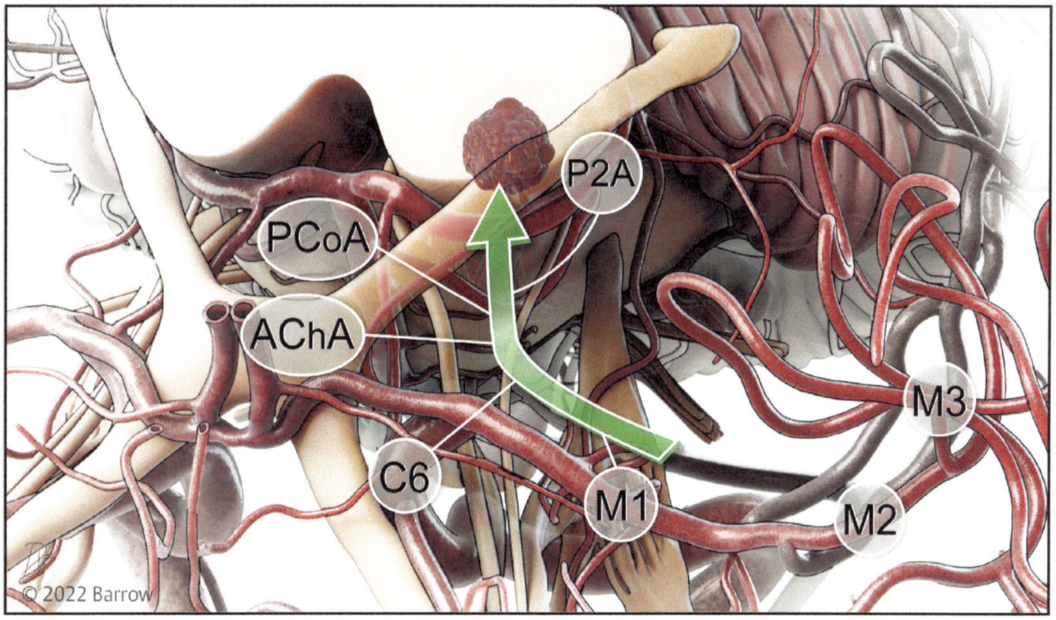

a

Fig. 4.10 Midbrain artery paths. Midbrain artery paths (*green arrows*), established by following arterial segments (*gray circles*) sequentially to reach targeted CMs (*red spheres*), are shown for **(a)** interpeduncular, peduncular,

(Continued)

Midbrain Artery Paths

Tegmental

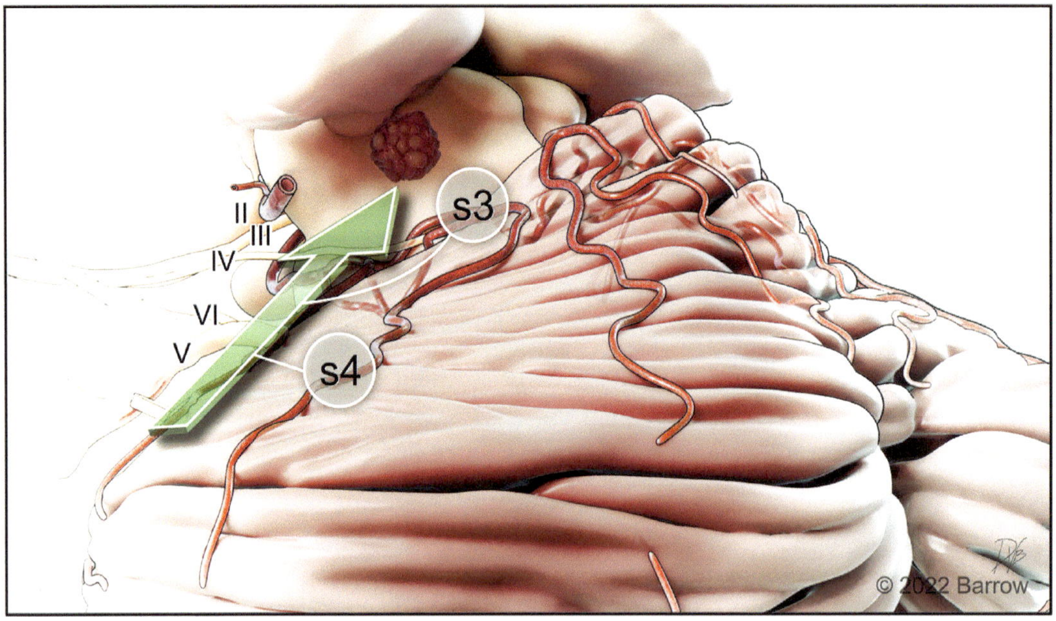

Quadrigeminal

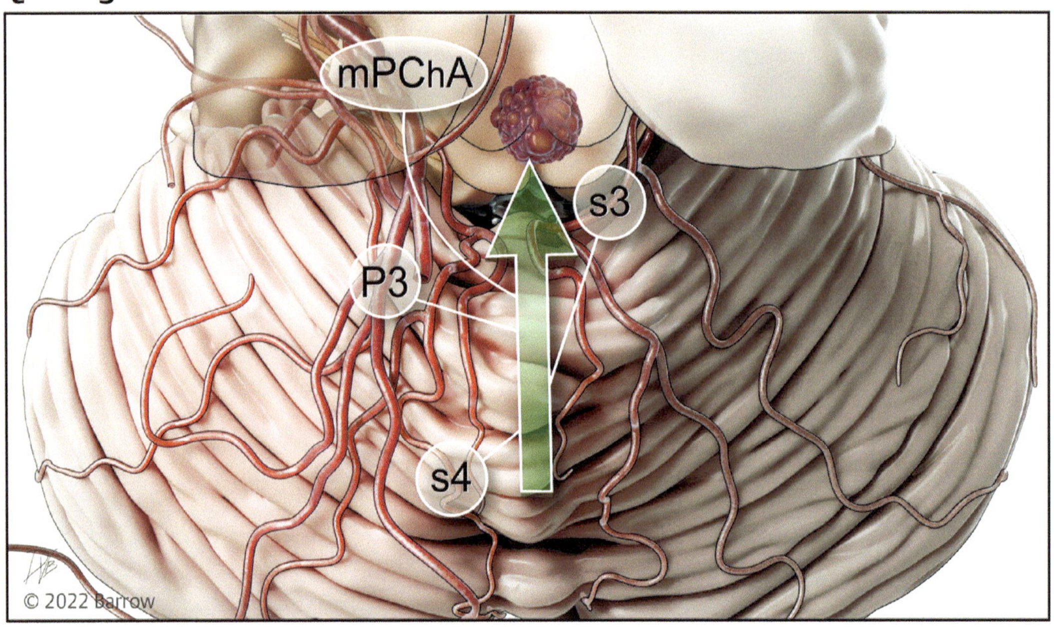

b

Fig. 4.10 *(Continued)* **(b)** tegmental, quadrigeminal, and

(Continued)

Midbrain Artery Paths

Periaqueductal

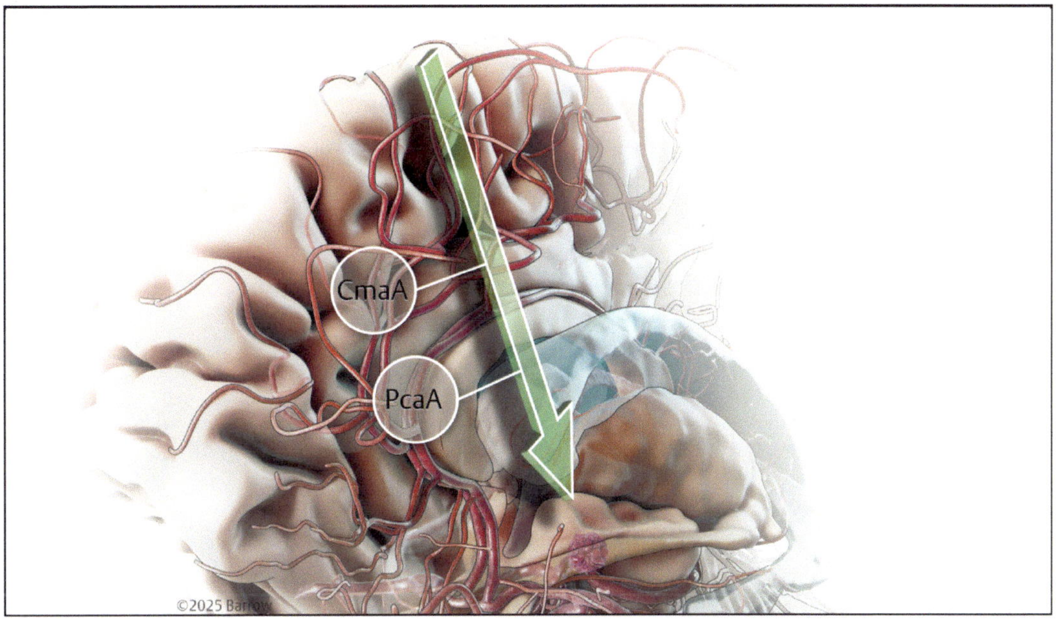

c

Fig. 4.10 *(Continued)* **(c)** periaqueductal CM subtypes. These arterial paths are summarized as dissection codes in ▶ Table 4.3. Roman numerals denote CNs. (Reproduced with permission from Barrow Neurological Institute, Phoenix, AZ.)

4

Pontine Artery Paths

Basilar

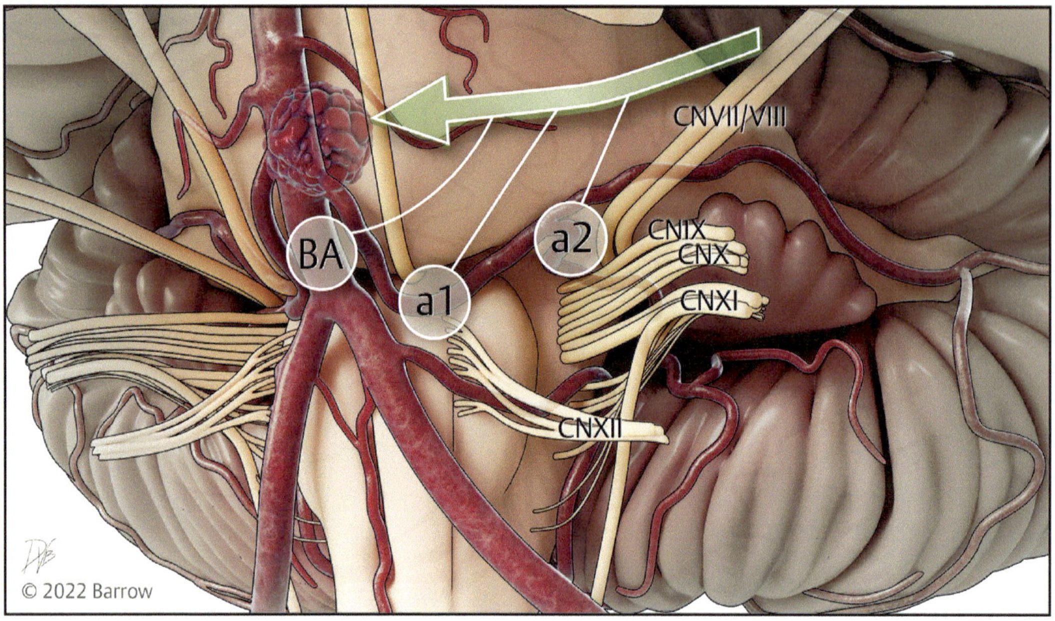

Peritrigeminal

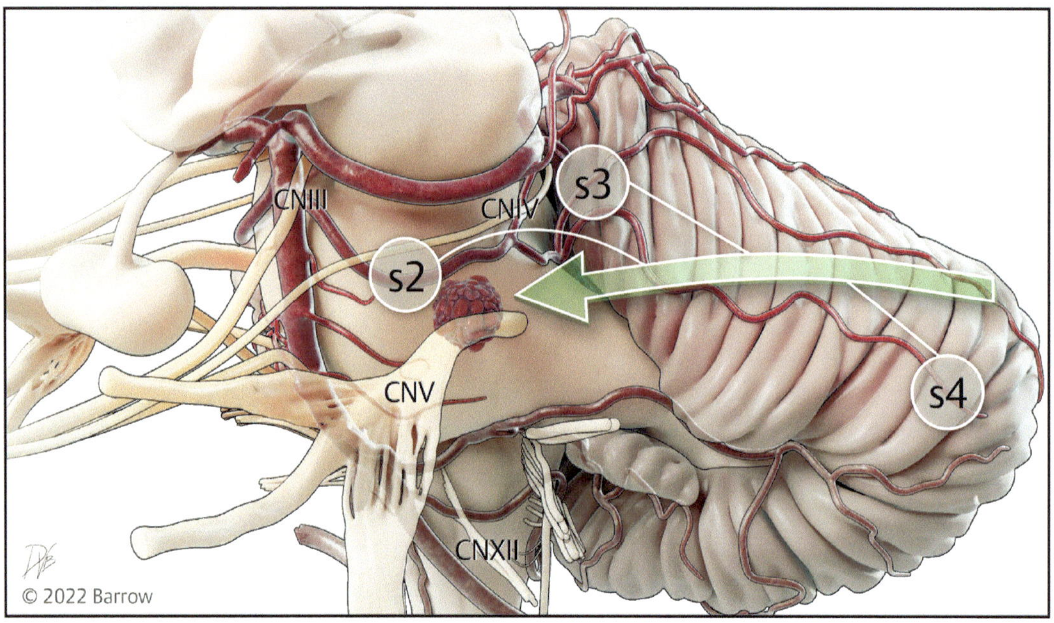

a

Fig. 4.11 Pontine artery paths. Pontine artery paths (*green arrows*), established by following arterial segments (*gray circles*) sequentially to reach targeted brainstem CMs (*red spheres*), are shown for **(a)** basilar, peritrigeminal,

(Continued)

Pontine Artery Paths

Rhomboid

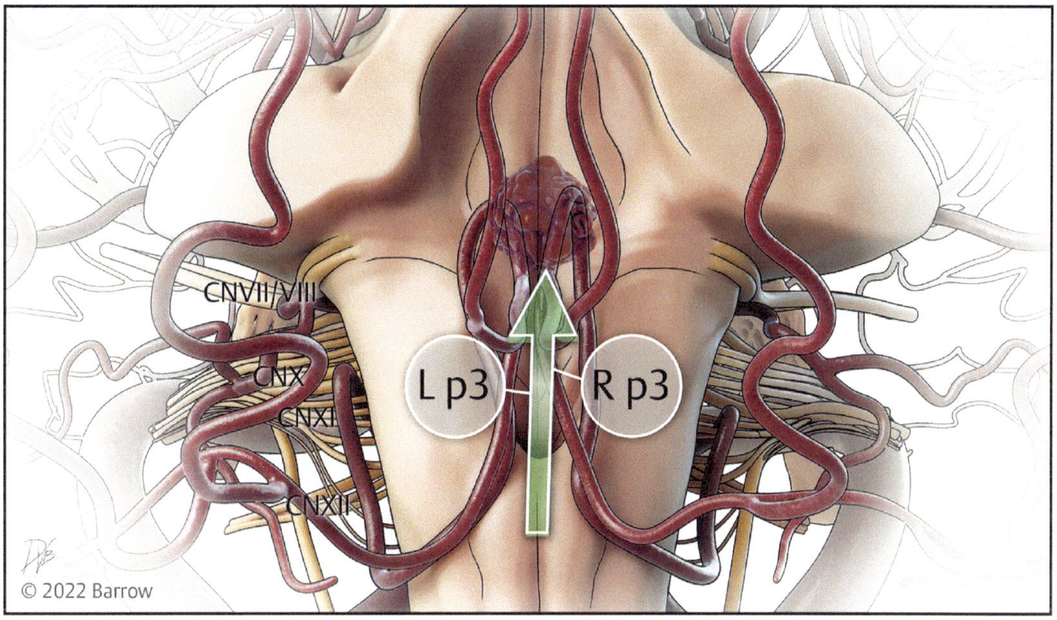

Supraolivary

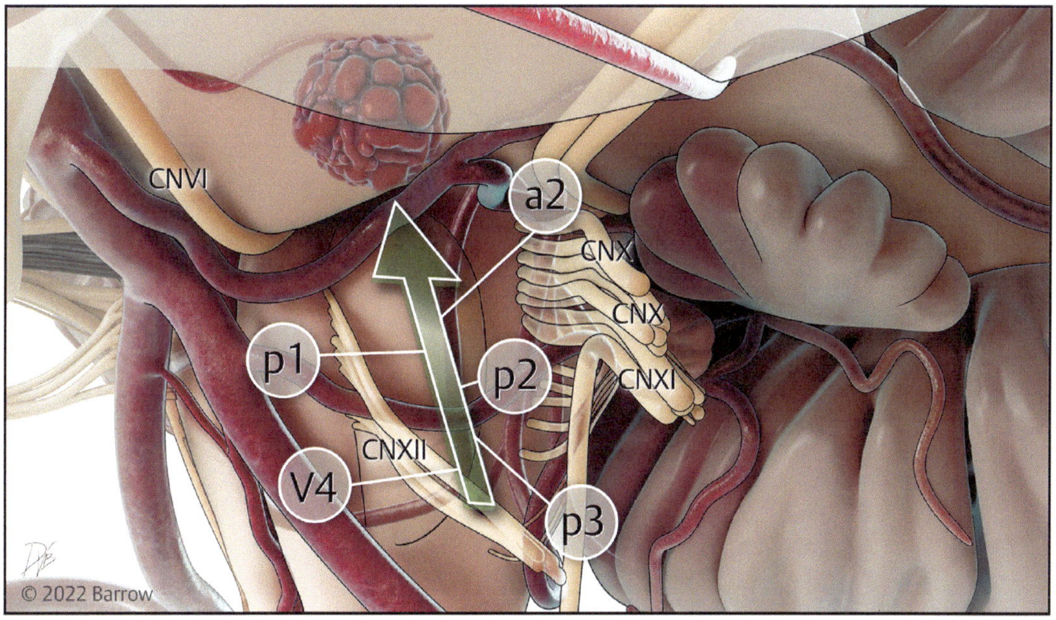

b

Fig. 4.11 *(Continued)* **(b)** rhomboid, supraolivary, and

(Continued)

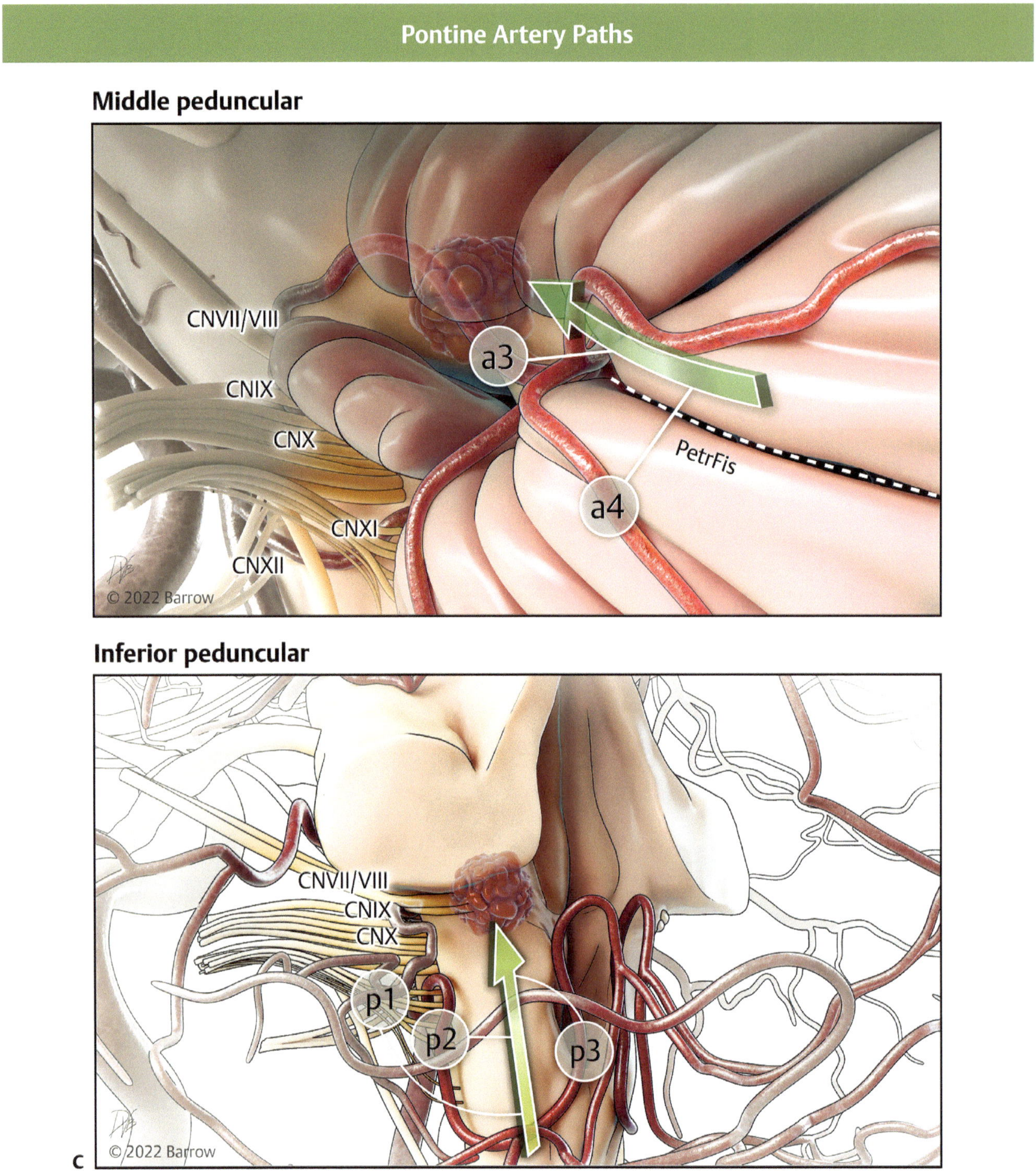

Fig. 4.11 *(Continued)* **(c)** middle and inferior peduncular CM subtypes. These arterial paths are summarized as dissection codes in ▸ Table 4.3. (Reproduced with permission from Barrow Neurological Institute, Phoenix, AZ.)

Medullary Artery Paths

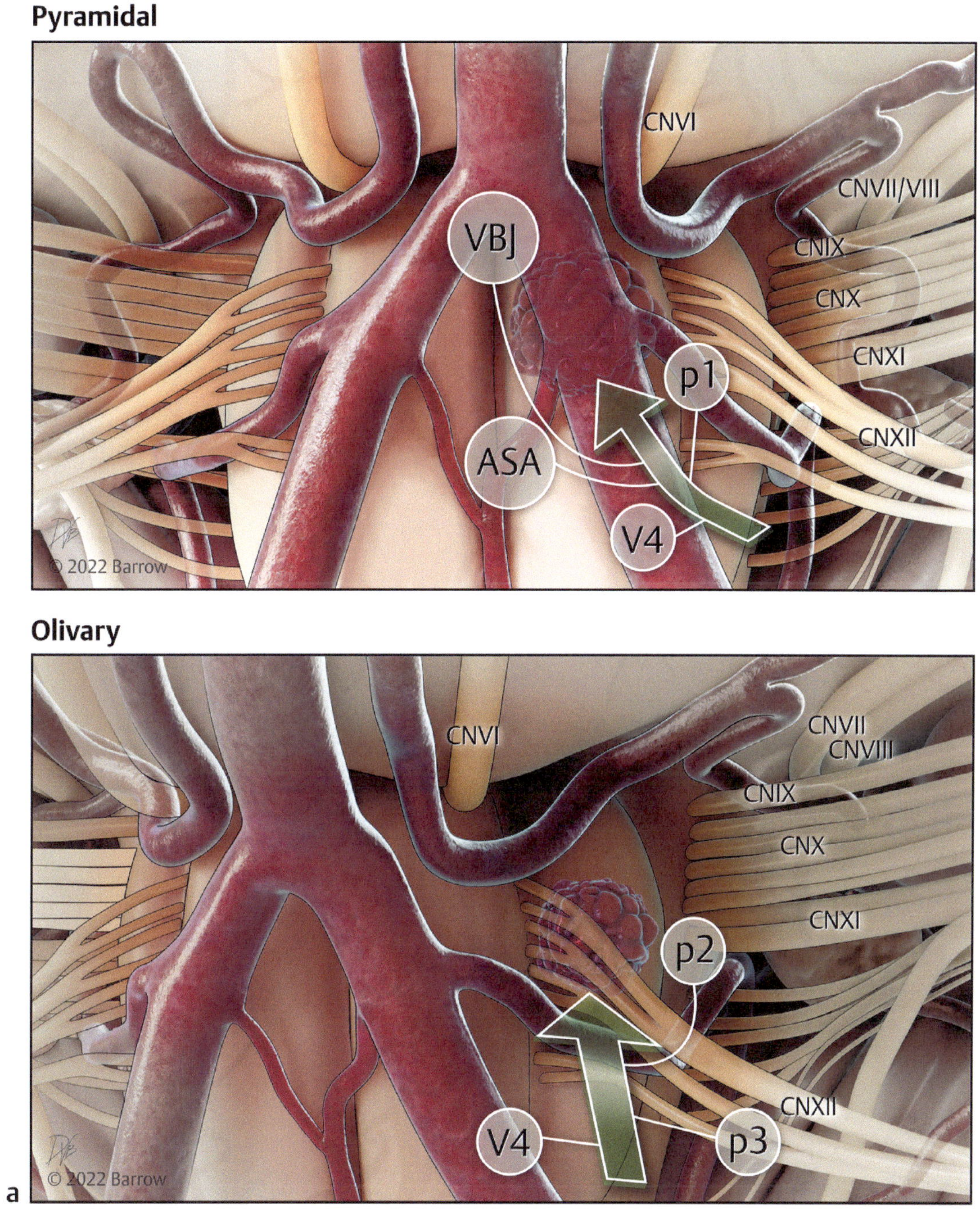

Fig. 4.12 Medullary artery paths. Medullary artery paths (*green arrows*), established by following arterial segments (*gray circles*) sequentially to reach targeted CMs (*red spheres*), are shown for **(a)** pyramidal, olivary,

(Continued)

4

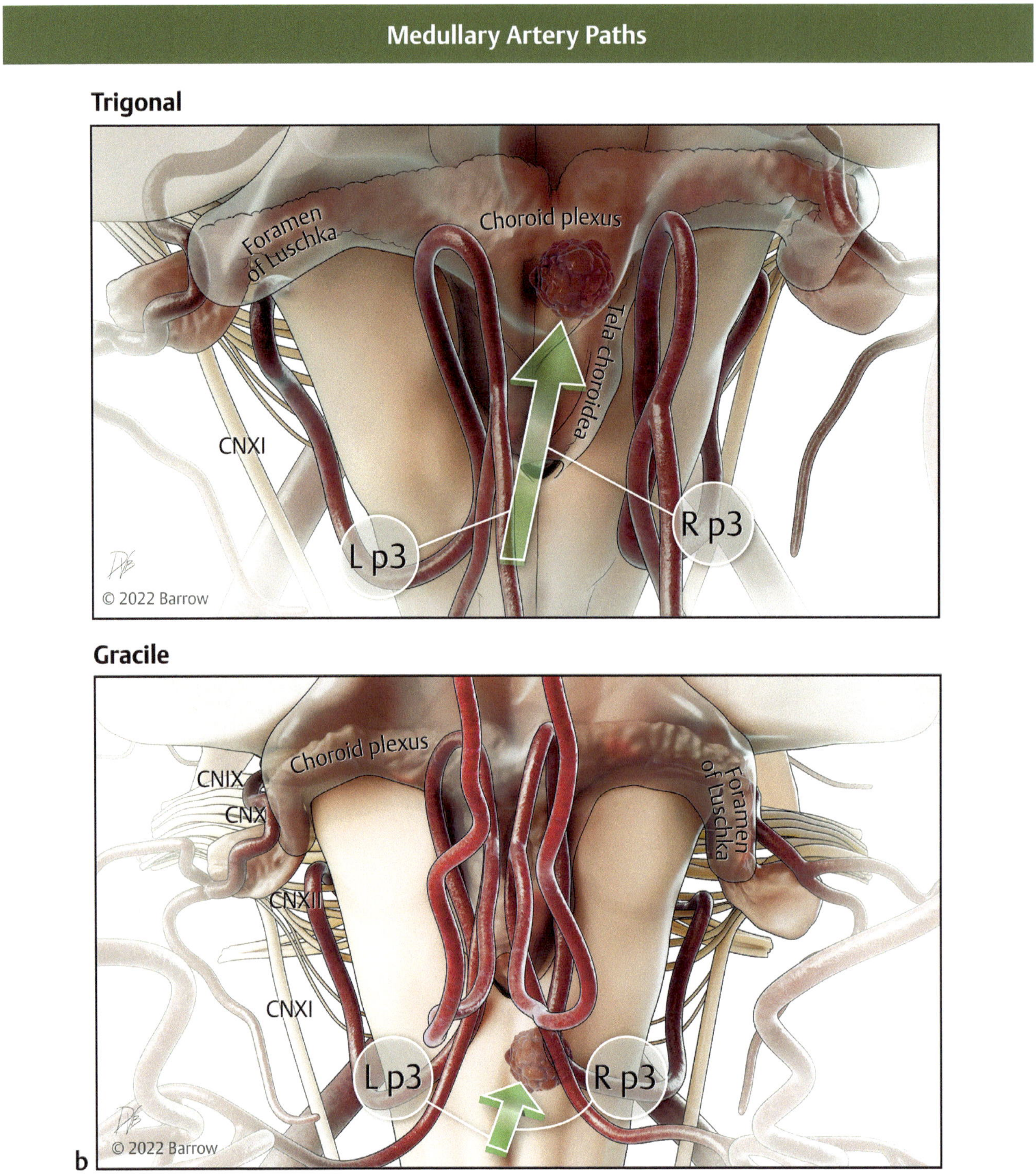

Fig. 4.12 *(Continued)* **(b)** trigonal, gracile, and

(Continued)

Medullary Artery Paths

Cuneate

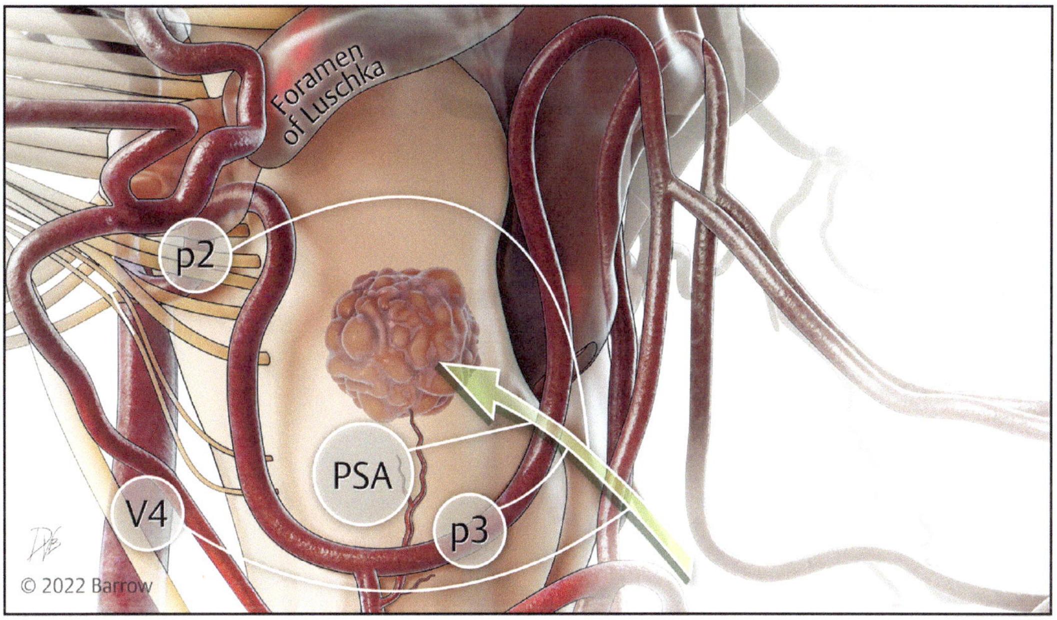

c

Fig. 4.12 *(Continued)* **(c)** cuneate CM subtypes. These arterial paths are summarized as dissection codes in ▶ Table 4.3. (Reproduced with permission from Barrow Neurological Institute, Phoenix, AZ.)

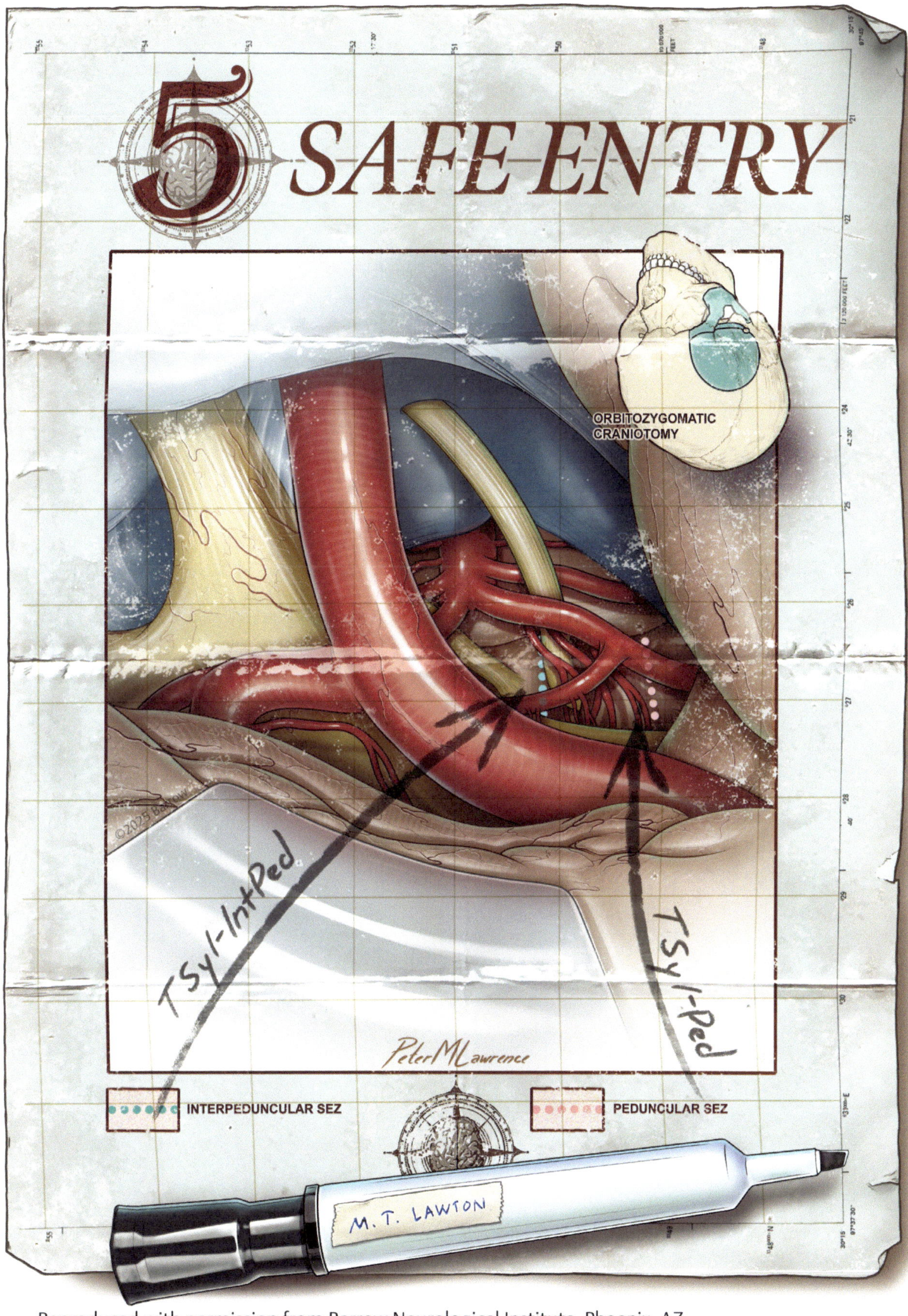
5
SAFE ENTRY
ORBITOZYGOMATIC
CRANIOTOMY
TSyl-IntPed
TSyl-Ped
PeterMLawrence
INTERPEDUNCULAR SEZ
PEDUNCULAR SEZ
M.T. LAWTON

5 Safe Entry Zones

Summary

In the recent past, neurosurgeons considered brainstem interventions too dangerous for the patient for most pathologies. However, vascular neurosurgeons considered cavernous malformations (CMs) suitable exceptions for microsurgical resection because they lacked a direct arterial supply, displaced rather than invaded the parenchyma, and could be removed piecemeal. Safe entry zones (SEZs) were introduced to grapple with microsurgical resection of CMs deep in the brainstem. The goal was to define anatomical approaches between or around eloquent nuclei and tracts to reach CMs in the brainstem and parenchyma with limited morbidity. Twenty-one SEZs are defined to guide neurosurgeons to CMs without causing substantial morbidity. Six SEZs are located in the midbrain, eight in the pons, and eight in the medulla (the median sulcus SEZ is used for both pontine and medullary lesions). Nonetheless, clinical experience with brainstem SEZs is limited. Case reports and small surgical series make it difficult to judge the safety of parenchymal transgression. However, clinical evidence shows that among 154 patients who underwent microsurgical brainstem resection of CMs and assessment of SEZ safety, the proportion of new postoperative permanent cranial nerve deficits in patients with superficial or exophytic CMs was equivalent (20%). The hypothesis that deep lesions result in worse outcomes than superficial and exophytic lesions was disproved. SEZs are indeed safe for accessing deep brainstem CMs. In patients with appropriately selected lesions, neurosurgeons can confidently offer microsurgical intervention.

Keywords: brainstem, cavernous malformation, cranial nerve, deep, exophytic, hemosiderin, neural tract, subtype, superficial, surgical approach

5.1 From Inoperable to Operable

Not long ago, neurosurgeons believed the brainstem was a surgical no man's land in which densely packed cranial nerve (CN) nuclei and ascending and descending neural tracts prevented operative transgression. Therefore, neurosurgeons considered brainstem intervention too dangerous for most pathologies. However, brainstem cavernous malformations (CMs) are more amenable to resection because they lack arterial input, displace rather than invade the parenchyma, and can be removed piecemeal. Vascular neurosurgeons who demonstrated that brainstem CMs were indeed operable lesions selected patients with preexisting deficits from prior hemorrhage and with lesions presenting to pial or ependymal surfaces. Microsurgical concepts such as the two-point method were developed to select the most strategic approach to the lesion. The superficial location of the pathology is implicit in this method. One point is placed where the lesion comes to a surgically accessible surface, and the other point is placed in the center of the lesion. The line connecting these points defines the optimal approach, which is then matched with a trajectory from available surgical options. However, some brainstem CMs lie beneath the pial or ependymal surface, and others appear superficial on preoperative magnetic resonance imaging (MRI) yet are beneath the surface intraoperatively due to radiological inaccuracies. In these instances, the neurosurgeon must decide whether to abort the operation or to transgress normal brainstem tissue to reach the lesion.

Safe entry zones (SEZs) were introduced to address deep brainstem CMs. The goal was to define anatomical locations between or around nuclei and tracts in which to incise the brainstem and transgress parenchyma to reach the lesion without significant morbidity. The use of brainstem SEZs enabled microsurgical management of brainstem CMs presenting to the brainstem surface and deep lesions below the brainstem surface with intervening parenchyma. This advancement doubled the number of patients who are eligible for surgery. However, the concept of SEZs is based mainly on anatomical studies in cadavers that demonstrate areas of access between or around critical nuclei and tracts without corresponding proof of safety. Brainstem CMs are rare, and few neurosurgeons have extensive surgical experience with them. Accordingly, clinical experience with brainstem SEZs is limited, and it consists of case reports and small surgical series, making it difficult to judge the safety of parenchymal transgression. A recent meta-analysis of 280 brainstem CM resections found 21 SEZs described in the literature, of which 5 were supported by credible evidence, defined as greater than 25 cases reported. These SEZs include the supra- and infracollicular, the supra- and infrafacial collicular, and the posterior median sulcus SEZs. The remaining SEZs were supported by limited evidence (7 SEZs, 6–24 cases) or case reports (10 SEZs, ≤5 cases). Brainstem transgression seems inherently morbid, and the safety of SEZs is still unclear.

5.2 Clinical Evidence

A cohort of 154 patients who underwent microsurgical brainstem CM resection was retrospectively examined over 23 years to assess the safety of SEZs for access to deep brainstem CMs. Lesions were characterized as exophytic, superficial, or deep based on preoperative MRI and intraoperative photographs or videos (▸ Table 5.1).

Resected brainstem CMs included 34 (22%) in the midbrain, 102 (66%) in the pons, and 18 (12%) in the medulla. Twenty-three (15%) were exophytic, 57 (37%) were superficial, and 74 (48%) were deep.

Established SEZs were used in 97% of deep lesions; the preferred SEZ for each lesion subtype was used in 91% of deep lesions. MRI accurately depicted exophytic brainstem CMs that did not require SEZ approaches (sensitivity of 96%) but overestimated the proximity of lesions superficial to brainstem surfaces (specificity of 67%), resulting in unanticipated SEZ use.

Outcomes were assessable in 97% (149/154) of patients. Final neurological outcomes were good in 80% of patients, and relative outcomes were stable or improved in 93% of patients.

Table 5.1 Patient demographics and brainstem CM characteristics according to surface proximity, as assessed by direct intraoperative visualization ($n = 154$)

Characteristic	Deep	Surface or exophytic	*p*-value
No. of patients	74	80	
CM location			
Midbrain	12 (16)	22 (28)	0.19
Pontine	54 (73)	48 (60)	
Medullary	8 (11)	10 (12)	
Mean ± SD age at operation (y)	42.6 ± 17.7	41.2 ± 4.8	0.60
Sex			
Female	36 (49)	47 (59)	0.21
Male	38 (51)	33 (41)	
Mean ± SD lesion size (mm)	1.9 ± 0.8	2.0 ± 1.7	0.48
Timing of last hemorrhage	71	78	
Acute	28 (39)	27 (35)	0.27
Subacute	20 (28)	16 (21)	
Chronic	23 (32)	35 (45)	
Unknown	3 (4)	2 (3)	
Preoperative brainstem CM bleed			
0	1 (1)	0 (0)	0.50
1	38 (51)	38 (48)	
≥2	35 (47)	42 (52)	
Associated DVA	28 (38)	35 (44)	0.46
Median (IQR) pre-op mRS score	2 (1–3)	2 (1–3)	0.85
No. of patients with follow-up	73	76	
Mean ± SD follow-up (mo)	18.7 ± 25.6	17.0 ± 20.2	0.61
CN deficits			
Pre-op	46 (62)	54 (68)	0.48
Discharge	38 (51)	49 (61)	0.21
Follow-up	29/73 (40)	38/76 (50)	0.23
Transient new CN deficit	25 (34)	25 (31)	0.73
Permanent new CN deficit	15/73 (21)	15/76 (20)	0.81
Mean overall change in CN deficits (min, max)	0 (−5, 3)	−1 (−4, 2)	0.65
Median (IQR) final mRS score	1 (0.5–2.5)	1 (1–2)	0.79
Final mRS score ≤ 2	53 (72)	66 (82)	0.10
mRS score stable/improved	67 (91)	72 (90)	0.91

Note: Data are reported as number (%) unless otherwise noted. Percentages may add to > 100% due to rounding.

Outcomes of patients with brainstem transgression through an SEZ did not differ from outcomes of patients with superficial or exophytic lesions that did not require SEZ use (final modified Rankin Scale score of ≤2 in 72% and 82%, respectively; $p = 0.10$). The proportion of permanent new CN deficits in patients with deep brainstem CMs and superficial or exophytic CMs was 20% in both groups ($p = 0.81$), and no significant change was seen in overall CN deficit (0 and −1; $p = 0.65$; ▶ Table 5.2). Neurological outcomes for deep brainstem CMs were equivalent to those for superficial or exophytic brainstem CMs, which validated the safety of SEZs for deep brainstem CMs. Because preoperative T1-weighted MRI can overestimate the lesion's surface proximity, detailed knowledge of SEZs is essential, as is readiness to use them in cases of radiological–microsurgical discordance. Most patients achieved favorable outcomes despite the transgression of eloquent brainstem tissue in and around SEZs.

5.3 The Safety of Safe Entry Zones

We dichotomized brainstem CMs into two groups, one comprising lesions at or protruding through the brainstem surface and the other comprising lesions below the brainstem surface. Parenchymal transgression within SEZs did not increase neurological morbidity, such that patients with deep brainstem CMs who required parenchymal transgression had the same neurological outcomes as did patients with exophytic or superficial brainstem CMs who did not require parenchymal transgression. It is difficult to imagine that entering the brainstem through normal tissue does not injure a tract or circuit of

Table 5.2 Neurological manifestations and CN deficits of patients undergoing brainstem CM resection according to surface proximity, deep versus superficial or exophytic

Characteristic	Deep						Surface or exophytic					
	Pre-op	Discharge	Follow-up	Transient	Permanent	Resolved	Pre-op	Discharge	Follow-up	Transient	Permanent	Resolved
Total no. of patients	74	74	73	25	15	66	80	80	76	25	15	55
mRS score ≥ 2	28 (38)	31 (42)	21 (29)	9	4	11	27 (34)	40 (50)	14 (18)	18	4	17
Hemiparesis	30 (41)	35 (47)	26 (36)	9	4	7	35 (44)	39 (49)	34 (45)	12	10	11
Hemisensory deficit	41 (55)	30 (41)	22 (30)	9	5	21	50 (62)	21 (26)	17 (22)	3	3	36
Dysmetria, ataxia	40 (54)	27 (36)	15 (21)	14	7	29	31 (39)	18 (22)	12 (16)	7	4	23
Dysphagia	8 (11)	9 (12)	1 (1)	4	0	6	2 (2)	8 (10)	1 (1)	7	1	2
Hydrocephalus	1 (1)	2 (3)	0 (0)	2	0	1	5 (6)	1 (1)	0 (0)	1	0	5
CN deficit												
III	7 (9)	8 (11)	5 (7)	5	3	5	8 (10)	10 (12)	7 (9)	3	2	3
IV	2 (3)	3 (4)	2 (3)	3	2	2	0 (0)	1 (1)	0 (0)	1	0	0
V	16 (22)	10 (14)	7 (10)	4	3	12	18 (22)	9 (11)	5 (7)	5	3	16
VI	20 (27)	20 (27)	11 (15)	7	4	12	29 (36)	30 (38)	23 (30)	8	7	13
VII	12 (16)	23 (31)	12 (16)	14	6	6	15 (19)	17 (21)	11 (14)	8	4	8
VIII	3 (4)	7 (9)	4 (5)	7	4	3	10 (12)	6 (8)	5 (7)	2	2	7
IX	5 (7)	3 (4)	2 (3)	3	2	5	3 (4)	1 (1)	1 (1)	0	0	2
X	6 (8)	3 (4)	3 (4)	2	2	5	4 (5)	1 (1)	0 (0)	1	0	4
XI	1 (1)	1 (1)	1 (1)	1	1	1	0 (0)	0 (0)	0 (0)	0	0	0
XII	3 (4)	3 (4)	1 (1)	3	1	3	2 (2)	1 (1)	1 (1)	1	1	2

importance. Nevertheless, we disproved the hypothesis that patients with deep lesions fare worse than those with superficial and exophytic lesions. SEZs are indeed safe for accessing deep brainstem CMs located beneath the surface, and in patients with appropriately selected lesions, we can confidently offer microsurgical intervention.

The relative safety of SEZs remains difficult to judge. Outcomes associated with the more frequently used SEZs were similar, suggesting that significant differences do not exist. However, additional experience is needed to make meaningful comparisons. In the meantime, the number of cases reported using a particular SEZ serves as a proxy for direct measures of safety. For example, the supra- and infracollicular, supra- and infrafacial collicular, and posterior median sulcus SEZs are reported most frequently in the medical literature and, consequently, are accepted as safe. In contrast, negative experiences reported with the intercollicular SEZ have made some neurosurgeons reluctant to use it. In our study, the middle cerebellar peduncle (MCP) SEZ was used most frequently, often traversing more than a few millimeters of parenchymal tissue. Excellent outcomes in these patients suggest that this SEZ might be the safest and most valuable.

5.4 The 21 Brainstem Safe Entry Zones

A total of 21 SEZs have been defined anatomically to incise the brainstem and transgress parenchyma to reach the lesion without significant morbidity (▸ Fig. 5.1). As SEZs are between or around nuclei and tracts, important neural structures are less prominent or more avoidable in and around these zones. Six SEZs are located in the midbrain, eight in the pons, and eight in the medulla (the median sulcus SEZ is used for both pontine and medullary lesions).

5.5 Midbrain Safe Entry Zones

The midbrain region contains tracts and nuclei involved in essential functions like motor coordination (red nucleus), eye movement (oculomotor nerve nucleus), visual processing (superior colliculi), and auditory processing (inferior colliculi; ▸ Fig. 5.2). A three-dimensional understanding of midbrain anatomy can aid the surgeon in SEZ selection (▸ Fig. 5.3; ▸ Video 5.1). Each SEZ is contained within an associated anatomical triangle and has a corresponding surgical approach (▸ Fig. 5.4, ▸ Fig. 5.5).

5.5.1 Interpeduncular Zone

The interpeduncular SEZ is a vertical line running in the midline of the interpeduncular fossa that splits the midbrain down the middle. It runs from the mamillary bodies superiorly to the pontomesencephalic sulcus inferiorly at the depth of the interpeduncular fossa, where the medial aspects of the cerebral peduncles intersect. This SEZ divides the posterior perforate substance where posterior thalamoperforating arteries from the basilar bifurcation and P1 posterior cerebral

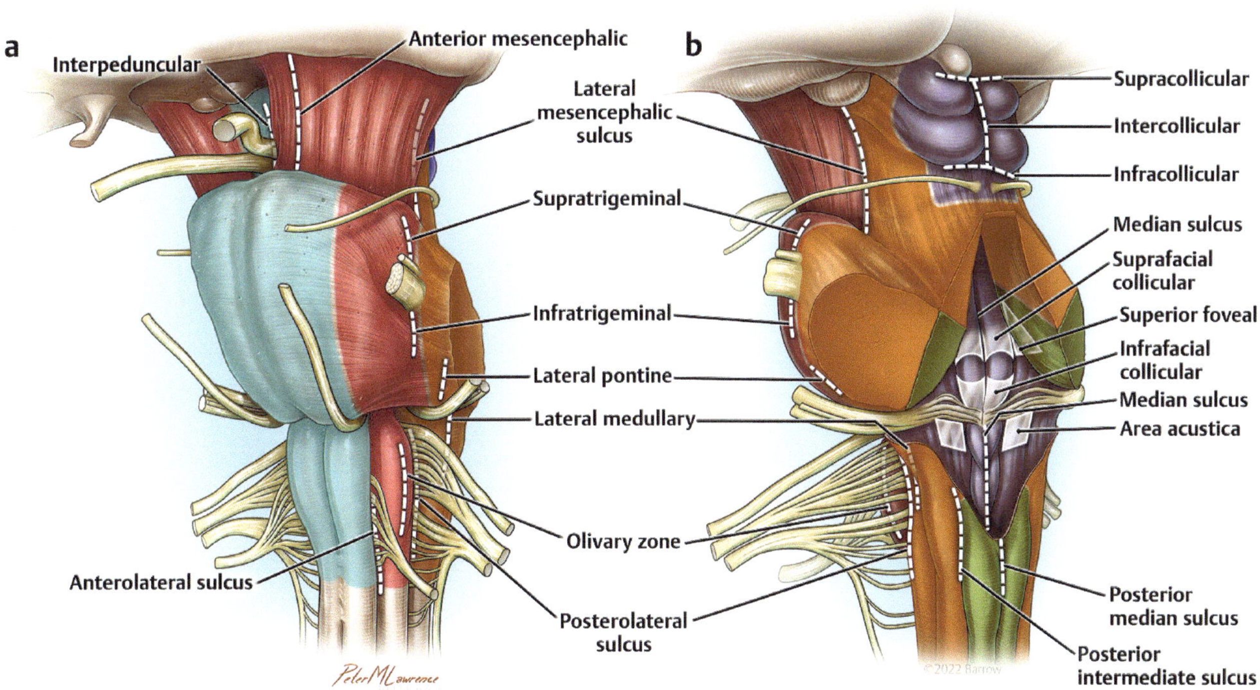

Fig. 5.1 The 21 SEZs of the brainstem (*dashed white lines*) are shown in **(a)** anterolateral and **(b)** posterolateral views. (Reproduced with permission from Barrow Neurological Institute, Phoenix, AZ.)

5

Midbrain Safe Entry Zones: Surgical Anatomy

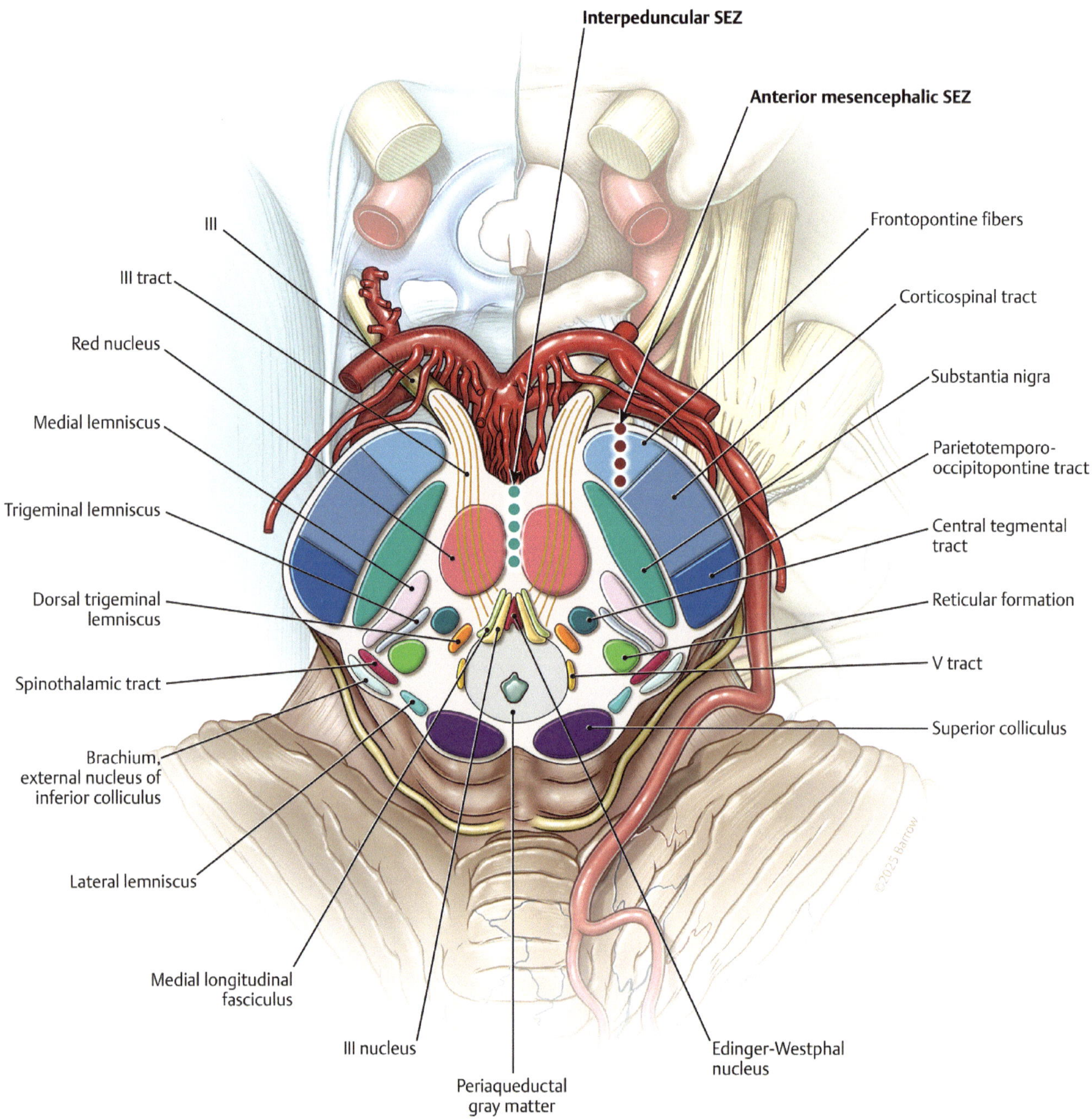

Fig. 5.2 The tracts and nuclei of the midbrain, shown in axial cross-section viewed from above, are involved in motor control (corticospinal tracts), motor coordination (red nucleus and substantia nigra), sensory processing (medial lemniscus and spinothalamic tracts), eye movement (oculomotor nerve nucleus), visual processing (superior colliculi), and auditory processing (inferior colliculi). The interpeduncular SEZ is shown as a *dotted teal line*, and the anterior mesencephalic SEZ is shown as a *dotted pink line*. Roman numerals denote CNs. (Reproduced with permission from Barrow Neurological Institute, Phoenix, AZ.)

Midbrain Safe Entry Zones

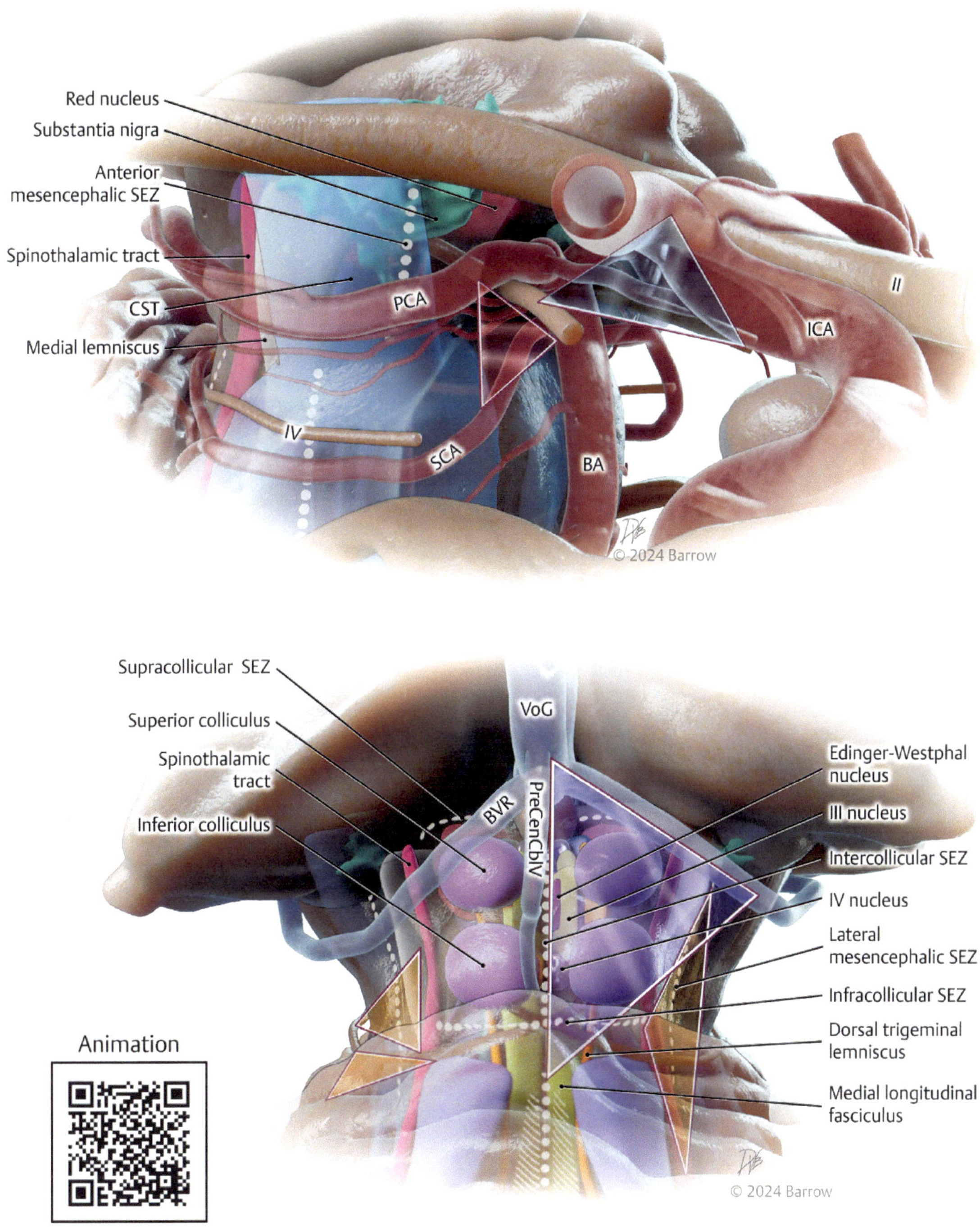

Fig. 5.3 The tracts and nuclei of the midbrain are shown three dimensionally from a right anterior oblique view (*upper*) and a posterior view (*lower*). Midbrain SEZs are shown as *dotted white lines*, and *anatomical triangles* are superimposed on the brainstem anatomy (animation; ▶ Video 5.1, Midbrain SEZs; QR code). Roman numerals denote CNs. (Reproduced with permission from Barrow Neurological Institute, Phoenix, AZ.)

Anterior Midbrain Safe Entry Zones: Surgical Approach

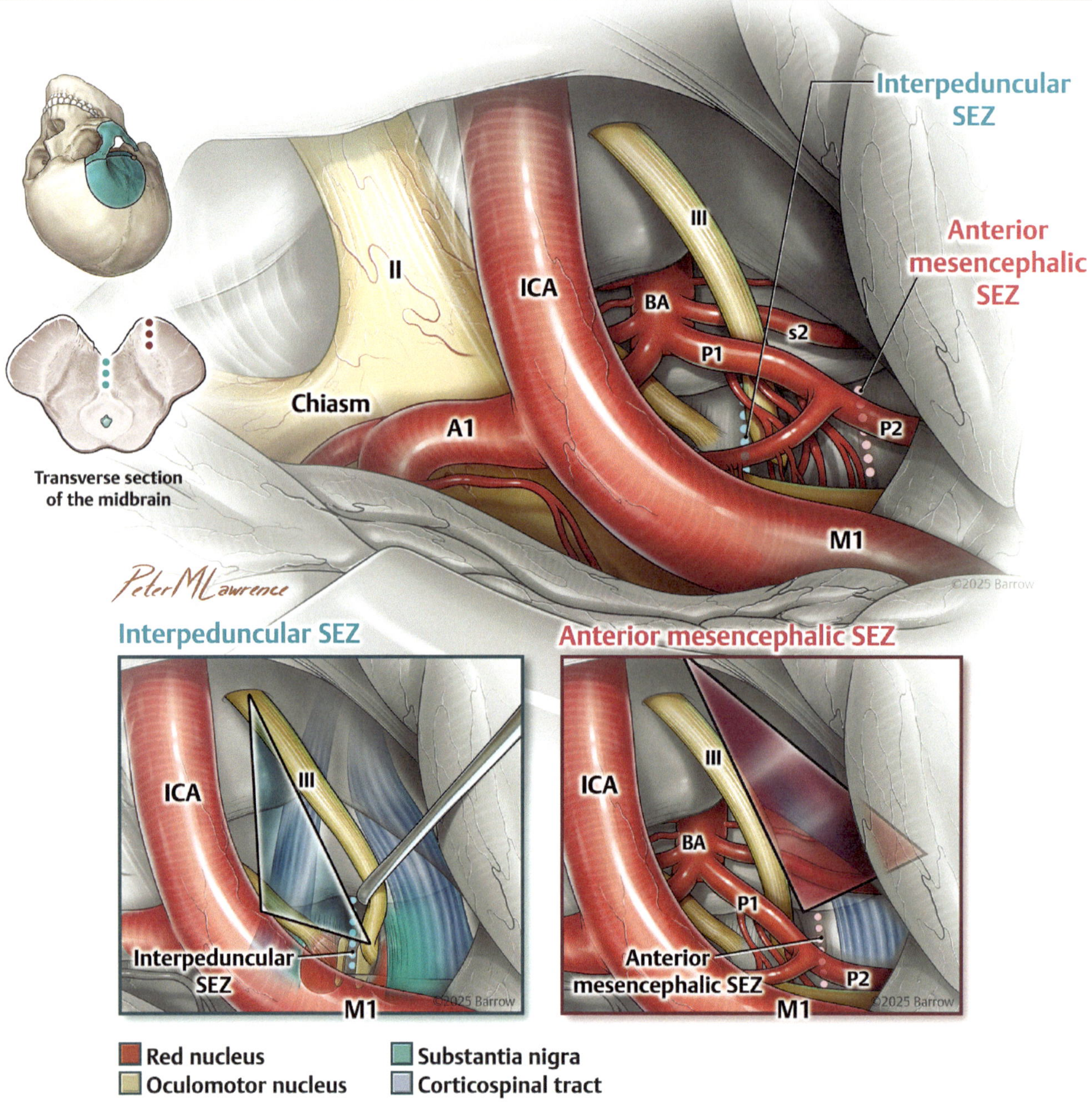

Fig. 5.4 The interpeduncular (*dotted teal line*) and anterior mesencephalic (*dotted pink line*) midbrain SEZs are depicted through the orbitozygomatic-pterional craniotomy (*upper left inset*; *teal*) and transsylvian approach. Entry trajectories are shown (*middle left inset*). The relationships between anatomical triangles, SEZs, and parenchymal tracts and nuclei are shown for interpeduncular (*lower left inset*) and anterior mesencephalic (*lower right inset*) SEZs. Roman numerals denote CNs. (Reproduced with permission from Barrow Neurological Institute, Phoenix, AZ.)

arteries (PCAs) enter the anterior midbrain. The cerebral peduncles, red nuclei, and exit zones of the oculomotor nerves are well off the midline, but oculomotor nerve nuclei, Edinger–Westphal nuclei, and medial longitudinal fasciculi (MLF) are adjacent to the midline posteriorly. The ventral and dorsal tegmental decussations course through the interpeduncular midline anteriorly and may be disrupted with this SEZ. The decussation of the superior cerebellar peduncles lies

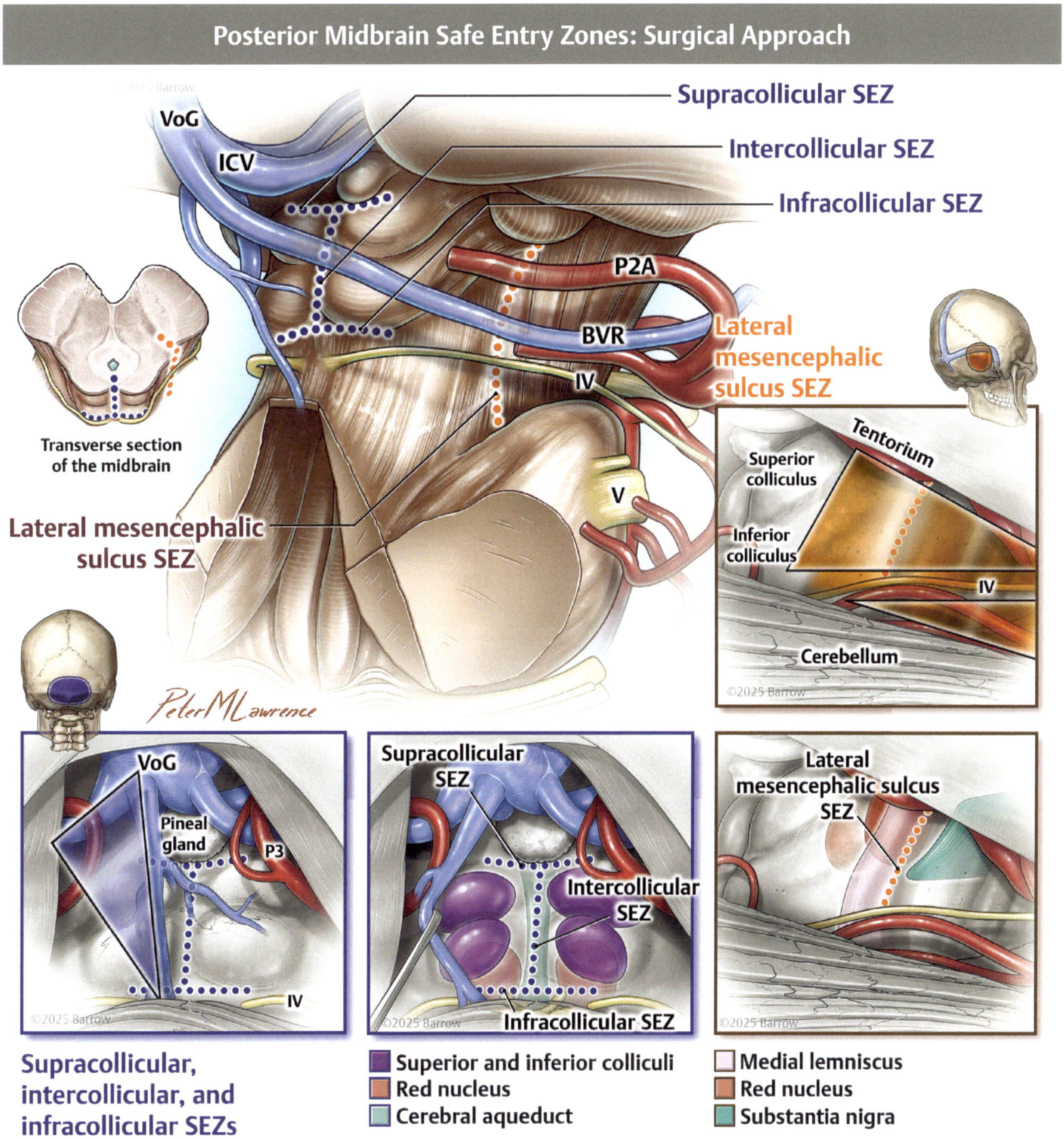

Fig. 5.5 The posterior midbrain SEZs are shown from a right posterior oblique view. Supra-, infra-, and intercollicular SEZs (*dotted purple lines*) are exposed through a torcular craniotomy (*middle left inset*) and midline supracerebellar-infratentorial approach in the sitting position. The lateral mesencephalic sulcus SEZ (*dotted orange line*) is exposed through a retrosigmoid craniotomy (*upper right inset*) and lateral supracerebellar-infratentorial approach, also in the sitting position. The relationships between anatomical triangles, SEZs, and parenchymal tracts and nuclei are shown for the supra-, infra-, and intercollicular SEZs (*lower left and lower middle insets*) and lateral mesencephalic sulcus SEZ (*middle right and lower right insets*). Entry trajectories are shown (*upper left inset*). Roman numerals denote CNs. (Reproduced with permission from Barrow Neurological Institute, Phoenix, AZ.)

at or below the level of the pontomesencephalic junction and is not at risk.

5.5.2 Anterior Mesencephalic Zone

The anterior mesencephalic SEZ, also known as the periocular SEZ, runs vertically in the medial aspect of the cerebral peduncle. Motor fibers in the corticospinal tracts occupy the middle third of the peduncle, and an incision in this SEZ transgresses the frontopontine tracts medially. The SEZ is outside the interpeduncular fossa and lateral to the oculomotor nerve. Although it extends from the optic tracts superiorly to the pontomesencephalic sulcus inferiorly, it lies deep to the distal P1 segment and P2A segment of the PCA and the s1 segment of the superior cerebellar artery, which limits the incision to the interval between these arteries. The substantia nigra lies deep and lateral to the SEZ, and the red nucleus lies deeper and medial to the SEZ. Temporo-parieto-occipito-pontine fibers occupying the lateral third of the cerebral peduncle, lateral to the corticospinal tract, are unaffected.

5.5.3 Lateral Mesencephalic Sulcus Zone

The lateral mesencephalic sulcus SEZ separates the peduncular surface of the midbrain anterolaterally from the tegmental surface posterolaterally, extending from the medial geniculate body of the thalamus superiorly to the pontomesencephalic sulcus inferiorly. This sulcus is a subtle depression in the tegmentum, and the lateral mesencephalic vein typically runs in the sulcus and is used to identify it. The sulcus descends in a posteromedial direction rather than purely vertical, and the entry incision deepens in an anteromedial direction perpendicular to the tegmental surface rather than purely medial. This trajectory thus skirts behind the substantia nigra and in front of the medial lemniscus. It courses anteriorly to the midbrain tegmentum and its sensitive structures, including the spinothalamic tract, ventral trigeminothalamic tract, reticular formation, central tegmental tracts, the brachium, and external nucleus of the inferior colliculus.

5.5.4 Intercollicular Zone

The intercollicular SEZ is a vertical line between the two superior and two inferior colliculi of the quadrigeminal plate or tectum in the posterior midbrain, from the pineal gland superiorly to the trochlear nerve exit zone inferiorly. The superior colliculi are involved in saccadic eye movements, visual fixation, and spatial attention and receive retinal inputs via the optic nerves, the optic tracts, the lateral geniculate nuclei, and the superior brachium. The inferior colliculi are involved in auditory processing. They receive inputs from the contralateral cochlear nuclei, the dorsal and ventral nuclei of the lateral lemniscus, and the superior olivary nuclei and relay outputs to the inferior brachium, the medial geniculate nucleus of the thalamus, and the primary auditory cortex. Commissural fibers crossing between the superior and inferior colliculi exist but are minimal and functionally insignificant, which makes this intercollicular transgression safe. However, the trochlear nerves decussate in the midline before exiting, which requires that intercollicular transgression stays above their root exit zone. The depth of transgression is limited to the posterior margin of the periaqueductal gray area.

5.5.5 Supracollicular and Infracollicular Zones

The supra- and infracollicular SEZs are transverse incisions immediately above the superior colliculi or below the inferior colliculi in the midline. Entry into this zone preserves collicular integrity by staying above or below the quadrigeminal plate. The pineal gland can obscure the supracollicular SEZ and can be mobilized upward. The decussation of the trochlear nerves is protected inferiorly by hugging the inferior aspect of the inferior colliculi. As with the intercollicular SEZ, the depth of transgression is limited to the posterior margin of the periaqueductal gray area.

5.6 Pontine Safe Entry Zones

The pons contains several CN nuclei and serves as a bridge to different regions of the nervous systems, contributing to key functions like balance (vestibular nuclei, superior cerebellar peduncle) and the transmission of major sensory and motor pathways (▶ Fig. 5.6). A three-dimensional understanding of midbrain anatomy can aid the surgeon in SEZ selection (▶ Fig. 5.7; ▶ Video 5.2). Each SEZ is contained within an associated anatomical triangle and has a corresponding surgical approach (▶ Fig. 5.8, ▶ Fig. 5.9).

5.6.1 Supratrigeminal and Infratrigeminal

The supra- and infratrigeminal SEZs are defined by the transtrigeminal line running vertically through the trigeminal nerve root. Technically, the supratrigeminal zone extends from the shoulder of the nerve root inferiorly to the pontomesencephalic sulcus superiorly. The infratrigeminal zone, also called the peritrigeminal zone, extends from the axilla of the nerve root to the pontomedullary sulcus (PMS) inferiorly. Practically, the tentorial incisura limits the upper extent of the supratrigeminal zone, and a large superior petrosal vein (Dandy's vein) may also restrict access. Similarly, the vestibulocochlear nerve complex may limit the lower extent of the infratrigeminal zone. Transgression along this line stays lateral to the descending corticospinal tract and anterior to the motor and sensory trigeminal nuclei and remains within the transverse pontine fibers coursing to the MCP.

Pontine Safe Entry Zones: Surgical Anatomy

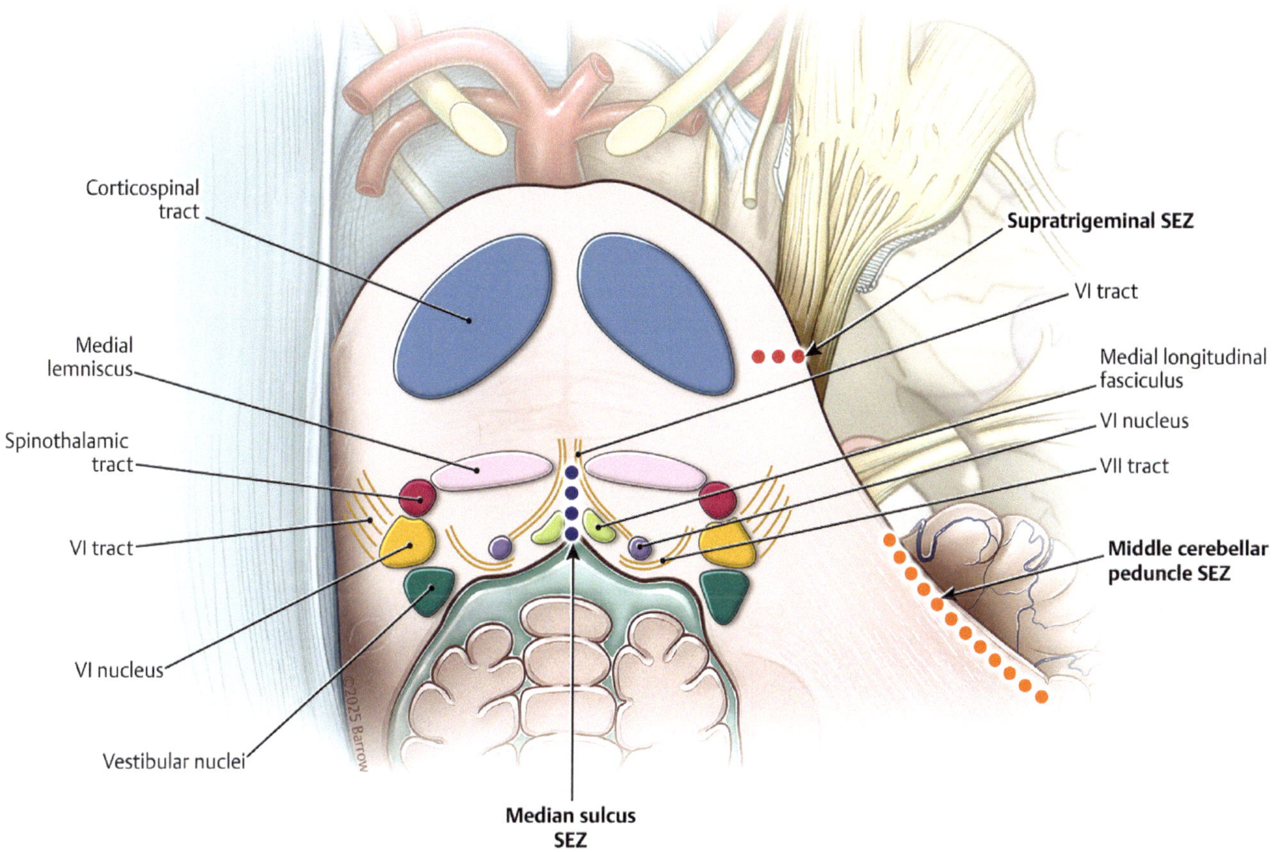

Fig. 5.6 The tracts and nuclei of the pons, shown in axial cross-section viewed from above, are involved in motor control (corticospinal tracts), motor coordination (superior cerebellar peduncle), sensory processing (medial lemniscus and spinothalamic tracts), eye movement (abducens nerve nucleus and medial longitudinal fasciculus), and balance (vestibular nuclei). Supratrigeminal (*red*), MCP (*orange*), and median sulcus (*purple*) SEZs are shown as *dotted lines*. Roman numerals denote CNs. (Reproduced with permission from Barrow Neurological Institute, Phoenix, AZ.)

5.6.2 Middle Cerebellar Peduncle or Lateral Pontine

The MCP SEZ lies in the cerebellopontine angle, where the superior and inferior semilunar lobules intersect lateral to the flocculus to form the interlobular triangle. After splitting the petrosal fissure along the course of the a3 segment of the anterior inferior cerebellar artery (AICA), the folia of these lobules peel away and uncover the lateral surface of the MCP. The revelation of this white matter zone provides entrance into the brachium pontis, in which an incision parallels the MCP's transverse pontine fibers. Deepening dissection through the peduncle accesses the lateral and central pons. This trajectory courses lateral and posterior to the trigeminal root entry zone and, more importantly, the corticospinal tract. The trajectory also must remain anterior to the pontine tegmentum, which contains the spinothalamic tract, the lateral lemniscus, the motor nucleus of the facial nerve, the spinal nucleus and tract of the trigeminal nerve, the ventral spinocerebellar tract, the rubrospinal tract, and the superior olivary nucleus.

5.6.3 Area Acustica

The area acustica is a rounded elevation in the floor of the lateral recess of the fourth ventricle, lateral to the sulcus limitans and between its superior and inferior foveae. The area acustica is localized best by the striae medullares, which are prominent white strands traversing the junctional part of the fourth ventricle's floor from the lateral recess to the sulcus limitans. The vestibular nuclei (superior, inferior, medial, and lateral) are located medially within the area acustica, and the cochlear nuclei are located laterally within the area acustica. The inferior cerebellar peduncle, or restiform body, runs lateral to vestibular nuclei and deep to cochlear nuclei.

Pontine Safe Entry Zones

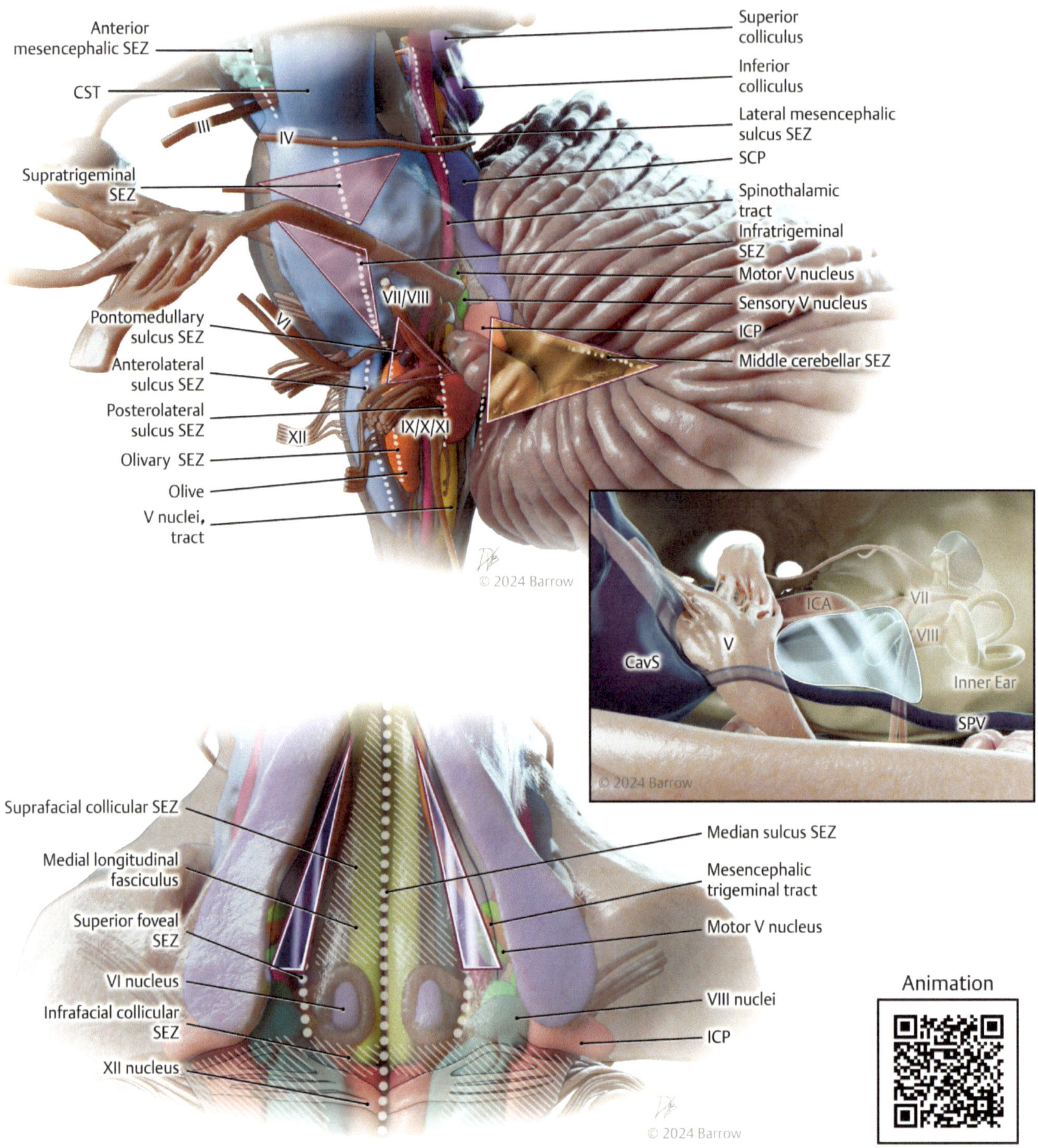

Animation

Fig. 5.7 The tracts and nuclei of the pons are shown three dimensionally from a left lateral view (above) and a posterior view (below). Pontine SEZs are shown as *dotted white lines*, and *anatomical triangles* are superimposed on the brainstem anatomy. The CN, vascular, and bony anatomy of the Kawase triangle (*teal quadrangle*) used to access basilar pontine cavernomas are shown in the *inset* (animation; ▶ Video 5.2, Pontine SEZs; QR code). Roman numerals denote CNs. (Reproduced with permission from Barrow Neurological Institute, Phoenix, AZ.)

Lateral Pontine Safe Entry Zones: Surgical Approach

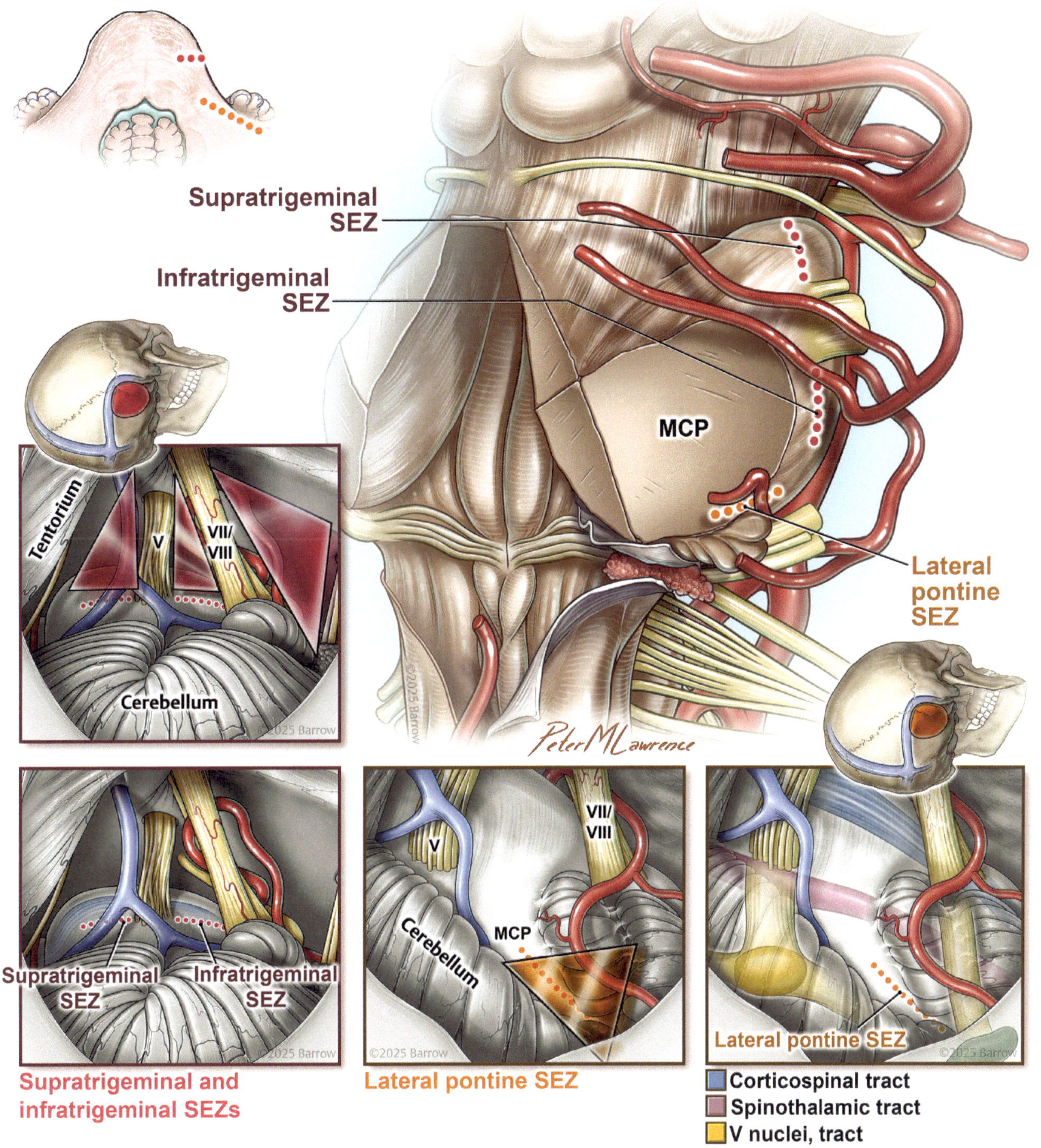

Fig. 5.8 The supra- and infratrigeminal SEZs (*dotted red line*) and the lateral pontine SEZ (*dotted orange line*) are depicted from a right posterior oblique view. Entry trajectories are shown (*uppermost left inset*). Supra- and infratrigeminal SEZs are exposed through the extended retrosigmoid craniotomy (*upper left inset*) and trans-cerebellopontine angle approach. The lateral pontine SEZ is also exposed through the extended retrosigmoid approach (*middle right inset*), but the approach is through the middle cerebellar peduncle. The relationships between anatomical triangles, SEZs, and parenchymal tracts and nuclei are shown for the supra- and infratrigeminal SEZs (*middle left and lower left insets*) and lateral pontine SEZ (*lower middle and lower right insets*). Roman numerals denote CNs. (Reproduced with permission from Barrow Neurological Institute, Phoenix, AZ.)

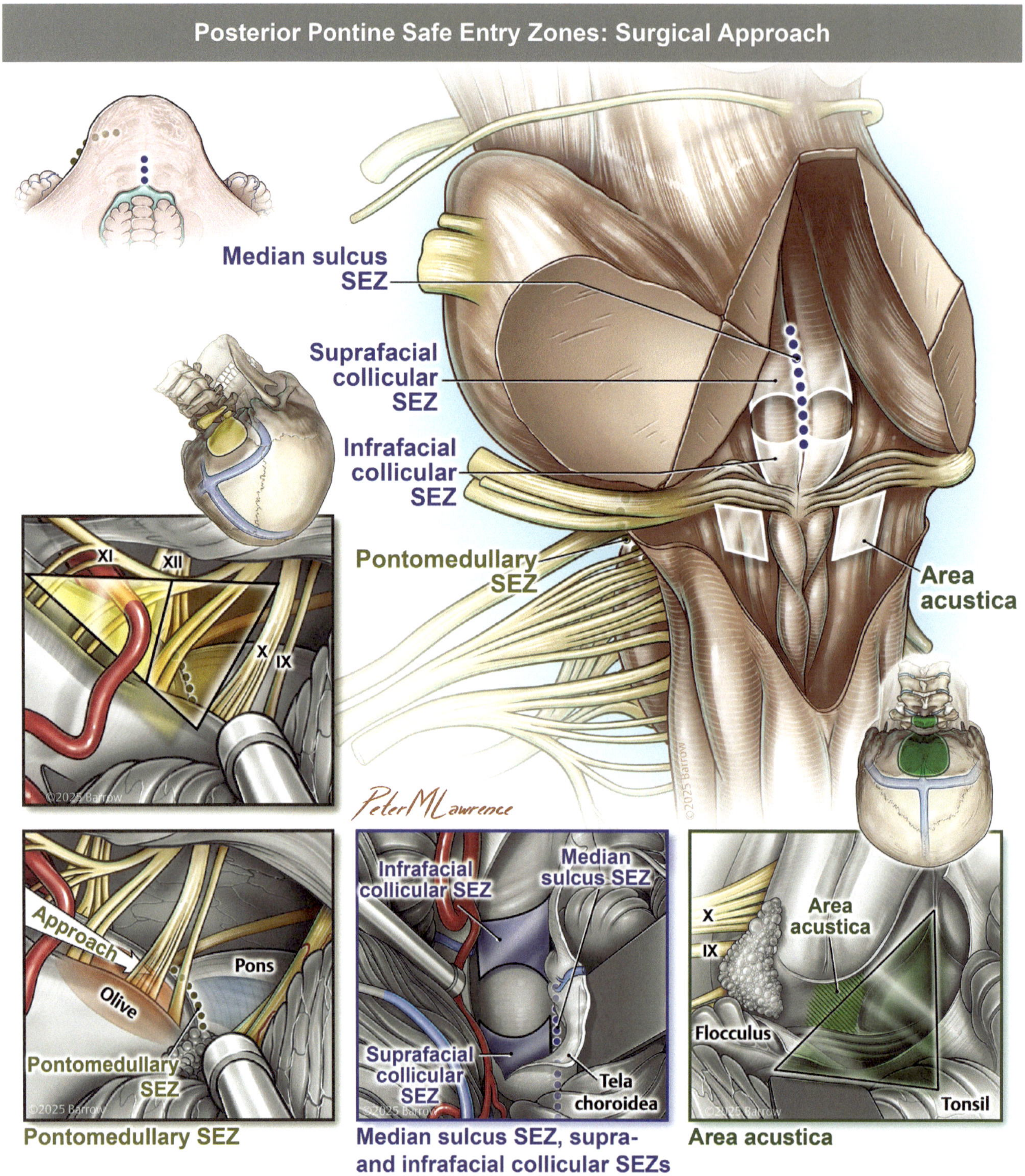

Fig. 5.9 The posterior pontine SEZs are shown from a left posterior oblique view. Entry trajectories are shown (*uppermost left inset*). The median sulcus SEZ (*dotted purple line*), area acustica, and supra- and infrafacial collicular SEZs (*white areas*) are all exposed through a suboccipital craniotomy with C1 laminectomy (*middle right inset*) and midline transventricular approach. The pontomedullary sulcus SEZ (*dotted yellow line*) is exposed through a far lateral craniotomy (*upper left inset*). The relationships between the anatomical triangle, SEZ, and parenchymal tracts and nuclei are shown for the pontomedullary sulcus SEZ (*middle left and lower left insets*). These relationships are shown for the median sulcus SEZ, area acustica, and supra- and infrafacial collicular SEZs (*lower middle and lower right insets*). Roman numerals denote CNs. (Reproduced with permission from Barrow Neurological Institute, Phoenix, AZ.)

5.6.4 Median Sulcus (Pons)

The median sulcus is the most prominent surface landmark on the fourth ventricular floor or rhomboid fossa, extending vertically in the midline from the cerebral aqueduct superiorly to the obex inferiorly. The median sulcus divides the floor longitudinally in the midline and is accentuated by the paramedian elevation of adjacent median eminences. The MLF parallel the median sulcus on both sides as they course between the oculomotor, trochlear, and abducens nerve nuclei. The median sulcus can be transgressed because there are few crossing fibers, but the proximity of the thin and delicate MLF puts it at risk during microdissection and retraction. Injury to the MLF would result in abnormalities in eye movement (internuclear ophthalmoplegia).

5.6.5 Suprafacial Collicular

The median eminence, which runs vertically alongside the more prominent median sulcus on the floor of the fourth ventricle, contains the facial colliculus in its pontine part and the three triangular parts of the calamus scriptorius in its medullary part, namely the hypoglossal trigone, the vagal trigone, and the area postrema. The sulcus limitans borders the median eminence laterally. The facial colliculus contains the abducens nucleus and the internal genu of the facial nerve as its fibers ascend from its nucleus and wrap around the abducens nucleus. The facial colliculus may not be evident anatomically, and stimulation is typically required to map its location. The suprafacial collicular zone is a triangular space bordered by the facial nerve inferiorly, the MLF medially, and the superior cerebellar peduncle superolaterally. This triangle is transgressed with a vertical incision that remains above the facial colliculus inferiorly and medial to the motor nucleus and mesencephalic tract of the trigeminal nerve laterally.

5.6.6 Superior Foveal

The superior and inferior foveae are dimples in the sulcus limitans; the superior fovea lies lateral to the facial colliculus in the pons, and the inferior fovea lies lateral to the hypoglossal trigone in the medulla. However, these landmarks are faint and difficult to see. The superior foveal triangle can be constructed with the sulcus limitans medially, the superior cerebellar peduncle superolaterally, and the vestibular area inferolaterally. Therefore, the superior foveal SEZ is best envisioned as a vertical incision at the level of and lateral to the facial colliculus. The lateral apex of the triangle approximates the top of the facial colliculus, and the zone is entered through a vertical incision in the inferior half of the triangle.

5.6.7 Pontomedullary Sulcus

The PMS demarcates the inferior border of the pons from the superior border of the medulla. It intersects midline structures, including the basilar sulcus of the pons and the anteromedian sulcus of the medulla, and courses laterally to the cerebellar peduncles. CNs VI to VIII originate from the superior aspect of the PMS, with CN VI originating at the level of the pyramidal tracts and CNs VII/VIII originating laterally to the inferior olive at the level of the retro-olivary (posterolateral) sulcus. The lower aspect of the inferior pons forms the superior border of the PMS, and the upper aspect of the inferior olive forms the inferior border of the PMS. The vertebral arteries join to form the basilar artery below the PMS in front of the medulla. The AICAs originate from the basilar trunk above the PMS and descend below CN VI and the PMS to course laterally across the upper aspect of the inferior olive. A transverse incision in the PMS is made above the olive, lateral to the pyramidal tracts, lateral to CN VI, and above the preolivary (anterolateral) sulcus and hypoglossal nerve rootlets. Entry is medial to CNs VII/VIII, CNs IX to XI, and the retro-olivary sulcus. An anterior trajectory is taken to reach lesions in the pontine underbelly, and a posterior trajectory is taken to reach lesions in the central pons.

5

5.7 Medullary Safe Entry Zones

Many ascending and descending nerve tracts pass through the medulla, carrying information between the brain and the spinal cord. Medullary nuclei perform vital functions such as the regulation of heart rate, blood pressure, and breathing (▸ Fig. 5.10). A three-dimensional understanding of midbrain anatomy can aid the surgeon in SEZ selection (▸ Fig. 5.11; ▸ Video 5.3). Each SEZ is contained within an associated anatomical triangle and has a corresponding surgical approach (▸ Fig. 5.12, ▸ Fig. 5.13).

5.7.1 Anterolateral Sulcus

The anteromedian fissure is the medulla's midline sulcus and runs vertically between the pyramids on its ventral surface. Although this essential landmark is inaccessible as an SEZ, the anterolateral sulcus can be reached through a far lateral exposure. The anterolateral sulcus, or preolivary sulcus, transmits the hypoglossal rootlets, which are easily identified by their relationship to the V4 segment of the vertebral artery and the hypoglossal canal. The SEZ extends from the PMS superiorly and the decussation of the pyramids inferiorly. A vertical incision between hypoglossal rootlets enters the medulla, and a bias laterally toward the olive will avoid the corticospinal tract medially.

5.7.2 Olive

The olivary nucleus is the medulla's most identifiable surface landmark, with a distinctive shape and nerve rootlets on either side. It lies between the anterolateral or preolivary sulcus from which the hypoglossal rootlets arise and the posterolateral or retro-olivary sulcus from which CN IX to XI rootlets arise. The olivary SEZ is a vertical incision that divides the olive between its superior pole at the PMS and CN VI and its inferior pole near the foramen magnum. Entry

5

Medullary Safe Entry Zones: Surgical Anatomy

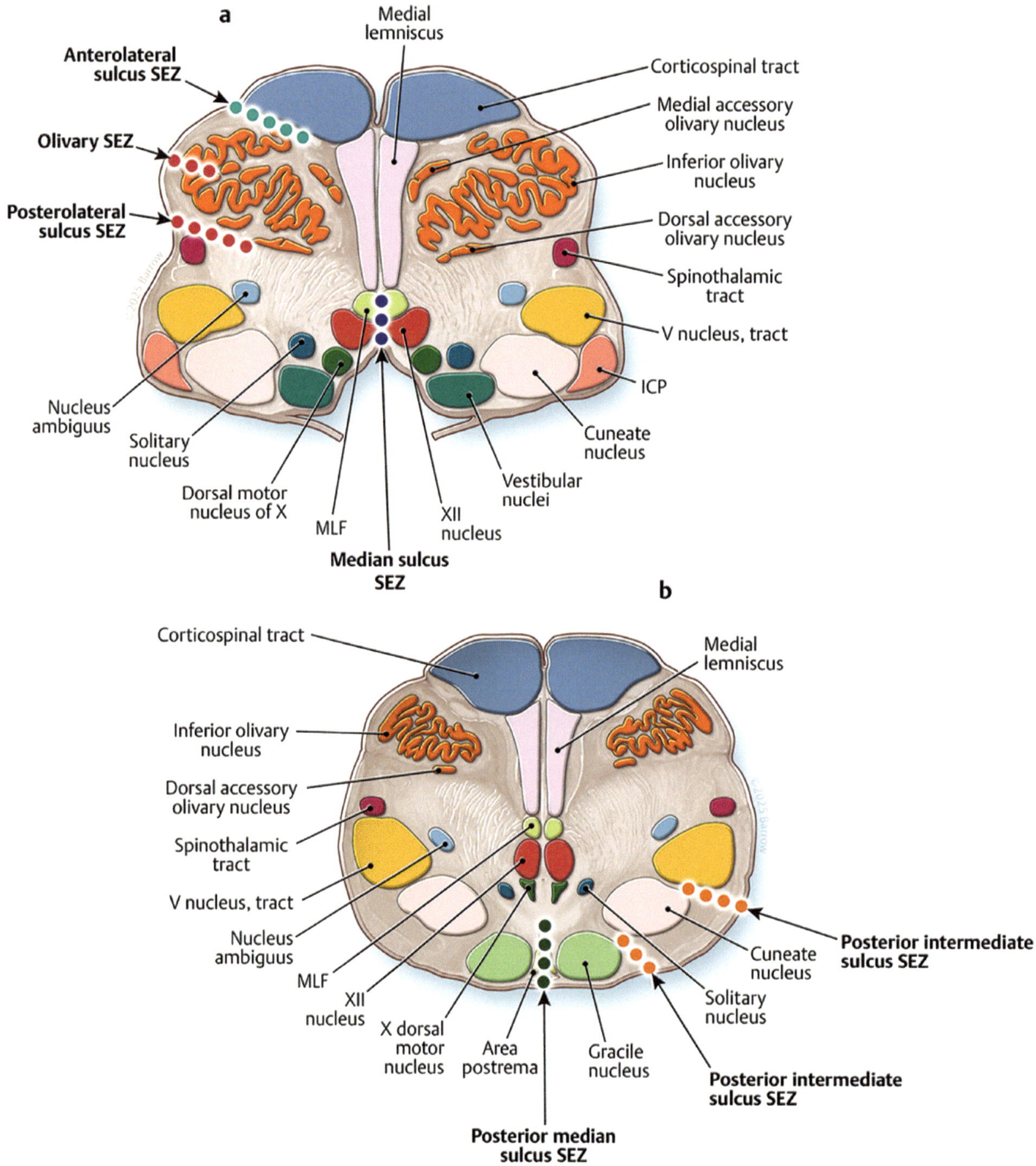

Fig. 5.10 The tracts and nuclei of the medulla, shown in axial cross-section **(a)** at the level of the fourth ventricle and **(b)** below the fourth ventricle, are involved in motor control (corticospinal tracts, hypoglossal nuclei, and nucleus ambiguus), motor coordination (spinocerebellar tract and vestibular nuclei), sensory processing (medial lemniscus, spinothalamic tracts, and gracile, cuneate, and solitary nuclei), autonomic function, and cardiovascular and respiratory control. Anterolateral sulcus (*teal*), olivary (*red*), posterolateral sulcus (*red*), median sulcus (*purple*), posterior median sulcus (*green*), and posterior intermediate sulcus (*orange*) SEZs are shown as *dotted lines*. Roman numerals denote CNs. (Reproduced with permission from Barrow Neurological Institute, Phoenix, AZ.)

Medullary Safe Entry Zones

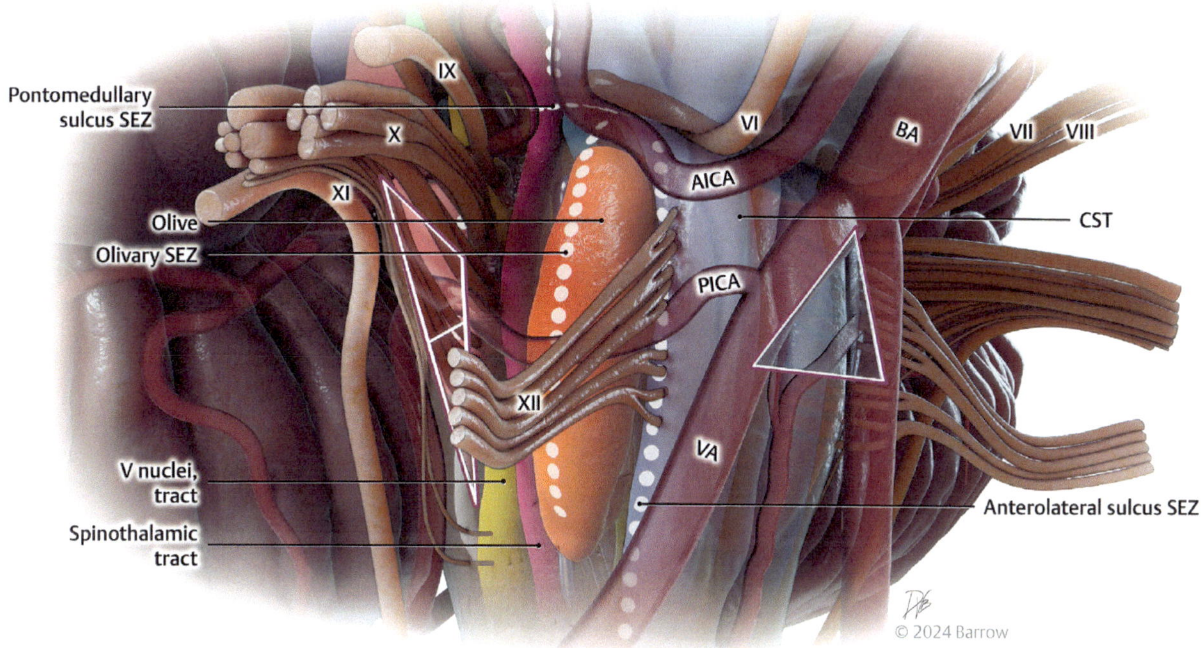

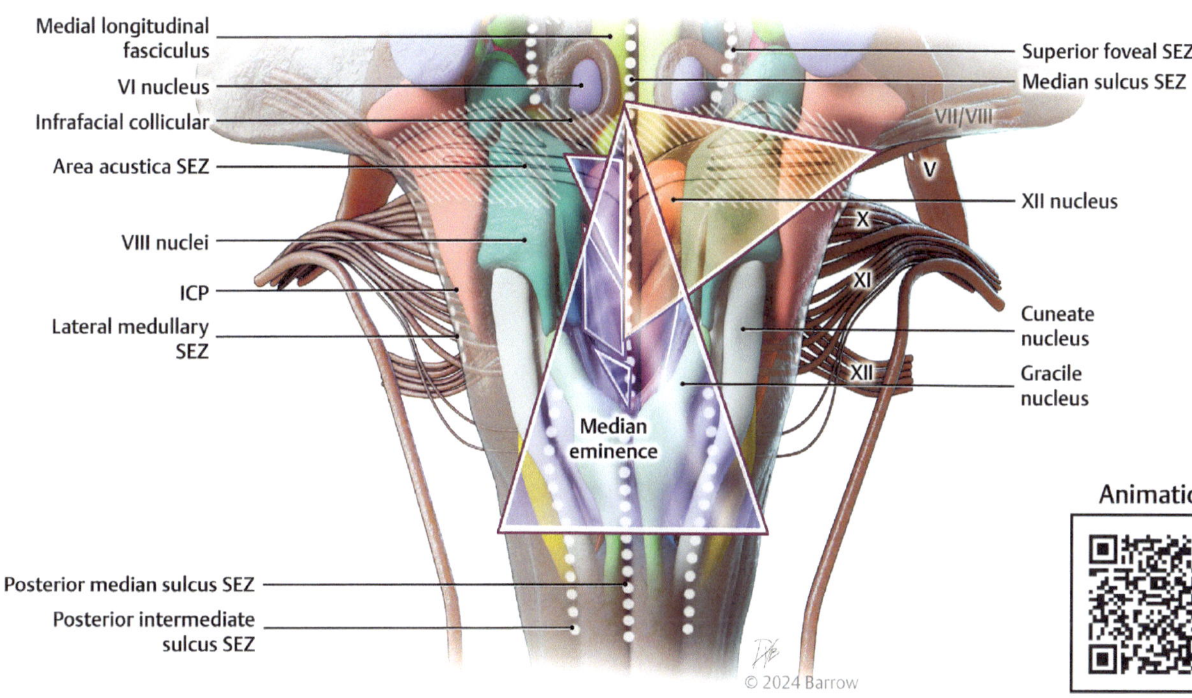

Animation

Fig. 5.11 The tracts and nuclei of the medulla are shown three dimensionally from a right anterior oblique view (*upper*) and a posterior view (*lower*). Medullary SEZs are shown as *dotted white lines*, and *anatomical triangles* are superimposed on the brainstem anatomy (animation; ▶ Video 5.3, Medullary SEZs; QR code). Roman numerals denote CNs. (Reproduced with permission from Barrow Neurological Institute, Phoenix, AZ.)

5

Anterolateral Medullary Safe Entry Zones: Surgical Approach

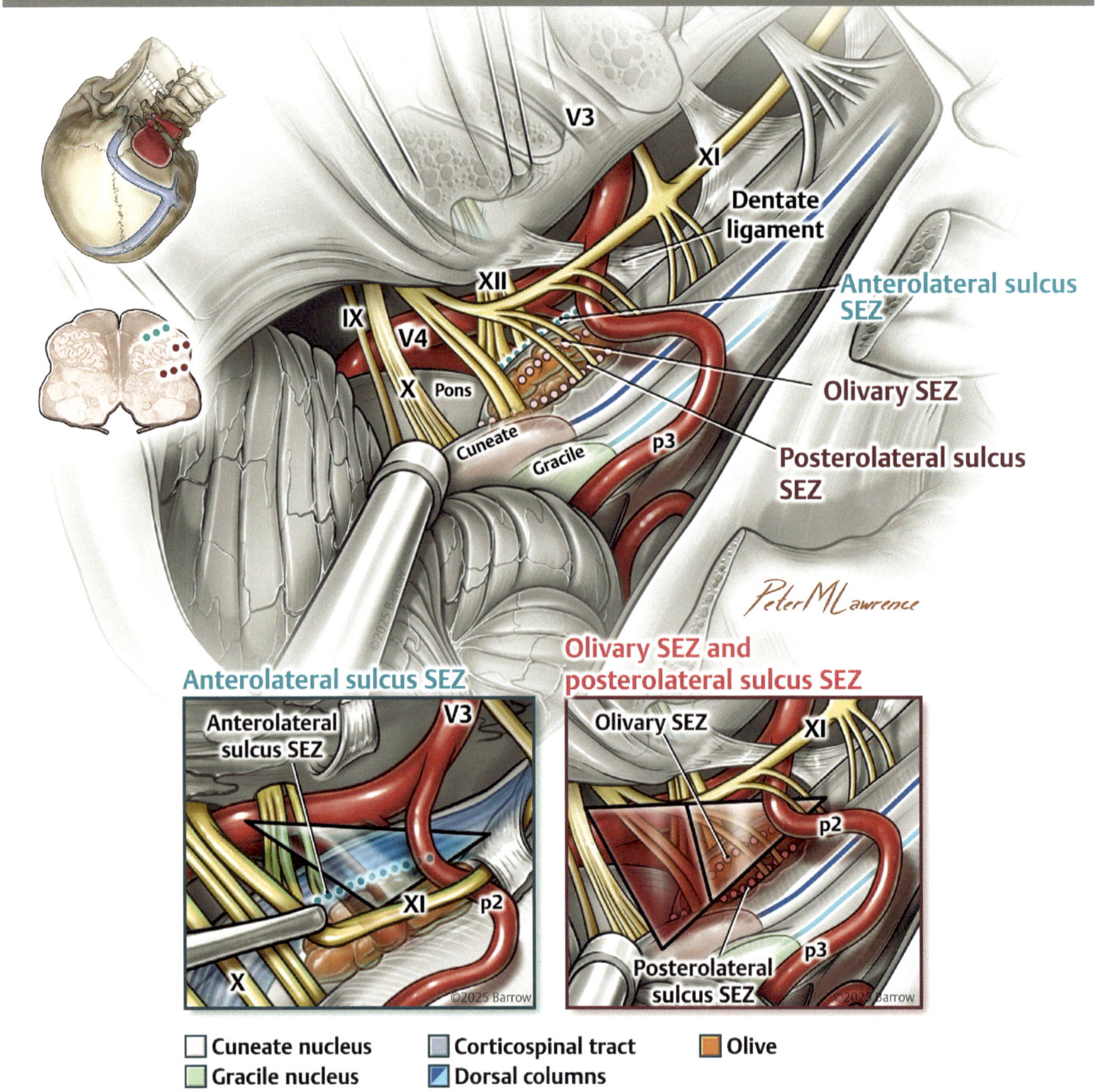

Fig. 5.12 The anterolateral sulcus SEZ (*dotted teal line*), olivary SEZ, and posterolateral sulcus SEZ (*dotted pink lines*) are depicted through the far lateral craniotomy with C1 laminectomy (*upper left inset*) and trans-cerebellomedullary cistern approach. The relationships between anatomical triangles, SEZs, and parenchymal tracts and nuclei are shown for the anterolateral sulcus (*lower left inset*) and olivary and posterolateral sulcus (*lower right inset*) SEZs. Entry trajectories are shown (*middle left inset*). Roman numerals denote CNs. (Reproduced with permission from Barrow Neurological Institute, Phoenix, AZ.)

Posterior Medullary Safe Entry Zones: Surgical Approach

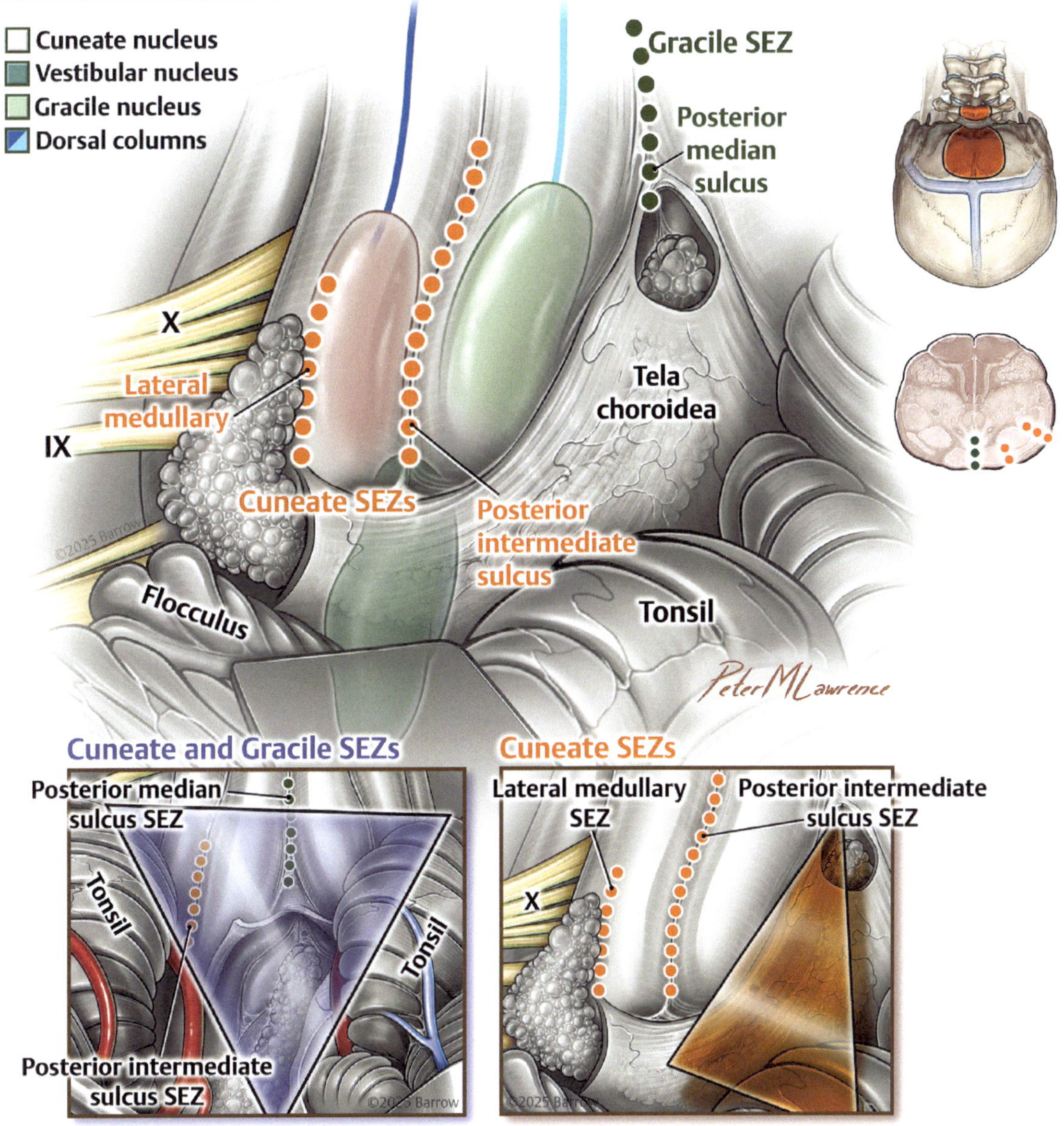

Fig. 5.13 The posterior medullary SEZs are shown from a right posterior view. The posterior median sulcus SEZ (*dotted green line*) and posterior intermediate sulcus and lateral medullary SEZs (*dotted orange lines*) are exposed through a suboccipital craniotomy with C1 laminectomy (*upper right inset*) and approaches through the cisterna magna. The relationships between anatomical triangles, SEZs, and parenchymal tracts and nuclei are shown for the posterior median sulcus SEZ (*lower left inset*) and posterior intermediate and lateral medullary SEZs (*lower right inset*). Entry trajectories are shown (*middle right inset*). Roman numerals denote CNs. (Reproduced with permission from Barrow Neurological Institute, Phoenix, AZ.)

perpendicular to the pial surface leads to the interior of the olivary nucleus. This approach avoids the posterior structures such as the vestibulospinal fibers, reticulospinal fibers, the ventral spinocerebellar tract, the spinothalamic tract, and the rubrospinal tract.

5.7.3 Posterolateral Sulcus and Lateral Medullary

The literature describes the posterolateral sulcus and lateral medullary SEZs as distinct, but they are difficult to differentiate because retro-olivary and posterolateral sulci are used interchangeably. Technically, these are two separate and distinct sulci. The retro-olivary sulcus is identified by the exiting medullary and spinal rootlets of the accessory nerve, whereas the posterolateral sulcus is identified lateral to the cuneate tubercle. The lateral funiculus of the medulla, or spinal nucleus, tract, and tubercle of the trigeminal nerve, lies between these two sulci but is indistinct, leaving the posterolateral medulla looking featureless and making these SEZs nearly synonymous. This region lies below and outside the lateral recess of the fourth ventricle and is the mirror image of the area acustica below the stria medullaris. The entry zone is a vertical incision in the retro-olivary sulcus between the rootlets of the accessory nerve or, more posteriorly, in the posterolateral sulcus along the cuneate tubercle. This space includes the inferior cerebellar peduncle, the trigeminal tubercle, and the spinothalamic tract.

5.7.4 Median Sulcus (Medulla)

The pontine portion of the median sulcus described above continues in the midline through the junctional and medullary parts of the fourth ventricular floor. The medullary portion of the median sulcus is more favorable than the pontine portion as an SEZ because the MLF end at the level of the abducens nucleus and stria medullaris, and extraocular eye movements are not at risk. The hypoglossal trigone, vagal trigone, and area postrema collectively form the calamus scriptorius in the caudal median eminence. They lack crossing fibers and are not as delicate as the MLF. Opening the medullary portion of the median sulcus is analogous to a midline myelotomy performed more cranially.

5.7.5 Infrafacial Collicular

The facial colliculus is located in the pontine part of the median eminence, and the nuclei of the calamus scriptorius are located in its medullary part. In between these inviolable structures is a small paramedian window to the pontomedullary junction. The infrafacial collicular SEZ is a rectangular space bordered by the facial nerve superiorly, the MLF medially, the stria medullaris inferiorly, and the sulcus limitans laterally. This zone is accessible in the widest part of the fourth ventricle and is transgressed with a vertical incision that remains below the facial colliculus. The facial colliculus might not be evident anatomically, and stimulation is typically required to map its location.

5.7.6 Posterior Median Sulcus

The posterior median sulcus courses between the gracile tubercles and fasciculi in the midline below the obex of the fourth ventricle. This sulcus is a continuation of the dorsal median sulcus of the spinal cord and, therefore, can be opened as in a midline myelotomy to access the posteroinferior aspect of the medulla outside of the fourth ventricle. This space requires no transgressing incision and only careful separation of a natural tissue plane defined by the perforating arteries and veins. Deep to the gracile tubercles lie the area postrema, the dorsal motor nucleus of the vagus nerve, the solitary nucleus and tract, and the dorsal longitudinal fasciculi.

5.7.7 Posterior Intermediate Sulcus

The posterior intermediate sulcus separates the gracile and cuneate tubercles, forming a natural division in the dorsal columns. Although described as a sulcus, it differs from the posterior median sulcus by being shallow and indistinct. The posterior median sulcus transmits arteries and veins that can be dissected to open the potential space, but the posterior intermediate sulcus lacks these vascular landmarks. Therefore, a vertically oriented transgressing incision is required with a deepening dissection between the gracile and cuneate nuclei.

5.8 Accuracy of Preoperative MRI in Determining Surface Proximity

The appearance of brainstem CMs on MRI makes these lesions easy to diagnose. The popcorn morphology, mixed signal intensities, hemosiderin ring, and their associations with developmental venous anomalies or venous malformations are pathognomonic. However, the assessment of surface proximity is more challenging. T2-weighted imaging intensifies the hemosiderin ring surrounding the pathology and overestimates surface proximity. Therefore, T1-weighted imaging provides better anatomical images and is the sequence of choice for evaluating surface proximity.

Exophytic and superficial brainstem CMs are more favorable for microsurgical resection because of their immediate accessibility, and surgery may be recommended to these patients based on surface proximity assessment on T1-weighted MRI. However, there is significant inaccuracy in differentiating superficial from deep CMs. MRI accurately depicted exophytic CMs that did not require an approach through an SEZ, as well as deep CMs that required an SEZ approach. Examples of radiological–microsurgical concordance are shown for exophytic (▶ Fig. 5.14) and deep (▶ Fig. 5.15) CMs. However, it overestimated the proximity of superficial lesions to brainstem surfaces. In our experience, 107 patients had CMs interpreted as superficial or exophytic on preoperative MRI, and 33 of them were found to have deep CMs intraoperatively (negative predictive value of 69%). Examples of radiological–microsurgical discordance are shown for superficial (▶ Fig. 5.16) and deep (▶ Fig. 5.17) CMs. Thus, our best radiological predictor of surface proximity favoring surgery will be

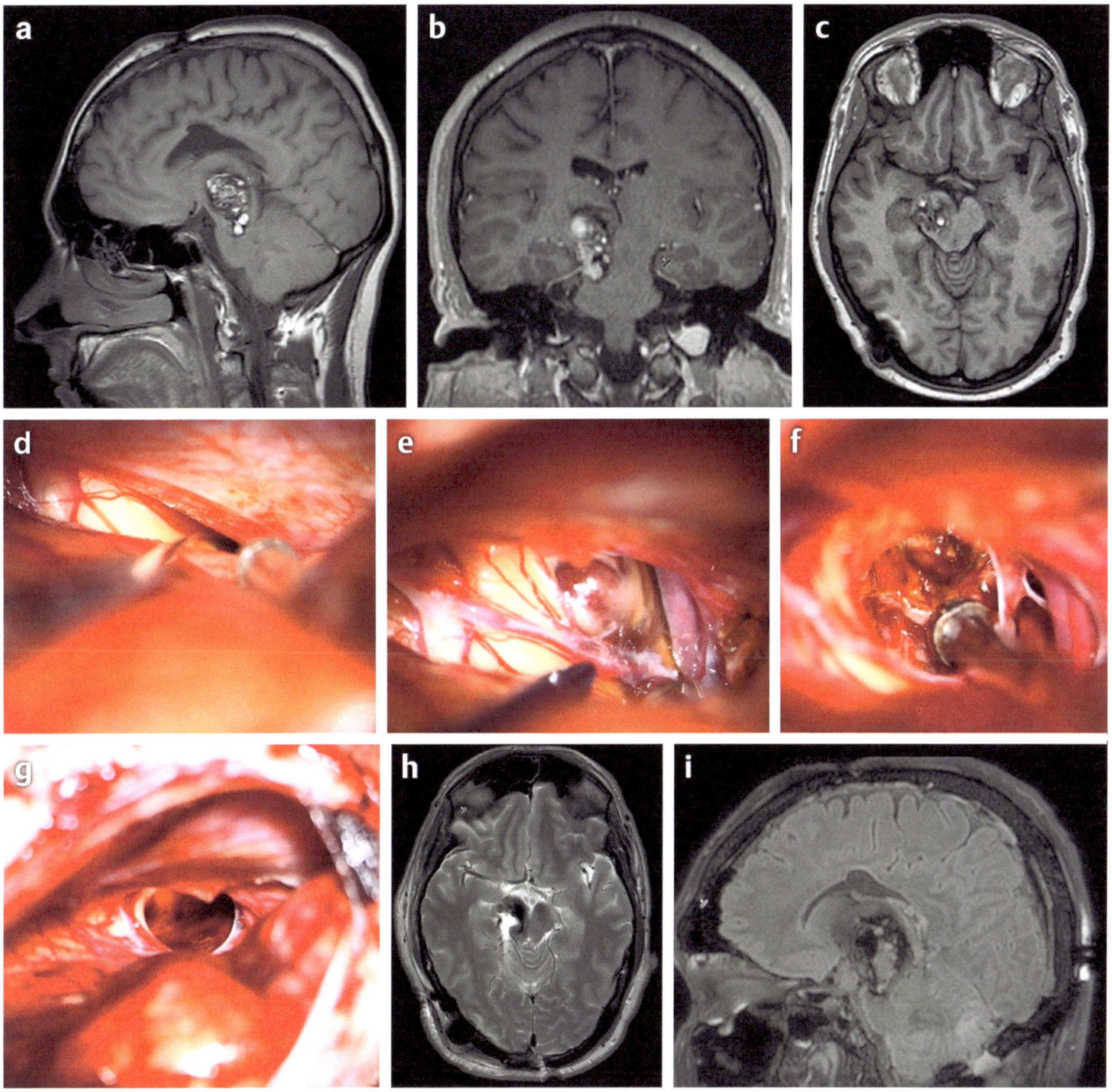

Fig. 5.14 Radiological–microsurgical concordance in a 32-year-old man with an exophytic tegmental midbrain CM extending superiorly into the central thalamus. Preoperative T1-weighted MRI suggested exophytic presentation in the right ambient cistern in **(a)** sagittal, **(b)** coronal, and **(c)** axial images. **(d)** A right lateral supracerebellar infratentorial approach was performed with the patient in the sitting position. **(e)** Intraoperatively, the CM was found bulging from the tegmentum into the ambient cistern. The CM was **(f)** circumferentially dissected and **(g)** completely resected. Postoperative **(h)** axial T2-weighted and **(i)** sagittal fluid-attenuated inversion recovery (FLAIR) MRI confirmed complete resection. (Reproduced with permission from Catapano JS, Benner D, Rhodenhiser EG, et al. Safety of brainstem safe entry zones: comparison of microsurgical outcomes associated with superficial, exophytic, and deep brainstem cavernous malformations. J Neurosurg 2022;139(1):113–123.)

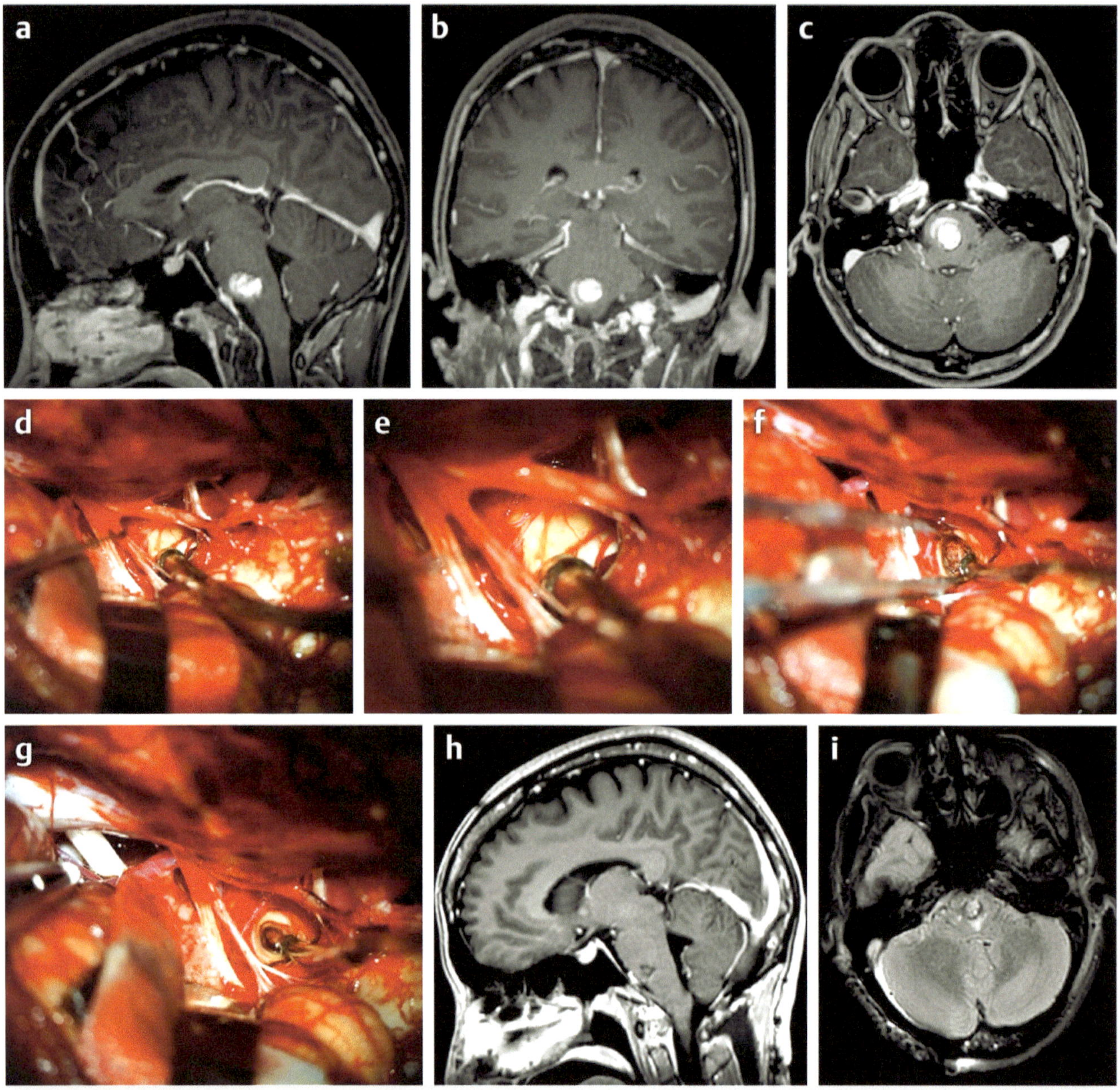

Fig. 5.15 Radiological–microsurgical concordance in a 30-year-old woman with a deep supraolivary pontine CM. Preoperative T1-weighted MRI suggested that the lesion was 2 to 3 mm below the right pontomedullary sulcus on **(a)** sagittal, **(b)** coronal, and **(c)** axial images. A right far lateral approach was performed, and intraoperative inspection through the vagoaccessory triangle confirmed the lesion's deep location with **(d)** low-magnification and **(e)** high-magnification views. **(f)** The pontomesencephalic sulcus SEZ was used to access and completely remove the lesion. **(g)** The relationship between the clean resection cavity and the cerebellopontine angle is shown. Postoperative **(h)** sagittal T1-weighted and **(i)** axial T2-weighted FLAIR MRI demonstrated complete resection. (Reproduced with permission from Catapano JS, Benner D, Rhodenhiser EG, et al. Safety of brainstem safe entry zones: comparison of microsurgical outcomes associated with superficial, exophytic, and deep brainstem cavernous malformations. J Neurosurg 2022;139(1):113–123.)

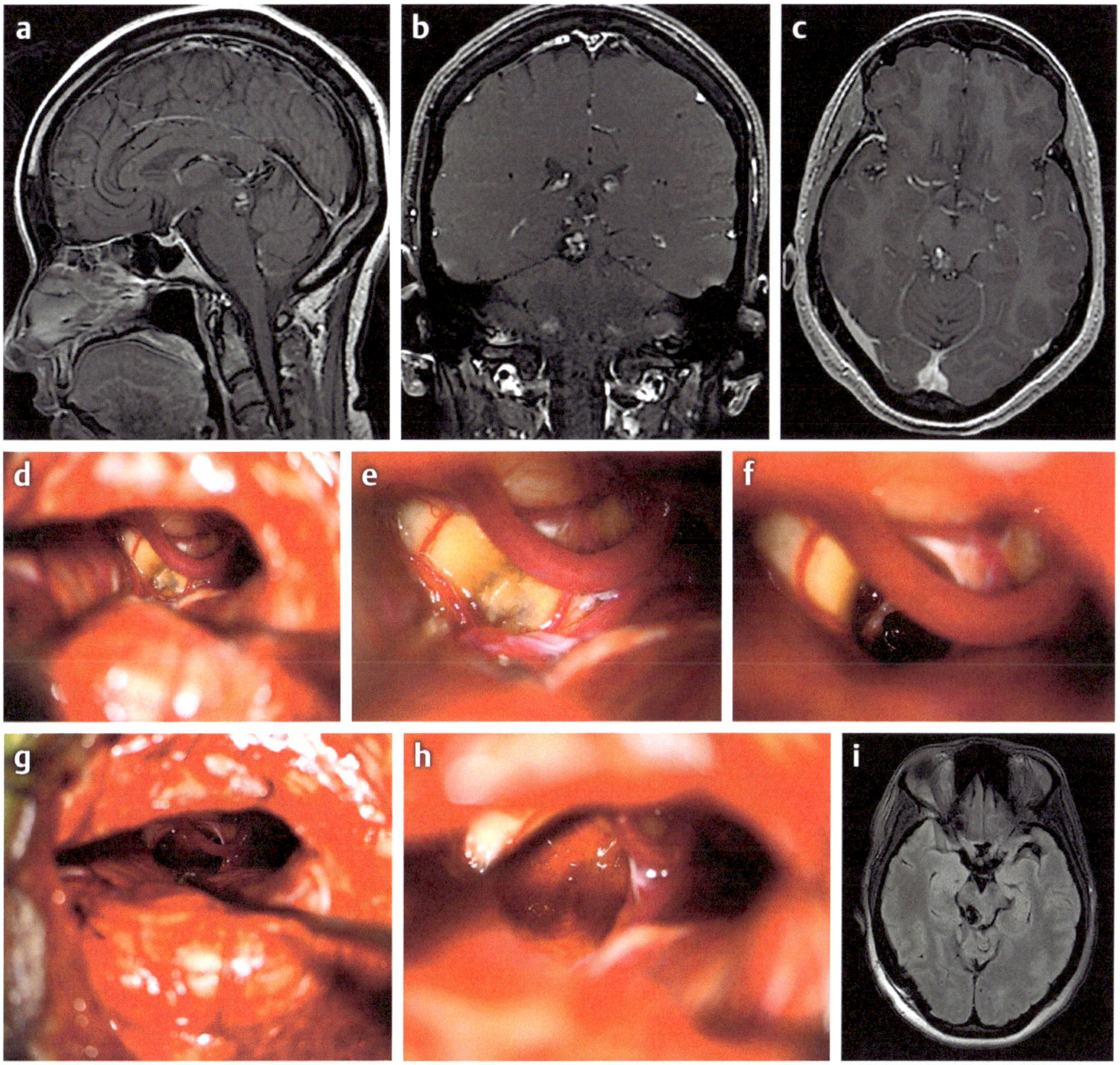

Fig. 5.16 Radiological–microsurgical concordance in a patient with a superficial quadrigeminal midbrain CM. Preoperative **(a)** sagittal, **(b)** coronal, and **(c)** axial T1-weighted MRI suggesting superficial presentation of the lesion to the right superior and inferior colliculi. A right paramedian supracerebellar infratentorial approach was performed with the patient in the sitting position. Intraoperatively, the CM presented to the surface of the tectum, as shown on **(d)** low-magnification and **(e)** high-magnification views. **(f)** The CM was just beneath the hemosiderin stain and was completely resected, as shown on **(g)** low-magnification and **(h)** high-magnification views. **(i)** Postoperative axial T2-weighted FLAIR image demonstrating complete resection. (Reproduced with permission from Catapano JS, Benner D, Rhodenhiser EG, et al. Safety of brainstem safe entry zones: comparison of microsurgical outcomes associated with superficial, exophytic, and deep brainstem cavernous malformations. J Neurosurg 2022;139(1):113–123.)

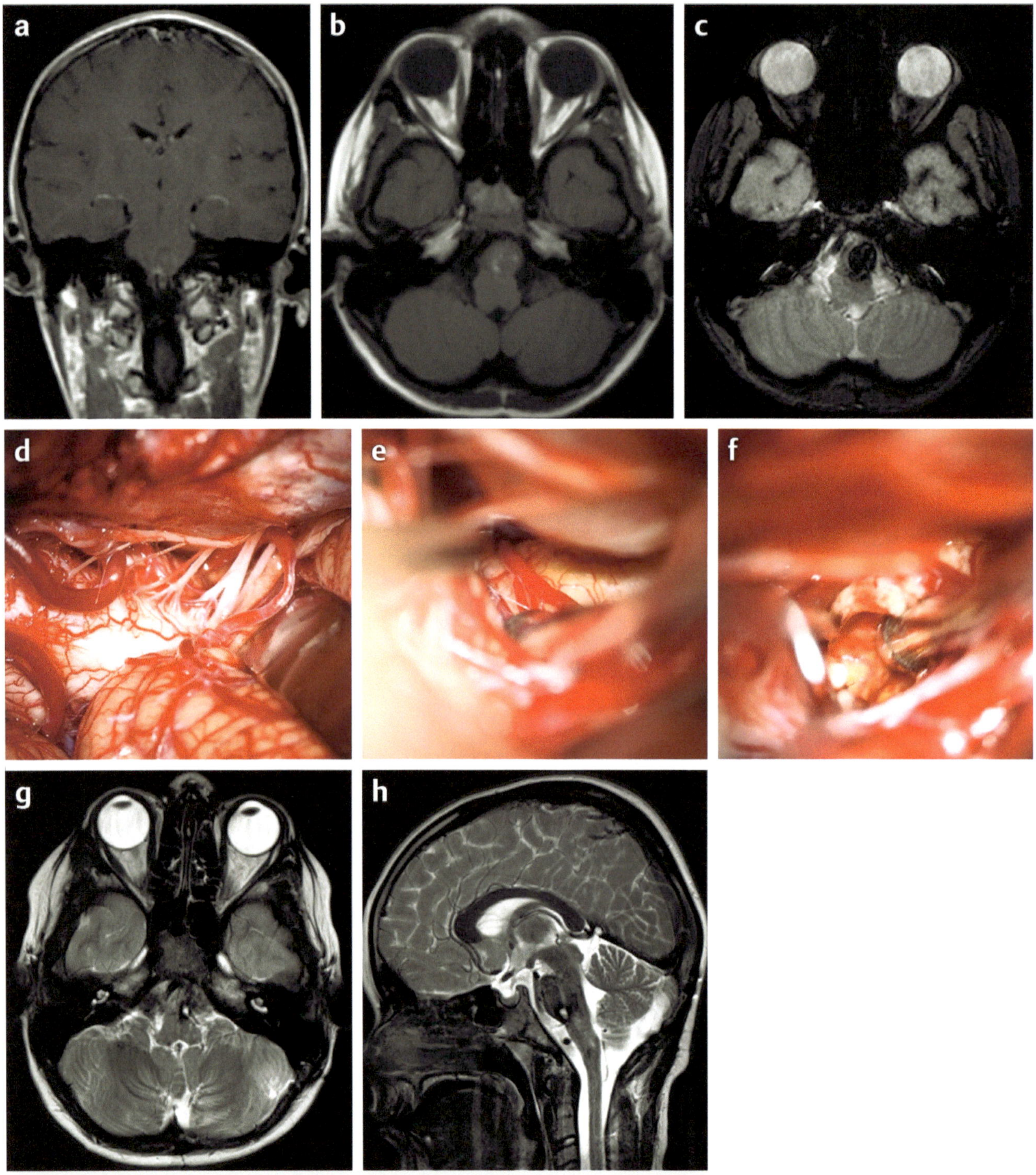

Fig. 5.17 Radiological–microsurgical discordance in a 9-year-old boy with a left supraolivary pontine CM. The lesion appeared to present superficially to the pontomedullary sulcus on preoperative MRI in T1-weighted **(a)** coronal and **(b)** axial images, as well as on a **(c)** T2-weighted axial image. **(d)** A left far lateral approach was performed, and **(e)** dissection through the vagoaccessory triangle revealed only a faint hemosiderin stain without a superficial cavernoma. **(f)** The lesion was accessed with an incision in the pontomedullary sulcus SEZ and dissection through 1 to 2 mm of parenchyma beneath the pial surface; the CM was completely resected. Postoperative T2-weighted MRI with **(g)** axial and **(h)** sagittal images confirmed complete resection. Radiological–microsurgical discordance resulted in the unanticipated use of the pontomedullary sulcus SEZ to reach a deep pontine brainstem CM that appeared to be superficial on preoperative MRI. (Reproduced with permission from Catapano JS, Benner D, Rhodenhiser EG, et al. Safety of brainstem safe entry zones: comparison of microsurgical outcomes associated with superficial, exophytic, and deep brainstem cavernous malformations. J Neurosurg 2022;139(1):113–123.)

Table 5.3 Comparison of radiological and microsurgical concordance and discordance: diagnostic accuracy of preoperative MRI was compared to the gold standard of intraoperative inspection for determining the brainstem CM surface proximity ($n = 154$)

MRI	Intraoperative verification		Diagnostic accuracy
	Deep, 74	Super/exo, 80	
Deep, 47	41	6	PPV: 87%
Superficial/exophytic, 107	33	74	NPV: 69%
	Sensitivity: 55%	Specificity: 93%	
	Superficial, 57	Deep/exophytic, 97	
Superficial, 80	48	32	PPV: 60%
Deep/exophytic, 74	9	65	NPV: 88%
	Sensitivity: 84%	Specificity: 67%	
	Exophytic, 23	Deep/superficial, 131	
Exophytic, 27	22	5	PPV: 81%
Deep/superficial, 127	1	126	NPV: 99%
	Sensitivity: 96%	Specificity: 96%	

Note: Data are number of CMs unless otherwise specified.

wrong in nearly one-third of cases and require the unanticipated use of SEZs (▶ Table 5.3).

This finding is striking for the inaccuracy of our best preoperative decision-making tool and the importance of knowing SEZs. Neurosurgeons surprised by the absence of the CM on the brainstem surface must choose between aborting the operation, relying on frameless stereotactic navigation, or resorting to SEZ use. Aborting the operation fails to accomplish the surgical mission, is disappointing for patients and neurosurgeons, and leaves pathology that could hemorrhage and further debilitate the patient. Complete reliance on stereotactic navigation can lead to errant transgressions into brainstem parenchyma if accuracy is compromised by brain shift, head motion, or baseline error. A thorough working knowledge of SEZs gives the neurosurgeon confidence to proceed with an unexpectedly deep lesion. Therefore, surgeons should adopt the SEZ concept, preoperatively study brainstem SEZ anatomy, and delicately dissect within these SEZs.

5.9 Neuronavigation, Hemosiderin Stain, and Neuromonitoring

SEZs rely on surface anatomy often distorted by hemorrhage, hematoma, edema, and the lesion. Therefore, additional techniques are crucial for reaching deep brainstem CMs when entering normal brainstem tissue. Stereotactic navigation is mandatory with all brainstem CMs and provides invaluable information about the entry site, trajectory, and proximity to the lesion. Even after reaching the target, navigation provides information about the extent of resection, the location of distant margins, and the adjacent intraparenchymal anatomy. Hemosiderin released after a CM hemorrhage creates a color gradient in normal tissue that can be tracked toward the lesions, with the intensity of golden-colored staining increasing as the lesion is neared. Stimulation mapping can also identify critical tracts (e.g., the corticospinal tract) and nuclei (e.g., the facial nucleus on the fourth ventricular floor). Intraoperative neurophysiological monitoring with motor evoked potentials, somatosensory evoked potentials, brainstem auditory evoked responses, and CN monitoring is also mandatory with brainstem CMs. However, monitoring tends to guide the progress and extent of resection rather than the approach to the lesion through normal parenchyma.

5.10 Brainstem CM Taxonomy and Associated SEZs

Brainstem CM taxonomy classifies lesions by their location in the brainstem, with type determined by the position in the midbrain, pons, or medulla, and subtype determined by the surface to which the lesion presents (i.e., anterior, posterior, lateral, anterolateral, or posterolateral). The 16 unique brainstem subtypes help guide surgical decision-making. Each CM subtype has a preferred or ideal surgical approach, and the identification of a particular CM subtype suggests the approach in those patients who opt for resection. Taxonomy also guides the surgical technique by associating a preferred or ideal SEZ with each CM subtype (▶ Table 5.4). The relationship between the brainstem CM subtype and SEZ further validates the clinical use of the taxonomy, adding insights into the approach and SEZ selection to improve patient outcomes.

Some variability exists in the choice of SEZ, especially when more than one SEZ is accessible through the preferred approach. Five brainstem CMs have multiple SEZs. Quadrigeminal brainstem CMs can be reached through the supracollicular, infracollicular, and intercollicular SEZs. Peritrigeminal brainstem CMs can be accessed through the supra- and infratrigeminal SEZs. Within the fourth ventricle, rhomboid pontine CMs are accessed through the median sulcus, suprafacial collicular, and superior foveal SEZs, whereas trigonal medullary CMs are accessed through the median sulcus and infrafacial collicular SEZs. Olivary medullary CMs can be exposed using the olivary zone, lateral medullary zone, and posterolateral sulcus SEZs. For these five brainstem CMs, SEZ options are suggested by the taxonomy, and the choice of a specific SEZ is dictated by the lesion's unique pathoanatomy. Taxonomy is not meant to govern the choice of SEZ but rather to equip the neurosurgeon with discrete options to be selected intraoperatively after surveying the pathology.

Table 5.4 Brainstem CM types and subtypes, preferred approach, and SEZ associated with each subtype, and the percentage of deep lesions that required the use of an SEZ

CM type	CM subtype	Total	Superficial or exophytic	Deep	Preferred approach	Preferred SEZ	SEZ abbreviation	SEZ used
Midbrain	Interpeduncular	1	1	0	TSyl-IntPed	Interpeduncular fossa	IPF	N/A
	Peduncular	10	4	6	TSyl-Ped	Anterior mesencephalic	AM	5 (83)
	Tegmental	15	11	4	SCIT-Lat	Lateral mesencephalic sulcus	LMS	3 (75)
	Quadrigeminal	5	3	2	SCIT-Mid	Inter-, supra-, infracol-licular	ICR, SC, IC	2 (100)
	Periaqueductal	3	3	0	TCal-TChor	None	None	N/A
Pontine	Basilar	4	3	1	Kaw	Supra-, infratrigeminal, peritrigeminal	ST, IT	1 (100)
	Peritrigeminal	7	2	5	xRS-CPA	Supra-, infra-, peritri-geminal	ST, IT	4 (80)
	Middle peduncular	40	12	28	xRS-MCP	Middle cerebellar peduncle/lateral pontine	MCP	27 (96)
	Inferior peduncular	13	4	9	SOcc-TeVe	Area acustica	AA	9 (100)
	Rhomboid	26	19	7	SOcc-Vent	Median sulcus, supra-facial collicular, supe-rior foveal	MS, SFC, SFo	5 (71)
	Supraolivary	12	8	4	FL-PMS	Pontomedullary sulcus	PMS	3 (75)
Medullary	Pyramidal	0	0	0	FL-PreMed	Anterolateral sulcus	ALS	N/A
	Olivary	13	7	6	FL-Med	Olivary zone, postero-lateral sulcus, lateral medullary	OZ, PLS, LM	6 (100)
	Trigonal	1	0	1	SOcc-Vent	Median sulcus, infrafa-cial collicular	MS, IFC	1 (100)
	Gracile	1	1	0	SOcc-Magna	Posterior median sulcus	PostMedS	N/A
	Cuneate	3	2	1	SOcc-TeVe	Posterior intermediate sulcus	PIS	1 (100)

Note: Numerical data are presented as number or number (%).

5

6 RESECTION

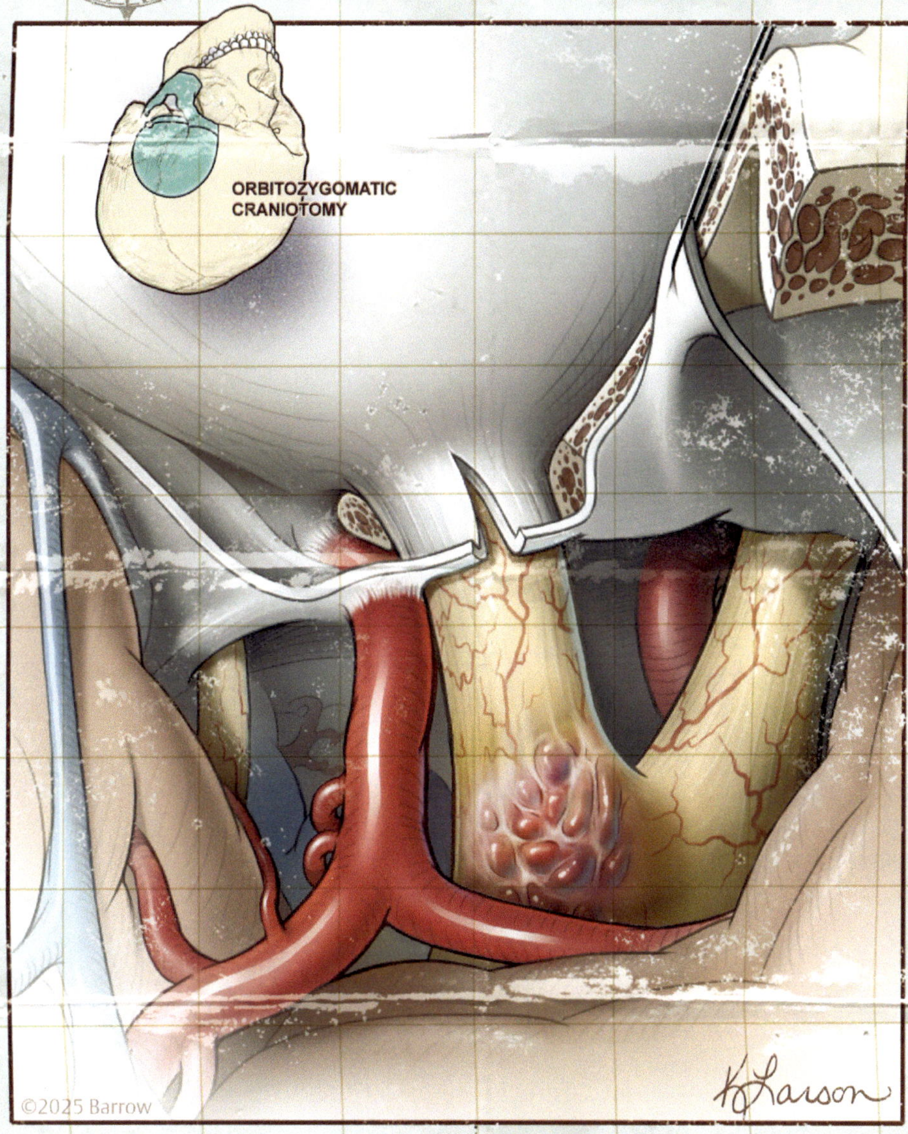

6 Resection Technique

Summary

Cavernous malformations (CMs) are compared to mulberries because of their similarity to the mulberry's drupelet morphology and purple-black coloration with irregular red areas. A mulberry consists of many drupelets, each containing a seed. Similarly, each CM cavern is filled with blood in various stages of hemoglobin degradation that can result in a mulberry appearance and telltale hemosiderin staining in surrounding brain tissue. This staining helps neurosurgeons locate the CM. With a superficial cerebral CM in the neurosurgeon's sight, the resection begins with circumferential cauterization of the capsule to shrink and move it toward the center to create a separation plane. Capsule preservation ensures that the CM can be removed en bloc without leaving any remnant. CMs deep to the surface require an approach through the brain parenchyma. In contrast to this extracapsular resection technique, an intracapsular resection technique is used for CMs in eloquent cerebral, deep cerebral, and brainstem locations. In the brainstem, transgression proceeds through one of the 21 safe entry zones (SEZs), such as the lateral pontine SEZ, which is located on the middle cerebellar peduncle at the bottom of the petrosal fissure. The CM is decompartmentalized internally, debulked piecemeal, and collapsed inward, with circumferential dissection of the capsule only after it has been imploded. Intracapsular resection removes pathology from within the capsule, with careful consideration of the eloquent fibers and tracts to achieve the best possible neurological outcome. This approach can reach lesions in several areas, depending on its trajectory. Safely transgressing brain parenchyma requires an *orienteering mentality*, with knowledge of the SEZ and the underlying tracts, nuclei, and trajectories needed to bypass them. In the future, neurosurgeons will have a virtual library of SEZs, individualized visible and invisible triangles, scaled and superimposed onto the surgical field as they operate. Until then, neurosurgeons must rely on their expert knowledge and operative skills to optimize patient outcomes.

Keywords: brain transgression, extracapsular, hemosiderin stain, intracapsular, invisible triangle, resection, technique

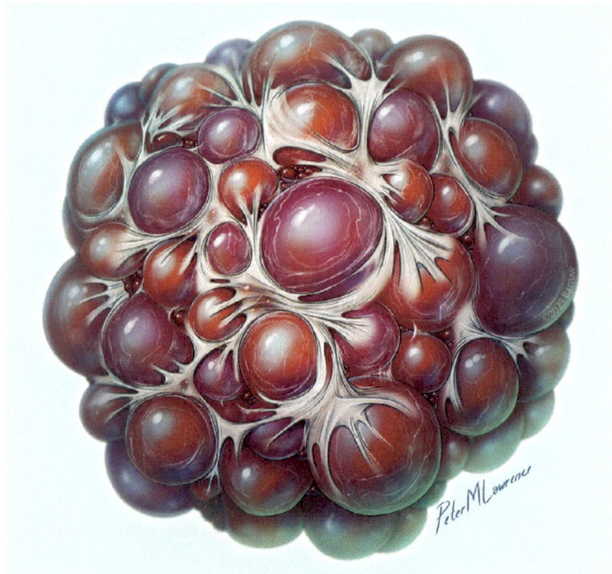

Fig. 6.1 CMs are compared to mulberries, which are drupelets, because of their purple-to-black coloration and patchy red areas. Each of the caverns of a CM contains blood of a differing age, with a spectrum of colors ranging from red to purple to brown to gold to clear, corresponding to the stages of hemoglobin degradation. (Reproduced with permission from Barrow Neurological Institute, Phoenix, AZ.)

6.1 The Mulberry

In botany, a drupe is a simple fruit, like a cherry, that contains a single seed or pit surrounded by fleshy fruit and wrapped in an outer skin. Drupelets are aggregates of individual drupes that form fruit like raspberries or blackberries. Cavernous malformations (CMs) are compared to mulberries, another drupelet, because of their purple-to-black coloration and patchy red areas (▶ Fig. 6.1). A cerebral CM is like a mulberry embedded in pudding. Each of its caverns contains blood of differing ages with a spectrum of colors ranging from red to purple to brown to gold to clear, corresponding to the stages of hemoglobin degradation. The compartmentalization of liquified blood within this aggregate of drupelets resembles a jewel that sparkles under the glare of the operating microscope. Exophytic or intraventricular cavernomas look like gems washed ashore, whereas parenchymal cavernomas look like gems buried in sand. Some cavernomas have thin skins that reveal their multicolored drupelets, and some have thick peels that separate them from the adjacent brain tissue. Entering and collapsing the lesion may release a thick chocolate fluid of subacute blood or the thin yellow liquid of a chronic hematoma; an adjacent compartment may sequester solid chunks of desiccated clot. Add to this picture the developmental venous anomaly or venous malformation whose caput medusa morphology almost grips the pathology like a hand in a glove. These surreal shapes, colors, and contrasts make the cavernoma a beautiful, albeit pathological, sight.

The other neuropathologies described as berries are not as serene as the cavernoma. Berry aneurysms resist intense hemodynamic forces, with throbbing walls often thinned by high shear stress and turbulent flows. Blood can be seen swirling inside the sac through these tenuous walls, and dissection of berry aneurysms is often in the setting of subarachnoid hemorrhage, an angry brain, and the threat of an intraoperative rupture. In contrast, cavernomas are still and calm, with negligible hemodynamics and no threat of rupture. There is no proximal or distal control, temporary clipping, or neck dissection. When the CM is seen, the operation's tension and uncertainty vanish. The target has been found, and all that remains is the resection. The hard part of cavernoma surgery is the journey to the CM: the approach, the dissection, and the identification of telltale signs that the target lies near. The rest of the operation, removing the mulberry, is calmer and more comfortable than removing other vascular lesions in the brain.

6.2 Extracapsular Resection Technique

Arrival at the CM's capsule marks the end of the approach phase and the beginning of the resection phase of the dissection (▸ Fig. 6.2). The capsule is cauterized to define and thicken it. Bipolar cautery applied to the pathology shrinks and mobilizes it toward its center. The separation plane between the

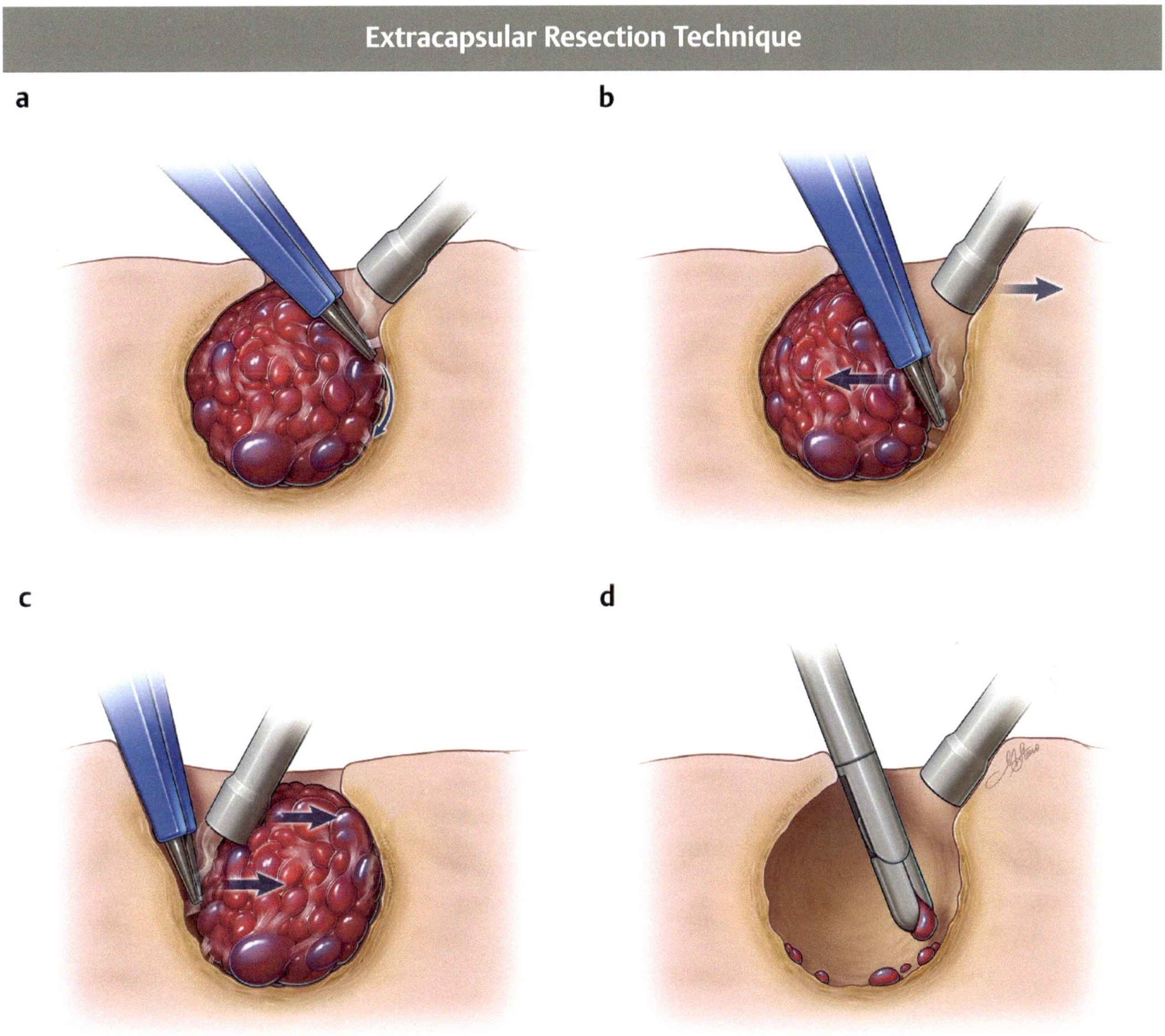

Fig. 6.2 Extracapsular resection technique. **(a)** The separation plane is developed by applying bipolar cautery to the CM to shrink and mobilize it toward its center. **(b)** Starting on the side opposite the bipolar forceps, the CM is mobilized toward the forceps and away from the suction tip, with the instruments pulling in opposite directions for traction-countertraction and cautery-retraction. **(c)** Working the lesion on the side of the bipolar forceps lessens the favorable traction-countertraction dynamic because the bipolar forceps and suction tip pull in the same direction, but this becomes easier later in the operation after shrinking the lesion and establishing the separation planes. **(d)** After the CM is removed en bloc or piecemeal, the resection cavity is inspected thoroughly to remove all remaining fragments. (Reproduced with permission from Barrow Neurological Institute, Phoenix, AZ.)

lesion and the surrounding brain is developed further with centripetal traction that pulls on the pathology rather than on the adjacent (sometimes eloquent) brain. Circumferential dissection encompasses all sides of the lesion. Ergonomically, starting on the side opposite the bipolar forceps and mobilizing the lesion toward the forceps (away from the suction tip) facilitates the early use of cautery to shrink the lesion and develop the separation plane. The bipolar forceps and suction tip are pulling in opposite directions for traction-countertraction and cautery-retraction. Working the lesion on the side of the bipolar forceps becomes easier later in the operation after shrinking the lesion and establishing the separation planes. The bipolar forceps and suction tip pull in the same direction, which lessens the favorable traction-countertraction dynamic. Capsule preservation ensures that every drupelet and all fragments of the CM are removed as one en bloc specimen, whereas piecemeal resection risks leaving remnants behind. However, piecemeal resection is necessary with large and giant CMs to debulk and maneuver around these lesions. Extracapsular hemorrhage and adjacent hematoma help establish the separation plane between the capsule and the surrounding brain. However, acute hemorrhage and secondary edema soften this plane and make circumferential dissection more traumatic, increasing the risk of surgery in the days following extracapsular hemorrhage. Retraction pressure on brain tissue is minimized, especially in patients with edematous brain tissue. Associated developmental venous anomalies or venous malformations are preserved during the resection to maintain venous drainage. Occasionally, the end branches or fingers of the venous malformation may need to be coagulated to liberate the cavernoma, which is well tolerated when the main trunk is preserved.

6.3 Intracapsular Resection Technique

The extracapsular resection technique described above is used with superficial cerebral CMs, but the intracapsular resection technique is used with CMs in eloquent areas and deep cerebral and brainstem CMs (▶ Fig. 6.3). The capsule is typically opened to evacuate liquified blood internally and debulk the lesion. The CM often has multiple compartments containing liquified blood that are interconnected, communicated, and evacuated. Internal decompression collapses the CM, pulling it into the resection cavity and establishing the separation plane between the capsule and the surrounding brain tissue. The dissection stays inside the capsule, resecting the core piecemeal and pulling the capsule inward toward the center. Bipolar cautery is not used as a dissection technique but only for hemostasis. The intracapsular technique is routinely used with brainstem CMs to minimize contact with the surrounding brainstem. The same rationale applies to eloquent areas like the sensorimotor cortex, visual cortex, and language areas.

Intracapsular piecemeal resection is slower than circumferential dissection and en bloc extracapsular resection and increases the risk of leaving a remnant. The right-angle method, discussed in a subsequent chapter, helps anticipate surgical blind spots, which drives meticulous inspection for remnants during surgery. The surgical axis, defined by a line connecting the superficial entrance into the operative corridor and the entry into the CM, is intersected by a perpendicular line from the surgical axis to the point on the lesion's capsule farthest from the axis. Perpendicular lines exceeding 1 cm in length drawn on axial, sagittal, and coronal magnetic resonance images help identify a potential blind spot. The surgical axis approximates the line of sight into the resection bed, which makes spots in the near corners more difficult to see than those in the far corners.

6.4 Brain Transgression

Brain tissue necessitating transgression lies between the target lesion and the hemosiderin stain or safe entry zone (SEZ) on an otherwise pristine pial surface. Superficial or exophytic CMs are accessed through their presenting components, but deeply seated lesions cannot be resected without transgression through normal brain tissue. This can be the most unsettling part of the operation because reaching the target is uncertain. Twenty-one SEZs provide access to deep brainstem CMs, but the transgression depth and trajectory beyond the SEZ influence the safety of resection and final neurological outcome. The trans-middle cerebellar peduncle (trans-MCP) approaches for brainstem CM resection illustrate the relationships between lesion location, surgical trajectory beyond the SEZ, and long-term clinical outcomes to understand the concept of safe passage through brain tissue.

The trans-MCP approach to the lateral and central pons is very versatile, and its well-tolerated SEZ has made it the most common approach for brainstem CMs; it was used in 17% (96/551) of patients with brainstem CMs in a recent 30-year (1990–2019), two-surgeon experience. The trans-MCP approach, or *petrosal fissure* approach, through the potential space between the cerebellum's superior and inferior semilunar lobules (interlobular triangle) uses the MCP's lateral extent for safe entry. Although conceptualized as a horizontal corridor to the lateral and central pons, the trans-MCP approach has a wider reach when the trajectory of tissue transgression is aimed vertically or posteriorly. Specifically, a rostral trajectory leads to pontine lesions extending into the midbrain, and a caudal trajectory leads to those extending into the medulla. Additionally, a more posterior trajectory accesses rhomboid pontine CMs that may not have breached the floor of the fourth ventricle and caused the stereotypical internuclear ophthalmoplegia observed in these patients. Correspondingly, increasing proportions of patients with pontine CMs with midbrain or medulla extension have undergone trans-MCP resection in recent years. With this evolution and broader application of the technique, SEZs are no longer just superficial points of entry but rather three-dimensional trajectories with associated tissue transgressions with neurological consequences.

6.5 Technical Overview of the Trans-MCP Approach

Trans-MCP approaches are initiated from an extended retrosigmoid (xRS) craniotomy, which widens the access corridor ventrally by skeletonizing the sigmoid sinus and mobilizing it anteriorly with tension on the dural flap, thereby allowing a more

Intracapsular Resection Technique

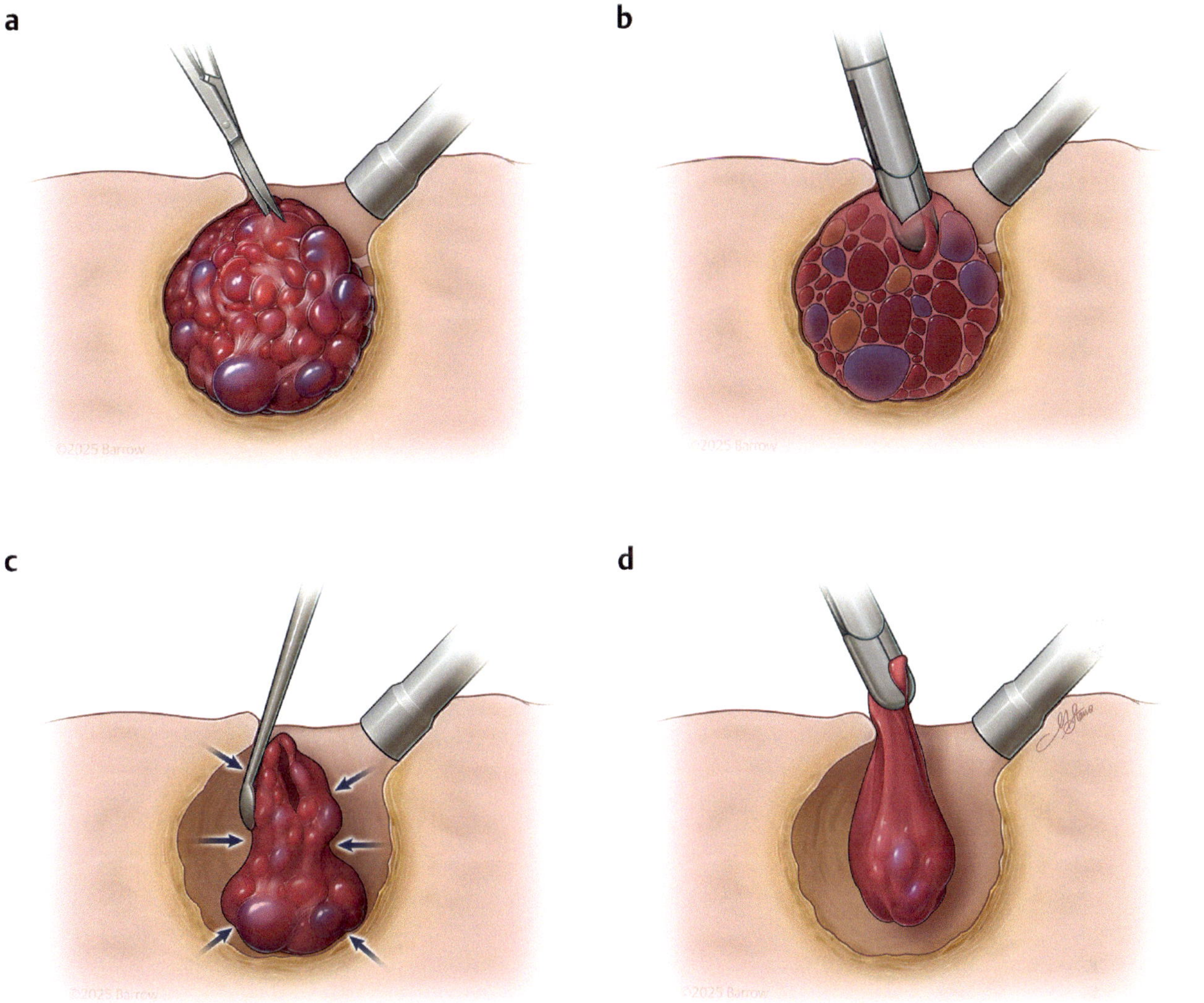

Fig. 6.3 Intracapsular resection technique. **(a)** The capsule is opened to evacuate liquified blood internally and debulk the CM. **(b)** The CM (seen in cross-section) often has multiple compartments containing liquified blood that are interconnected and communicated. These compartments are evacuated. Portions of the solid CM are removed piecemeal with a pair of grasping forceps, staying inside the capsule to protect the adjacent eloquent brain. **(c)** After the CM is internally debulked, its capsule collapses, pulling it into the resection cavity; a round knife is used to establish the separation plane between the capsule and the surrounding brain tissue. **(d)** After complete separation of the capsule from the adjacent brain, the deflated CM is removed. (Reproduced with permission from Barrow Neurological Institute, Phoenix, AZ.)

direct trajectory into the MCP (▸ Fig. 6.4a). The xRS craniotomy also provides additional exposure inferiorly, which is critical when carrying the resection superiorly for CMs in the midbrain. After the craniotomy and dural opening, the release of cerebrospinal fluid from the lateral cerebellomedullary cistern and the wide opening of the cerebellopontine cistern reveal the petrosal (horizontal) fissure along the ventrolateral cerebellum between the superior and inferior semilunar lobules (▸ Fig. 6.4b). The deep arachnoid overlying cranial nerves V, VII, and VIII can be left in place, which reduces the risk of accidental heat or traction injury (▸ Fig. 6.4c). Sharp arachnoid dissection is used to widely split the petrosal fissure, proceeding from posterolateral to anteromedial until an optimal entry point is identified along the lateral margin of the MCP, typically superolateral to the vestibulocochlear root entry zone (▸ Fig. 6.4d). Opening the petrosal fissure is akin to a classic sylvian fissure split: a4 branches take the place of M4 branches in guiding dissection, and the semilunar lobules are separated instead of the frontal and temporal lobes. The interlobular triangle is opened as the corridor to the MCP, which provides the corridor's insula-like floor.

Once the petrosal fissure has been opened, neuronavigation guides entry point optimization, and a trajectory is

6

Trans-MCP Approach Overview

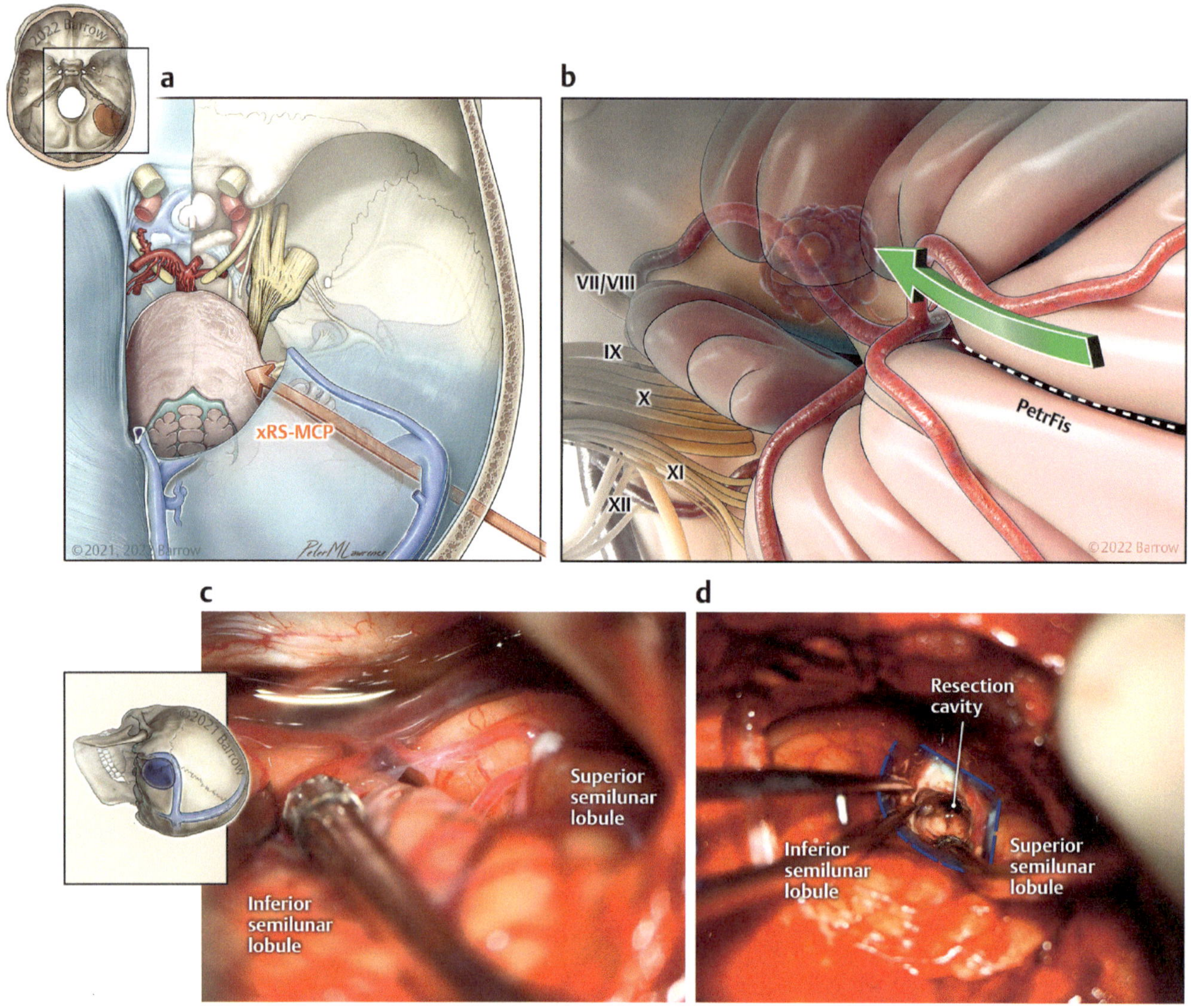

Fig. 6.4 Neuroanatomical and technical overview of the trans-MCP approach for brainstem CM resection. **(a)** Illustration of the superior overview of the surgical trajectory of the xRS trans-MCP approach (*orange arrow*). The *upper left inset* shows the location of the xRS craniotomy. **(b)** Illustration of the left lateral view of the PetrFis, a potential space between the cerebellum's superior and inferior semilunar lobules through which the a3 (flocculopeduncular) segment of the anterior inferior cerebellar artery runs and can be dissected to open the petrosal fissure to reach the CM (*green arrow*). **(c)** Intraoperative view of the left petrosal fissure between the superior and inferior semilunar lobules, as seen through an xRS craniotomy (*lower left inset*). Note the preservation of the arachnoid in the cerebellopontine angle cistern, which protects the lower CNs medially. **(d)** The corridor of the trans-MCP approach is shown inside the interlobular triangle (*blue outline*). The MCP entry point is selected laterally on the MCP, away from CNs VII/VIII. Roman numerals denote CNs. (Reproduced with permission from Barrow Neurological Institute, Phoenix, AZ.)

aligned with the long axis of the brainstem CM. The pial surface is cauterized and opened sharply, after which gentle bimanual spreading dissection with lighted bipolar forceps and a long, microscopic suction tip is used to fashion a narrow corridor to the lesion. Once the CM capsule is identified and opened, hematoma pockets are evacuated, and internal debulking collapses the capsule inward. The separation plane between the CM capsule and the adjacent brainstem is circumferentially dissected, and the lesion is resected (▶ Fig. 6.4d).

Tissue transgression through the MCP that parallels these transverse pontine fibers and remains in the ventral two-thirds of the pons should avoid the corticospinal tracts (CSTs) anteriorly and the pontine tegmentum posteriorly. The most common new or persistent deficit after trans-MCP resection is dysmetria or ataxia, typically attributable to disruption of the afferent cerebellar circuits inhabiting the basis pontis and MCP (▶ Fig. 6.5, ▶ Fig. 6.6). These deficits are typically mild and well tolerated, and they almost always improve with time and therapy (▶ Table 6.1, ▶ Table 6.2).

6.6 Superomedial Trajectory Beyond the SEZ: Superior Cerebellar Peduncle

In contrast to the mild, transient deficits described above, major deficits including severe dysmetria and ataxia, hemiparesis, dysarthric speech, dysphagia, and a decline in modified Rankin Scale score have been observed in a small but important subgroup of patients. The strongest predictor of this unfavorable clinical outcome is the involvement of the contralateral midbrain (▶ Table 6.3). Excursion into the contralateral midbrain requires a steep superomedial trajectory adjacent to the ascending dentatorubral tract in the superior cerebellar peduncle (SCP), which is the major outflow tract of the cerebellum traveling to the thalamus and motor cortex (▶ Fig. 6.7a). Even when the trajectory skirts below the SCP, arrival at the midline transgresses tissue in the axilla of the decussating fibers of the SCP. Anatomically, the inferior pole of the red nucleus resides just above the level of the pontomesencephalic junction, which places the decussation of the SCP in the upper pons (▶ Fig. 6.7b). Therefore, a superomedial trajectory through the MCP can easily intersect the crossing SCP from the opposite side with contralateral dissection of a pontomesencephalic brainstem CM. The low-lying position of the SCP's decussation and its exquisite eloquence explain the association of this trajectory with increased neurological risk.

Unlike subarachnoid dissection, which involves anatomical landmarks, waypoints, and triangles that enable safe and informed travel to deep targets, transparenchymal brainstem dissection offers nothing but white matter. From the SEZ to the CM, neuronavigation and perhaps some hemosiderin staining are the only guides. Diffusion tensor imaging and tractography superimpose neuroanatomical information onto the surgical field, but their accuracy is diminished by CM hemorrhage, surrounding edema, and distortion of tracts by the CM. Neurophysiologic monitoring offers intraoperative feedback, but the SCP cannot be monitored or stimulated directly, and conductive changes in the motor system can be detected only after a costly transgression has been made. Therefore, tissue transgression beyond the SEZ requires heightened anatomical knowledge and spatial awareness of extremely eloquent structures like the SCP.

The SCP is part of the Guillain–Mollaret triangle and comprises the ipsilateral red nucleus, inferior olive, and contralateral dentate nucleus in the cerebellum. Collectively, these structures form the dentato-rubro-olivary pathway, with the SCP connecting the ipsilateral dentate and contralateral red nuclei. Damage within the Mollaret triangle interrupts afferent input to the olivary nucleus with loss of inhibition and hypertrophy followed by atrophy over a 6-month period. This hypertrophic olivary degeneration presents with palatal or oculopalatal myoclonus and lacks an effective treatment. Damage to the SCP can cause Holmes tremor, a rare but well-described phenomenon in which disabling motor symptoms arise after midbrain CM resections, including technically flawless, uncomplicated operations with strict adherence to SEZ principles. This tremor can leave patients dependent and nonfunctional. Lesions that cross the midline require neurosurgeons to cross the midline, which increases the risk of causing bilateral deficits, violating decussating structures, or harming midline fasciculi. This reality was recognized and incorporated in the brainstem CM grading scale, with a point assigned for lesions crossing the axial midpoint. Crossing the SCP represents the greatest risk associated with trans-MCP approaches, and climbing into the axilla of its decussation to reach pontomesencephalic CMs should be done with extreme caution.

6.7 Posteromedial Trajectory Beyond the SEZ: Pontine Tegmentum

The CST is a more recognized determinant of functional outcome than the SCP. It is equally present in the territory of the trans-MCP approach, yet it was not at risk in my surgical

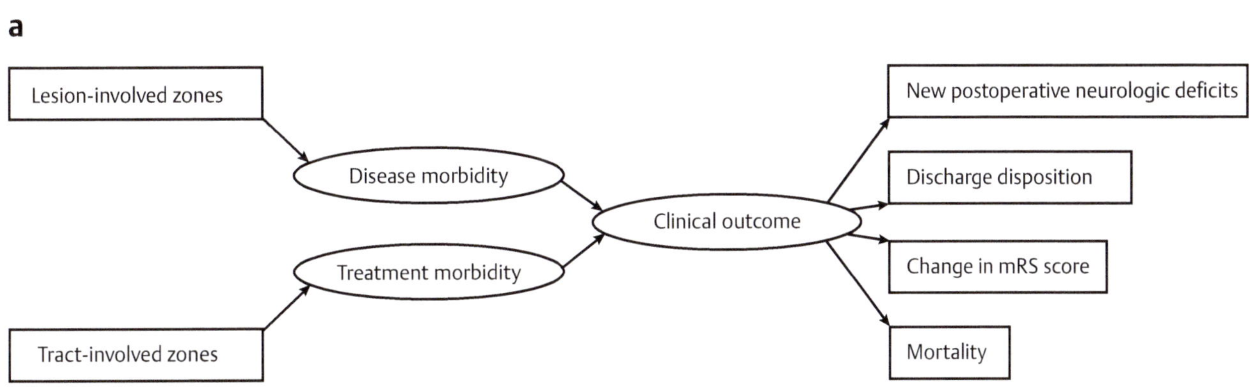

Fig. 6.5 Structural equation modeling and regions of interest (ROIs) for CM involvement. **(a)** Directed acyclic graph for the structural equation modeling analysis of clinical outcomes after trans-MCP resections of brainstem CMs.

(Continued)

6

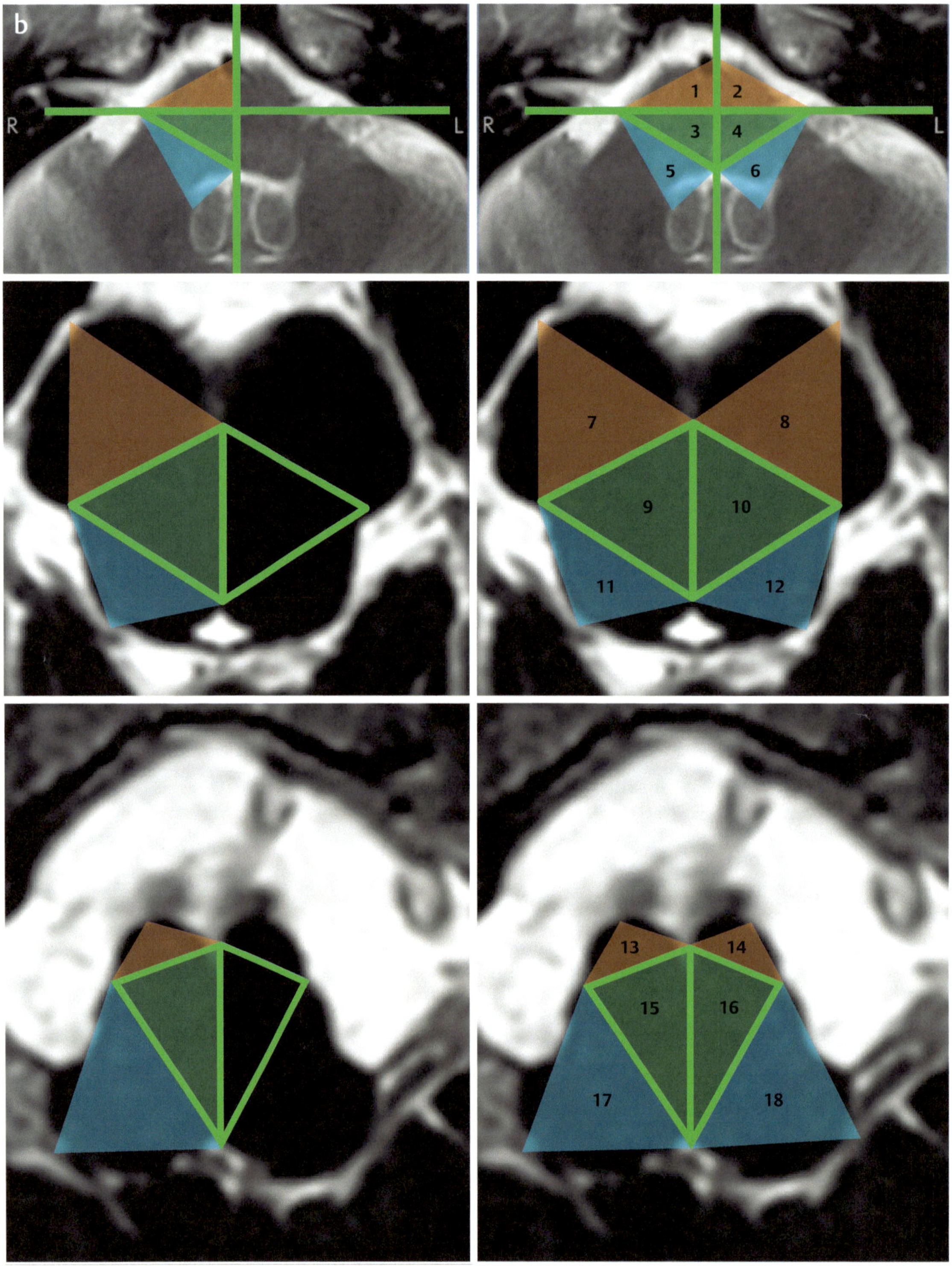

Fig. 6.5 *(Continued)* **(b)** ROIs for assessment of brainstem CM or tract involvement. Six ROIs at each of the three brainstem levels (e.g., pons, midbrain, medulla) were defined in the axial plane using reproducible anatomical landmarks: two each at the anterior (*brown shading*), medial (*green shading*), and posterior (*blue shading*) regions. ROIs for pontine lesions (*upper panels*) were defined by a midline sagittal line, a line between the posterior lip of the internal auditory canals, and lines between the CN VII/VIII root entry zone and the midpoint of the fourth ventricular floor bilaterally (*upper left panel*). Pontine ROIs are numbered 1 to 6 (*upper right panel*). ROIs for pontomesencephalic lesions (*middle panels*) were defined by a midline sagittal line, lines between the lateral mesencephalic sulcus and the interpeduncular midline bilaterally, and lines between the lateral mesencephalic sulcus and the midpoint of the fourth ventricular floor bilaterally (*middle left panel*). Pontomesencephalic ROIs are numbered 7 to 12 (*middle right panel*). ROIs for pontomedullary lesions (*lower panels*) were defined by a midline sagittal line, lines between the preolivary sulcus and the anterior median fissure bilaterally, and lines between the preolivary sulcus and the midpoint of the fourth ventricular floor bilaterally (*lower left panel*). Pontomedullary ROIs are numbered 13 to 18 (*lower right panel*). (Reproduced with permission from Graffeo CS, Srinivasan VM, Scherschinski L, et al. Expanding the reach of the trans-middle cerebellar peduncle approach: pontine cavernous malformations, tissue transgression beyond the safe entry zone, and the invisible triangle. J Neurosurg 2023;140(5):1344–1356.)

a

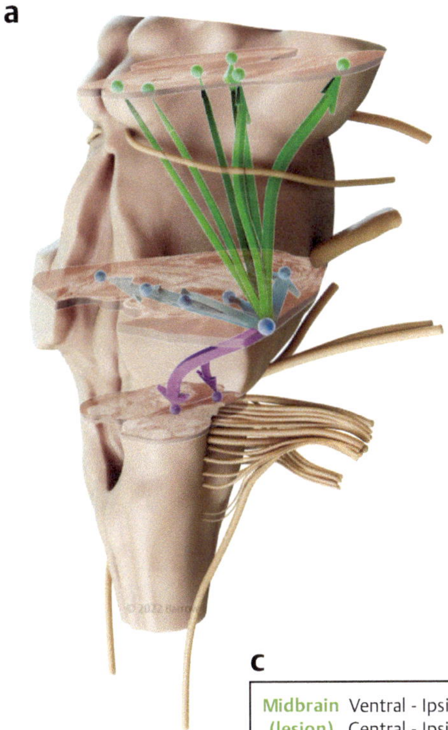

b

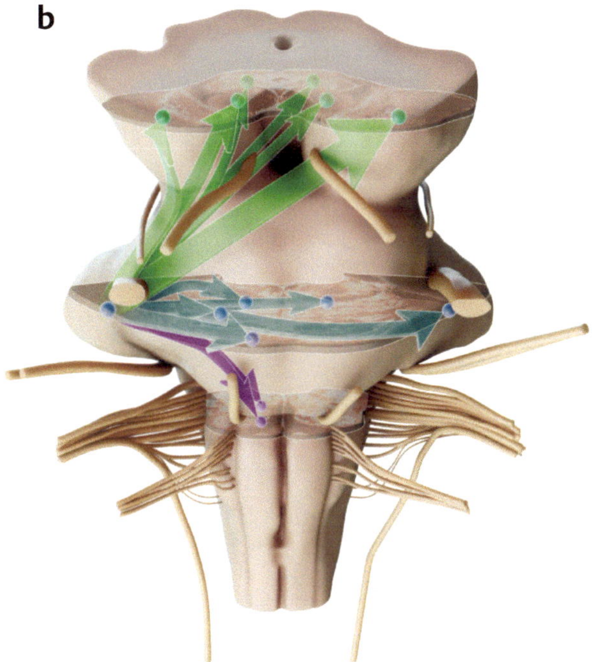

c

Midbrain (lesion)	Ventral - Ipsilateral	11	1	Ventral - Contralateral
	Central - Ipsilateral	13	2	Central - Contralateral
	Dorsal - Ipsilateral	5	1	Dorsal - Contralateral
Pons (lesion)	Ventral - Ipsilateral	18	10	Ventral - Contralateral
	Central - Ipsilateral	25	15	Central - Contralateral
	Dorsal - Ipsilateral	20	2	Dorsal - Contralateral
Medulla (lesion)	Ventral - Ipsilateral	7	1	Ventral - Contralateral
	Central - Ipsilateral	7	4	Central - Contralateral
	Dorsal - Ipsilateral	3	0	Dorsal - Contralateral

d

Lesion		mRS decline		Diplopia		Trigeminal dysfunction		Facial weakness		Hearing loss		Dysarthria		Hemiparesis		Hemisensory deficit		Dysmetria, ataxia		Headache	
		Ipsi	Contra	Ipsi	Contra	Ipsi	Contra	Ipsi	Contra	Ipsi	Contra	Ipsi	Contra	Ipsi	Contra	Ipsi	Contra	Ipsi	Contra	Ipsi	Contra
Midbrain	Ventral	2	0	4	0	4	0	6	0	0	0	3	0	3	0	5	0	8	0	1	0
	Central	2	1	3	1	5	1	5	1	0	0	3	1	3	0	6	1	7	2	1	0
	Dorsal	2	0	1	0	1	0	2	0	0	0	1	0	2	0	1	0	4	0	1	0
Pons	Ventral	2	2	5	3	3	2	8	5	3	0	2	1	5	4	4	3	11	10	4	2
	Central	4	2	8	4	6	3	12	7	3	1	4	1	6	4	8	4	16	10	2	2
	Dorsal	3	1	4	0	2	0	8	1	3	0	2	0	6	1	5	1	12	3	3	0
Medulla	Ventral	2	1	1	0	0	0	4	1	1	0	1	0	4	1	2	0	9	1	0	0
	Central	2	2	2	1	0	0	5	3	1	1	1	0	4	3	3	1	10	8	1	0
	Dorsal	1	0	2	0	0	0	3	0	1	0	0	0	1	0	2	0	6	0	1	0

e

Tract		mRS decline		Diplopia		Trigeminal dysfunction		Facial weakness		Hearing loss		Dysarthria		Hemiparesis		Hemisensory deficit		Dysmetria, ataxia		Headache	
		Ipsi	Contra	Ipsi	Contra	Ipsi	Contra	Ipsi	Contra	Ipsi	Contra	Ipsi	Contra	Ipsi	Contra	Ipsi	Contra	Ipsi	Contra	Ipsi	Contra
Midbrain	Ventral	0	0	0	0	0	0	0	0	0	0	0	0	0	0	0	0	0	0	0	0
	Central	1	0	1	0	0	0	1	0	0	0	1	0	1	0	1	0	1	0	0	0
	Dorsal	0	0	0	0	0	0	0	0	0	0	0	0	0	0	0	0	0	0	0	0
Pons	Ventral	0	0	0	0	0	0	0	0	0	0	0	0	0	0	0	0	0	0	0	0
	Central	0	0	1	0	0	0	0	0	0	0	0	0	0	0	0	0	2	0	0	0
	Dorsal	1	0	3	1	4	0	3	1	1	1	2	0	1	0	3	0	5	0	1	0
Medulla	Ventral	0	0	0	0	0	0	0	0	0	0	0	0	0	0	0	0	0	0	0	0
	Central	0	0	0	0	0	0	0	0	0	0	0	0	0	0	0	0	0	0	0	0
	Dorsal	1	0	0	0	0	0	3	0	1	0	1	0	3	0	1	0	3	0	0	0

Fig. 6.6 Semitransparent three-dimensional images of brainstem neuroanatomy and heat maps of lesions or tracts and postoperative neurological deficits. **(a)** Lateral and **(b)** anteroposterior neuroanatomy with superimposed major axes of a brainstem CM, defined as the longest distance from the MCP entry point to the farthest brainstem region involved with the lesion. *Arrow sizes* correspond to the number of lesions with that major axis. Colors correspond to lesions with dominant involvement of the midbrain (*green*), pons (*blue*), or medulla (*lavender*). **(c)** Simple heat map depicts the number of lesions in each brainstem region, with lower incidences of involvement colored *green* and higher incidences colored *red*. **(d)** Contingency heat map depicts the coincidence of postoperative neurological deficits with involvement of the lesion. **(e)** Corresponding contingency heat map of postoperative neurological deficits with involvement of a tract and no lesion. (Images a and b are reproduced with permission from Barrow Neurological Institute, Phoenix, AZ. Images c–e are reproduced with permission from Graffeo CS, Srinivasan VM, Scherschinski L, et al. Expanding the reach of the trans-middle cerebellar peduncle approach: pontine cavernous malformations, tissue transgression beyond the safe entry zone, and the invisible triangle. J Neurosurg 2023;140(5):1344–1356.)

Table 6.1 Demographic and clinical data of patients ($n = 31$) in a single-surgeon cohort study who underwent brainstem CM resection with a primary trans-MCP approach from July 1, 2017, to June 30, 2021

Parameter	Value
Age at surgery (y), median (IQR)	50 (24–49)
Sex	
Women	19 (61)
Men	12 (39)
Symptomatic CM hemorrhage	29 (94)
Familial cerebral CM syndrome	7 (23)
CM grade, median (range)	4 (1–6)
Gross total resection	29 (94)
Discharge disposition	
Home	19 (61)
Rehabilitation	9 (29)
Skilled nursing facility	3 (10)
Hemorrhage from CM remnant	1 (3.2)
Total follow-up duration (mo), median (IQR)	9 (6–37)

Note: Data are n (%) unless otherwise indicated.

6

Table 6.2 Preoperative and postoperative neurological symptoms among patients ($n = 31$) in a single-surgeon cohort study who underwent brainstem CM resection with a primary trans-MCP approach from July 1, 2017, to June 30, 2021

Parameter	Preoperative	Postoperative	Δ
Diplopia	14 (45)	9 (29)	−5 (−16)
Trigeminal dysfunction	9 (29)	6 (19)	−3 (−10)
Facial weakness	9 (29)	13 (42)	+4 (+13)
Hearing loss	2 (6)	6 (19)	+4 (+13)
Dysphagia or dysarthria	4 (13)	4 (13)	0
Hemiparesis	15 (48)	7 (23)	−8 (−26)
Hemisensory deficit	18 (58)	8 (26)	−10 (−32)
Dysmetria or ataxia	14 (45)	19 (61)	+5 (+16)
mRS score ≤ 2	7 (23)	9 (29)	+2 (+6)
Headache	9 (29)	4 (13)	−5 (−16)
Composite neurological status at last follow-up			
0	N/A	12 (39)	N/A
1	N/A	10 (32)	N/A
2	N/A	5 (16)	N/A
3	N/A	2 (7)	N/A
4	N/A	1 (3)	N/A
5	N/A	0 (0)	N/A
6	N/A	1 (3)	N/A

Note: Data are presented as n (%) unless otherwise indicated.

series of 31 patients who underwent brainstem CM resection with a primary trans-MCP approach from July 1, 2017, to June 30, 2021. This finding was attributed to the importance of the CST in surgical planning. Preoperative magnetic resonance imaging and diffusion tensor imaging tractography localize the CST and facilitate MCP transgression posterior to it. Among 31 patients, hemiparesis was observed in 15 (48%) preoperatively and only 7 (23%) at follow-up, indicating informed avoidance of the CST. However, the looming presence of the CST and its extreme eloquence can redirect tissue transgression more posteriorly through the MCP and result in tissue transgression in the pontine tegmentum, with serious neurological sequelae. Although few, these patients were more likely to have cranial neuropathies involving the facial, abducens, trigeminal, and vestibulocochlear

Table 6.3 Radiographic predictors of unfavorable neurological outcome among patients in a single-surgeon cohort study who underwent brainstem CM resection with a primary trans-MCP approach from July 1, 2017, to June 30, 2021 ($n = 31$)

Lesion and tract location	Involvement			
	Ipsilateral		Contralateral	
	Odds ratio (OR)	*p*-value	OR	*p*-value
Lesion				
Midbrain				
Ventral	0.78	0.63	0.30	0.41
Central	1.85	0.34	7.14	**0.04**
Dorsal	0.36	**0.04**	0.30	0.41
Pons				
Ventral	0.78	0.63	0.79	0.66
Central	1.85	0.34	0.57	0.26
Dorsal	0.36	**0.04**	1.44	0.73
Medulla				
Ventral	0.81	0.73	0.85	0.91
Central	1.17	0.79	1.97	0.37
Dorsal	3.66	0.13	N/A	N/A
Tract				
Midbrain				
Ventral	1.52	0.19	N/A	N/A
Central	1.37	0.26	12.18	**<0.001**
Dorsal	1.05	0.89	N/A	N/A
Pons				
Ventral	0.92	0.75	0.79	0.54
Central	1.51	0.19	0.89	0.66
Dorsal	0.85	0.62	0.73	0.63
Medulla				
Ventral	0.79	0.54	N/A	N/A
Central	0.73	0.41	N/A	N/A
Dorsal	1.31	0.55	N/A	N/A

Note: Bold *p*-values indicate statistical significance ($p < 0.05$).

nerves, in addition to the expected dysmetria or ataxia, corresponding to tissue transgression without a corresponding lesion in the pontine tegmentum (▶ Fig. 6.6; ▶ Table 6.3).

The pontine tegmentum is the dorsal portion of the pons lying between the medial lemniscus and the fourth ventricular floor. In addition to containing the nuclei of cranial nerves V, VI, VII, and VIII, the pontine tegmentum is home to the medial longitudinal fasciculus, paramedian pontine reticular formation, central tegmental tract, reticular formation, tectospinal tract, and medial margin of the SCP, among other structures. Certain patients with symptomatic hemorrhages from middle peduncular CMs that extended into the rhomboid pontine territory were selected for trans-MCP approaches. These patients typically had a thin layer of intact fourth ventricular floor overlying the lesion and lacked the internuclear ophthalmoplegia that accompanies classic rhomboid pontine CMs. The recommended exposure for a purely rhomboid CM, a suboccipital craniotomy with a transventricular approach, would transgress a functional fourth ventricular floor, which could cause morbidity to extraocular eye movements. Instead, the xRS craniotomy with a trans-MCP approach was taken, with a posteromedial trajectory through the pons. These patients did well. They had favorable outcomes associated with posteromedial pontine CM resections, including decreased risk of persistent postoperative deficits and an increased probability of preoperative deficits resolving after surgery. Therefore, middle peduncular or central pontine CMs extending into the rhomboid pontine territory can be well managed with a posteromedially directed trans-MCP approach that cautiously avoids transgressing the pontine tegmentum. Transgressing a greater distance through the MCP (> 1 cm) may be safer than transgressing a lesser distance through the fourth ventricular floor (1–2 mm) when the lesion does not breach the ependymal layer.

6.8 Invisible Triangles

Many safe courses can be charted through the brainstem from a common point of origin on the lateral MCP at the base of the petrosal fissure. The trans-MCP approach is an established

6

Invisible Triangle Anatomy

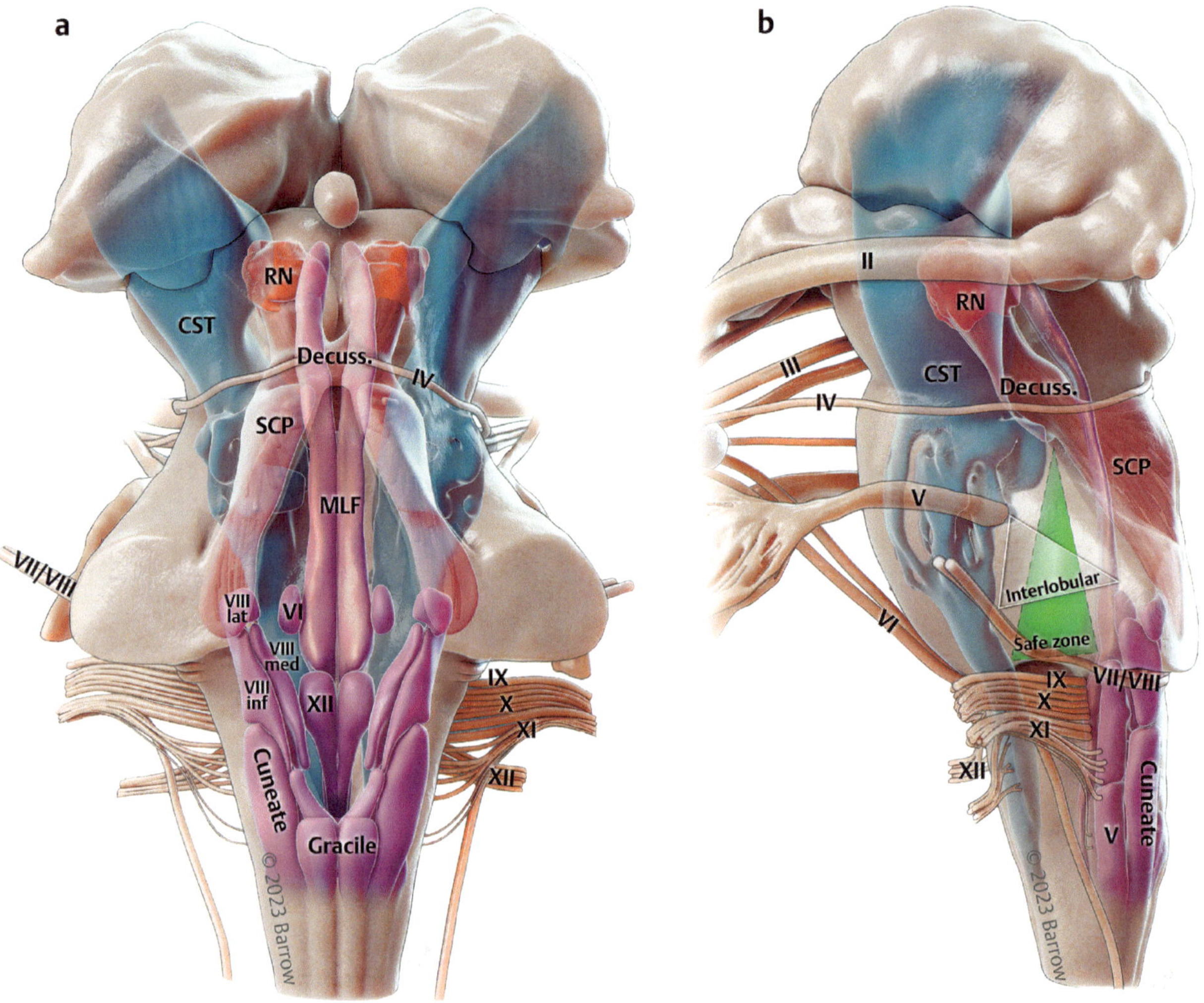

Fig. 6.7 Overview of invisible triangle safe zone. **(a)** Posterior and **(b)** left lateral illustrated neuroanatomical views of the CST (*blue*), dentatorubral tract (*orange*), and nuclei and tracts of the pontine tegmentum (*lavender*). The interlobular triangle defines the surgical corridor through the subarachnoid space, whereas the invisible triangle, depicted as a safe zone (*green triangle*), defines the surgical corridor through the parenchymal white matter. The CST borders this invisible triangle anteriorly, the pontine tegmentum posteromedially, and the SCP and its decussation superomedially. Note that the low-lying position of the axilla of the SCP decussation in the upper pons makes these tracts vulnerable to transgression with superomedial trajectories to reach pontomesencephalic CMs. In addition, the pontine tegmentum occupying the dorsal third of the pons makes its nuclei and tracts vulnerable to transgression with posteromedial trajectories to reach pontine CMs near the fourth ventricular floor. Roman numerals denote CNs. (Reproduced with permission from Barrow Neurological Institute, Phoenix, AZ.)

workhorse for CMs in the lateral and central pons, and this accessible, laterally situated SEZ opens an extraordinary range of trajectories through superior, inferior, and posterior angulations. Most deep pontine CMs, including large lesions, those with contralateral or posterior extension, and others extending into the midbrain and medulla, can be resected safely with the trans-MCP approach. Three critical boundaries for tissue transgression associated with neurological sequela have been identified: the CST anteriorly, the SCP superomedially, and the pontine tegmentum posteromedially. Together, these structures form a surgical triangle within the pontine white matter that represents a safe zone, outside of which is a no-transgression zone (▸ Fig. 6.7b). Iatrogenic harm can happen when the trans-MCP approach is pushed to these limits, with tissue transgression at the boundaries of this invisible triangle (▸ Fig. 6.8).

The CST-SCP-tegmentum triangle resides within the white matter, unlike other triangles in the system of brainstem CM triangles. It lacks visible anatomical landmarks, making it akin to the Mollaret rather than Kawase triangle. Unfortunately, novel waypoints could not be devised for this corridor using its surface anatomy, like the trigeminal root entry zone and flocculus. Neurosurgeons should embrace the trans-MCP approach

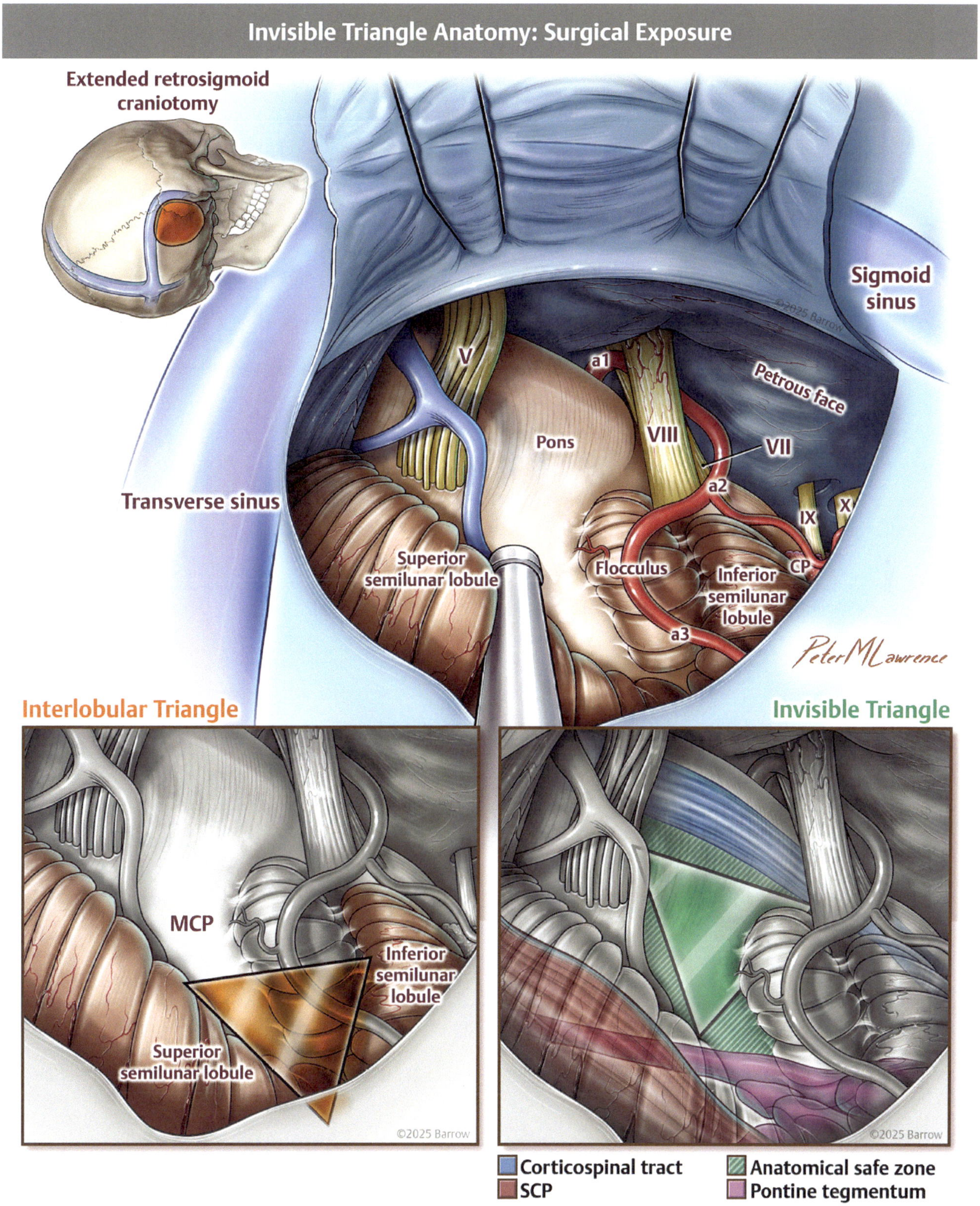

Fig. 6.8 Anatomy of the invisible, or CST-SCP-tegmentum triangle. Overview of the surgical exposure of the xRS craniotomy and trans-MCP approach, as seen in this right-sided exposure (*upper left inset*). The MCP SEZ is laterally located and accessed through the interlobular triangle (*lower left inset*; *orange triangle*). Once the middle peduncular white matter is entered, tissue transgression must respect the boundaries of the invisible triangle (*lower right inset*; *green triangle*), namely the corticospinal tract anteriorly (*blue*), pontine tegmentum posteromedially (*purple*), and the SCP and its decussation superomedially (*orange*). The flocculus anatomy varies and forms the inferior border of this space. Although this CST-SCP-tegmentum space (*lined green area*) is not triangular, the lack of visible anatomical landmarks within the white matter mandates confinement within the invisible triangle to keep safe distances from these eloquent structures. Roman numerals denote CNs. (Reproduced with permission from Barrow Neurological Institute, Phoenix, AZ.)

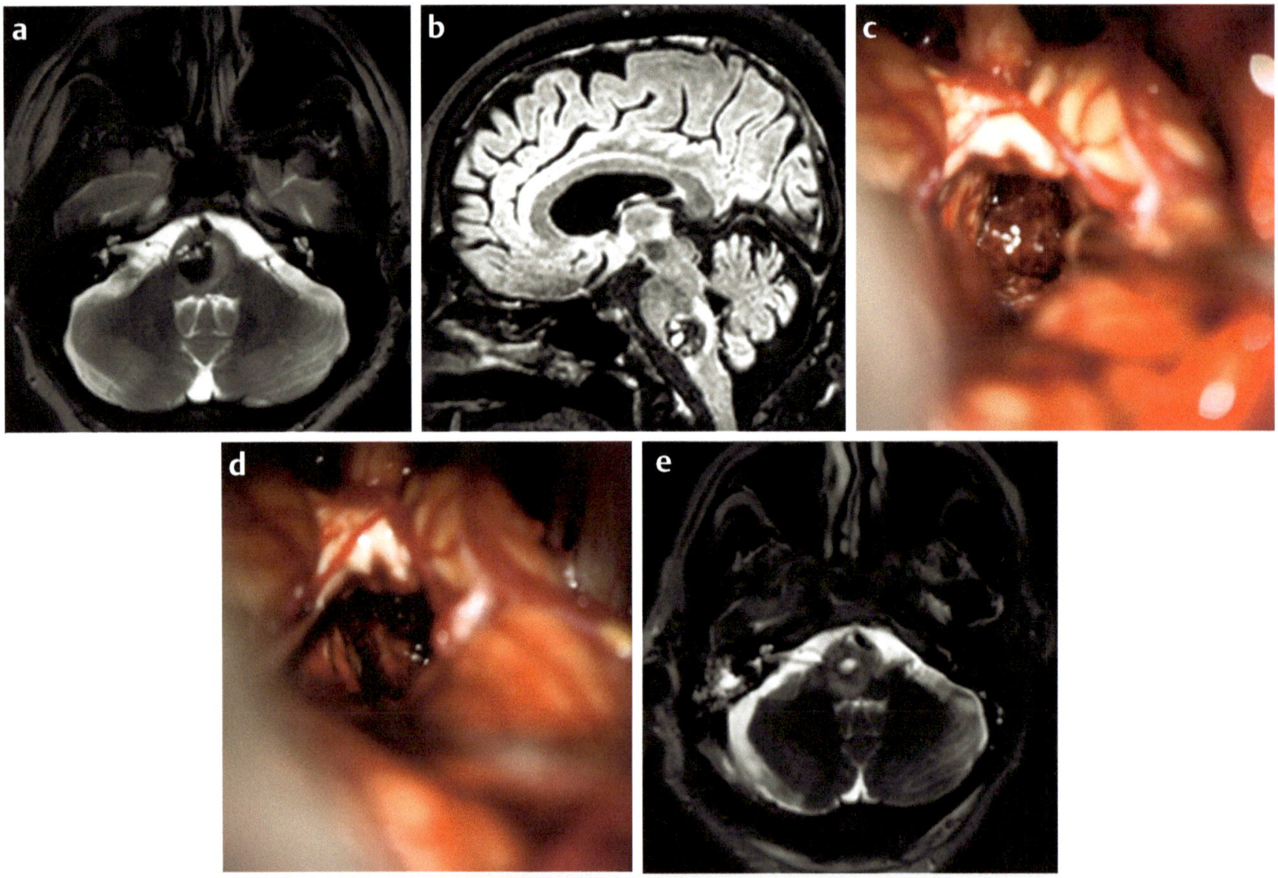

Fig. 6.9 Illustrative case 1. T2-weighted **(a)** axial and **(b)** sagittal fluid-attenuated inversion recovery magnetic resonance imaging demonstrates a heterogeneous, mixed-intensity mass lesion involving the central aspects of the inferior pons and superior medulla. Intraoperative still photographs highlight the trans-MCP corridor into **(c)** the CM and **(d)** the resection cavity after removal of the CM. **(e)** Gross total resection was radiographically confirmed, as shown on T2-weighted axial MRI. (Reproduced with permission from Graffeo CS, Srinivasan VM, Scherschinski L, et al. Expanding the reach of the trans-middle cerebellar peduncle approach: pontine cavernous malformations, tissue transgression beyond the safe entry zone, and the invisible triangle. J Neurosurg 2023;140(5):1344–1356.)

and meticulously study the neuroanatomy of the CST, SCP, and pontine tegmentum. They must steer the transgressive corridor centrally through the triangle toward the MCP's transverse pontine fibers to reach targeted CMs. The dissection task is to work the peripheral margins of the lesion into the central corridor of the triangle rather than transgress the tissue close to these margins. The extreme eloquence of the CST should not push neurosurgeons out of the safe zone of the basis pontis and too far posteriorly into the pontine tegmentum (▶ Fig. 6.9). Neurosurgeons should beware of crossing the SCP when reaching upward toward midbrain CMs (▶ Fig. 6.10). Finally, neurosurgeons should beware of entering the pontine tegmentum when reaching posteriorly to the rhomboid portion of these lesions.

6.9 Orienteering Beyond

This detailed discussion of the trans-MCP approach emphasizes the importance of what happens between the SEZ and cavernoma resection. SEZs are described in exquisite anatomical detail as linear incisions in the brainstem. However, the transgression through tissue beyond the SEZ significantly affects the outcome. Unlike subarachnoid dissection, which is conducted in an air medium with illumination and perspective, transparenchymal dissection is conducted through white matter with no landmarks or perspective. Brain transgression is at the opposite end of the spectrum from subarachnoid dissection, without natural corridors, obvious triangles, and arterial waypoints. Consequently, safely transgressing brain tissue requires an orienteering mentality, which means knowledge of an SEZ that includes the incision line, the underlying tracts and nuclei, and the trajectory needed to evade those tracts and nuclei. False competence comes from learning the SEZs; true competence comes from knowing the anatomy beneath the SEZ and how to navigate through that tissue. Neuronavigation lacks this anatomical detail.

The invisible triangle is a powerful idea because it is a construct in the mind of the neurosurgeon. Technology cannot inject this image into the neurosurgeon's ocular display or project it onto the surgical field. Neurosurgeons must create these

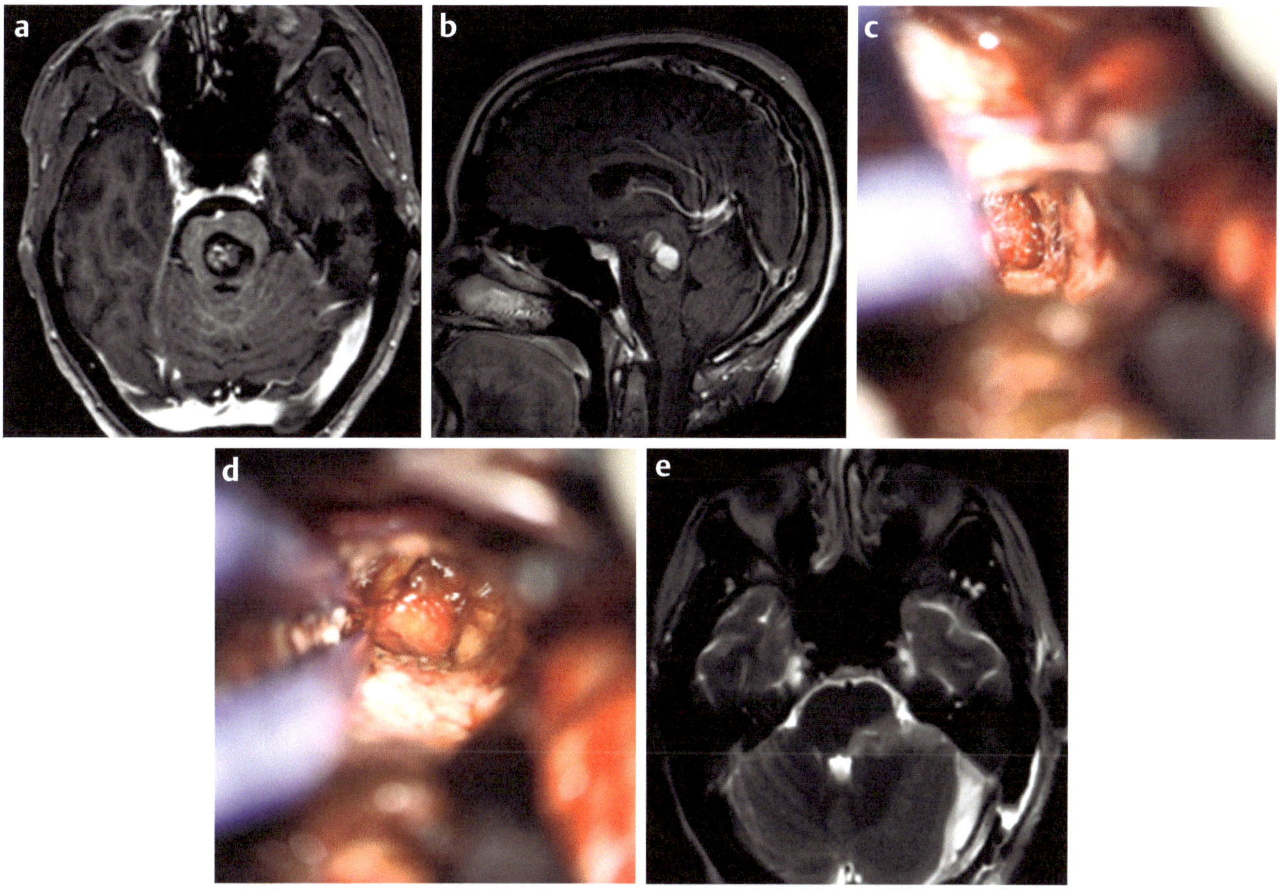

Fig. 6.10 Illustrative case 2. T1-weighted contrast-enhanced **(a)** axial and **(b)** sagittal MRI slices demonstrate a heterogeneous, mixed-intensity, partially enhancing mass lesion involving the central aspects of the superior pons and inferior midbrain. **(c)** Intraoperative still photographs highlight the trans-MCP corridor into the CM and **(d)** the resection cavity after removal of the CM. **(e)** Gross total resection was radiographically confirmed, as shown on T2-weighted axial MRI. (Reproduced with permission from Graffeo CS, Srinivasan VM, Scherschinski L, et al. Expanding the reach of the trans-middle cerebellar peduncle approach: pontine cavernous malformations, tissue transgression beyond the safe entry zone, and the invisible triangle. J Neurosurg 2023;140(5):1344–1356.)

triangles and no-transgression zones in their mind's eye and beware when operating without seeing them. This orienteering mentality goes well beyond the practice of following arrows and lines on navigation displays. This chapter focuses on the trans-MCP approach and the CST-SCP-pontine tegmentum triangle within the pontine white matter as an example of this point, but there are other constructs elsewhere in the brain and more to be discovered. These insights about safe tissue transgression elevate cavernoma resection beyond simple subarachnoid dissection. The day will come when technology does this work for us with augmented reality built into our operating microscopes. Neurosurgeons will have the library of visible and invisible triangles scaled and superimposed onto the surgical field as they operate. For now, we must work diligently to discern and comprehend this anatomy and build mental constructs that make us better neurosurgeons to optimize patient outcomes.

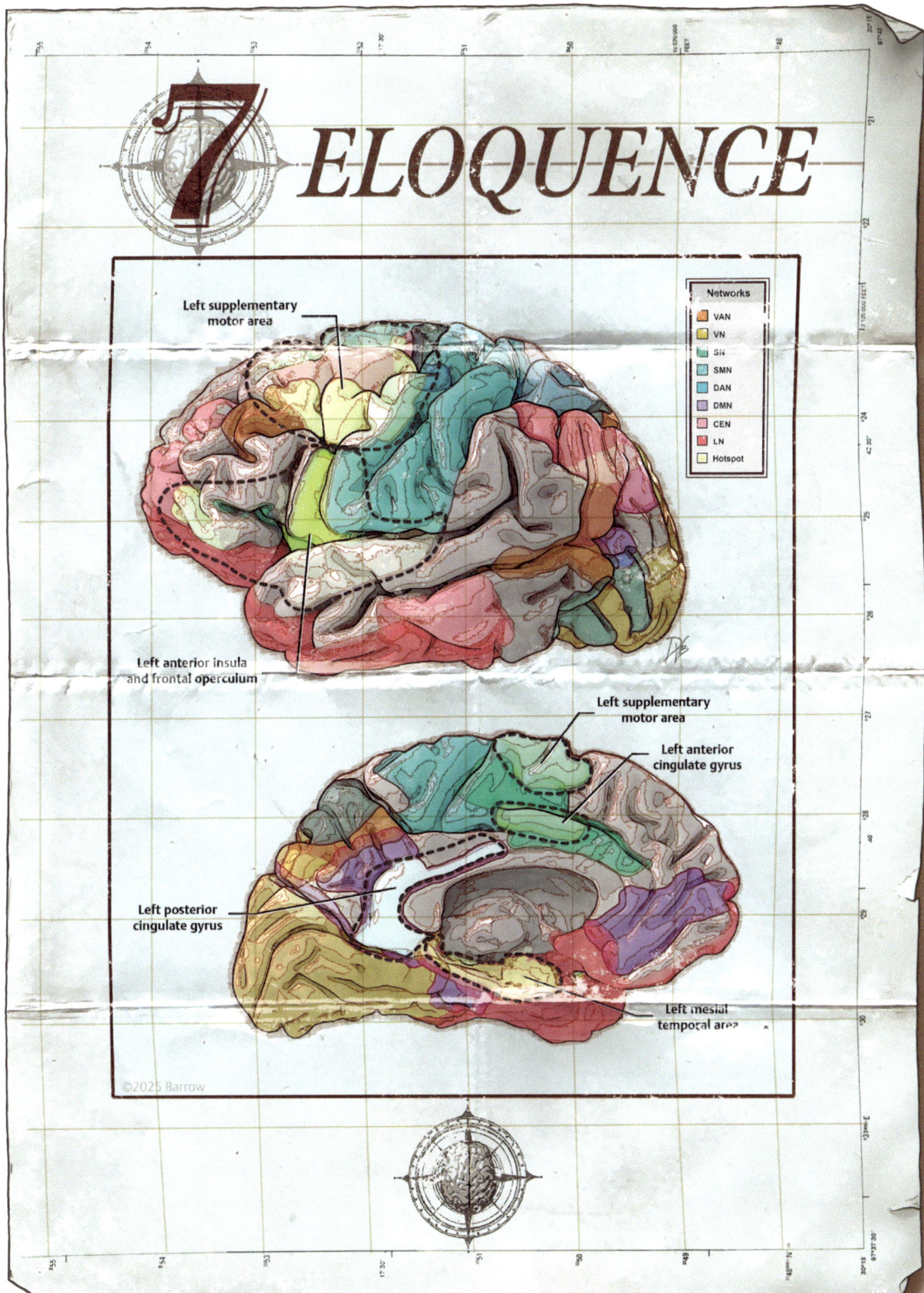

Reproduced with permission from Barrow Neurological Institute, Phoenix, AZ.

7 Eloquent Noneloquence

Summary

"Humans use only 10% of their brains" is an often quoted but misguided saying. As inaccurate as this 10% myth seems to neurosurgeons, our concept of brain eloquence is strikingly similar. The Human Connectome Project has transformed our understanding of brain circuitry and led to the discovery of large-scale brain networks, including the (1) default mode network, (2) central executive network, (3) salience network, (4) dorsal attention network, (5) sensorimotor network, (6) visual network, and (7) limbic/paralimbic network. Mapping suggests that the entire cerebrum is involved in cognitive function, contradicting our neurosurgical conception of eloquence. Today, we must ask: Are areas long considered noneloquent truly eloquent, and is any cortex noneloquent? The answers have a profound bearing on surgical strategy. We should be able to improve our microsurgical techniques and patient outcomes by minimizing transgression through these hotspots of *eloquent noneloquence*. Microsurgical cavernous malformation (CM) resection provides a unique opportunity to study these hotspots. In a recent study, postoperative outpatient clinic records of 362 CM resections were analyzed for cognitive deficits. Machine learning analyses of lesion objects and trajectory cylinder mapping identified seven hotspots of novel eloquent noneloquence: the (1) supplementary motor area (bilateral), (2) anterior cingulate cortex (bilateral), (3) posterior cingulate cortex (bilateral), (4) anterior insula (left), (5) frontal pole (right), (6) mesial temporal lobe (left), and (7) occipital cortex (right). The imperative not to transgress the eloquent cortex led to transgression of these hotspots, contributing to poor outcomes based on modified Rankin Scale scores. The seven hotspots long considered by neurosurgeons to be noneloquent cerebral safe entry zones are, in fact, eloquent and unsafe for transgression. These hotspots redefine our neurosurgical conception of eloquence and suggest more refined transcortical dissection techniques are needed to maximize transsulcal dissection, intracapsular resection, and tissue preservation for better patient outcomes.

Keywords: cavernous malformation, central executive network, default mode network, Human Connectome Project, limbic network, paralimbic network, sensorimotor network, supplementary motor area, visual network

7.1 Ten Percent Myth

The often-quoted statement that "humans use only 10% of their brains" is a false attribution to Albert Einstein or a misinterpretation of William James's work. This misguided saying suggests that parts of the brain with distinct and important functions, like the primary motor, sensory, and visual cortexes, are islands in the sea of an otherwise-unused brain. As inaccurate as this 10% myth may seem to neurosurgeons, our concept of brain eloquence is strikingly similar. When Spetzler and Martin incorporated the eloquence of the brain adjacent to an arteriovenous malformation (AVM) as one of three variables in their grading system for predicting the risk of microsurgical AVM resection, only the sensorimotor, visual, and language cortexes were included in their definition of eloquent cortex. Implicit in this definition was that other cortical areas are noneloquent and could be transgressed with impunity.

The Human Connectome Project transformed our understanding of brain circuitry by mapping short- and long-range bundles of nerve fibers interconnecting regions of the brain structurally and functionally in over 1,000 human participants using sophisticated imaging technologies like high-resolution magnetic resonance imaging (MRI), resting-state and task-based functional MRI (fMRI), diffusion MRI, magnetoencephalography, and electroencephalography (EEG). The Human Connectome Project and connectomics led to the discovery of large-scale brain networks, which are widespread, seemingly unrelated brain regions or parcels anatomically wired together with synchronized activity. Many large-scale brain networks have been identified: (1) the default mode network (DMN), (2) the salience network (SN), (3) the dorsal attention network (DAN), (4) the central executive network (CEN), (5) the sensorimotor network (SMN), (6) the visual network (VN), and (7) the limbic and paralimbic network (LN). Cognition can be understood not as individual parcels working in isolation but as multiple parcels in a network firing together and multiple networks working with orchestrated interactivity. Higher cognitive function may result from tightly coordinated electrical signaling between these networks. Conversely, neuropsychiatric disorders such as depression, anxiety, autism, and schizophrenia may be the result of dyscoordination and disruption of signaling between networks.

Surveying the map of large-scale brain networks suggests that every cortical parcel is part of a network, and the entire cerebrum is involved in cognitive function. This finding is at odds with our neurosurgical conception of eloquence and raises questions: Is any cortex noneloquent, and for neurosurgeons, are areas long considered noneloquent truly eloquent? The answers have a profound impact on surgical strategy, and consequently, technology has emerged to integrate brain networks into preoperative planning and intraoperative navigation. Quicktome (Omniscient Neurotechnology) is an example that uses resting-state MRI to build patient-specific brain maps, including network templates, constrained spherical deconvolution-based tractography, and structural connectivity atlases. Informed neurosurgical decision-making that preserves brain networks during transcortical procedures is a step toward modernizing our conception of eloquence and incorporating it into contemporary neurosurgical practice.

7.2 Eloquent Noneloquence

Cerebral cavernous malformations (CMs) are pathological lesions that cause discrete cortical disruption with hemorrhage, and the transcortical resection of these lesions can cause additional iatrogenic disruption. Therefore, a collection of microsurgically treated CMs provides a unique opportunity to study areas of *eloquent noneloquence*. Neurosurgeons plan their resections to avoid transgressing eloquent brain tissue, instead selecting alternative routes through noneloquent tissue that reach the target. An assessment of neurological and cognitive morbidity in these patients could identify areas thought to be cortical safe entry zones (SEZs) that are not safe but eloquent. Like established SEZs for brainstem CMs, cortical SEZs must be areas of true noneloquence that can be transgressed to access the pathology.

Can cortical SEZs be established for cerebral CMs as the areas around and away from eloquent noneloquence? Recently, results from a large patient series of superficial cerebral CMs that Robert F. Spetzler and I resected microsurgically at two large institutions were analyzed using a combination of traditional neurological outcome measures, additional measures to detect functional decline, Quicktome algorithms, and sophisticated machine learning techniques. The neurosurgical conception of eloquence can be redefined by mapping hotspots or cortical areas of eloquence in areas formerly considered to be noneloquent. Perhaps we can improve our microsurgical techniques and patient outcomes by minimizing transgression through these hotspots of eloquent noneloquence.

7.3 Clinical Evidence

Patients from a consecutive microsurgical series of superficial cerebral CMs at our center over a 13-year period (November 2008 through June 2021) were retrospectively analyzed. Neurological outcomes were measured with the modified Rankin Scale (mRS), and new, permanent neurological or cognitive symptoms not detected by changes in mRS scores were measured as additional functional decline. Symptoms indicating functional decline included new sensory, motor, cranial nerve, and speech deficits. Cognitive deficits in learning, memory, motor planning, attention, and social function were identified in outpatient clinic records by any of the following: (1) the need for rehabilitation or physical therapy beyond 6 weeks postoperatively, (2) additional MRI after the routine 6-month surveillance, (3) additional office visits after the routine 6-month follow-up, and (4) referrals to neuropsychologists or psychiatrists. Virtual object models for CMs and approach trajectories to subcortical lesions were merged into a template brain model for subtyping and Quicktome connectomic analyses. Parcellation outputs from the models were analyzed for regional cerebral clustering.

Overall, 362 superficial cerebral CMs were resected in 346 patients, and convexity subtypes were the most common (132/362, 36.5%; ▶ Table 7.1). Relative to the preoperative mRS score, 327 of 362 cases (90.3%) improved or remained stable, 35 (9.7%) worsened, and 47 (13.0%) had additional functional decline. Machine learning analyses of lesion objects (▶ Fig. 7.1) and trajectory cylinder mapping (▶ Fig. 7.2) identified seven

Table 7.1 Cerebral CM subtypes by patient outcome status

Subtype	Total CMs (*n* = 362)	CMs by patient outcome				
		Improved/unchanged	Worsened	Additional decline	Unfavorable	Favorable
Frontal	155/362 (42.8)	140/327 (42.8)	15/35 (42.9)	18/47 (38.3)	33/82 (40.2)	122/280 (43.6)
Medial	42/155 (27.1)	38/140 (27.1)	4/15 (26.7)	6/18 (33.3)	10/33 (30.3)	32/122 (26.2)
Convexity	56/155 (36.1)	52/140 (37.1)	4/15 (26.7)	7/18 (38.9)	11/33 (36.7)	45/122 (36.9)
Basal	34/155 (21.9)	29/140 (20.7)	5/15 (33.3)	2/18 (11.1)	7/33 (21.2)	27/122 (22.1)
Sylvian	23/155 (14.8)	21/140 (15.0)	2/15 (13.3)	3/18 (16.7)	5/33 (15.2)	18/122 (14.8)
Parietal	89/362 (24.6)	76/327 (23.2)	13/35 (37.1)	10/47 (21.3)	23/82 (28.0)	66/280 (23.6)
Medial	24/89 (27.0)	22/76 (28.9)	2/13 (15.4)	2/10 (20.0)	4/23 (17.4)	20/66 (30.3)
Convexity	32/89 (36.0)	27/76 (35.5)	5/13 (38.5)	5/10 (50.0)	10/23 (43.5)	22/66 (33.3)
Sylvian	33/89 (37.1)	27/76 (35.5)	6/13 (46.2)	3/10 (30.0)	9/23 (39.1)	24/66 (36.4)
Occipital	31/362 (8.6)	29/327 (8.9)	2/35 (5.7)	2/47 (4.3)	4/82 (4.9)	27/280 (9.6)
Medial	5/31 (16.1)	5/29 (17.2)	0/2 (0)	0/2 (0)	0/4 (0)	5/27 (18.5)
Convexity	14/31 (45.2)	13/29 (44.8)	1/2 (50)	1/2 (50.0)	2/4 (50)	12/27 (44.4)
Basal	12/31 (38.7)	11/29 (37.9)	1/2 (50)	1/2 (50.0)	2/4 (50)	10/27 (37.0)
Temporal	87/362 (24.0)	82/327 (25.1)	5/35 (14.3)	17/47 (36.2)	22/82 (26.8)	65/280 (23.2)
Medial	7/87 (8.0)	6/82 (7.3)	1/5 (20.0)	2/17 (11.8)	3/22 (13.6)	4/65 (6.2)
Convexity	30/87 (34.5)	28/82 (34.1)	2/5 (40.0)	2/17 (11.8)	4/22 (18.2)	26/65 (40.0)
Basal	26/87 (29.9)	26/82 (31.7)	0/5 (0)	9/17 (52.9)	9/22 (40.9)	17/65 (26.2)
Sylvian	24/87 (27.6)	22/82 (26.8)	2/5 (40.0)	4/17 (23.5)	6/22 (27.3)	18/65 (27.7)
Total	362/362 (100)	327/362 (90.3)	35/362 (9.7)	47/362 (13.0)	82/362 (22.7)	280/362 (77.3)

Note: All data are presented as proportion (%).

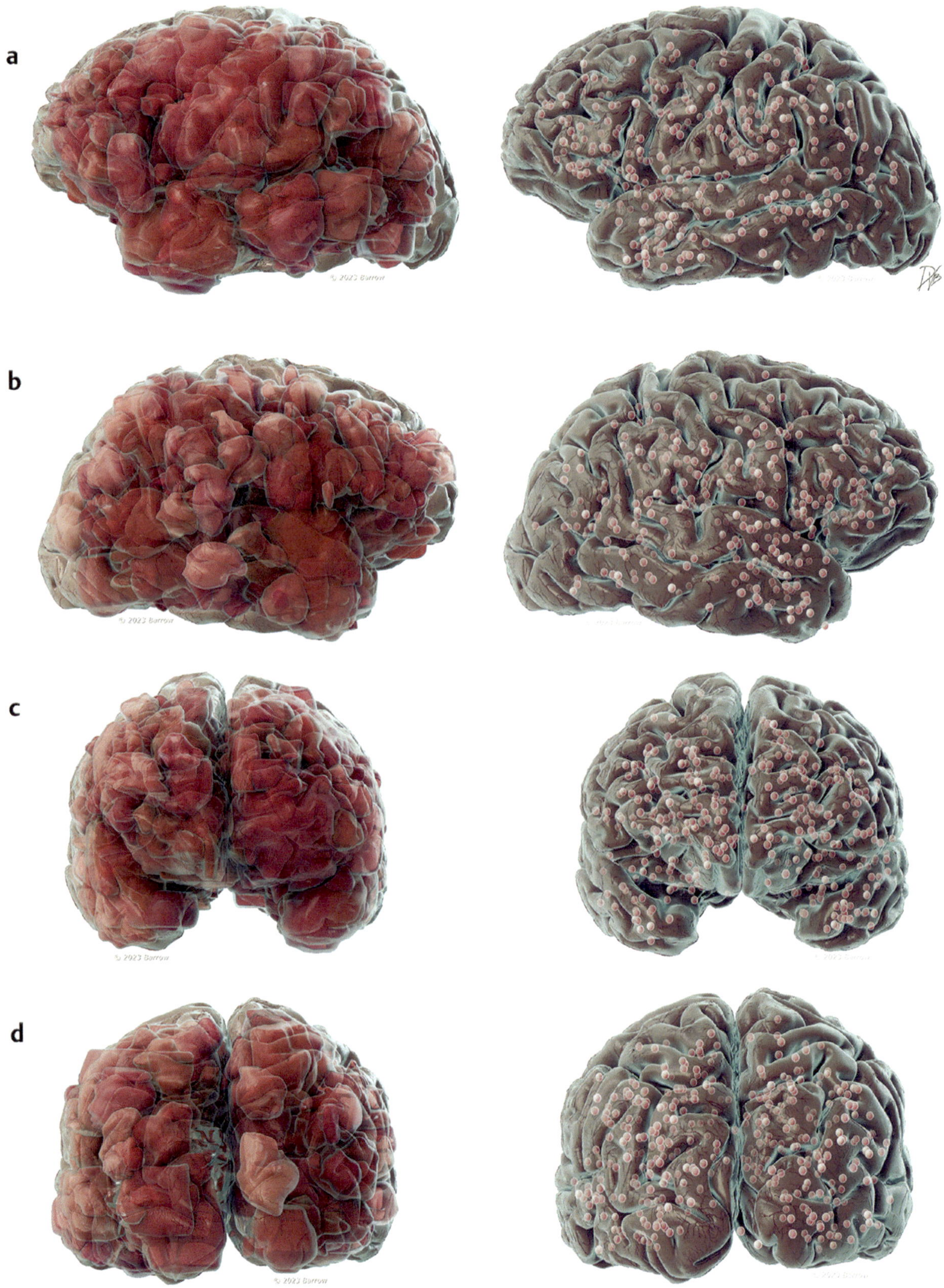

Fig. 7.1 Cerebral CM mapping. **(a)** Left and **(b)** right lateral views and **(c)** anterior and **(d)** posterior views showing individual virtual cerebral CMs mapped to the cerebral model template. *Left*: Volumetric extent of each CM. *Right*: Location of each CM as shown by uniform spheres. (Reproduced with permission from Barrow Neurological Institute, Phoenix, AZ.)

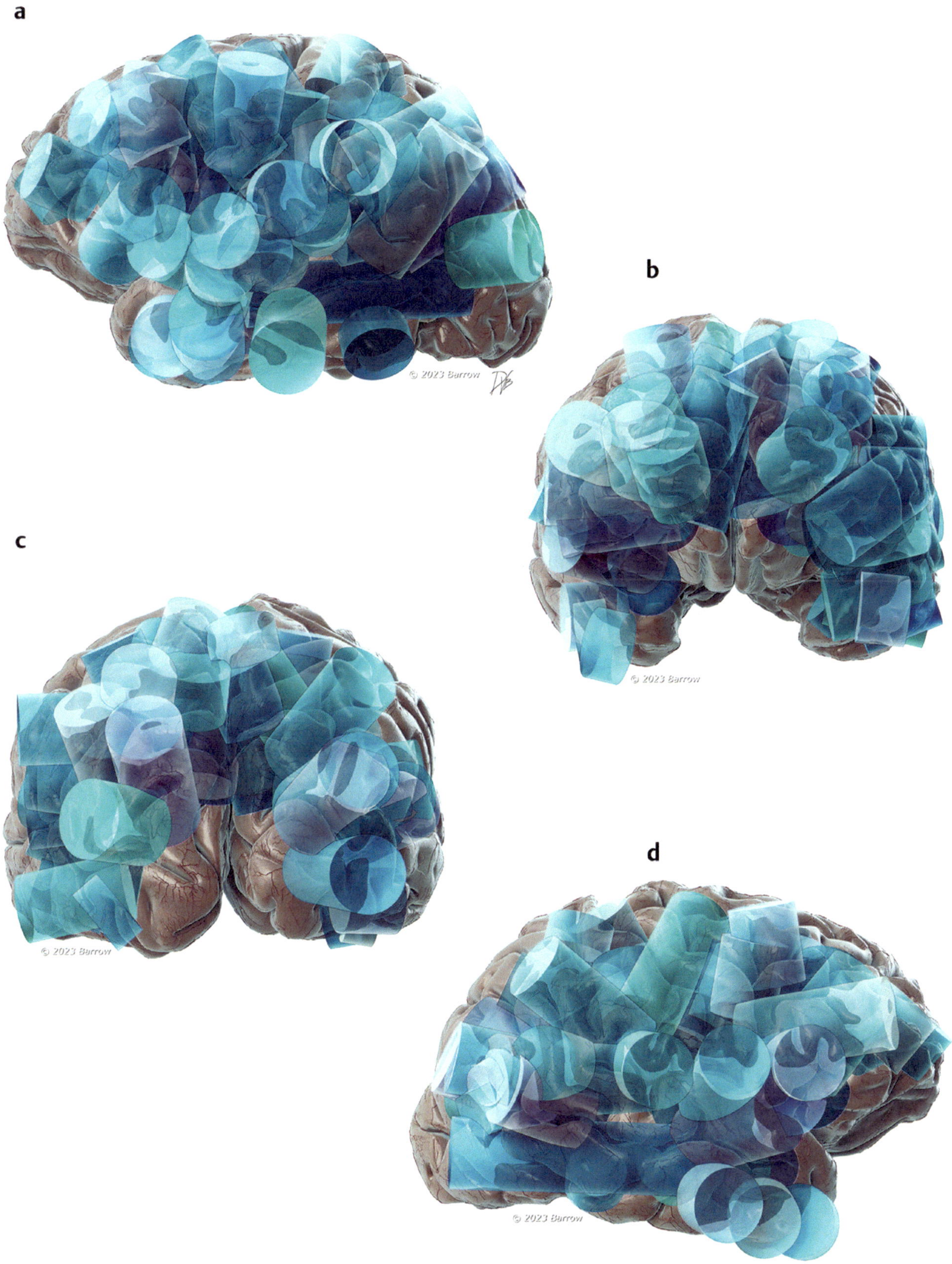

Fig. 7.2 Cerebral approach mapping. **(a)** Left lateral, **(b)** anterior, **(c)** posterior, and **(d)** right lateral views showing the deep CM approach trajectories. Each approach is represented as a cylinder with a diameter of 2 cm. (Reproduced with permission from Barrow Neurological Institute, Phoenix, AZ.)

hotspots of novel eloquence (▶ Fig. 7.3): the (1) supplementary motor area (SMA, bilateral), (2) anterior cingulate cortex (bilateral), (3) posterior cingulate cortex (bilateral), (4) anterior insula (left), (5) frontal pole (right), (6) mesial temporal lobe (left), and (7) occipital cortex (right).

7.4 Eloquent Cortex

Eloquence is defined as discourse marked by force and persuasiveness or the art of using such discourse. The cortex that directly controls a distinct and important function like motion or language and whose damage produces a focal neurological deficit is also described as eloquent. Although brain tissue is incapable of forceful discourse per se, the concept of the eloquent cortex is deeply engrained in the neurosurgical lexicon. Korbinian Brodmann used Nissl staining to define 52 cortical regions based on cytoarchitecture, associating eloquent functions like speech with areas 44 and 45 (Broca's area) and areas 39 and 40 (Wernicke's area). Wilder Penfield mapped the cerebral cortex with direct electrical stimulation of the brain and demonstrated that motor and sensory function was organized somatotopically in the cortex to an extent that varied in proportion to its importance and complexity, as captured by the homunculus. Spetzler and Martin incorporated eloquence in their AVM grading system, including sensorimotor, visual, and language cortex in their definition of eloquent cortex. These memorable heuristics are so engrained that neurosurgeons have a heightened awareness of these classically eloquent regions and, consequently, plan transcortical surgery to avoid their transgression. Neurosurgeons who transgress these eloquent regions quickly learn from their mistakes and avoid them next time. Our experience with superficial cerebral CMs demonstrated strict avoidance of classically eloquent cortex with, for example, only 16 of 362 (4.4%) approaches through pre- or postcentral gyrus or central sulcus. Instead, routes were selected further anteriorly or posteriorly. Alternatively, patients with CMs in classically eloquent areas were observed.

Despite the imperative not to transgress the eloquent cortex, we observed poor outcomes based on mRS scores in 6.9% of cases (25/362) and worsened outcomes in 9.7% (35/362) cases. To uncover the broader impact of CM resection, we included another 13.0% (47/362) of cases with additional functional decline, raising the overall unfavorable outcome rate to 22.7% (82/362). With this more critical assessment of outcomes, a more extensive cerebral parcel map was constructed that better identified areas of microsurgical risk or eloquent noneloquence. It is widely accepted that brainstem CM surgery is performed optimally by maximizing subarachnoid dissection to determine where the CM comes to a pial surface to minimize brain tissue transgression. Similarly, cerebral CM surgery is optimized by maximizing transsulcal dissection, shortening the distance to the CM, and minimizing the extent of cortical transgression. We can extrapolate our experience in the brainstem and define cortical SEZs when tissue transgression is unavoidable. We found that cortical SEZs are fewer in number and less safe than expected. Thus, many supposedly noneloquent areas were, in fact, eloquent. The inadequacies of bedside assessments and traditional outcome measures have created a false sense of safety in transcortical surgery. fMRI and connectomics now inform us that large-scale brain networks occupy domains previously considered noneloquent. Dissection through these regions may not be the safe passage previously expected, and flawed or outdated notions of eloquence may explain the functional and cognitive consequences observed in our patients.

7.5 Large-Scale Brain Networks

Large-scale brain networks (▶ Fig. 7.4), or intrinsic brain networks, are collections of regions throughout the brain connected structurally and functionally as demonstrated by fMRI BOLD (blood oxygen level–dependent) signal or other modalities like positron emission tomography, magnetoencephalography, or EEG. These widespread parcellations or nodes have interconnecting white matter tracts and exhibit synchronized activity during complex tasks. Large-scale brain networks include seven major networks (DMN, CEN or control, SN, DAN, SMN, VN, and LN) as well as other networks (ventral attention network [VAN], language, accessory language, auditory, multiple demand, and medial temporal networks). The areas of unexpected surgical morbidity in our cerebral parcel map for eloquence may appear random (▶ Table 7.2, ▶ Table 7.3) but are understandable from the perspective of large-scale network disruption. Parcellations with high feature importance are parts of the central core of key networks or connect that network to others (i.e., hubness; ▶ Table 7.4, ▶ Table 7.5, ▶ Table 7.6).

The DMN is one of the largest networks based on cortical territory and is active when the individual is awake, at rest, and engaged in the internal activity of the mind, which includes daydreaming, passive sensory processing, envisioning, and memory retrieval. This network is one of the most active, working when the individual is not engaged in external tasks (task-negative system) or focused on external visual signals. The DMN is centered in the medial frontoparietal cortex, but its parcellations extend throughout all lobes and surfaces.

The CEN initiates and modulates cognitive control and is associated with intelligence, thought, decision-making, and executive function. This network works when the individual is engaged in external tasks (task-positive system) and is inversely associated with the activity of the DMN. External thinking during active tasks, planning, and problem-solving requires working memory and attention, thereby engaging other key networks simultaneously. The CEN is located in the bilateral frontal and parietal convexities.

The SN monitors the significance of external and internal inputs, directing engagement by identifying important biological activity and cognitive events. The SN acts as a switch that transitions between the resting state of the DMN and the active state of the CEN, activating and deactivating these two key networks. The SN monitors the external world to decide how other networks react to new information and stimuli. Pain sensation, emotions, and motivational states are surveyed, and the activity of other networks is modulated accordingly to establish the brain's reaction to these inputs. The SN is centered in the anterior cingulate cortex and anterior insula.

The DAN actively orients and holds attention during goal-directed tasks and executive functions. Top-down processing is the intentional control of behavior or performance that enables the individual to focus on an activity and ignore environmental or biological stimuli or noise. In contrast, bottom-up processing

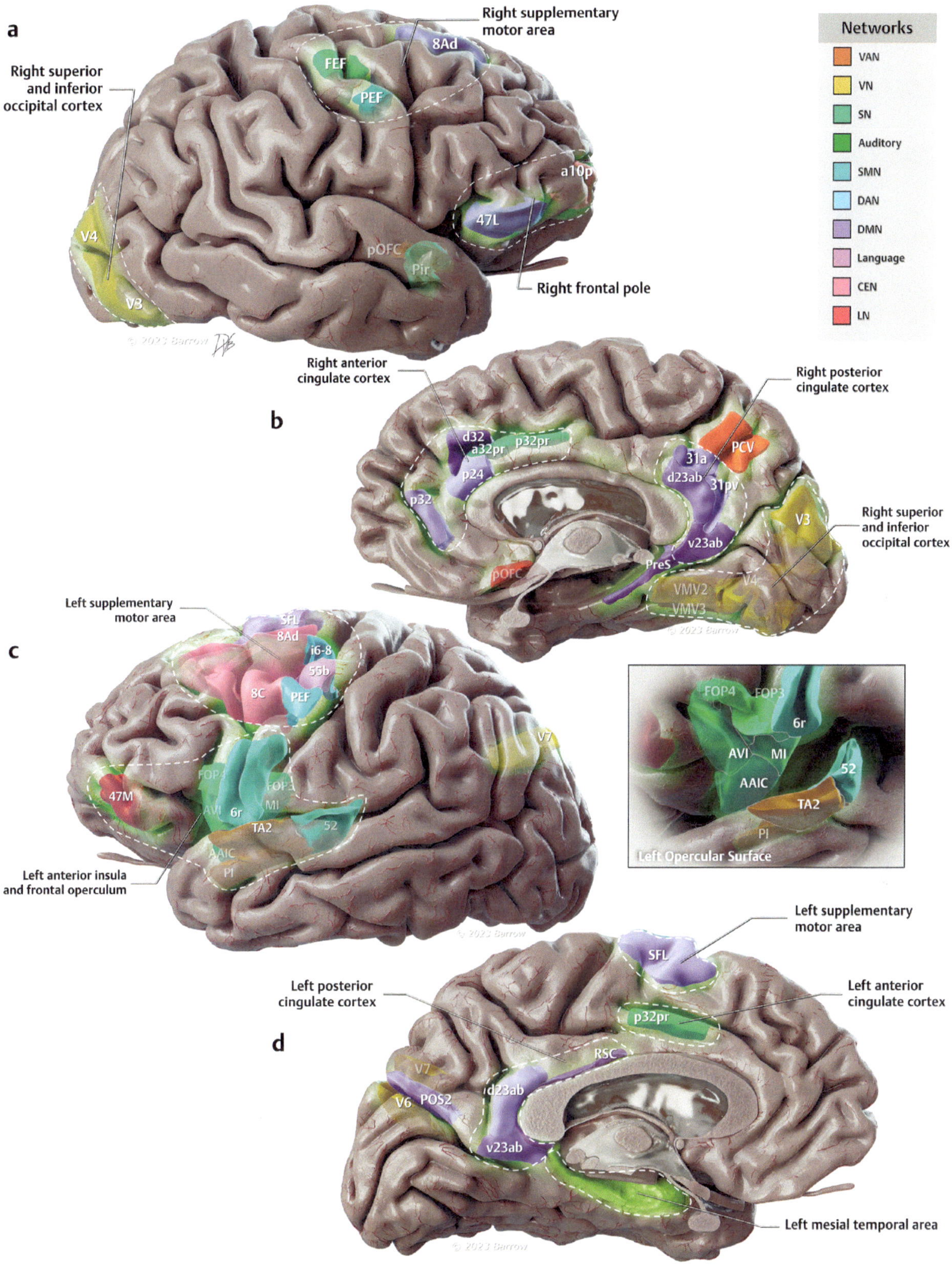

Fig. 7.3 Parcel map of cerebral eloquence with seven key hotspots: SMA (bilateral), anterior cingulate cortex (bilateral), posterior cingulate cortex (bilateral), anterior insula (left), frontal pole (right), mesial temporal lobe (left), and occipital cortex (right). Images show the anatomical locations of the seven hotspots of functional risk as *dashed shapes* encircling the clusters of parcels in the model. **(a)** Right lateral, **(b)** right medial, **(c)** left lateral, and **(d)** left medial views. The *inset* depicts parcels in the left anterior insula, which is one of the seven key hotspots. (Reproduced with permission from Barrow Neurological Institute, Phoenix, AZ.)

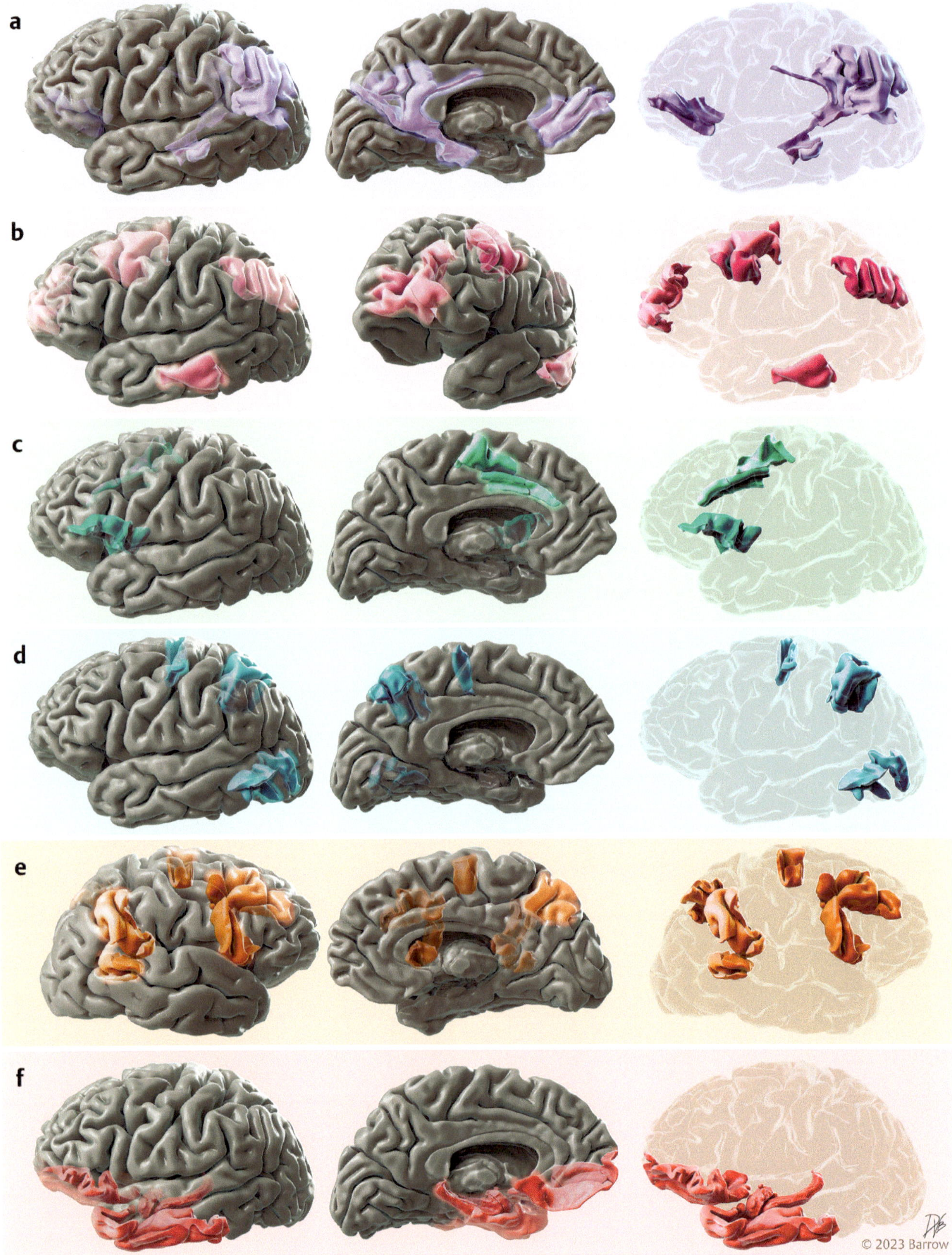

Fig. 7.4 Large-scale brain networks include seven major networks, including the DMN, CEN, SN, DAN, SMN, VN, and LN, along with the VAN, language, accessory language, auditory, multiple demand, and medial temporal networks. Six key brain networks are shown: **(a)** DMN, **(b)** CEN, **(c)** SN, **(d)** DAN, **(e)** VAN, and **(f)** LN. (Reproduced with permission from Barrow Neurological Institute, Phoenix, AZ.)

Table 7.2 Feature importance for the lesion object mapping strategy that leveraged a support vector classification machine learning model to predict which patients experienced neurocognitive decline after cerebral CM resection

Hemisphere	Functional region address	Feature importance	Primary network
Left	6r	1.010931	SMN
Left	SFL	1	DMN
Right	52	1	SMN
Right	Pir	1	SMN
Right	v23ab	1	DMN
Right	PreS	0.883181	DMN
Left	AAIC	0.862412	SN
Left	Ventral diencephalon	0.840592	Subcortical
Left	MI	0.77123	SN
Left	RSC	0.733324	DMN
Left	POS2	0.723708	DMN
Right	p24	0.712424	DMN
Right	V3	0.681034	VN
Right	V4	0.681034	VN
Right	VMV2	0.681034	VN
Right	VMV3	0.681034	VN
Left	V6	0.658699	VN
Left	V7	0.658699	VN
Right	PEF	0.658558	DAN
Right	pOFC	0.543881	LN
Right	Pallidum	0.520327	Subcortical
Left	v23ab	0.510635	DMN
Right	p32	0.5	DMN
Left	Putamen	0.476663	Subcortical
Left	Hippocampus	0.459302	Subcortical
Left	Amygdala	0.424823	Subcortical
Left	Pallidum	0.424823	Subcortical
Right	a32pr	0.414532	SN
Right	8Ad	0.351071	CEN
Right	p32pr	0.331403	SN
Left	8C	0.310431	CEN
Right	d32	0.271205	DMN
Right	FEF	0.239835	DAN

Note: The machine learning model achieved excellent performance (area under the curve = 0.81; accuracy = 93%).

is the response to environmental or biological stimuli that switches attention to important signals and often interrupts higher cognitive activity. The VAN calls attention to these other sensory stimuli and noises. The VAN is often inhibited during top-down focused attention to prevent distraction by irrelevant stimuli. The DAN is located bilaterally in the intraparietal sulci and frontal eye fields, and the VAN is in the right-sided temporoparietal junction and ventral frontal cortex.

7.6 Seven Hotspots of Cerebral Eloquence

The context of large-scale brain networks explains the surgical morbidity we observed with the resection of superficial cerebral CMs, with seven hotspots in the parcel map corresponding to the transgression in key regions of major networks (▶ Fig. 7.5). The SMA, the first of these hotspots, occupies the posterior third of the superior frontal gyrus and helps plan and initiate movement. Because the SMN is one of the most important networks, with three of the top five parcellations with feature importance on lesion mapping, the neurosurgeons rarely approached target CMs through the pre- or postcentral gyri or the central sulcus (16/362, 4.4%). However, alternative approaches were taken through the adjacent SMA (e.g., precentral sulcus, superior frontal sulcus, superior frontal gyrus, inferior frontal sulcus) to protect the SMN from transgression. The SMA was exploited as an anterior route to CMs in the motor networks, but it emerged as an eloquent hotspot. The SMA syndrome, or transient hemiplegia and mutism after cortical transgression or resection in the medial or convexity

Table 7.3 Feature importance for the transcerebral trajectory mapping strategy that leveraged a support vector classification machine learning model to predict which patients experience neurocognitive decline after cerebral CM resection

Hemisphere	Functional region address	Feature importance	Primary network
Right	47l	0.56691	VAN
Left	FOP4	0.500019	SN
Left	Putamen	0.457555	Subcortical
Left	8Ad	0.412382	CEN
Left	PEF	0.387531	DAN
Right	31a	0.357876	DMN
Right	PCV	0.357876	VAN
Left	PI	0.334497	Auditory
Left	TA2	0.334497	Auditory
Right	d23ab	0.331781	DMN
Right	31pv	0.329698	DMN
Left	p32pr	0.301525	SN
Left	47m	0.288694	LN
Left	AVI	0.288694	SN
Left	d23ab	0.23895	DMN
Right	a10p	0.23573	CEN
Right	Accumbens	0.221352	Subcortical
Left	55b	0.217872	Language
Left	i6–8	0.217872	DAN
Left	FOP3	0.211325	SN

Note: The machine learning model achieved excellent performance (area under the curve = 0.93; accuracy = 75%).

Table 7.4 Categorical binary breakdown of clinical deficits among 82 cases with unfavorable outcomes

Clinical deficit	Cases (%)
Motor	17 (20.7)
Sensory	20 (24.4)
Neuropathic pain	15 (18.3)
Visual disturbance	16 (19.5)
Language	24 (29.3)
Cognitive	19 (23.2)
Cranial nerve palsy	6 (7.3)
Seizure	10 (12.2)
Ataxia	4 (4.9)
Vertigo	2 (2.4)
Miscellaneous	4 (4.9)

portions of the superior frontal gyrus, shows the interconnectedness or hubness of networks in this region. Six parcellations with feature importance in the left SMA belong to five networks, and their white matter tracts, including the frontal aslant tract, link the SMA to premotor areas, Broca's area, and the SN for motor and speech initiation.

The anterior and posterior cingulate gyri also emerged as eloquent hotspots, which can explain their importance to the DMN and SN. Nine parcellations in the DMN and four in the SN had feature importance in lesion mapping, and four in the DMN and SN had feature importance in trajectory mapping. The anterior and posterior cingulate gyri are noneloquent areas straddling the leg sensorimotor cortex. Consequently, interhemispheric approaches to medial frontal and parietal CMs often transgressed these areas. Gravity-assisted dissection of the interhemispheric fissure, with the midline

Table 7.5 Feature importance for the lesion object mapping model

Regional address	Feature importance
L_6r	1.010931
L_SFL	1
R_52	1
R_Pir	1
R_v23ab	1
R_PreS	0.883181
L_AAIC	0.862412
L_VentralDC	0.840592
L_MI	0.77123
L_RSC	0.733324
L_POS2	0.723708
R_p24	0.712424
R_V3	0.681034
R_V4	0.681034
R_VMV2	0.681034
R_VMV3	0.681034
L_V6	0.658699
L_V7	0.658699
R_PEF	0.658558
R_pOFC	0.543881
R_Pallidum	0.520327
R_p32	0.5
L_v23ab	0.480635
L_Putamen	0.476663
L_H	0.459302
L_Amygdala	0.424823
L_Pallidum	0.424823
R_a32pr	0.414532
R_8Ad	0.351071
R_p32pr	0.331403
L_8C	0.310431
R_d32	0.271205
R_FEF	0.239835
L_Pol2	0.130973
R_IFJa	0.124972
R_IFJp	0.124972
R_PHA2	0.122248
R_PHA3	0.122248
L_Cerebellum	0.1
L_52	0.079134
R_31pv	0.048281
L_FST	0.037198
L_PHT	0.037198
L_i6-8	0.016049
R_13l	1.67E-16
L_10d	0
L_10r	0
L_13l	0
L_2	0
L_23d	0
L_24dv	0

(Continued)

Table 7.5 (*Continued*) Feature importance for the lesion object mapping model

Regional address	Feature importance
L_25	0
L_31a	0
L_3a	0
L_5L	0
L_5m	0
L_6ma	0
L_6mp	0
L_7AL	0
L_7Am	0
L_7PC	0
L_7Pm	0
L_9a	0
L_9p	0
L_a24	0
L_Accumbens	0
L_AIP	0
L_FEF	0
L_FOP2	0
L_Ig	0
L_OP2-3	0
L_p10p	0
L_p24	0
L_p24pr	0
L_p32	0
L_PFcm	0
L_PFop	0
L_PH	0
L_Pir	0
L_pOFC	0
L_PSL	0
L_s32	0
L_SCEF	0
L_STSva	0
L_STSvp	0
L_TA2	0
L_TE1p	0
L_TGd	0
L_TPOJ3	0
L_V3	0
L_V3B	0
L_V4	0
L_VMV3	0
L_VVC	0
R_10d	0
R_10r	0
R_24dd	0
R_24dv	0
R_43	0
R_47m	0
R_6mp	0

(Continued)

Table 7.5 (*Continued*) Feature importance for the lesion object mapping model

Regional address	Feature importance
R_9-46d	0
R_FOP2	0
R_H	0
R_IFSa	0
R_IFSp	0
R_Ig	0
R_LO1	0
R_OP1	0
R_PF	0
R_PFop	0
R_PFt	0
R_PSL	0
R_STSva	0
R_TGv	0
R_V3CD	0
R_V6	0
R_VVC	0
R_V2	−0.0003
R_ProS	−0.00037
L_Thalamus	−0.00138
L_Hippocampus	−0.00694
L_6a	−0.0156
L_1	−0.02101
L_IP2	−0.02427
L_LIPv	−0.02427
L_VIP	−0.02427
R_8BM	−0.02669
R_2	−0.02913
R_31a	−0.02913
R_31pd	−0.02913
R_5mv	−0.02913
R_7AL	−0.02913
R_LIPv	−0.02913
R_PCV	−0.02913
R_POS2	−0.02913
L_6d	−0.03165
R_55b	−0.04556
R_OP2-3	−0.04556
R_OP4	−0.04556
R_d23ab	−0.04779
R_IP0	−0.05754
R_IPS1	−0.05754
R_LO3	−0.05754
R_MT	−0.05754
R_PGi	−0.05754
R_PGp	−0.05754
R_V3B	−0.05754
L_TPOJ2	−0.07411
R_Putamen	−0.09667
R_11l	−0.09729

(*Continued*)

Table 7.5 (*Continued*) Feature importance for the lesion object mapping model

Regional address	Feature importance
R_47s	−0.09729
L_IP0	−0.10259
L_MT	−0.10259
L_PBelt	−0.11131
L_STSdp	−0.11131
R_a9-46v	−0.12493
R_p47r	−0.12493
R_23d	−0.1252
R_p24pr	−0.1252
R_45	−0.12948
R_AVI	−0.12948
L_AVI	−0.13759
L_FOP5	−0.13759
R_23c	−0.15433
L_8BL	−0.163
L_IFJp	−0.16976
L_44	−0.19128
L_3b	−0.20141
L_POS1	−0.20167
R_47l	−0.20419
R_A5	−0.20419
R_STGa	−0.20419
L_a32pr	−0.21344
R_6r	−0.21906
R_6d	−0.22866
L_33pr	−0.22927
R_Thalamus	−0.23285
L_p32pr	−0.23669
R_6a	−0.23984
R_a10p	−0.24992
L_31pd	−0.25269
L_31pv	−0.25269
L_d23ab	−0.25269
L_PCV	−0.25269
L_PreS	−0.25438
L_PHA3	−0.2581
R_PoI1	−0.25816
R_PoI2	−0.25816
R_EC	−0.26383
R_STSdp	−0.26396
L_MST	−0.26473
L_VMV1	−0.26668
L_46	−0.26668
L_p47r	−0.26668
L_6v	−0.26954
L_TPOJ1	−0.27345
R_PHA1	−0.27553
R_9p	−0.27822
R_7m	−0.28182
R_i6-8	−0.29657

(*Continued*)

Table 7.5 (*Continued*) Feature importance for the lesion object mapping model

Regional address	Feature importance
R_6ma	−0.29789
R_SCEF	−0.29789
R_SFL	−0.29789
L_8Ad	−0.29803
L_10pp	−0.30086
L_10v	−0.30086
L_OFC	−0.30086
R_10pp	−0.30086
R_33pr	−0.3034
L_IFJa	−0.31024
R_VMV1	−0.31897
L_IPS1	−0.3413
R_AAIC	−0.34403
R_MI	−0.34403
L_A1	−0.34569
L_MBelt	−0.34569
L_OP1	−0.34569
L_MIP	−0.36557
L_V1	−0.36926
R_p10p	−0.37484
L_8BM	−0.37644
L_9m	−0.37644
L_d32	−0.37644
L_VMV2	−0.37799
L_DVT	−0.37888
R_10v	−0.39815
R_OFC	−0.39815
R_PFcm	−0.39982
R_RI	−0.39982
R_FST	−0.40389
R_MST	−0.40389
R_Amygdala	−0.40554
R_Hippocampus	−0.40554
R_DVT	−0.40563
L_PHA2	−0.45108
R_POS1	−0.45155
R_25	−0.45612
R_TPOJ2	−0.46143
R_PI	−0.46235
R_STSda	−0.46235
R_TA2	−0.46235
L_47m	−0.46653
L_47s	−0.46653
L_11l	−0.46653
L_a10p	−0.46653
R_3b	−0.46822
R_FOP4	−0.48167
R_9m	−0.49167
R_AIP	−0.49265
R_IP2	−0.49265

(*Continued*)

Table 7.5 (*Continued*) Feature importance for the lesion object mapping model

Regional address	Feature importance
R_PFm	−0.49265
L_OP4	−0.5
L_TE1m	−0.5
R_a24	−0.5
R_PeEc	−0.50887
R_LIPd	−0.52178
L_PFm	−0.53765
L_FOP3	−0.57518
R_8Av	−0.57915
L_45	−0.57967
R_a24pr	−0.58415
R_44	−0.61115
L_PI	−0.62074
L_FFC	−0.62907
L_8Av	−0.64037
L_IFSa	−0.64119
R_Accumbens	−0.64238
R_46	−0.65539
R_p9−46v	−0.65539
R_FFC	−0.66638
L_23c	−0.66667
L_24dd	−0.66667
L_5mv	−0.66667
L_STGa	−0.66667
L_STSda	−0.66667
L_TE1a	−0.66667
R_TE2p	−0.66676
L_STV	−0.67552
L_PHA1	−0.67573
R_8C	−0.68935
R_3a	−0.69688
R_TPOJ3	−0.73059
R_6v	−0.76235
L_TE2p	−0.77586
L_47l	−0.77878
L_ProS	−0.78179
L_PGi	−0.78683
L_9−46d	−0.79974
R_STV	−0.80009
L_FOP4	−0.81931
L_RI	−0.82709
R_4	−0.83451
L_PeEc	−0.8659
R_s6−8	−0.87269
L_a9−46v	−0.93335
L_PEF	−0.9504
R_8BL	−0.95255
L_V2	−0.95549
L_TF	−0.96603
L_PF	−0.98935

(*Continued*)

Table 7.5 (*Continued*) Feature importance for the lesion object mapping model

Regional address	Feature importance
L_PFt	−0.98935
L_43	−1
L_a24pr	−1
L_A5	−1
L_FOP1	−1
L_IP1	−1
R_9a	−1
R_A1	−1
R_LBelt	−1
R_MBelt	−1
R_PBelt	−1
R_TE2a	−1
R_TGd	−1
L_LIPd	−1.02427
L_s6-8	−1.06134
L_a47r	−1.06668
R_s32	−1.09729
R_Cerebellum	−1.11682
R_FOP5	−1.12948
L_LBelt	−1.17278
L_7m	−1.18768
R_TPOJ1	−1.19991
L_IFSp	−1.22894
R_IP1	−1.26916
R_TF	−1.33315
R_VentralDC	−1.3486
R_Caudate	−1.35768
L_55b	−1.35968
R_a47r	−1.37484
L_PoI1	−1.37874
L_Caudate	−1.46596
Brain-Stem	−1.49089
L_A4	−1.5
L_TE2a	−1.5
R_RSC	−1.54763
L_4	−1.73012
L_p9-46v	−1.73362
R_V1	−1.9997
R_p32	1.5664
L_MI	1.085095
L_8Ad	1.065608
L_8BL	0.883051
R_d23ab	0.866939
R_31pv	0.832355
R_Pir	0.825921
R_FEF	0.759765
L_VentralDC	0.735945
L_SFL	0.696317
L_45	0.689008
L_Hippocampus	0.68544

(*Continued*)

Table 7.5 (*Continued*) Feature importance for the lesion object mapping model

Regional address	Feature importance
L_1	0.684455
L_i6-8	0.656121
L_H	0.643841
R_Amygdala	0.627189
R_pOFC	0.612888
L_TPOJ2	0.575115
L_PHT	0.575115
L_FST	0.575115
L_PHA2	0.568671
R_p24	0.53621
R_33pr	0.518138
R_a24	0.500688
R_PEF	0.498985
R_6r	0.477192
L_Putamen	0.457444
L_PoI2	0.456903
L_PreS	0.446212
L_POS2	0.437981
R_11l	0.433162
R_6a	0.408187
L_46	0.402423
R_EC	0.348129
L_6v	0.325343
L_IFJp	0.277738
L_POS1	0.266295
L_6r	0.263519
R_IFJa	0.236957
R_p32pr	0.211398
R_8Ad	0.211398
R_Thalamus	0.19491
R_a24pr	0.193326
R_IFJp	0.18591
R_8C	0.172924
R_VMV3	0.158357
R_VMV2	0.158357
R_a32pr	0.152445
R_VVC	0.15184
R_52	0.15184
L_44	0.146426
R_Pallidum	0.133098
L_DVT	0.124573
R_PHA3	0.119284
R_PHA2	0.119284
L_9-46d	0.118497
R_V4	0.095838
R_V3	0.095838
R_8BM	0.074494
L_IFJa	0.070807
Brain-Stem	0.067306
R_OFC	0.067191

(*Continued*)

Table 7.5 (*Continued*) Feature importance for the lesion object mapping model

Regional address	Feature importance
L_Pol1	0.067183
R_Caudate	0.067085
L_Cerebellum	0.059677
R_VMV1	0.034766
R_TGd	0.03356
R_47s	0.03356
R_V1	0.026219
R_Cerebellum	0.020105
R_PreS	0.018391
R_v23ab	0.010062
R_V6	0
R_V3B	0
R_TPOJ3	0
R_TPOJ2	0
R_TPOJ1	0
R_TGv	0
R_TE2a	0
R_STV	0
R_STGa	0
R_RI	0
R_PSL	0
R_PGp	0
R_PGi	0
R_PFt	0
R_PFop	0
R_PFm	0
R_PFcm	0
R_PF	0
R_PBelt	0
R_p47r	0
R_p10p	0
R_OP4	0
R_MT	0
R_MST	0
R_MI	0
R_LO3	0
R_LBelt	0
R_IPS1	0
R_IP2	0
R_IP1	0
R_IP0	0
R_IFSa	0
R_FST	0
R_FOP5	0
R_AVI	0
R_AIP	0
R_AAIC	0
R_a9–46v	0
R_A5	0
R_A1	0

(Continued)

Table 7.5 (*Continued*) Feature importance for the lesion object mapping model

Regional address	Feature importance
R_6mp	0
R_47m	0
R_47l	0
R_45	0
R_43	0
R_3b	0
R_24dd	0
R_10r	0
R_10d	0
L_VIP	0
L_V7	0
L_TGd	0
L_TE1p	0
L_TE1m	0
L_s32	0
L_pOFC	0
L_Pallidum	0
L_p32	0
L_p24	0
L_p10p	0
L_Amygdala	0
L_A4	0
L_a32pr	0
L_a24	0
L_a10p	0
L_9p	0
L_9a	0
L_7Pm	0
L_7Am	0
L_7AL	0
L_6mp	0
L_5mv	0
L_5m	0
L_5L	0
L_25	0
L_24dd	0
L_23d	0
L_13l	0
L_11l	0
L_10r	0
L_10d	0
R_10v	−0.00011
R_10pp	−0.00011
L_OFC	−0.00011
L_10v	−0.00011
L_10pp	−0.00011
R_PeEc	−0.00011
L_8C	−0.00361
R_POS1	−0.00929
R_DVT	−0.00929

(Continued)

Table 7.5 (*Continued*) Feature importance for the lesion object mapping model

Regional address	Feature importance
L_RSC	−0.01489
L_p24pr	−0.01807
L_33pr	−0.01807
R_p9–46v	−0.01891
R_IFSp	−0.01891
L_v23ab	−0.02344
R_6d	−0.02677
R_3a	−0.02677
R_TE2p	−0.03143
R_TA2	−0.03143
R_STSva	−0.03143
R_STSdp	−0.03143
R_STSda	−0.03143
R_Pol1	−0.03143
R_PI	−0.03143
R_MBelt	−0.03143
R_H	−0.03143
R_FFC	−0.03143
R_POS2	−0.03551
R_PCV	−0.03551
R_LIPv	−0.03551
R_LIPd	−0.03551
R_7AL	−0.03551
R_5mv	−0.03551
R_31a	−0.03551
R_2	−0.03551
R_PHA1	−0.03892
L_VVC	−0.04107
L_VMV3	−0.04107
L_V4	−0.04107
L_V3B	−0.04107
L_TPOJ3	−0.04107
L_PSL	−0.04107
L_PH	−0.04107
L_PFm	−0.04107
L_PFcm	−0.04107
L_PCV	−0.04107
L_PBelt	−0.04107
L_MT	−0.04107
L_MIP	−0.04107
L_LIPv	−0.04107
L_LIPd	−0.04107
L_IP2	−0.04107
L_IP1	−0.04107
L_IP0	−0.04107
L_FFC	−0.04107
L_d23ab	−0.04107
L_AIP	−0.04107
L_A1	−0.04107
L_7PC	−0.04107

(Continued)

Table 7.5 (*Continued*) Feature importance for the lesion object mapping model

Regional address	Feature importance
L_31pv	−0.04107
L_31pd	−0.04107
L_31a	−0.04107
L_23c	−0.04107
L_PFop	−0.04161
L_OP4	−0.04161
L_FOP2	−0.04161
L_3a	−0.04161
L_2	−0.04161
L_3b	−0.04847
L_6d	−0.04847
L_STGa	−0.06182
L_Pir	−0.06182
L_p47r	−0.06182
L_FOP5	−0.06182
L_AVI	−0.06182
L_a47r	−0.06182
L_47s	−0.06182
L_47m	−0.06182
R_V3CD	−0.06252
R_LO1	−0.06252
R_Putamen	−0.06624
R_OP2–3	−0.06996
R_OP1	−0.06996
R_Ig	−0.06996
R_FOP2	−0.06996
L_TE2a	−0.07301
L_TE1a	−0.07301
L_STSva	−0.07301
L_STSda	−0.07301
L_VMV2	−0.07457
L_VMV1	−0.07457
L_d32	−0.07795
L_9m	−0.07795
L_OP1	−0.08268
L_Ig	−0.08268
R_23d	−0.09199
R_ProS	−0.09737
R_Pol2	−0.10139
L_TE2p	−0.11408
L_STSvp	−0.11408
L_STSdp	−0.11408
L_PHA3	−0.11408
L_MBelt	−0.11408
L_52	−0.11408
L_OP2–3	−0.11462
L_43	−0.11462
R_23c	−0.1275
L_Thalamus	−0.1278
L_Caudate	−0.15185

(Continued)

Table 7.5 *(Continued)* Feature importance for the lesion object mapping model

Regional address	Feature importance
R_V2	−0.1564
R_d32	−0.15994
L_V6	−0.16516
L_V3	−0.16516
L_IPS1	−0.16516
R_7m	−0.16764
R_31pd	−0.16764
L_RI	−0.1695
L_LBelt	−0.1695
R_Hippocampus	−0.17161
L_FEF	−0.17939
L_8Av	−0.18285
L_4	−0.18625
L_Accumbens	−0.18778
L_V1	−0.20671
L_PEF	−0.21076
R_25	−0.21303
L_AAIC	−0.22053
R_RSC	−0.23043
L_A5	−0.23172
R_a47r	−0.23443
R_a10p	−0.23443
R_9p	−0.23443
R_9m	−0.23443
R_9a	−0.23443
R_9–46d	−0.23443
R_SFL	−0.24023
R_SCEF	−0.24023
R_6ma	−0.24023
R_55b	−0.24023
R_46	−0.24023
R_24dv	−0.24023
L_SCEF	−0.25348
L_24dv	−0.25348
L_55b	−0.25381
L_8BM	−0.25702
L_a24pr	−0.25831
R_FOP4	−0.26078
L_FOP3	−0.2659
L_FOP1	−0.2659
R_44	−0.27969
R_4	−0.28755
L_TA2	−0.29354
L_6ma	−0.30368
L_PFt	−0.30868
L_PF	−0.30868
L_IFSa	−0.31099
L_47l	−0.31099
L_TF	−0.31509
L_PI	−0.31509

(Continued)

Table 7.5 *(Continued)* Feature importance for the lesion object mapping model

Regional address	Feature importance
R_8BL	−0.31819
L_V2	−0.32373
L_6a	−0.33451
L_p9–46v	−0.33527
R_p24pr	−0.3503
L_STV	−0.38382
R_TF	−0.3888
R_Accumbens	−0.40081
L_TPOJ1	−0.42489
L_PGi	−0.42489
L_MST	−0.42489
R_13l	−0.43329
R_s32	−0.43369
L_7m	−0.43793
L_a9–46v	−0.45389
L_FOP4	−0.48643
L_IFSp	−0.49527
R_8Av	−0.50226
R_6v	−0.50389
L_PHA1	−0.55492
R_s6–8	−0.56505
R_i6–8	−0.56505
L_ProS	−0.61347
L_PeEc	−0.63234
R_VentralDC	−0.80356
L_s6–8	−0.8159
L_p32pr	−1.23583

Table 7.6 Feature importance for the transcerebral trajectory mapping model

Regional address	Feature importance
R_47l	0.56691
L_FOP4	0.500019
L_Putamen	0.457555
L_8Ad	0.412382
L_PEF	0.387531
R_31a	0.357876
R_PCV	0.357876
L_PI	0.334497
L_TA2	0.334497
R_d23ab	0.331781
R_31pv	0.329698
L_p32pr	0.301525
L_47m	0.288694
L_AVI	0.288694
L_d23ab	0.23895
R_a10p	0.23573

(Continued)

7

Table 7.6 (*Continued*) Feature importance for the transcerebral trajectory mapping model

Regional address	Feature importance
R_Accumbens	0.221352
L_55b	0.217872
L_i6-8	0.217872
L_FOP3	0.211325
R_Pallidum	0.19453
L_9m	0.187412
L_d32	0.187412
R_FOP4	0.180729
L_PFt	0.16966
L_6mp	0.169354
L_Ig	0.162274
L_9p	0.158599
R_p10p	0.153982
L_6a	0.152176
L_a32pr	0.149349
L_11l	0.144324
L_45	0.144324
L_47l	0.144324
R_47m	0.144184
L_PFop	0.128136
L_24dv	0.114114
L_46	0.098155
L_9-46d	0.098155
R_FOP5	0.095746
L_24dd	0.074372
L_MI	0.049991
R_10pp	0.048438
R_13l	0.048438
R_47s	0.048438
R_OFC	0.048438
R_Pir	0.048438
R_pOFC	0.048438
R_TGd	0.048438
R_Putamen	0.039115
R_Caudate	0.02053
L_6d	0.015813
R_EC	0.013802
R_VentralDC	0.013802
L_DVT	0.009483
L_IP0	0.009483
L_IP1	0.009483
L_IPS1	0.009483
L_MIP	0.009483
L_PGp	0.009483
L_PGs	0.009483
L_POS1	0.009483
L_POS2	0.009483
L_V1	0.009483
L_V2	0.009483
L_V3	0.009483

(Continued)

Table 7.6 (*Continued*) Feature importance for the transcerebral trajectory mapping model

Regional address	Feature importance
L_V3A	0.009483
L_V3B	0.009483
L_V4	0.009483
L_V6	0.009483
L_V6A	0.009483
L_V7	0.009483
L_OP2-3	0.007527
L_4	0.00027
L_FEF	0
L_FST	0
L_MST	0
L_PeEc	0
L_PGi	0
L_PH	0
L_PHA2	0
L_PHA3	0
L_ProS	0
L_TPOJ2	0
L_V8	0
L_VMV1	0
L_VMV2	0
L_VMV3	0
L_VVC	0
R_8Ad	0
R_8Av	0
R_8BL	0
R_8C	0
R_9p	0
R_A1	0
R_Cerebellum	0
R_FFC	0
R_i6-8	0
R_LBelt	0
R_LO1	0
R_LO3	0
R_MST	0
R_MT	0
R_OP1	0
R_OP2-3	0
R_PFcm	0
R_PFm	0
R_PGi	0
R_RI	0
R_STV	0
R_TPOJ1	0
R_TPOJ2	0
R_TPOJ3	0
R_VMV1	0
R_VMV2	0
R_VVC	0

(Continued)

Table 7.6 (*Continued*) Feature importance for the transcerebral trajectory mapping model

Regional address	Feature importance
R_AVI	−0.00342
R_SCEF	−0.00481
L_5m	−0.00526
R_5m	−0.00526
R_SFL	−0.02062
L_3a	−0.02577
L_3b	−0.02577
L_IFJp	−0.02836
R_6mp	−0.0341
R_52	−0.03464
R_MBelt	−0.03464
R_PHA2	−0.03464
R_PHA3	−0.03464
R_PI	−0.03464
R_PoI1	−0.03464
R_PreS	−0.03464
R_STSda	−0.03464
R_STSdp	−0.03464
R_STSva	−0.03464
R_STSvp	−0.03464
L_2	−0.03553
R_33pr	−0.03806
R_8BM	−0.03806
R_a24pr	−0.03806
R_a32pr	−0.03806
R_p32pr	−0.03806
L_7m	−0.03905
L_52	−0.04152
L_A1	−0.04152
L_LBelt	−0.04152
L_MBelt	−0.04152
L_OP1	−0.04152
L_PBelt	−0.04152
L_PFcm	−0.04152
R_23d	−0.04539
R_IFSa	−0.04803
L_7Pm	−0.04853
R_7Am	−0.04853
R_7m	−0.04853
R_7Pm	−0.04853
R_ProS	−0.04853
R_v23ab	−0.04853
L_H	−0.04905
L_Hippocampus	−0.04905
L_PF	−0.04905
L_PHT	−0.04905
L_PSL	−0.04905
L_RI	−0.04905
L_STSdp	−0.04905
L_STV	−0.04905

(Continued)

Table 7.6 (*Continued*) Feature importance for the transcerebral trajectory mapping model

Regional address	Feature importance
L_TPOJ1	−0.04905
L_6r	−0.06076
R_10r	−0.0653
L_43	−0.06904
L_23c	−0.07539
L_Caudate	−0.07539
L_6v	−0.07657
R_PGp	−0.07918
R_PGs	−0.07918
R_V1	−0.07918
R_V2	−0.07918
R_V3	−0.07918
R_V3A	−0.07918
R_V3B	−0.07918
R_V3CD	−0.07918
R_V4	−0.07918
R_V6	−0.07918
R_V6A	−0.07918
R_V7	−0.07918
R_9a	−0.0846
R_p24pr	−0.08658
L_IFSa	−0.08926
L_p9–46v	−0.08926
R_AAIC	−0.09916
L_33pr	−0.10376
L_a24pr	−0.10376
R_24dv	−0.10854
R_11l	−0.11333
L_OP4	−0.11809
R_IP2	−0.12101
R_LIPd	−0.12101
R_LIPv	−0.12101
R_MIP	−0.12101
R_VIP	−0.12101
L_Pir	−0.12306
L_STGa	−0.12306
L_STSda	−0.12306
L_STSva	−0.12306
L_TE1a	−0.12306
L_TGd	−0.12306
L_31a	−0.12418
R_4	−0.12693
L_31pd	−0.13188
R_6a	−0.14089
L_23d	−0.14135
L_31pv	−0.14136
L_5L	−0.14136
L_7Am	−0.14136
L_PCV	−0.14136
R_5L	−0.14136

(Continued)

7

Table 7.6 (*Continued*) Feature importance for the transcerebral trajectory mapping model

Regional address	Feature importance
R_24dd	−0.14275
R_IFSp	−0.14284
R_p9–46v	−0.14284
L_p10p	−0.14437
R_43	−0.1476
R_44	−0.1476
R_6r	−0.1476
R_A4	−0.1476
R_FOP1	−0.1476
R_FOP2	−0.1476
R_FOP3	−0.1476
R_Ig	−0.1476
R_MI	−0.1476
R_OP4	−0.1476
R_PBelt	−0.1476
R_TA2	−0.1476
R_RSC	−0.15236
R_25	−0.15542
R_a24	−0.15542
R_d32	−0.15542
R_p24	−0.15542
R_3a	−0.16018
R_3b	−0.16018
R_p47r	−0.16177
L_44	−0.1623
L_A4	−0.16458
L_A5	−0.16458
L_PoI1	−0.16458
R_31pd	−0.16954
R_POS1	−0.16954
R_A5	−0.18224
R_PoI2	−0.18224
R_AIP	−0.18358
L_SFL	−0.18379
L_Thalamus	−0.18462
L_IFSp	−0.19112
R_Thalamus	−0.19613
R_IP0	−0.20019
R_IP1	−0.20019
R_IPS1	−0.20019
R_POS2	−0.20019
R_1	−0.20346
R_2	−0.20346
R_6d	−0.20346
L_7PC	−0.20519
L_AIP	−0.20519
L_IP2	−0.20519
L_LIPd	−0.20519
L_LIPv	−0.20519
L_PFm	−0.20519

(Continued)

Table 7.6 (*Continued*) Feature importance for the transcerebral trajectory mapping model

Regional address	Feature importance
L_VIP	−0.20519
R_5mv	−0.20871
L_8Av	−0.21777
L_FFC	−0.21892
L_TE2p	−0.21892
R_Amygdala	−0.22836
R_Hippocampus	−0.22836
R_PeEc	−0.22836
R_a47r	−0.23544
L_a47r	−0.23772
L_p47r	−0.23772
L_FOP1	−0.2387
L_FOP2	−0.2387
R_TE2a	−0.24216
R_TGv	−0.24216
R_DVT	−0.24872
L_7AL	−0.25372
L_5mv	−0.26028
L_8C	−0.26194
L_STSvp	−0.26797
L_TE1p	−0.26797
R_10d	−0.26915
L_1	−0.27423
R_H	−0.27679
R_TE2p	−0.27679
R_TF	−0.27679
R_46	−0.28661
L_SCEF	−0.30272
L_FOP5	−0.30667
R_9–46d	−0.31718
R_a9–46v	−0.31718
L_RSC	−0.32598
R_23c	−0.32764
L_TE1m	−0.34198
L_TE2a	−0.34198
L_TF	−0.34198
L_s6–8	−0.36263
L_8BL	−0.37188
L_8BM	−0.37188
L_p24pr	−0.38376
L_6ma	−0.40711
L_PoI2	−0.41081
R_9m	−0.41293
R_p32	−0.41293
L_IFJa	−0.43519
L_a9–46v	−0.44249
R_45	−0.47116
L_a10p	−0.52641
L_9a	−0.55523

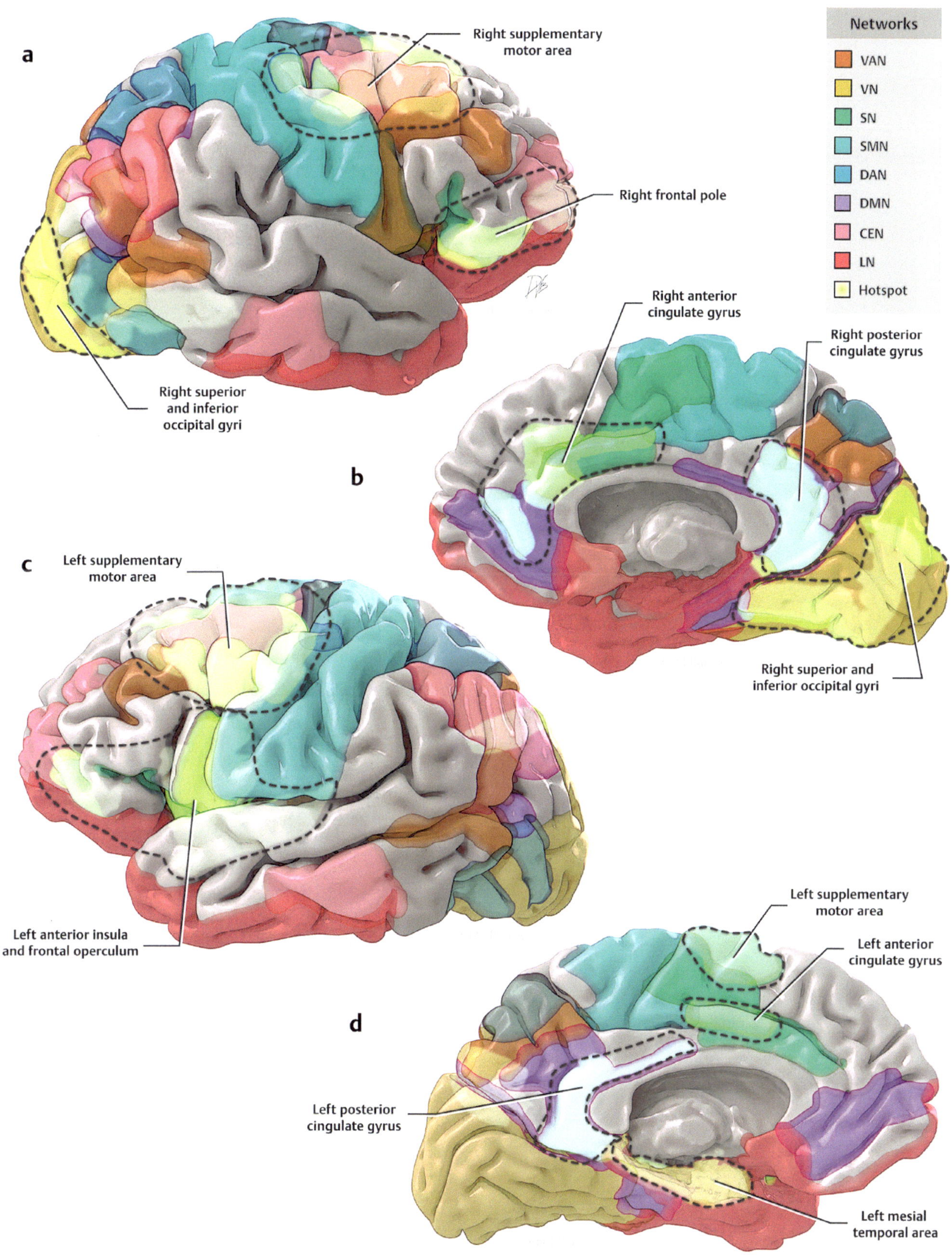

Fig. 7.5 Large-scale brain networks are shown with an overlay of the seven hotspots (*black dashed outlines*) identified in the study. Large-scale brain networks include the VAN, VN, SN, SMN, DAN, DMN, CEN, and LN. The graphic shows the right cerebral hemisphere from the **(a)** lateral and **(b)** medial perspectives, as well as the left cerebral hemisphere from the **(c)** lateral and **(d)** medial perspectives. (Reproduced with permission from Barrow Neurological Institute, Phoenix, AZ.)

of the head positioned horizontally for gravity retraction of the dependent hemisphere, made this route a frequent choice for medial CM subtypes. An underappreciation of the DMN and SN could have contributed to their surgical disruption. Gravity-assisted interhemispheric approaches should remain the first-line exposures for medial CMs, along with more transsulcal dissection to reach the target and greater respect for these two core networks.

The left anterior insula emerged as an eloquent hotspot partly because of its proximity to 6r, the parcellation with the highest feature importance on lesion mapping and part of the SMN involved in speech. In addition, two parcellations in the auditory network had high feature importance on trajectory mapping, indicating the significance of the auditory cortex on the temporal side of the sylvian fissure. Anterior insular CMs are not included with superficial cerebral CMs but are deep cerebral CMs because they abut the caudate nucleus and putamen. However, sylvian CMs are included with superficial cerebral CMs and require transsylvian dissection for their resection. Anterior insular eloquence requires meticulous dissection technique when transsylvian routes are taken on the dominant side, especially when the M2 insular segments of the middle cerebral artery are intimately involved in the dissection.

The right frontal pole was the hotspot with the least expected eloquence. This nondominant frontal pole is often considered noneloquent because its removal does not cause hemiparesis, aphasia, or coma. However, it participates in behavior, socialization, and impulse control. Frontal pole parcels with feature importance belonged to the CEN and VAN. Overall, the CEN has just two parcellations with feature importance in lesion mapping and two in trajectory mapping. CEN transgressions might have been detected in high-functioning patients due to the inclusion of additional functional decline.

In contrast to the right frontal pole, the left mesial temporal and right occipital hotspots are less surprising for their eloquence, given their recognized involvement in memory function and visual perception, respectively. Notably, the hippocampus is not included in the definition of eloquence in the Spetzler–Martin AVM grading system. The side of the mesial temporal hotspot suggests that functional decline may be due to effects on verbal memory. Functional declines in the right-sided occipital hotspot are thought to be due to its role in visuospatial processing.

7.7 Expanding the Concept of Cerebral Eloquence

An accurate and expanded definition of cortical SEZs is needed to guide the transgression of cortical tissue, avoid eloquent areas, and reduce unfavorable outcomes, as with the 21 brainstem SEZs. We consider the seven cortical hotspots as *unsafe* entry zones. These hotspots further our conceptualization of eloquence when added to the motor and sensory strips, visual cortex, Broca's and Wernicke's areas, and the auditory areas on the cortical map. It would be erroneous to conclude that all areas outside classical eloquence and the seven hotspots are cortical SEZs, but this simplistic view significantly expands our concept of cerebral eloquence.

Increasing the extent of subarachnoid and transgyral dissection and performing intracapsular rather than extracapsular resections could improve outcomes associated with cerebral CM resection. As discussed in Chapter 6, superficial cerebral CMs in classically noneloquent cortex are resected using an extracapsular technique that circumferentially dissects the lesion rather than an intracapsular technique that internally collapses and then separates the lesion from the adjacent brain. A more expansive concept of cerebral eloquence encourages broader use of the intracapsular technique, but the consequences of this technical modification require further study. The benefits of minimalistic, tissue-sparing techniques are clear from the positive results of the recently released ENRICH (Early Minimally Invasive Removal of Intracerebral Hematoma) trial demonstrating improved functional outcomes in the surgical group relative to medical management, especially in the context of previously negative results from the STICH (Surgical Trial in Intracerebral Hemorrhage) trial.

We included large-scale brain networks in our interpretation of this experience because human connectomics helps us understand our outcomes and improve our microsurgical technique. This sophisticated analysis depended on the Quicktome machine learning algorithm (Omniscient Neurotechnology) for parcel designation, tissue transgression analysis, and calculation of feature importance. Although these methods and metrics are unfamiliar to most neurosurgeons, they are validated by the literature in related disciplines like computational neurosciences. Our methodology emphasizes the size of the parcel and network disruption (collisions) rather than the location of that disruption within a network (centrality) or the interconnections with other networks (hubness), which may be important factors. Our database included a large cohort of highly selected surgical patients with robust radiographic imaging. We were particularly interested in cognitive outcomes, but detailed neuropsychological test results were unavailable. Conventional neurological outcomes measured by mRS scores were augmented by the additional functional decline factor as a real-world surrogate for cognitive outcomes. Still, this crude metric might not correlate with neuropsychological metrics. Complete pre- and postoperative neuropsychological and cognitive testing are needed to assess the surgical outcomes.

The microsurgical management of superficial cerebral CMs has relied on transgyral and transsulcal resections that circumvent areas of traditional eloquence and navigate areas presumed to be noneloquent. Seven areas of the brain long considered by neurosurgeons to be noneloquent SEZs are, in fact, eloquent and unsafe for transgression, including (1) the SMA (bilateral), (2) anterior cingulate cortex (bilateral), (3) posterior cingulate cortex (bilateral), (4) anterior insula (left), (5) frontal pole (right), (6) mesial temporal lobe (left), and (7) the occipital cortex (right). These eloquent noneloquent areas redefine our neurosurgical conception of eloquence and suggest more refined transcortical dissection techniques are needed to maximize transsulcal dissection, intracapsular resection, and tissue preservation. Human connectomics, awareness of large-scale brain networks, and prioritization of cognitive outcomes require an updated concept of cortical eloquence and the incorporation of this information into our surgical strategies and navigational tools.

8 RECURRENCE

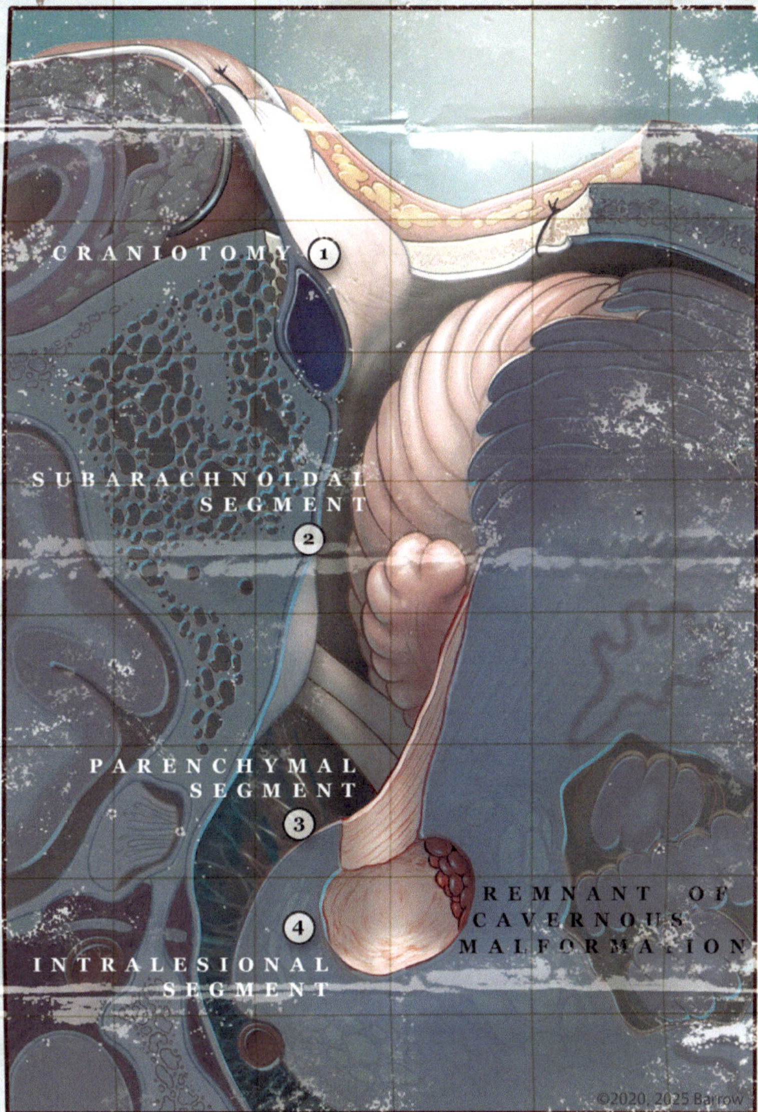

Peter M Lawrence
Mark Schornak

8 Residual and Recurrent Cavernous Malformations

Summary
Successful resection of cavernous malformations (CMs) is measured first by the complete removal of the lesion and second by the absence of new permanent neurological deficits. Research suggests that completely resected CMs do not recur de novo in the same location. This concept implies that, in recurrent cases, some residual CM or remnant was present and poorly visualized immediately after resection. A blind spot in the operative corridor is the most common cause of residual brainstem CMs. Anatomical obstacles can also hide CM remnants. Blind spots are areas in the surgical corridor with compromised views. Corridors to brainstem CMs have small openings, long lengths, and limited views of the resection bed. Neurosurgeons must conceptualize the blind spots and deliberately inspect them at the end of the resection, even after the resection seems complete. Careful approach selection to align the lesion's axis with the surgical axis results in good visualization of the lesion in the resection cavity. When these axes do not align, visualization is impaired. The right-angle method helps anticipate blind spots and drives meticulous inspection of the resection cavity for CM remnants. The fine lines between complete resection and residual lesion, safe and harmful resection, and heeding and ignoring neuromonitoring make this operation one of the most challenging in neurosurgery. We must constantly work toward an acceptable balance of safety and resection completeness to optimize patient outcomes.

Keywords: blind spot, brainstem, cavernoma, cavernous malformation, hemorrhage, neurological deficit, rebleeding, remnant, resection, right-angle method, two-point method

8.1 Problem of Recurrence

When resecting cavernous malformations (CMs) in any location, success is measured first by the complete removal of the symptomatic lesion and second by the absence of new permanent neurological deficits. Curative resection at the time of the index surgery rids the patient of the offending lesion and eliminates the risk of future deterioration caused by rehemorrhage, at least in the sporadic form of the disease. Surgical success is common with most CMs in the cerebral and cerebellar hemispheres, but resection of deep cerebral (basal ganglia and thalamus) and brainstem CMs is challenging. The proximity of these cavernomas to the descending and ascending tracts and cranial nerve nuclei makes it costly to transgress any normal tissue or disrupt normal tissue adjacent to the lesion in the separation plane. This interplay between tissue sensitivity and extreme eloquence makes it difficult to avoid leaving a remnant, if not impossible. In the largest institutional surgical case series by a single neurosurgeon, Spetzler reported a rate of residual or recurrent brainstem CMs of 11% (29 of 260 patients).

Brainstem CM recurrence is associated with many difficulties. For the patient, it is a clinical setback that can generate frustration, disappointment, and additional morbidity. For neurosurgeons, recurrence can rattle self-confidence, cause embarrassment, and diminish the trust of patients and colleagues. Symptomatic recurrences require operative intervention, which can increase morbidity, lengthen recovery, and add to overall hospitalization and rehabilitation costs. Although rare, this problem deserves special attention.

8.2 Clinical Evidence

Over a 21-year period (October 1, 1997, through November 30, 2018), 14 of 213 patients (6.6%) underwent a second surgical resection for a recurrent brainstem CM after primary surgical resection (▶ Table 8.1). Twelve patients were clinically symptomatic at the time of the recurrent hemorrhage; two patients had asymptomatic recurrences detected on surveillance magnetic resonance imaging (MRI) at their 6-month follow-up visit. Thirty-four hemorrhagic events were observed among these 14 patients over 576 patient-years (recurrent hemorrhage rate: 5.9% per year; median discrete hemorrhagic events: 2; median time to rehemorrhage: 897 days). The recurrence was in the pons in 10 cases, the midbrain in 2 cases, and the medulla in 2 cases. Twelve of the 14 patients underwent primary surgical treatment in an acute (0–3 weeks) or subacute (3–8 weeks) time frame. A blind spot in the operative corridor was the most common cause of residual brainstem CMs and occurred in nine patients (▶ Fig. 8.1, ▶ Fig. 8.2). An anatomical obstacle hid the remnant in two patients (a developmental venous anomaly in one and cranial nerves IX and X in another). In another two patients, the tissue at the depth of the cavity was misinterpreted as normal brainstem rather than a remnant of the lesion (▶ Fig. 8.3). In one patient, the recurrence was thought to be a satellite lesion immediately adjacent to the main brainstem CM (▶ Fig. 8.4). All recurrent CMs were completely removed. Two patients required two operations to treat recurrences.

Overall, 12 patients had unchanged or improved modified Rankin Scale scores at the last clinical evaluation compared with admission, and 2 patients had worse scores (▶ Table 8.2). Recurrence was more common among patients who underwent resection in the first versus the second half of the series (8.5 vs. 4.7%), suggesting that increased surgeon experience may be associated with lower recurrence rates (▶ Fig. 8.5).

8.3 Detection

The 6.6% rate of recurrence and rebleeding requiring reoperation an average of 2.5 years after the primary surgical resection suggests the difficulty of detecting remnants. With the management protocol at my institution, postoperative MRI is performed within 48 hours after resection to identify remnants, and those patients with positive imaging findings are returned to the operating room to complete the resection. There was no immediate return to the operating room in this

Table 8.1 Characteristics of patients with recurrent brainstem CMs requiring reoperation

Patient	Age (y)	Sex	No. of events	Total no. of operations	Years between operations	Days to rebleeding[a]	Timing to operation	Clinical presentation at rehemorrhage	Location	Volume (mm^3)	Maximum diameter (mm)	Depth to pia	Surface	Cross axial midline	CM grade[b]
1	41	F	4	2	2.1	707	Subacute	No	Pons	N/A	N/A	Superficial	Dorsal	Yes	4
2	37	F	2	2	0.1	7	Acute	No	Pons	9,472	29.5	Deep	Dorsal	Yes	2
3	22	F	2	2	0.0	1	Acute	No	Medulla	2,033	17.2	Superficial	Ventral	Yes	1
4	56	M	2	2	0.1	21	Acute	Yes	Pons	15,497	33.5	Deep	Ventral	Yes	5
5	38	F	2	2	5.7	2,082	Subacute	Yes	Pons	2,098	16.9	Superficial	Dorsal	Yes	3
6	67	F	3	2	2.3	838	Acute	Yes	Pons	2,077	16.9	Deep	Dorsal	No	3
7	39	F	3	3[c]	8.9	3,249	Acute	Yes	Pons	3,710	27.4	Superficial	Ventral	Yes	2
8	26	F	2	2	5.9	2,159	Acute	Yes	Midbrain	3,093	29.3	Deep	Ventral	No	2
9	32	F	2	2	2.8	1,005	Acute	Yes	Medulla	1,320	15.2	Deep	Ventral	Yes	2
10	26	F	3	2	0.4	127	Acute	No	Pons	271	8.5	Exophytic	Dorsal	Yes	1
11	37	F	2	2	4.5	1,620	Acute	Yes	Pons	3,316	19.3	Deep	Dorsal	No	1
12	39	F	2	2	1.2	430	Acute	Yes	Pons	546	10.7	Exophytic	Ventral	No	1
13	43	F	3	2	3.2	1,113	Acute	No	Midbrain	1,116	11.7	Superficial	Dorsal	No	3
14	40	F	2	3[d]	0.7	957	Subacute	Yes	Pons	383	10.2	Superficial	Ventral	Yes	3

[a]Days to rebleed represents the time from last surgery to clinical or radiographic evidence of rehemorrhage.
[b]Brainstem CM grade was measured by five factors: size of cavernoma (0–2 cm, 0 points; > 2 cm, 1 point), crossing axial midpoint (no, 0 points; yes, 1 point), presence of developmental venous anomalies (no, 0 points; yes, 1 point), age (0–40 years, 0 point; > 40 years, 2 points), and hemorrhage timing (acute [0–3 weeks], 0 points; subacute [3–8 weeks], 1 point; or chronic [> 8 weeks], 2 points).
[c]Patient underwent three operations.
[d]Patient presented with slowly progressive evidence of deterioration and elected to undergo a third surgery.

8

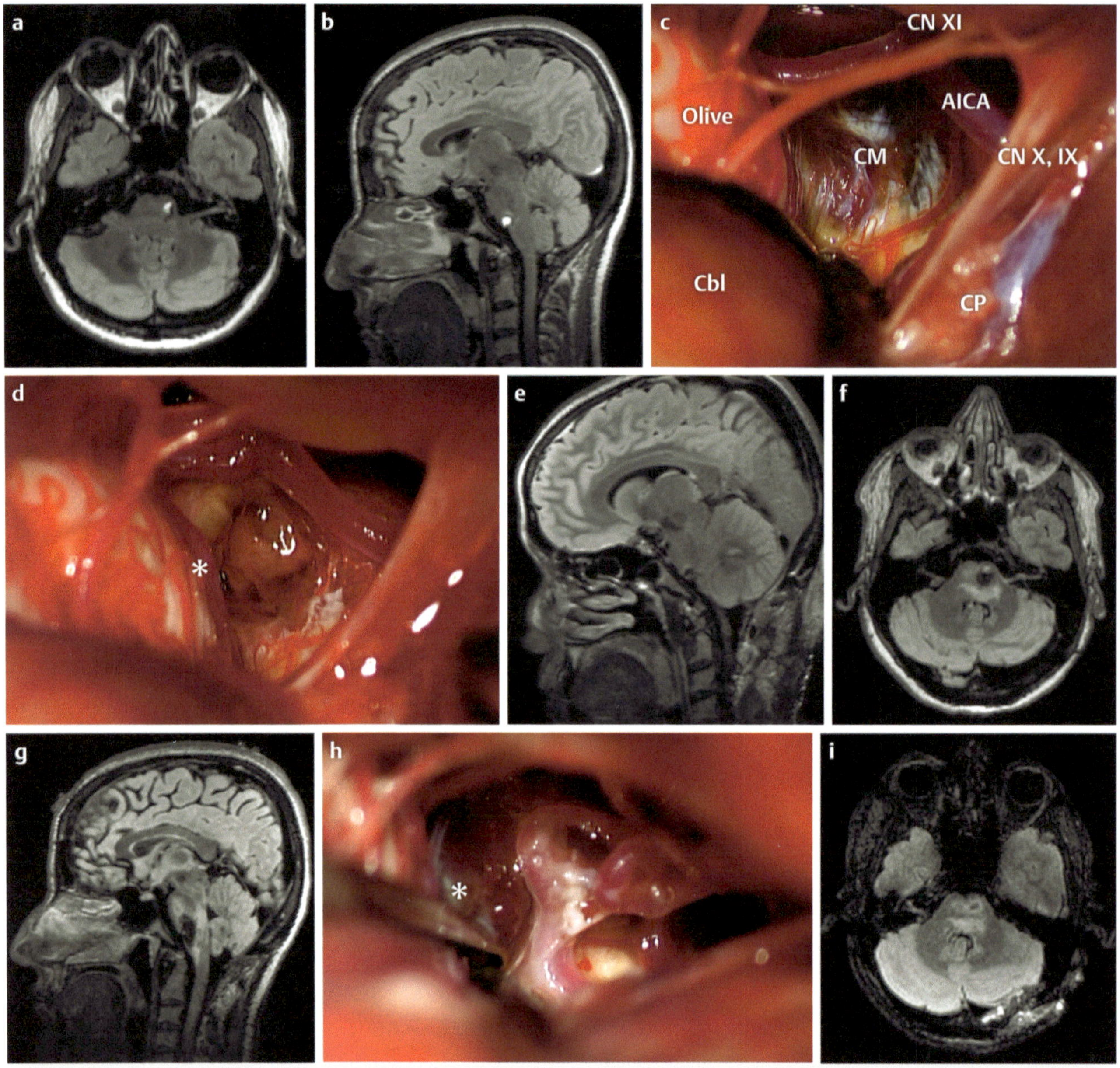

Fig. 8.1 Illustrative case 1. A 39-year-old woman (patient 12) presented with diplopia and blurred vision. A residual pontine CM was hidden in the inferior blind spot of a left far lateral craniotomy with trans-pontomedullary sulcus approach behind the olivary nucleus. The initial lesion had been diagnosed on T2 fluid-attenuated inversion recovery (FLAIR) MRI: **(a)** axial and **(b)** sagittal views. **(c)** A far lateral craniotomy exposed the lesion in the vagoaccessory triangle between the vagus nerve (CN X), spinal accessory nerve (CN XI), and olivary nucleus (Olive). **(d)** This exophytic lesion was resected through a trans-pontomedullary sulcus approach, but the residual lesion remained inferiorly behind the olivary nucleus (*asterisk*). **(e)** No residual lesion was seen on postoperative T2 FLAIR MRI (sagittal view), but the patient presented 14 months later with symptomatic rehemorrhage. Evidence of hemorrhage was seen on T2 FLAIR MRI: **(f)** axial and **(g)** sagittal views. **(h)** At reoperation through the same left far lateral craniotomy, the CM (*asterisk*) was found inferiorly in the previous resection cavity, behind the olivary nucleus. **(i)** The lesion was removed completely, as confirmed with postoperative axial T2 FLAIR MRI, and the patient recovered with no new neurological deficits. (Images **a, b, e–g, and i** are reproduced with permission from Garcia RM, Oh T, Cole TS, Hendricks BK, Lawton MT. Recurrent brainstem cavernous malformations following primary resection: blind spots, fine lines, and the right-angle method. J Neurosurg 2020;135(3):671–682. Images **c, d, and h** are reproduced with permission from Barrow Neurological Institute, Phoenix, AZ.)

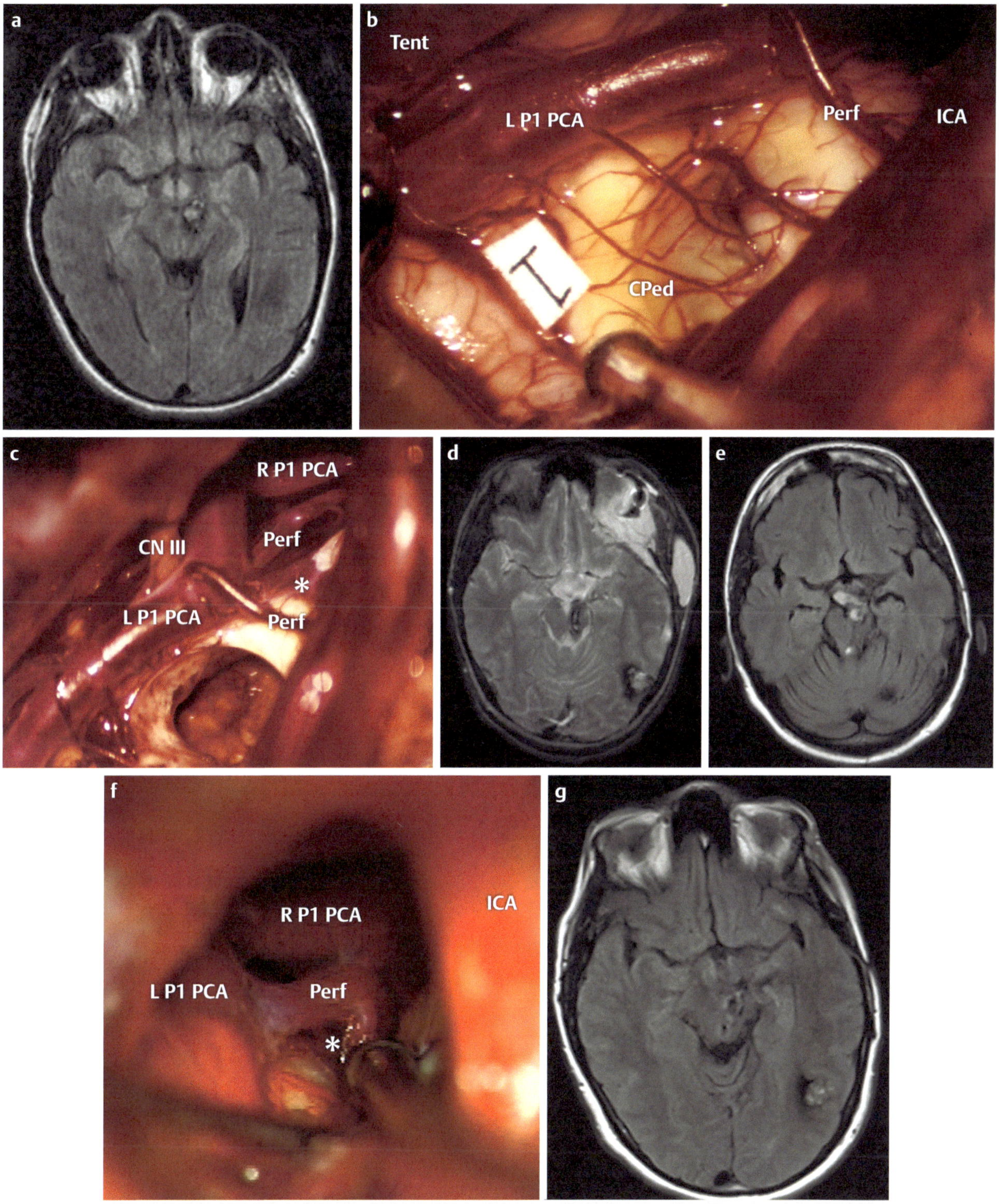

Fig. 8.2 Illustrative case 2. A 26-year-old woman (patient 8) presented with diplopia, hemiparesis, and hemianesthesia. A residual midbrain CM was found hidden in the medial blind spot under the cerebral peduncle after a left orbitozygomatic-pterional craniotomy with a transsylvian approach. **(a)** The initial lesion had been diagnosed on axial T2 fluid-attenuated inversion recovery (FLAIR) MRI. **(b)** Through a left orbitozygomatic-pterional craniotomy and transsylvian approach, the cerebral peduncle was exposed and mapped to identify the descending motor tract (1). **(c)** The lesion was resected medial to the motor tract through the hemosiderin stain on the cerebral peduncle. The lesion was accessed between the thalamoperforators (Perf), but the residual lesion remained medially (*asterisk*). **(d)** No residual lesion was seen postoperatively on T2 FLAIR MRI (axial view), but the patient presented 6 years later with symptomatic rehemorrhage. **(e)** Evidence of hemorrhage was seen on T1-weighted axial MRI. **(f)** At reoperation through the same left orbitozygomatic-pterional craniotomy with a transsylvian approach, the recurrent CM was found medial to the previous resection cavity, underneath a more medial thalamoperforator trunk (*asterisk*). **(g)** The lesion was removed completely, as confirmed postoperatively with axial T2 FLAIR MRI, and the patient recovered with no new neurological deficits. (Images **a, d, e, and g** are reproduced with permission from Garcia RM, Oh T, Cole TS, Hendricks BK, Lawton MT. Recurrent brainstem cavernous malformations following primary resection: blind spots, fine lines, and the right-angle method. J Neurosurg 2020;135(3):671–682. Images **b, c, and f** are reproduced with permission from Barrow Neurological Institute, Phoenix, AZ.)

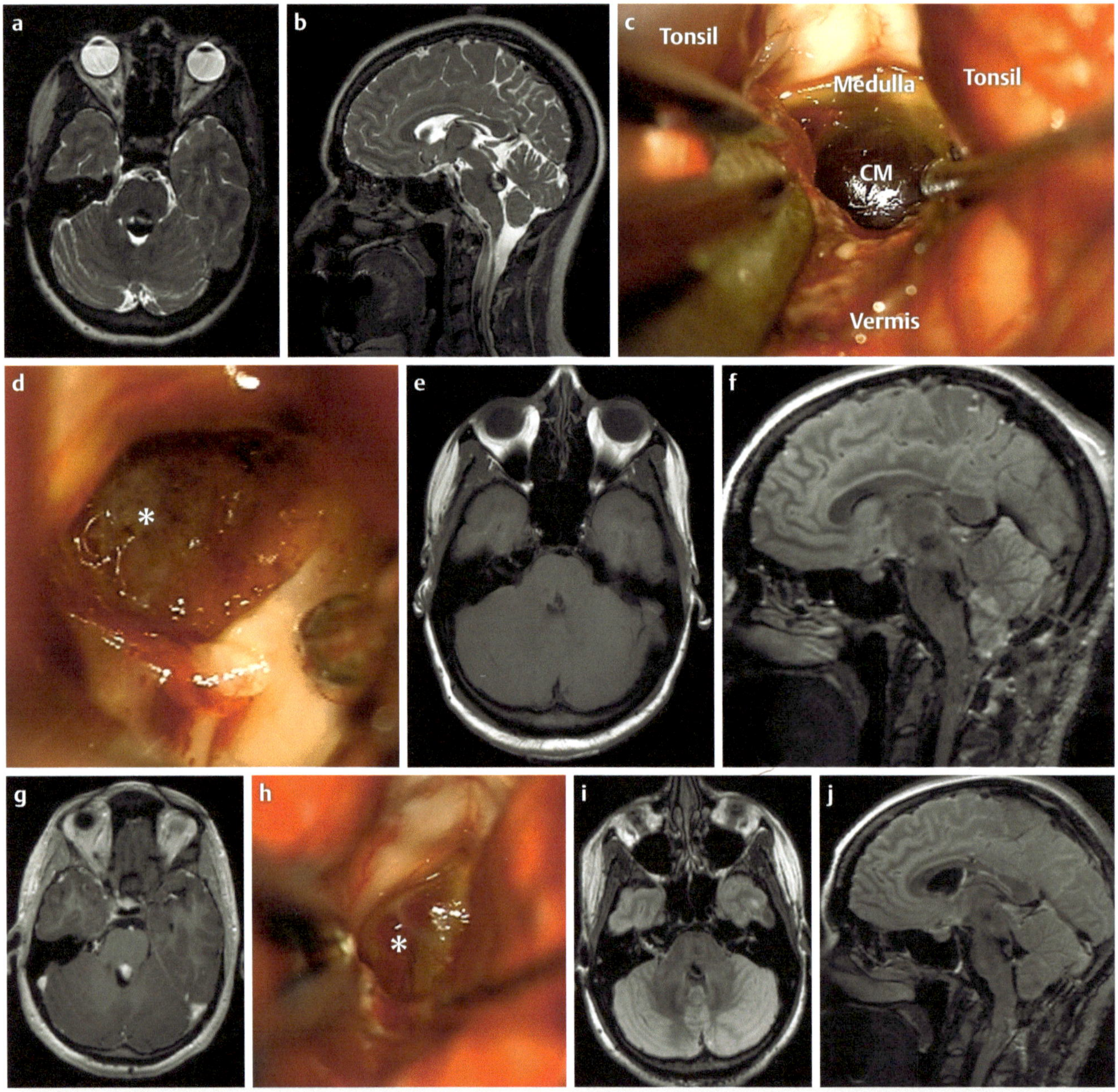

Fig. 8.3 Illustrative case 3. A 26-year-old woman (patient 10) presented with headache and diplopia. Her initial brainstem CM was found on T2-weighted MRI: **(a)** axial and **(b)** sagittal views. **(c)** A suboccipital craniotomy and transventricular approach easily exposed the lesion in the floor of the fourth ventricle. **(d)** After what was thought to be a complete resection, the deep wall of the resection cavity was interpreted as gliotic pons (*asterisk*). The recurrence in this case resulted from a misinterpretation of the deep margin of the CM. Postoperative MRI did not suggest any residual CM: **(e)** T1-weighted axial and **(f)** T2 fluid-attenuated inversion recovery (FLAIR) sagittal views. However, the patient presented 4 months later with rehemorrhage. **(g)** Evidence of hemorrhage was seen on T1-weighted axial MRI. **(h)** At reoperation through the same suboccipital craniotomy, recurrent CM was found at the depths of the previous resection cavity (*asterisk*). Deeper dissection into the cavity exposed the residual lesion, and it was removed completely, as confirmed postoperatively with **(i)** axial and **(j)** sagittal T2 FLAIR MRI. The patient recovered with no new neurological deficits. (Images **a, b, e–g, i, and j** are reproduced with permission from Garcia RM, Oh T, Cole TS, Hendricks BK, Lawton MT. Recurrent brainstem cavernous malformations following primary resection: blind spots, fine lines, and the right-angle method. J Neurosurg 2020;135(3):671–682. Images **c, d, and h** are reproduced with permission from Barrow Neurological Institute, Phoenix, AZ.)

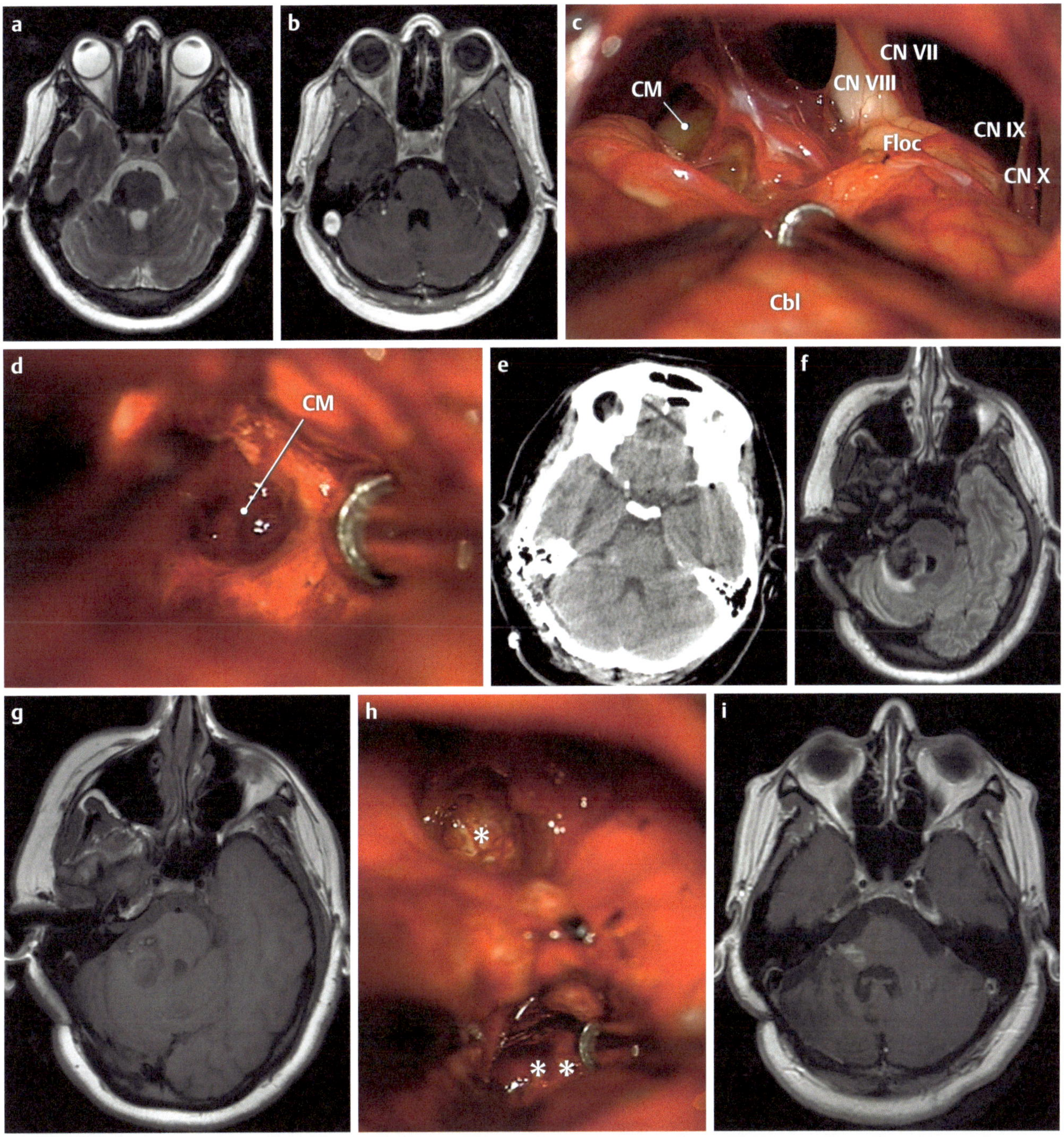

Fig. 8.4 Illustrative case 4. A 32-year-old woman (patient 11, first operation) presented with right facial numbness, and MRI showed a brainstem CM in the right lateral pons at the level of the trigeminal root entry zone, as seen on **(a)** axial T2-weighted and **(b)** axial T1-weighted gadolinium-enhanced images. Note the satellite CM lateral to the pontine lesion in the middle cerebellar peduncle (MCP). **(c)** An extended retrosigmoid craniotomy and dissection into the cerebellopontine angle exposed the greenish hemosiderin stain on the lateral pontine surface, superior to the facial (CN VII) and vestibular nerves (CN VIII). **(d)** The lesion was identified in the lateral pons and removed. **(e)** Postoperative imaging with computed tomography and MRI (not shown) did not have findings suggestive of residual lesion. The patient returned 4.5 years later with a new hemorrhage at the site of the prior surgery, as seen on axial **(f)** T2 fluid-attenuated inversion recovery and **(g)** T1-weighted MRI. The hematoma was contiguous with the previously unresected satellite lesions in the MCP. **(h)** At reoperation through an extended retrosigmoid craniotomy, the satellite lesion was resected through a transfloccular/trans-MCP approach (*double asterisk*), and a small recurrence was resected at the previous resection cavity in the lateral pons (*asterisk*). **(i)** Postoperative axial T1-weighted MRI confirmed complete resection, and the patient recovered with no new neurological deficits. (Images **a, b, e–g, and i** are reproduced with permission from Garcia RM, Oh T, Cole TS, Hendricks BK, Lawton MT. Recurrent brainstem cavernous malformations following primary resection: blind spots, fine lines, and the right-angle method. J Neurosurg. 2020;135(3):671–682. Images **c, d, and h** are reproduced with permission from Barrow Neurological Institute, Phoenix, AZ.)

Table 8.2 Outcomes of patients with brainstem CMs requiring reoperation

		Preop neurologic deficits			Last clinical evaluation deficits			Patient parameters					
Patient	Preop symptoms	Cranial nerve, *n*	Motor, *n*	Other	Cranial nerve, *n*	Motor, *n*	Other	Surgical approach	DVA	Preop mRS score	Last mRS score	Follow-up (mo)	Length of stay (d)
1	Motor weakness, paresthesia, imbalance, slurred speech, dizziness	3	4+/5	Hemianesthesia	3	None	None	Suboccipital transvermian	No	3	2	66	6
2	Headache, nausea, vomiting, dysarthria, weakness	3	4+/5	Hemianesthesia	1	None	None	Suboccipital transvermian	No	4	2	10	13
3	Vertigo, diplopia, numbness, dysphagia	2	4+/5	Hemianesthesia, ataxia	2	None	Ataxia	Right far lateral	No	2	2	5	6
4	Obtunded	5	0/5	None	2	2/5	Hemianesthesia	Left extended retrosigmoid	Yes	4	5	93	19
5	Motor weakness, facial numbness	1	3/5	Hemianesthesia	1	None	None	Suboccipital transvermian	Yes	4	2	13	6
6	Motor weakness	2	3/5	Hemianesthesia	5	None	Hemianesthesia	Suboccipital transventricular	Yes	3	3	31	8
7	Paresthesia, diplopia, facial numbness and droop, vertigo	2	None	Hemianesthesia	1	None	Hemianesthesia	Translabyrinthine; right extended retrosigmoid	No	1	1	39	10
8	Diplopia, motor weakness	1	4+/5	None	1	None	None	Left orbitozygomatic/pterional	Yes	2	1	17	12
9	Headache, diplopia	1	None	Hemianesthesia	1	None	None	Right extended retrosigmoid	Yes	2	1	6	7
10	Headache, diplopia	0	None	None	1	None	None	Suboccipital transventricular	No	1	1	6	5
11	Facial numbness, spastic leg	2	None	None	1	None	Ataxia	Right extended retrosigmoid	Yes	3	2	95	8
12	Diplopia, blurry vision	0	None	None	1	None	None	Left far lateral	Yes	1	1	38	11
13	Headache, paresthesia, facial numbness, diplopia	1	None	Hemianesthesia	1	None	Hemianesthesia	Left lateral suboccipital, supracerebellar-infratentorial	Yes	1	1	52	3
14	Motor weakness, paresthesia	0	None	None	0	4+/5	Hemianesthesia	Right extended retrosigmoid (2)	Yes	1	3	41	1

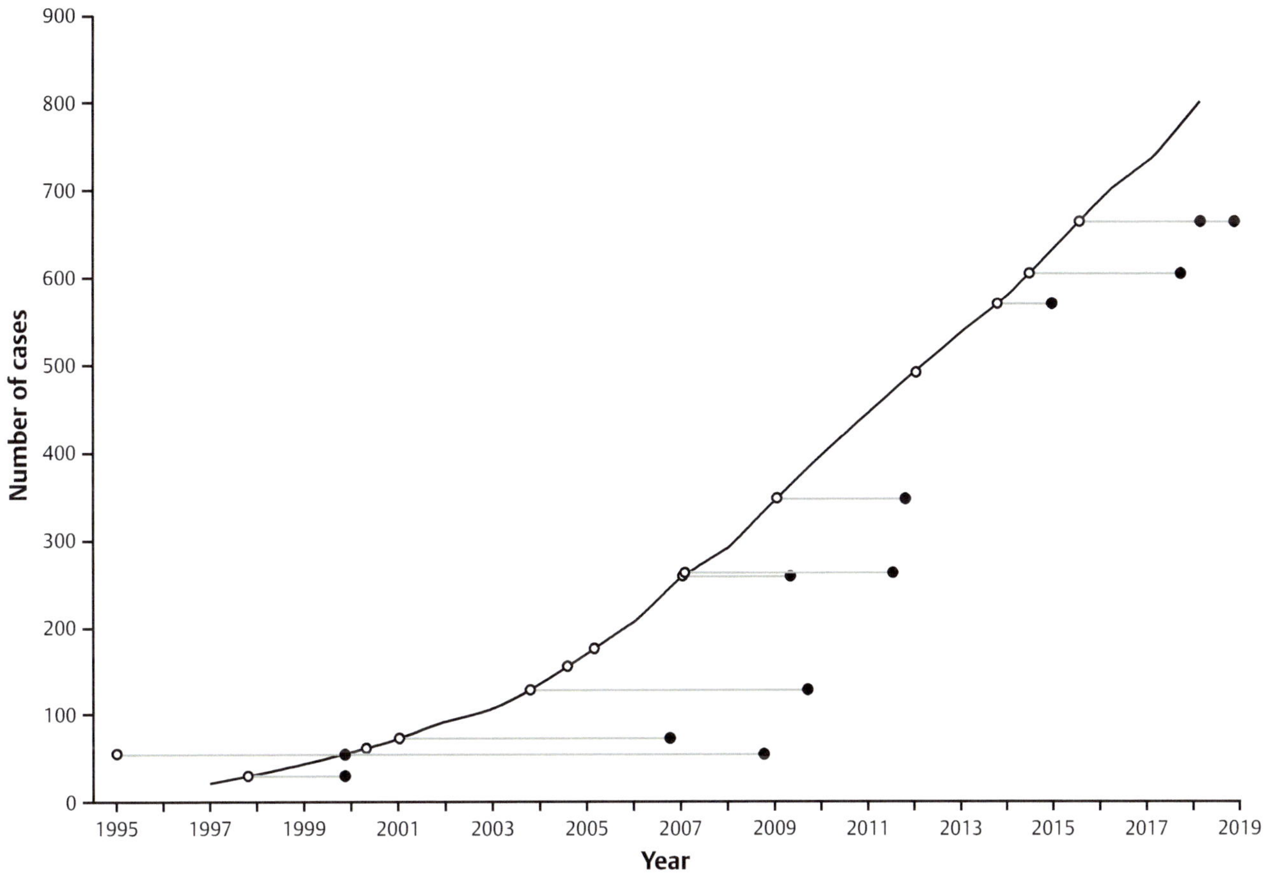

Fig. 8.5 Effect of neurosurgeon experience on the incidence of residual or recurrent brainstem CM. The cumulative case volume of all cerebral CMs resected by the author during an approximately 20-year period is plotted. Patients with residual or recurrent CMs are superimposed chronologically as horizontal lines, with the line beginning at the time of the first operation and ending at the time of the last operation. Initial operations are indicated with a *white dot*, and operations to treat residual or recurrent brainstem CM are indicated with a *black dot*. If the second operation occurred less than 6 months after the initial operation, both operations are indicated with a single *white dot*. Two patients underwent three operations. For one of these patients, the initial operation was performed by another surgeon in 1995. Recurrence was more common among patients who underwent resection in the first versus the second half of the series (8.5 vs. 4.7%), suggesting that increased surgeon experience may be associated with lower recurrence rates. (Reproduced with permission from Garcia RM, Oh T, Cole TS, Hendricks BK, Lawton MT. Recurrent brainstem cavernous malformations following primary resection: blind spots, fine lines, and the right-angle method. J Neurosurg 2020;135(3):671–682.)

surgical experience. If no residual brainstem CM is found in the immediate postoperative period, a follow-up MRI is done at 6 months to evaluate the cavity after the blood has been resorbed and the tissues have healed. In this surgical experience, two patients returned to the operating room after positive findings on surveillance imaging. This vigilant protocol failed to identify residual or recurrent lesions in 12 of the 14 patients with recurrence, reflecting the difficulty of detecting tiny remnants in the perioperative period and suggesting that, in many cases, new hemorrhages must occur before detection is possible. Tissue edema, hemostatic agents, and pooled blood in the resection cavity can hide a remnant. Thus, I meticulously pursue hemostasis with bipolar cautery, avoid oxidized cellulose products inside the cavity or on its walls, and fill the resection bed with irrigant before closing.

A 93.4% complete resection rate is consistent with other reports in the literature. Still, some of the 199 patients who were not operated on who were deemed cured may have had asymptomatic recurrences that had not yet bled or been diagnosed. Therefore, the 6.6% recurrence rate in our study could be underestimated. In addition, patients with recurrent brainstem CMs who opted to forego repeat surgery were difficult to identify retrospectively. Although I do not know of such patients in this series, they would not have been included in the study. The bleeding behavior of recurrent brainstem CMs in this experience, namely the 5.9% annual hemorrhage risk, is consistent with that reported for brainstem CMs that are not operated on and appears to be associated with a similar clinical course.

8.4 Surgical Blind Spots

Blind spots, or areas in the surgical corridor with a compromised or inadequate view, were identified as the most common cause of incomplete brainstem CM resection. The inherent depth of lesions in the brainstem and the length of the surgical

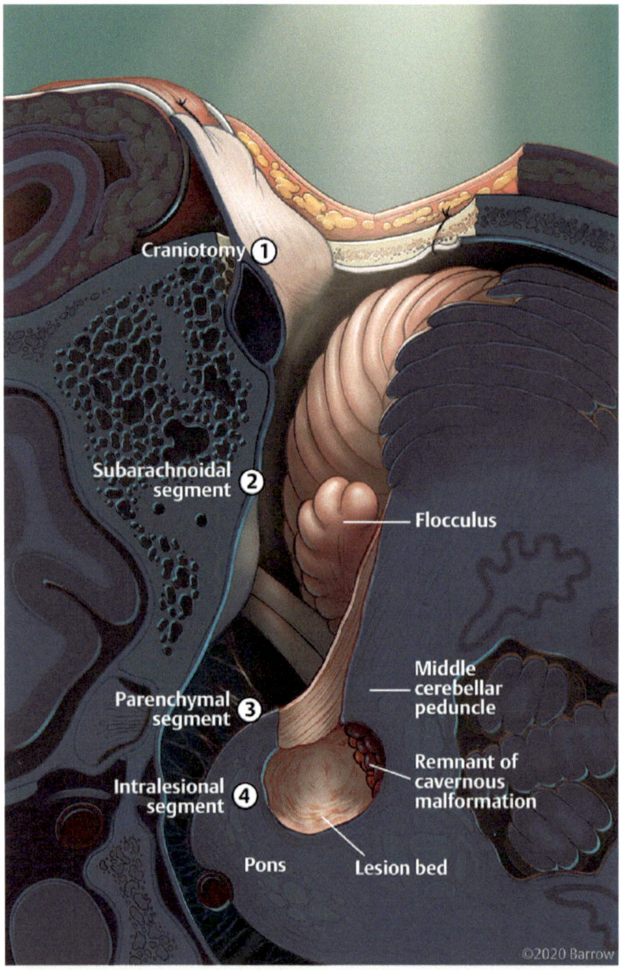

Fig. 8.6 Illustration of the anatomy of the blind spot. The inherent depth of a brainstem CM and the length of the corridor required to reach it make blind spots inevitable. The surgical corridor comprises (1) the craniotomy; (2) a subarachnoid, cisternal, or ventricular segment; (3) a parenchymal segment; and (4) an intralesional segment. With a brainstem CM, the small keyhole opening into the lesion is displaced to the end of a long corridor that limits the viewing angles, decreases visualization, and creates blind spots where a remnant can be hidden. (Reproduced with permission from Barrow Neurological Institute, Phoenix, AZ.)

corridor make blind spots inevitable. The surgical corridor comprises (1) the craniotomy, (2) a subarachnoid or ventricular segment, (3) a parenchymal segment, and (4) an intralesional segment (▶ Fig. 8.6). Each component adds length and limits visualization. For example, the trans-middle cerebellar peduncle approach to a middle peduncular pontine CM has a corridor made up of the retrosigmoid craniotomy, subarachnoid dissection into the cerebellopontine angle, a tunnel through the middle cerebellar peduncle, and entrance into the lesion. The view of the lesion through this 6-cm corridor can be obscured by the edges of the craniotomy, a prominent flocculus, the collapsing white matter of the middle cerebellar peduncle, or the corners at the interface between the middle cerebellar peduncle and the lesion laterally. Corridors to brainstem CMs have small openings, long lengths, and limited viewing angles, which are the opposite of the keyhole concept, in which a small opening plus a wide range of views still enable good visualization of the lesion. With brainstem CMs, the keyhole is displaced to the end of an already long corridor without a wide range of viewing angles, which decreases visualization and requires the lesion to be mobilized into the viewing axis. The blind spots created by this geometry force possible blind dissection and hide the pathology. One must conceptualize the blind spots and deliberately inspect these spaces at the end of the resection, even after the resection seems complete.

This difficult geometry is compounded by darkness, swollen brain tissue, and poor approach selection. Lighted instruments (bipolar forceps and suction tips) in long corridors are invaluable. Endoscopes are sometimes useful to inspect the cavity after resection. Brain edema can narrow the corridor and make the walls more susceptible to injury with manipulation and retraction. Delaying surgery for 1 to 2 weeks after a hemorrhage allows time for the edema to resolve and the associated hematoma to liquefy, making it easier to develop and dissect the brainstem CM separation planes. Dynamic retraction is important within deep corridors because it slightly shifts the tissues, viewing axis, and illumination with each move to glimpse potential blind spots. Fixed retraction is rarely helpful to see within the resection cavity and often obstructs the dissection maneuvers.

8.5 Right-Angle Method

The "two-point method" helps guide the selection of approaches to brainstem CMs. The first point is placed where the CM comes to a pial or ependymal surface, the second point is placed at the center of the lesion, and the line connecting these two points defines the lesion's axis. The two-point method is a heuristic that matches the lesion's axis with the surgical axis, which is the trajectory of the operative corridor. When these axes align, the lesion is well visualized within the resection cavity; visualization is impaired when these axes do not align.

One way to conceptualize blind spots is with another method: the "right-angle method." The surgical axis is defined by two points: one at the superficial entrance into the operative corridor (corridor entry, point 1) and one at the entry into the brainstem CM (front wall, point 2; ▶ Fig. 8.7). The surgical axis is drawn by connecting these points and extending this line through the lesion to its back wall (point 3). With the right-angle method, a perpendicular line is drawn from the surgical axis to the point on the lesion's capsule farthest from the axis. Lobulations and compartments often make these lesions irregular and asymmetric rather than spherical. Perpendicular lines drawn on axial, sagittal, and coronal MRI identify multiple potential blind spots, and any perpendicular line exceeding 1 cm in length identifies a potential blind spot. The surgical axis approximates the line of sight into the resection bed, which makes spots in the near corners more difficult to see than those in the far corners. A line of sight down a long corridor cannot make right turns, which transforms ledges of eloquent tissue in the near field into blind spots. The right-angle method helps anticipate these blind spots, which drives meticulous inspection for CM remnants during the operation (▶ Fig. 8.7).

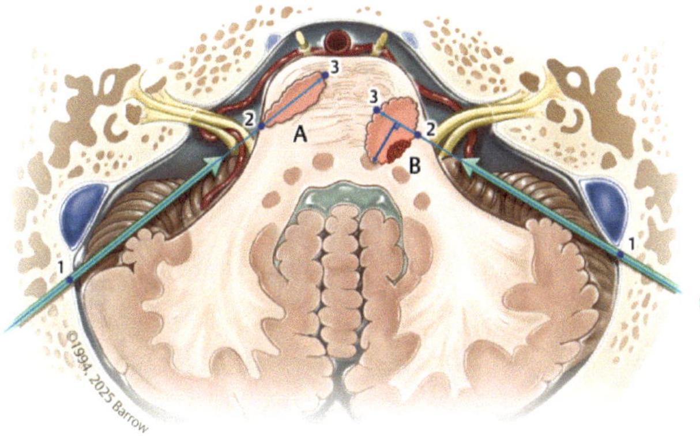

Fig. 8.7 Illustration of the right-angle method. The surgical axis is defined by two points: one at the superficial entrance into the operative corridor (corridor entry, point 1) and one at the entry into the brainstem CM (front wall, point 2). The surgical axis is drawn by connecting these points and extending this line through the lesion to its back wall (point 3). The right-angle method draws a perpendicular line from the surgical axis to the point on the lesion's capsule farthest from the axis. Any perpendicular line exceeding 1 cm in length is a potential blind spot. This illustration shows two pontine CMs, each exposed through an extended retrosigmoid craniotomy with trans-middle cerebellar peduncle approach. The long axis of lesion A aligns with the surgical axis, and the right-angle method identifies no blind spot. In contrast, the long axis of lesion B does not align with the surgical axis, and the right-angle method identifies a posterolateral blind spot hiding a remnant (*red*) of the CM. (Reproduced with permission from Barrow Neurological Institute, Phoenix, AZ.)

8.6 Fine Line

After blind spots, misinterpretation of the resection cavity contents was the next most common cause of residual or recurrent lesions. Every resection requires the painstaking evaluation of the plane that separates the CM from the brain or brainstem. In other words, overcoming blind spots and obtaining proper views bring the greater challenge of dissection at the border between the lesion and the parenchyma, between morbidity and cure. Direct visualization and cautious dissection define these differences. Sometimes, color, contour, and texture make this distinction obvious, with mulberry-like lesions embedded in hemosiderin-stained parenchyma or a thick capsule that peels away cleanly from the brainstem. Other times, the hemorrhagic parenchyma blends indistinctly with the pathology, particularly in the cases where the remnant was not in a blind spot but left behind in plain sight. The brainstem's supreme eloquence can make neurosurgeons cautious. Conservatism keeps operations safe and patients intact, whereas probing deeper and pushing further can be essential or devastating. At these moments of uncertain interpretation, completeness and morbidity pull at each other like a tug-of-war in the neurosurgeon's mind. A fine line separates complete resection from recurrence and good outcomes from new deficits.

The capsule is the key to safe and complete lesionectomy. A small opening into the capsule is necessary to drain the liquified hematoma and reduce the lesion's size. Caverns are opened and decompartmentalized internally to explore the different portions of the lesion. Capsular preservation keeps the lesion whole and protects the brainstem from the neurosurgeon's maneuvers. Gradually, the capsule pulls away from the parenchyma. The dissection then switches from intracapsular to extracapsular, freeing adhesions circumferentially and collapsing the capsule inward to reveal the remaining points of adhesion. Ideally, circumferential dissection liberates the brainstem CM with its capsule intact, except for the initial entry site. Sharp dissection is performed with round knives of varying sizes and angles and rarely with microscissors. Delicate traction with a grasping instrument and countertraction with the suction tip finally deliver the lesion.

Neurophysiological monitoring identifies areas of highest eloquence, like the facial colliculus in the fourth ventricular floor or the pyramidal tract in the cerebral peduncle of the midbrain. Neuromonitoring warns the neurosurgeon when the dissection is too rough or strays into monitored tracts and nerves. Although these alarms help redirect or modulate the dissection, they can also derail the neurosurgeon. A sudden signal change elicits worry and hesitation, often at the end of a resection when the borders of the lesion have been reached. Too much caution at the finish line can easily lead to leaving a brainstem CM remnant. Small diminutions of signals should not deter the pursuit of curative resection because they often translate to transient deficits postoperatively. The information must be processed without impeding progress to complete resection. Neuromonitoring has become the standard of care for this operation but requires a steeled mindset to press onward when neurophysiological signals change, representing another fine line to be managed.

The fine lines between complete resection and recurrence, safe and harmful resection, and heeding and ignoring neuromonitoring make this operation one of the most challenging in neurosurgery. It lacks the drama of intraoperative rupture or the elegance of deep bypasses, but it demands circumspection at every step, from the approach selection to the exposure to each maneuver during the resection. It demands constant calculation regarding how hard to pull, how deep to probe, and how thoroughly to search. Other challenging operations happen in subarachnoid spaces or deep cisterns, but the resection of a CM is within the brain or brainstem, which raises the stakes to the highest level. Even extensive neurosurgical experience does not eliminate the problem of incomplete resection. Residual lesions were observed less frequently with increasing experience, which reflects the maturation of technique, comfort working within the brainstem, awareness of blind spots, and a feel for separation planes. However, recurrences were still observed late in this surgical experience of more than 800 cerebral CMs. One of the greatest benefits of experience is that it reduces the uncomfortable dissonance created by walking these fine lines. The enduring problem of brainstem CM remnants, despite extensive experience, highlights the need for a neurosurgeon to constantly modulate between an aggressive approach associated with undue operative morbidity and a conservative approach associated with high rates of recurrence. We must constantly work toward an acceptable balance of safety and completeness, yielding a recurrence rate of about 5% of cases.

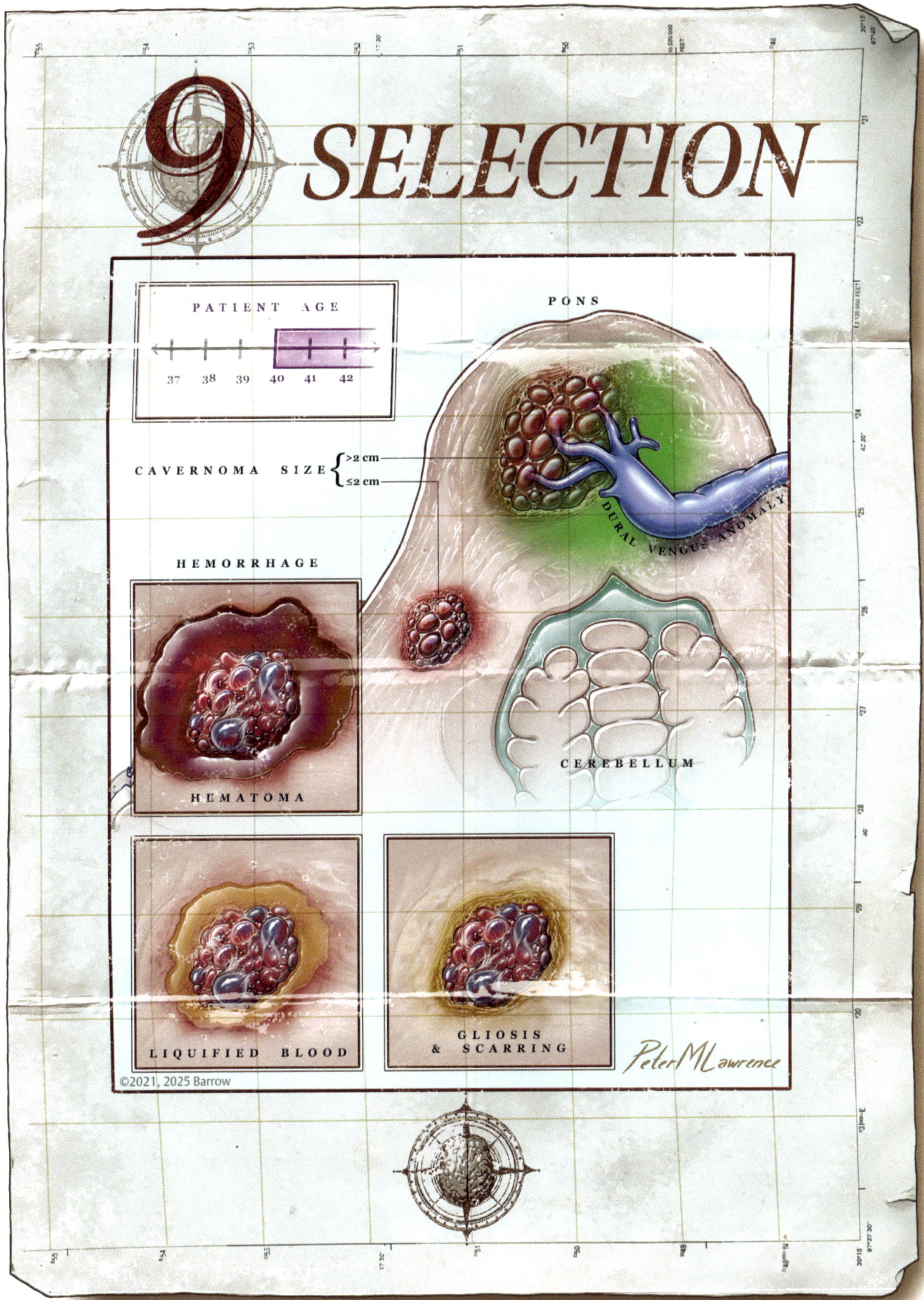

Reproduced with permission from Barrow Neurological Institute, Phoenix, AZ.

9 Patient Selection

Summary

Neurosurgeons have been historically reluctant to operate on brainstem cavernous malformations (CMs). Today, brainstem CMs are surgically managed with good outcomes in most patients. Patient selection is a critical determinant of these results. At Barrow Neurological Institute, we developed a 7-point brainstem CM grading system that combines anatomical factors of lesion size, eloquence, and venous anatomy with clinical factors of age and hemorrhagic presentation. This scoring system can predict long-term functional outcomes and guide clinical decision-making. The grading system was externally validated in a 277-patient group. Outcomes were predicted by brainstem CM grade, with good outcomes observed in 47 of 54 patients (87%) with low-grade brainstem CMs (grades 0–II), 135 of 181 patients (75%) with intermediate-grade brainstem CMs, and 21 of 42 patients (50%) with high-grade brainstem CMs (grades VI–VII). Conversely, rates of neurological deterioration increased with increasing brainstem CM grade, with worsening observed in 2 of 54 patients (4%) with low-grade brainstem CMs, 29 of 181 patients (16%) with intermediate-grade brainstem CMs, and 17 of 42 patients (40%) with high-grade brainstem CMs. The difficult analysis of innumerable variables was simplified by the grading system to assigning points in a formula and establishing categories of low-, intermediate-, and high-grade brainstem CMs. The brainstem CM grading system facilitates the selection of surgery for patients with low-grade CMs and observation for patients with high-grade CMs, but the boundary of operability lies somewhere within the intermediate grades. Each neurosurgeon must calibrate this boundary to their unique abilities, practices, and outcome results.

Keywords: arteriovenous malformation, brainstem, cavernous malformation, developmental venous anomaly, grading scale, hemorrhage, outcome, risk assessment

9.1 Rationale for a Brainstem Cavernous Malformation Grading Scale

Cavernous malformations (CMs) in the cerebral and cerebellar hemispheres can be resected safely, and surgery is indicated when young age, neurological symptoms, mass effect, hemorrhagic behavior, accessible location, and low operative risk compare favorably to natural history risks. These decisions are straightforward and rarely require tools like grading systems to advise patients. In contrast, treatment of patients with brainstem CMs is challenging due to the lesion's rarity, the technical difficulty of surgery near critical anatomy, and significant associated operative risks. Brainstem CMs account for 15 to 18% of intracranial CMs, and their hemorrhage rates appear to be more than twice those of other intracranial CMs. Neurosurgeons have been reluctant to operate on these lesions, and brainstem CMs are now aggressively managed with an early postoperative neurological morbidity rate of 45%; a long-term, permanent morbidity rate of 14%; and good outcomes (improved or unchanged) in 84% of patients. Patient selection remains a critical determinant of these results and has been inadequately addressed in the literature. The recommendation for surgery is a difficult decision that depends on patient presentation, lesion size, accessibility, distance to the pial or ependymal surface, hemorrhage history, and surgeon expertise, among other factors, and would be facilitated by a grading system.

Rational patient selection is derived from the identification of measurable preoperative factors that correlate with operative morbidity and neurological outcomes. These clinical or anatomical factors are often packaged in grading scales that simplify this arduous task of patient selection and make surgical risk assessment formulaic. Hernesniemi and colleagues proposed the first grading system for CMs, but their system applied to all CMs, including those in the spinal cord, rather than just to those in the brainstem. This system would characterize all brainstem CMs as high-risk grade 3 lesions, with a 54% chance of long-term disability after surgery, and would thus fail to differentiate good surgical candidates from poor surgical candidates. A grading system designed specifically for brainstem CMs that predicts outcomes associated with microsurgical resection might be a valuable clinical tool for neurosurgeons wrestling with patient selection. Such a grading system would differentiate patients with brainstem CMs who might expect more favorable surgical outcomes and offer guidance in patient selection.

Rather than consider all CMs and develop a broadly applicable grading system that was weak for brainstem CMs, my colleagues and I focused on brainstem CMs to serve the patients who would most benefit from a grading system. In 2015, we published a study that identified the critical predictors in a 15-year experience with brainstem CMs in 104 patients, representing the fourth largest experience reported in the literature. Informed by a considerable experience with arteriovenous malformations (AVMs), we took a similar approach in developing a new grading system to predict outcomes for CMs. We combined anatomical factors like size, eloquence, and venous anatomy with clinical factors like age and hemorrhagic presentation to produce a meaningful new grading system for brainstem CMs that predicted long-term functional outcomes and guided clinical decision-making (▶ Table 9.1, ▶ Table 9.2, ▶ Table 9.3). The Lawton brainstem CM grading scale was born out of this effort.

9.2 Lawton Brainstem CM Grading Scale

A brainstem CM grading system, the so-called Lawton or Lawton-Garcia brainstem CM grading system, was constructed using the five significant variables identified in the multivariable model (▶ Fig. 9.1). Analogous to AVM grading systems, this grading system consists of five variables with a total of 7 possible points assigned for size (maximum axial diameter ≤ 2 vs. > 2 cm), lesion crossing the brainstem axial midpoint, presence of a venous malformation or developmental venous anomaly (DVA), patient age (≤ 40 vs. > 40 years), and time from most recent hemorrhage to surgery. A total of 7 points can be assigned because, first, age was weighted by coefficients in the multivariable model, resulting in two points for patients older

Table 9.1 Brainstem CM grading in 277 patients by brainstem location

Variable	Points	Patients, *n* (%)			
		Midbrain (*n* = 77)	Pons (*n* = 160)	Medulla (*n* = 40)	Total (*N* = 277)
Size (cm)					
≤ 2	0	54 (70)	101 (63)	37 (92)	192 (69)
> 2	1	23 (30)	59 (37)	3 (8)	85 (31)
Crossing axial midpoint					
No	0	36 (47)	69 (43)	15 (38)	120 (43)
Yes	1	41 (53)	91 (57)	25 (62)	157 (57)
DVA					
No	0	40 (52)	55 (34)	27 (68)	122 (44)
Yes	1	37 (48)	105 (66)	13 (32)	155 (56)
Age (y)					
≤ 40	0	33 (43)	89 (56)	21 (52)	143 (52)
> 40	2	44 (57)	71 (44)	19 (48)	134 (48)
Hemorrhage[a]					
Acute (< 3 wk)	0	13 (17)	33 (21)	8 (20)	54 (19)
Subacute (3–8 wk)	1	12 (16)	21 (13)	4 (10)	37 (13)
Chronic (> 8 wk)	2	52 (68)	106 (66)	28 (70)	186 (67)

[a]Percentages may total less than 100% or greater than 100% due to rounding.

Table 9.2 Surgical approaches to brainstem CMs in 277 patients by location

Surgical approach	Patients, *n*/total (%)
Midbrain	
All patients	77/277 (28)
Transcallosal-transchoroidal	13/77 (17)
Orbitozygomatic-transsylvian	3/77 (4)
Supracerebellar-infratentorial	
Midline and paramedian	34/77 (44)
Lateral	23/77 (30)
Other	4/77 (5)
Pons	
All patients	160/277 (58)
Extended retrosigmoid	
Trans-cerebellopontine angle and trans-middle cerebellar peduncle	90/160 (56)
Suboccipital-transventricular	29/160 (18)
Suboccipital-telovelar	16/160 (10)
Far lateral-trans-pontomedullary sulcus	16/160 (10)
Subtemporal-transtentorial	1/160 (1)
Kawase/anterior transpetrous	7/160 (4)
Posterior transpetrous	1/160 (1)
Medulla	
All patients	40/277 (14)
Suboccipital-transventricular	19/40 (48)
Far lateral-trans-cerebellomedullary cistern	17/40 (42)
Suboccipital-telovelar	2/40 (5)
Extended retrosigmoid–trans-cerebellopontine angle	2/40 (5)

than 40 years. Second, the time between hemorrhage and surgery has three intervals: acute (< 3 weeks), which is assigned 0 points; subacute (3–8 weeks), which is assigned 1 point; and chronic (> 8 weeks) or unruptured, which is assigned 2 points. Points are added, and grades are assigned ranging from 0 to 7 points. Neurological outcomes are predicted by brainstem CM grade, with the chances of an unfavorable outcome and increasing surgical morbidity with increasing CM grade.

This grading system embraces the predictive power of age and early surgery after the most recent hemorrhage; DVAs also

Table 9.3 Absolute and relative outcomes by brainstem CM grade

Brainstem CM grade	No. patients	Outcome		mRS score	
		Good	Poor	Same or improved	Worse
		mRS score ≤ 2	mRS score > 2		
0	1	1 (100)	0 (0)	1 (100)	0 (0)
I	13	12 (92)	1 (8)	13 (100)	0 (0)
II	40	34 (85)	6 (15)	38 (95)	2 (5)
III	62	50 (81)	12 (19)	57 (92)	5 (8)
IV	65	51 (78)	14 (22)	54 (83)	11 (17)
V	54	34 (63)	20 (37)	41 (76)	13 (24)
VI	29	17 (59)	12 (41)	19 (66)	10 (34)
VII	13	4 (31)	9 (69)	6 (46)	7 (54)
All (0–VII)	277	203 (73)	74 (27)	229 (83)	48 (17)

Note: Data are presented as n (%) unless otherwise indicated.

contribute to the predictability of the outcome. Size and a location that crossed the axial midpoint also contributed to the predictability of the outcome. Outcome predictors for brainstem CMs and AVMs are strikingly similar, even though their pathobiology and pathophysiology are quite different. The predictors used in the Spetzler-Martin grading system include size, eloquence, and venous drainage. The predictors for the Lawton–Young AVM grading system include age, hemorrhagic presentation, and compactness. These six variables are routinely combined into a supplemented Spetzler–Martin score for AVMs. Except for compactness or diffuseness, which applies to AVMs and not to CMs because the latter have a discrete capsule and a clear demarcation from the parenchyma, predictors that appear to affect brainstem CM outcomes are remarkably similar to those associated with AVM outcomes. This indicates that many of the same surgical factors that influence AVM outcomes also influence brainstem CM outcomes. This insight might offer a new, analogous methodology for preoperative risk assessment at the bedside.

9.3 Elements of the Brainstem CM Grading System

Patient selection for microsurgical treatment of brainstem CMs is a critical determinant of treatment success. The Lawton brainstem CM grading system was developed to assist in selecting those patients who are most likely to benefit from surgery. Each of the five variables that make up the Lawton brainstem CM grading system, including lesion size, location relative to the brainstem axial midpoint, presence of a DVA, patient age, and hemorrhage status, is discussed in detail below.

9.3.1 Size

Size is an obvious factor in resecting brain AVMs and brainstem CMs but does not always emerge as a statistically significant factor because conservative biases may influence patient selection with brainstem lesions at either extreme. Larger lesions might not be associated with worse outcomes because of exophytic pial presentation or shorter distances beneath pial surfaces, larger operative cavities, larger hematoma, and greater separation of fiber tracts through which to work. As with AVMs, lesion size is an important intuitive, if not statistical, consideration and was built into our brainstem CM grading system. Larger lesions have more contact area with surrounding brainstem tissue, which increases circumferential dissection, tissue manipulation, the risk to perforators, bleeding, the likelihood of leaving residual lesion, and the need for reoperation.

9.3.2 Crossing the Axial Midpoint

The concept that some areas are more critical and inviolable than others is important in AVM surgery and is captured by the term *eloquence*. However, the entire brainstem is considered eloquent, making eloquence meaningless in a brainstem CM grading system. We captured this concept for brainstem CMs by assessing whether they crossed the axial midpoint, with the idea that such lesions are more deeply embedded in the brainstem than those on the periphery, might require more parenchymal transgression, are closer to more vital central tracts and nuclei, and can incur bilateral brainstem morbidity. Furthermore, central brainstem CMs are associated with greater technical challenges, including longer surgical corridors, reduced visualization, more blind spots in the resection cavity, and limited maneuverability of instruments. Other measures of brainstem eloquence were considered, like depth below the pial or ependymal surface, ventral location, or crossing the midline, but whether a CM crossed the axial midpoint proved to be a simple and reproducible approximation for eloquence.

9.3.3 Developmental Venous Anomaly

Although some authors observe DVAs with all brainstem CMs, we found them radiographically and intraoperatively in slightly more than half of our patients. Surprisingly, and for the first time, we found an association between DVAs and neurological outcomes (univariable analysis, $p = 0.03$; multivariable analysis, odds ratio [OR] = 4.01; 95% confidence interval [CI]: 1.04–15.40; $p = 0.04$). The preservation of DVAs is an established practice because they are part of the normal venous circulation, and their compromise can cause venous ischemia or infarction. DVAs were meticulously preserved in this operative experience, and therefore, their association with the outcome was not due

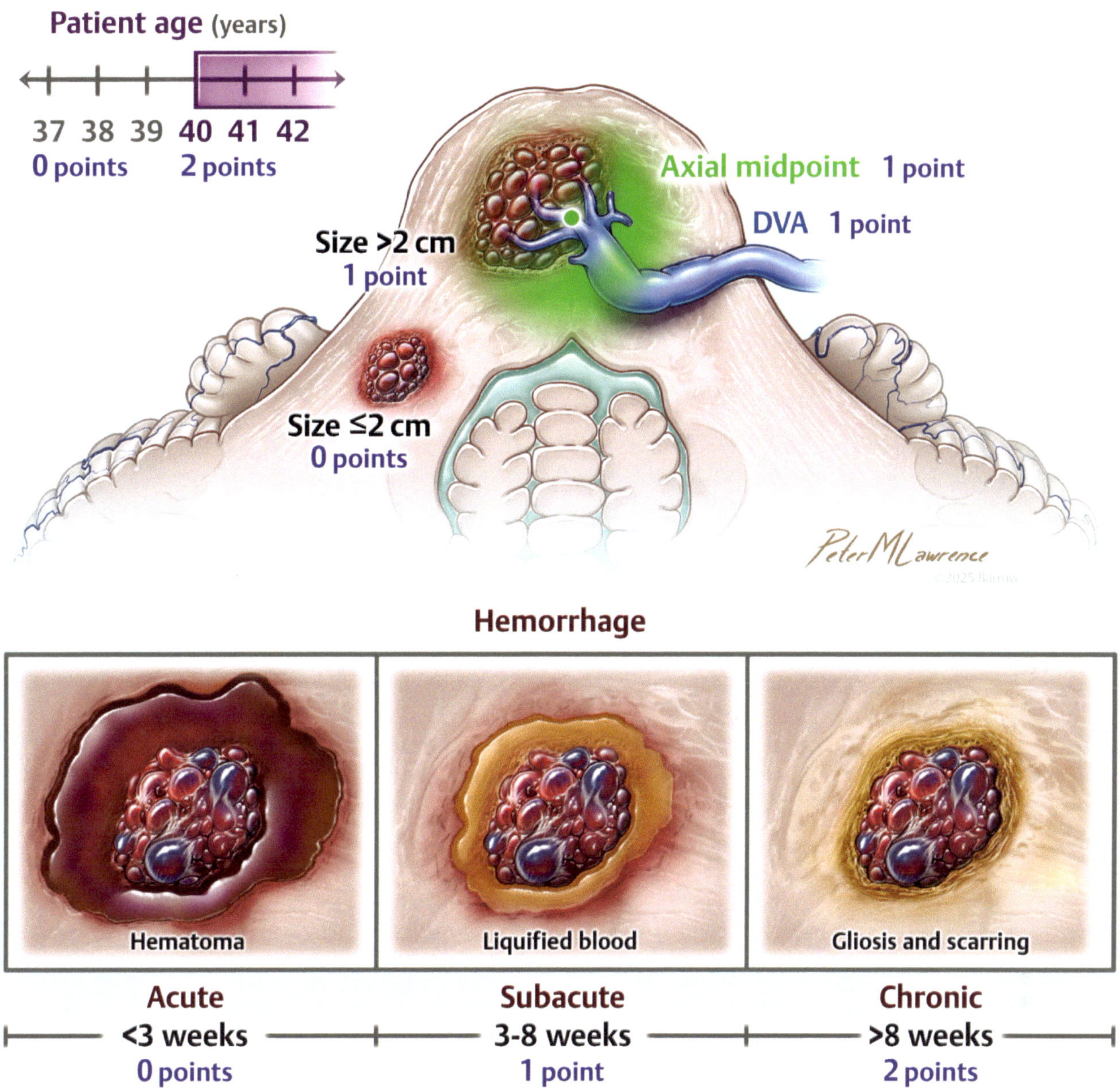

Fig. 9.1 The Lawton brainstem CM grading system consists of five variables with points assigned for size (maximum axial diameter ≤ 2 vs. > 2 cm), lesions that cross the axial midpoint, a venous malformation or DVA, patient age, and time since the most recent hemorrhagic event. With the brainstem CM grading system, 7 points can be assigned because age is weighted with 2 points for patients ≥ 40 years old, and the time between hemorrhage and surgery has three intervals: acute (< 3 weeks), subacute (3–8 weeks), and chronic (> 8 weeks) or unruptured. The grading system categorizes patients into eight grades (0–VII) because it is possible for patients to have no points assigned. (Reproduced with permission from Barrow Neurological Institute, Phoenix, AZ.)

to their sacrifice or venous complications. We speculate that DVAs increase the overall complexity of brainstem CM resection, often creating obstacles in the surgical corridor, brisk bleeding during resection, or generating satellite lesions in the brainstem. In the Spetzler–Martin grading system, deep venous drainage is a surrogate measure of deep AVM location and does not relate directly to venous physiology. In the Lawton brainstem CM grading system, DVAs have no relation to lesion depth and can course in many directions, deep or superficial to the lesion. Points are assigned based on preoperative magnetic resonance imaging (MRI) and apply only to those DVAs large enough to be radiographically visible.

9.3.4 Age

Age is the only factor that predicts outcome in all major brainstem CM experiences, including ours ($p = 0.002$ in the univariable and $p = 0.001$ in the multivariable analyses). Age was also identified as a significant factor for predicting outcomes after AVM surgery and is incorporated into the Lawton–Young supplementary grading system. Like that grading system, this brainstem CM grading system used an arbitrary 40-year cutoff as a dividing line between young and old patients. These findings indicate the importance of neural plasticity in recovery, rehabilitation, and general resilience after brainstem CM resection, particularly among pediatric patients (< 20 years of age). These findings also indicate the negative effects of increasing comorbidities beyond 40 years for general anesthetic and surgical risks, recoverability, and overall outcome.

9.3.5 Hemorrhage

The supplementary grading system for AVMs recognizes the surgical advantages of hemorrhage by scoring a point for patients presenting with unruptured AVMs. Hemorrhage facilitates surgery by separating the AVM from the adjacent brain, and hematoma evacuation creates working space around the nidus that can minimize brain transgression or access a deep nidus that might otherwise have been unreachable. These advantages apply to brainstem CMs, which explains the predictive power of early surgery after the most recent hemorrhage. Early surgery allows time to stabilize the patient's condition, reduce edema around the lesion, and capitalize on the liquefied hematoma around or within the brainstem CM. Although the topic has not been rigorously studied, in our experience, this liquefied hematoma remains for approximately 8 weeks; accordingly, we chose this endpoint for the subacute time window in our grading system. In the chronic phase, the liquid of the hematoma is absorbed, and the brainstem CM adheres to the surrounding parenchyma with gliosis, scar tissue, and hematoma organization, making it more difficult to remove safely and cleanly. A brainstem CM's ease of separation from the brainstem is critically important from a technical standpoint, and an acute or subacute hematoma helps the neurosurgeon peel the lesion gently away. Therefore, this hemorrhage variable measures the time interval from hemorrhage to surgery, capturing this surgical nuance. Forty percent of our patients underwent surgery acutely, and 64% underwent surgery within 8 weeks. Others have shown the number of hemorrhagic events patients experienced to have influenced the surgical outcome. However, it was insignificant in our experience and excluded from the brainstem CM grading system. The number of brainstem CM hemorrhages is beyond the surgeon's control and is very difficult to assess. Some events are likely not captured by the patient or physician. In contrast, the timing of surgery relative to the hemorrhage can be orchestrated by the neurosurgeon and used in the selection process.

9.4 Validation of the Brainstem CM Grading System

Risk prediction models should be externally validated before integration into patient care. The brainstem CM grading system was developed and internally validated from a retrospective analysis of 104 patients. An external validation cohort comprised patients with brainstem CMs resected since the publication of the brainstem CM grading system and those resected by Dr. Robert F. Spetzler over a 16-year period (▶ Fig. 9.2). A total of 277 patients were included in the study. The average brainstem CM grade was 3.9, and most brainstem CMs (181 patients, 65%) were intermediate grade (grades III–V; ▶ Fig. 9.3). Outcomes were predicted by brainstem CM grade, with good outcomes observed in 47 of 54 patients (87%) with low-grade brainstem CMs (grades 0–II), 135 of 181 patients (75%) with intermediate-grade brainstem CMs, and 21 of 42 patients (50%) with high-grade brainstem CMs (grades VI–VII; ▶ Fig. 9.4). Conversely, rates of neurological deterioration increased with increasing brainstem CM grade, with worsening observed in 2 of 54 patients (4%) with low-grade brainstem CMs, 29 of 181 patients (16%) with intermediate-grade brainstem CMs, and 17 of 42 patients (40%) with high-grade brainstem CMs. In the chi-squared analysis, high-grade brainstem CMs were associated with increased odds of neurological worsening compared to low- and intermediate-grade brainstem CMs (OR = 5.0; 95% CI: 2.4–10.4; $p < 0.001$). The receiver operating characteristic analysis demonstrated acceptable discrimination for predicting unfavorable functional outcomes (modified Rankin Scale [mRS] score > 2) with an area under the curve (AUC) of 0.74 (95% CI: 0.68–0.80; $p < 0.001$; ▶ Fig. 9.5), which is comparable to that of other grading systems in widespread use, including the Spetzler–Martin grading system (AUC = 0.69) and the supplemented Spetzler–Martin grading system (AUC = 0.75) for brain AVMs.

Two other studies demonstrated the generalizability of the brainstem CM grading system to low- and medium-volume centers. Lashkarivand and colleagues found that, in a consecutive series of 22 patients treated microsurgically over 10 years, the Lawton brainstem CM grading system correlated with mRS

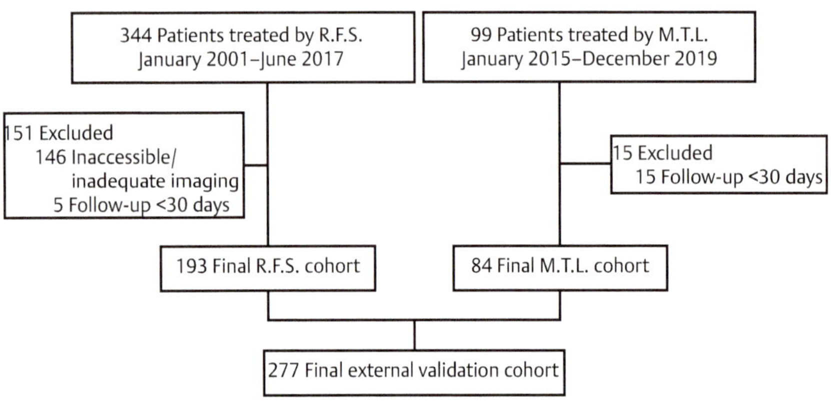

Fig. 9.2 Flowchart of patient selection for external validation cohort for the Lawton brainstem CM grading scale. (Reproduced with permission from Catapano JS, Rutledge C, Rumalla K, et al. External validation of the Lawton brainstem cavernous malformation grading system in a cohort of 277 microsurgical patients. J Neurosurg 2021;136(5):1231–1239.)

9

scores and results of the 36-Item Short-Form Health Survey. Similarly, Santos and colleagues analyzed 67 patients with brainstem CMs treated surgically over a 16-year period. They found the Lawton brainstem CM grading system to be a strong predictor of patient outcome, with an AUC of 0.72.

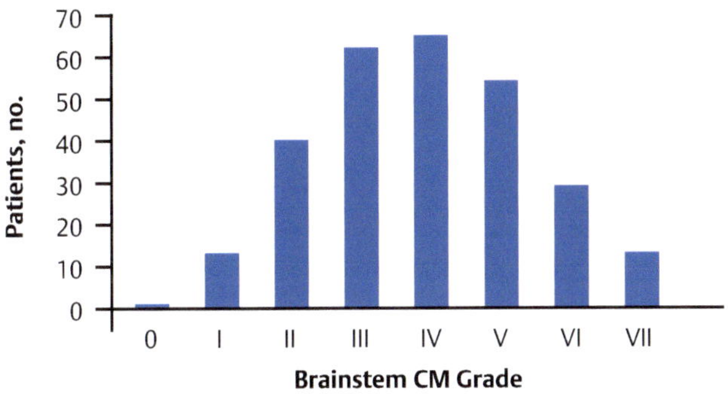

Fig. 9.3 Bar graph showing the bell-shaped distribution of brainstem CM grades among 277 patients. Most brainstem CMs (181 patients, 65%) were intermediate grade (grades III–V). (Reproduced with permission from Catapano JS, Rutledge C, Rumalla K, et al. External validation of the Lawton brainstem cavernous malformation grading system in a cohort of 277 microsurgical patients. J Neurosurg 2021;136(5):1231–1239).

9.5 Clinical Application

Patient selection has been inadequately addressed in the neurosurgery literature but remains a critical determinant of outcomes in brainstem CM microsurgery. Rational patient selection is derived from the identification of measurable preoperative factors correlated with operative morbidity and neurological outcomes and packaging them with clinical and anatomical factors into a memorable grading system. The difficult analysis of innumerable variables is simplified to assigning points in a formula and establishing categories of low-, intermediate-, and high-grade brainstem CMs. The original article proposing the brainstem CM grading system included only six patients with high-grade brainstem CMs and precluded the definition of a clear operative threshold. The 42 patients with high-grade brainstem CMs in our external validation have brought that dividing line into relief: surgery in these patients is associated with significantly increased odds of poor outcome (OR = 3.4; $p < 0.001$) and neurological worsening (OR = 5.0; $p < 0.001$). Therefore, brainstem CM grading defines a boundary of operability at brainstem CM grade V.

Consequently, brainstem CM grading clarifies a management algorithm for a complex and highly variable group of patients. A proactive surgical posture can be justified for low-grade brainstem CMs (grade 0–II) based on good outcomes in 87% of patients and worsening in only 4%. Conversely, a conservative posture can be justified for high-grade brainstem

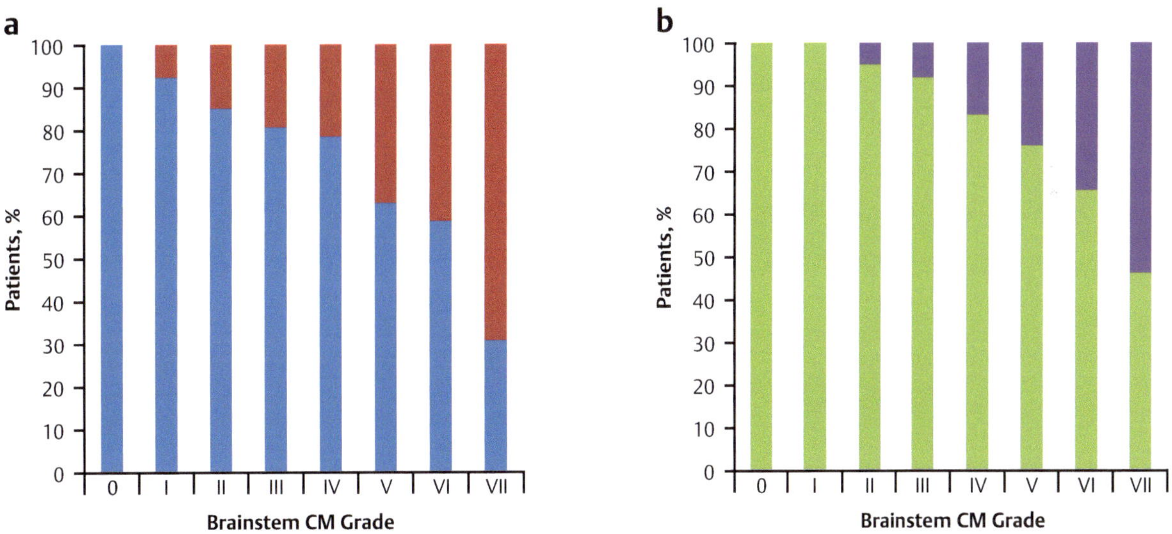

No. of patients	1	13	40	62	65	54	29	13
Outcome								
Poor	0	1	6	12	14	20	12	9
Good	1	12	34	50	51	34	17	4

■ Poor outcome ■ Good outcome

No. of patients	1	13	40	62	65	54	29	13
mRS score								
Worsened	0	0	2	5	11	13	10	7
Same or improved	1	13	38	57	54	41	19	6

■ mRS score worsened ■ mRS score same or improved

Fig. 9.4 Absolute and relative patient outcomes after CM resection by brainstem CM grade. **(a)** Absolute and **(b)** relative outcomes of patients with brainstem CMs after microsurgical resection plotted as percentages of patients in tables below bar graphs. Percentages of poor neurological outcomes and neurological deterioration increased with higher brainstem CM grades. (Reproduced with permission from Catapano JS, Rutledge C, Rumalla K, et al. External validation of the Lawton brainstem cavernous malformation grading system in a cohort of 277 microsurgical patients. J Neurosurg 2021;136(5):1231–1239).

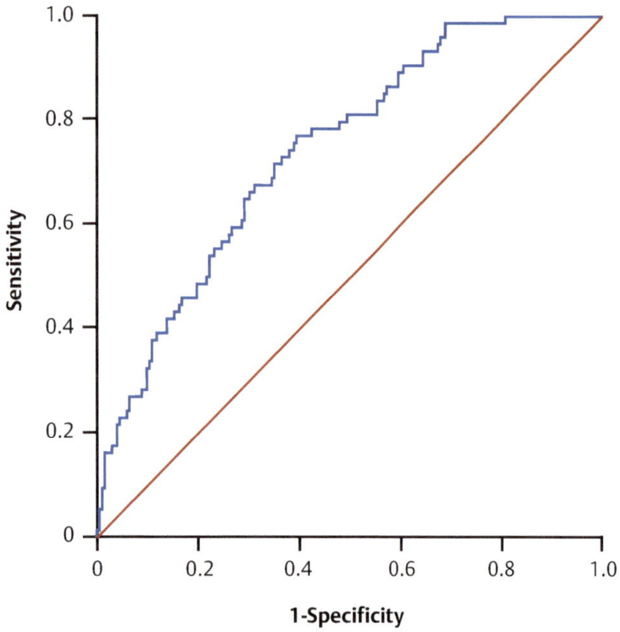

Fig. 9.5 Receiver operating characteristic curve indicating the predictive accuracy of brainstem CM grades for unfavorable neurological outcomes (modified Rankin Scale score > 2) with area under the receiver operating characteristic curve of 0.74 (95% CI: 0.68–0.80; $p < 0.001$). (Reproduced with permission from Catapano JS, Rutledge C, Rumalla K, et al. External validation of the Lawton brainstem cavernous malformation grading system in a cohort of 277 microsurgical patients. J Neurosurg 2021;136(5):1231–1239).

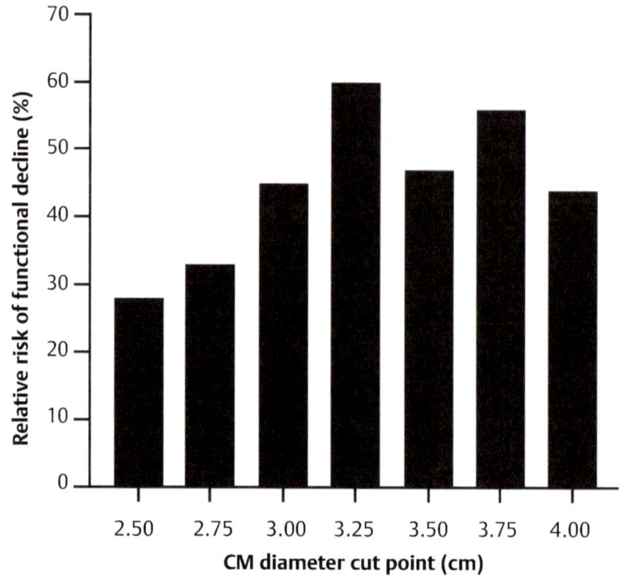

Fig. 9.6 Postoperative rate of severe functional decline (≥ 2-point increase in modified Rankin Scale score) by cerebral CM diameter cut point. CMs in the database were grouped according to different cerebral CM diameter cut points in 0.25-cm increments. A statistically significant change was noted in the relative risk of postoperative functional decline at 3.0 cm in diameter (OR = 4.5; 95% CI: 1.2–16.9; $p = 0.02$). (Reproduced with permission from Srinivasan VM, Karahalios K, Rumalla K, Shlobin NA, Rahmani R, Scherschinski L, Benner D, Catapano JS, Labib MA, Graffeo CS, Lawton MT. Giant cerebral cavernous malformations: redefinition based on surgical outcomes and systematic review of the literature. J Neurosurg 2022;137(6):1733–1741.)

CMs (grades VI-VII) based on good outcomes in 50% of patients and worsening in 40%. These patients are monitored clinically and radiographically with surveillance MRI annually or biannually. In addition, they may benefit from medical management with beta-blockers (e.g., propranolol) or emerging pharmacologic agents designed to reduce hemorrhagic activity. Patients with intermediate-grade brainstem CMs have acceptable surgical results (good outcomes in 75% of patients and worsening in 16%) and should also be carefully considered for microsurgical resection.

Although the brainstem CM grading system facilitates the selection of surgery for patients with low-grade CMs and the observation of patients with high-grade CMs, the boundary of operability may lie somewhere within the intermediate grades for most neurosurgeons. Each neurosurgeon must calibrate this boundary to their unique abilities, practices, and outcome results. The purpose of a grading system is to guide the analysis of a particular patient's condition, but treatment recommendations must be individualized. No grading system can replace a thorough and thoughtful assessment of the clinical and emotional condition of each patient, the anatomy of the lesion, and the technical ability of the neurosurgeon. Brainstem CM grading is a basic tool for patient selection, and patients should be fully informed of possible risks, as their tolerances may differ from those of their neurosurgeons. Therefore, the grading system empowers patients with essential information to make the best decisions.

9.6 Giant Cavernomas

The Lawton CM grading system is a surgical risk predictor for brainstem CMs but is silent on cerebral CMs. Large or giant size may be one such predictor for cerebral lesions. Giant cerebral CMs have been referred to in the literature without a clear definition of the term *giant*. For other pathologies, the term is well defined and used consistently. For example, giant aneurysms have a cross-sectional diameter of at least 25 mm, and giant pituitary adenomas are defined as having a diameter of at least 40 mm. Giant CMs are rarely reported. Many cases are managed conservatively, and others are treated surgically without being reported in the literature. An accepted definition of giant CMs would be valuable for accurate reporting and as a predictor of the risk associated with microsurgical resection. The term *giant*, as applied to cerebral CMs, should identify the size threshold at which the pathology becomes more complex, or its treatment becomes more technically difficult. In addition, this size threshold could be defined by surgical outcome, specifically by determining the CM diameter at which operative risk showed the greatest increase.

In our institutional cohort of 179 patients with large cerebral CMs, the mean (standard deviation [SD]) CM size was 2.38 (0.89) cm in diameter and 5.98 (8.91) cm^3 in volume. CM maximum diameter of ≥ 3 cm was associated with a greater risk of severe postoperative decline (≥ 2 points increase in mRS score; ▶ Fig. 9.6). After adjusting for age and deep versus superficial location, a size ≥ 3 cm strongly predicted a severe postoperative decline (OR = 4.5; 95% CI: 1.1–18.5). Therefore, we proposed a 3-cm diameter as the definition of a giant CM on the basis of the inflection point for functional and neurological outcomes. This definition establishes clarity and consistency in the discourse and reporting of CMs.

In a case reported in 2004, I resected a giant CM in the right frontoparietal lobes measuring 13 cm in diameter and noted no clear definition of giant CMs. My coauthors and I suggested defining giant CMs as ≥ 6 cm in diameter, an arbitrary selection. However, few lesions meet this threshold, and neurosurgeons need a more relevant definition. Such a definition could be based on the incidence, an arbitrary size similar to the method used to define other giant lesions, or some outcome measure. Giant aneurysms account for approximately 5% of aneurysms in most surgical series, and a similar threshold could be established for giant CMs. In our combined Barrow Neurological Institute database of approximately 2,000 supratentorial CMs from 2 neurosurgeons (Michael T. Lawton and Robert F. Spetzler), we found 94 lesions ≥ 2 cm in diameter. Therefore, assuming a 5% incidence of giant cerebral CMs, we would define giant size as approximately 2 cm in diameter. If we arbitrarily applied the 2.5-cm threshold for giant aneurysms to CMs, the incidence of giant CMs would be halved, or approximately 2.5%. Instead, we based our proposed definition on functional outcomes and logistic regression.

The maximal diameter alone, rather than complex volumetric analyses, was sufficient for outcome prediction and facilitated clinical application. Our proposed definition of giant CMs having a diameter of ≥ 3 cm is evidence based and clinically relevant. Overall, 34 patients had CMs that exceeded this threshold, with a mean diameter of 3.8 cm (▸ Fig. 9.7). These giant CMs accounted for 19% (34 of 179) of large CMs and approximately 2% (34 of approximately 2,000) of all CMs in our cohort. This overall incidence may be lower than that observed with other giant lesions, such as giant aneurysms. However, it is higher than that

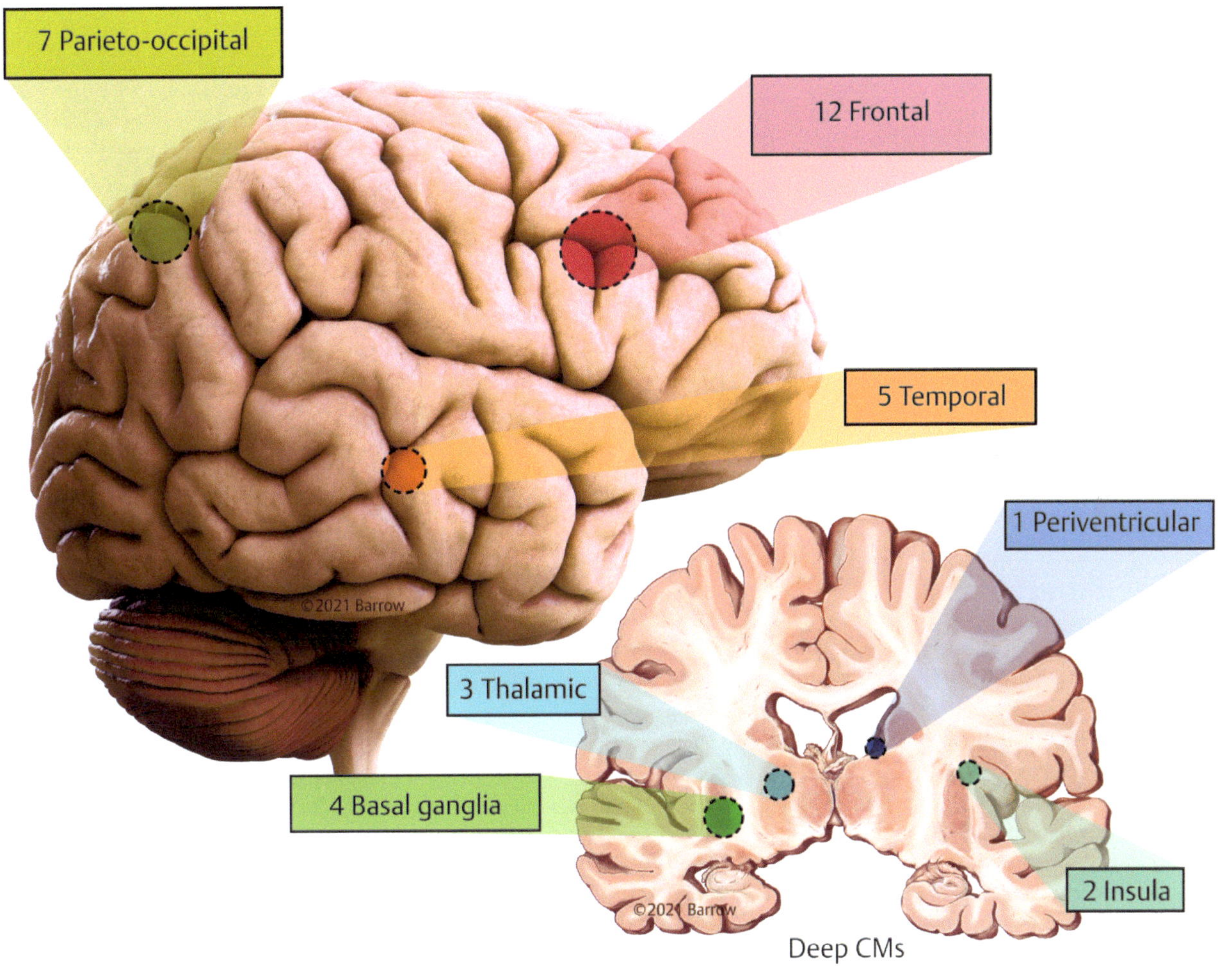

Fig. 9.7 Institutional series of giant cerebral CMs, defined as ≥ 3.0 cm in diameter. Locations of the cerebral CMs were determined on the basis of radiographic appearance, intraoperative descriptions, intraoperative photographs, and operative videos. Frontal lesions (12) were most common, followed by parieto-occipital (7), temporal (5), basal ganglia (4), thalamic (3), insula (2), and periventricular (1) lesions, for a total of 34 giant cerebral CMs. (Reproduced with permission from Barrow Neurological Institute, Phoenix, AZ.)

9

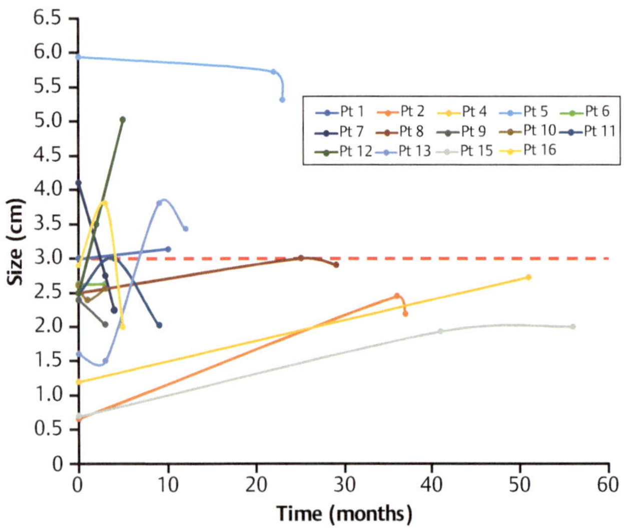

Fig. 9.8 Natural history of large and giant cerebral CMs. The graph shows the size variation of large and giant cerebral CMs in the data set. The *red dashed line* indicates the proposed definition of giant cerebral CMs as those with a diameter ≥ 3 cm. These patients had multiple time points of radiographic measurements before their immediate preoperative measurement, which is the rightmost data point on the graph for each line. Some lesions showed dramatic growth (e.g., patient 13), whereas others experienced growth that was slower and more linear. In addition, lesions sometimes crossed the inflection point of 3 cm. Two patients (patients 3 and 14) were omitted from the graph for visualization purposes. Both patients had long courses with minimal lesion growth. (Reproduced with permission from Srinivasan VM, Karahalios K, Rumalla K, et al. Giant cerebral cavernous malformations: redefinition based on surgical outcomes and systematic review of the literature. J Neurosurg 2022;137(6):1733–1741 and Catapano JS, Rutledge C, Rumalla K, et al. External validation of the Lawton brainstem cavernous malformation grading system in a cohort of 277 microsurgical patients. J Neurosurg 2021;136(5):1231–1239.)

observed with the previously suggested definition of 6 cm and is still clinically relevant.

We observed that giant CMs changed in size over time, with growth from repeated hemorrhage and shrinkage from hematoma absorption (▶ Fig. 9.8). Some had dramatic increases in size over short periods, and others had slow growth over the years due to multiple small hemorrhages or a single significant hemorrhage. Although most giant CMs tend to enlarge over time, they can regress from giant to large, albeit rarely, unlike tumors or aneurysms, which do not decrease in size over time. The dynamic nature of CMs makes radiographic surveillance an essential part of the conservative management and longitudinal evaluation of these patients.

Importantly, the 3-cm threshold identifies a CM as giant and serves as a warning signal that surgical intervention may be associated with increased risk. This proposed definition is not meant as a contraindication to microsurgical management. Patients with giant CMs may be the most in need of surgery to relieve mass effects or protect from natural history risk (▶ Fig. 9.9), just as giant aneurysms have a risk of rupture and cause significant and intolerable symptoms that demand intervention.

9.7 Hannegan's Sign

The message of this chapter is that successful cavernoma surgery depends on careful patient selection. Choosing the right surgical patients is as important as the surgical techniques discussed in previous chapters, yet little time is spent analyzing patient selection. The brainstem CM grading system and giant size definition are novel heuristics to guide these tough decisions. Another one is Hannegan's sign.

This book is dedicated to Lisa Hannegan, who was my clinical nurse practitioner from the first day of my neurosurgical practice after residency to my last day at the University of California, San Francisco, 20 years later (▶ Fig. 9.10). She accompanied me on my learning curve, from my first to my 5,000th aneurysm, from rookie mistakes to milestone achievements, from assistant professor to vice chairman, and on every step along my early career journey. Lisa spent the first half of her career as a clinical nurse practitioner for Dr. Charlie Wilson, caring for his pituitary, vascular, and tumor patients. She was dubbed one of *Charlie's Angels*. I was blessed to have had someone trained by a neurosurgery legend as my clinical partner. Together, we grew vascular neurosurgery from an anemic service dominated by a world-renowned interventional neuroradiology group into a robust program with five operating room blocks per week, 400 surgeries per year, and strong collaborations with the stroke and neurocritical care neurology and interventional neuroradiology groups. We cofounded The Aneurysm and AVM Foundation, a monthly support group for recovering aneurysm and AVM patients that expanded into patient advocacy, fundraising, and grant funding for vascular research. Together, Lisa, Alfredo Quinones-Hinojosa, April Sabangan, and Will Aarsheim cofounded Mission:BRAIN, a nonprofit organization that provides neurosurgical expertise and resources to patients, caregivers, and health care providers in underserved areas throughout the world to *treat, educate, and empower*. Lisa embodied the ideals of the nursing profession with her caring, generosity, and selflessness.

Hannegan's sign originated in my neurosurgical clinic, where Lisa accompanied me each week for new patient visits, postoperative checks, and follow-up appointments. She interviewed and examined patients first, while I reviewed charts and imaging studies before seeing the patients. New and challenging patients would capture my attention and prompt prolonged screen time. I would linger over the large thalamic CM deep to the posterior limb of the internal capsule but surfacing posteriorly near the lateral geniculate body in the ambient cistern. I would linger over the central pontine CM surrounded by

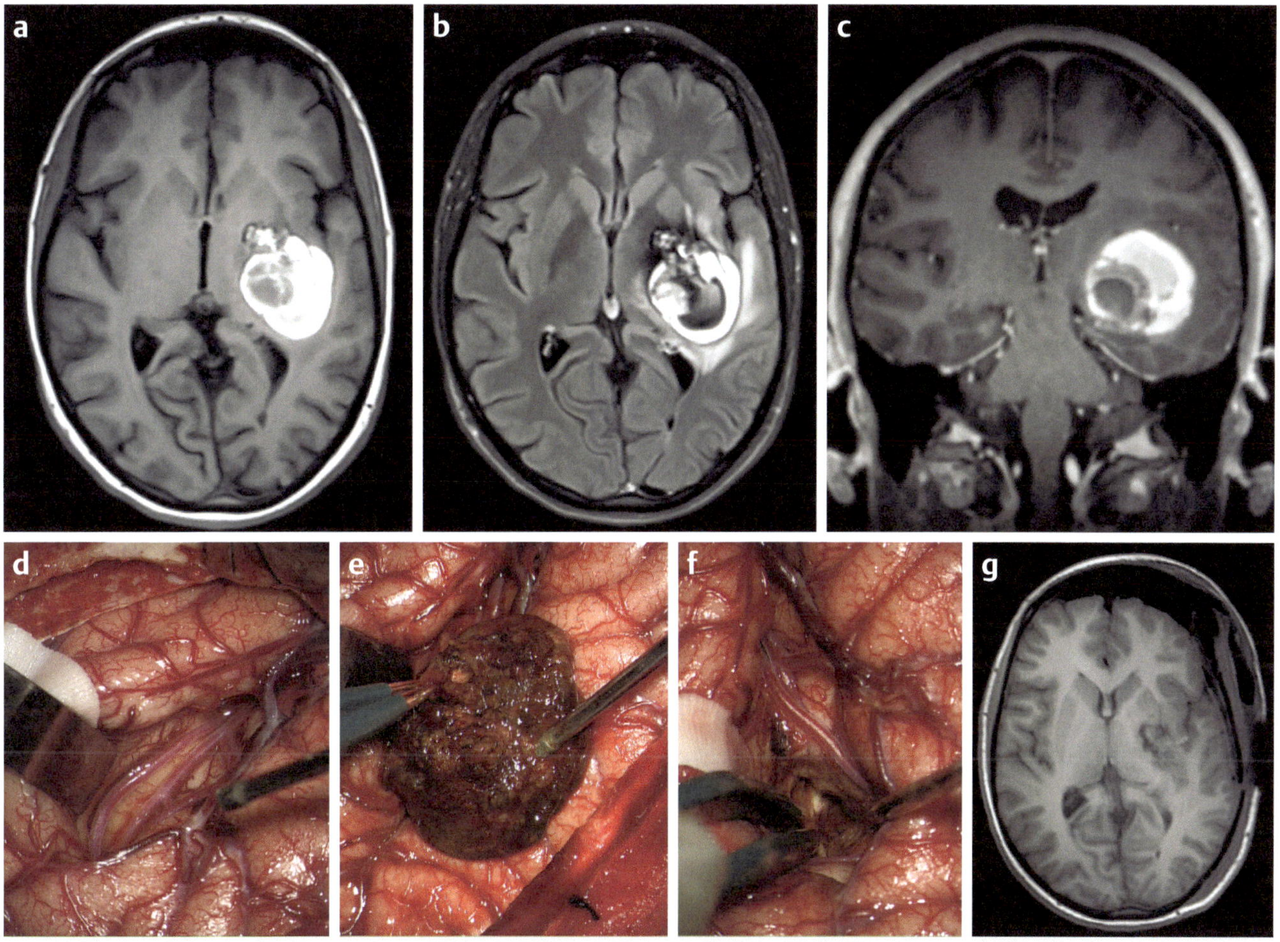

Fig. 9.9 MRI of a representative patient with a left insular giant cerebral CM. The patient was in their mid-20 s and presented with right quadrantanopia and headaches. **(a)** Preoperative axial T1-weighted MRI shows a 4.8 × 3.7-cm left insular giant cerebral CM with surrounding edema and brain compression due to a left to right midline shift. **(b)** Preoperative axial fluid-attenuated inversion recovery imaging and **(c)** coronal T1-weighted contrast-enhanced MRI show the heterogeneous lesion and its hematoma cavity. **(d)** A transsylvian approach was used to perform a gross total resection of the giant cerebral CM. The insula is exposed in this intraoperative photograph. **(e)** The giant cerebral CM was removed en bloc after internal decompression of the hematoma. **(f)** The cavity within the insula was carefully inspected to ensure no residual tissue remained. **(g)** Gross total resection was confirmed on postoperative axial T1-weighted MRI. Postoperatively, the patient had right-dominant hemiparesis, right neglect, a right-sided hemisensory deficit, and continuing right quadrantanopia. At the 6-month postoperative follow-up, the patient had largely regained right-sided strength and motion but continued to have some right-sided weakness and quadrantanopia. The imaging studies remained negative for residual or recurrent cerebral CM. (Images **a–c and g** are reproduced with permission from Srinivasan VM, Karahalios K, Rumalla K, et al. Giant cerebral cavernous malformations: redefinition based on surgical outcomes and systematic review of the literature. J Neurosurg 2022;137(6):1733–1741. Images **d–f** are reproduced with permission from Barrow Neurological Institute, Phoenix, AZ.)

brainstem but surfacing anterolaterally at the pontomedullary sulcus. I would scour the images, searching for the right approach and a microsurgical option to offer the patient, while the clinic schedule backed up and Lisa waited impatiently. Then, she would say, "When you have to stare at the images for longer than 5 minutes trying to decide whether and how to operate, you probably should not." This wisdom became known as Hannegan's sign.

Hannegan's sign is easier to remember than grading scales, and a positive sign may be predictive of poor neurological outcomes, although it has not been analyzed or externally validated. It is an indicator of noise inside the head, warning of the struggle between wanting to tackle a challenging case and worrying about its complexity. It reflects neurosurgeon intuition, screaming that substantial risk is involved. Hannegan's sign marks a surgical boundary as it is reached. It was always difficult for me to acknowledge these boundaries, but that knowing look from Lisa, that rolling of her eyes, assured me that all neurosurgeons have limits, and it was okay for me to accept mine. Hannegan's sign embodies the

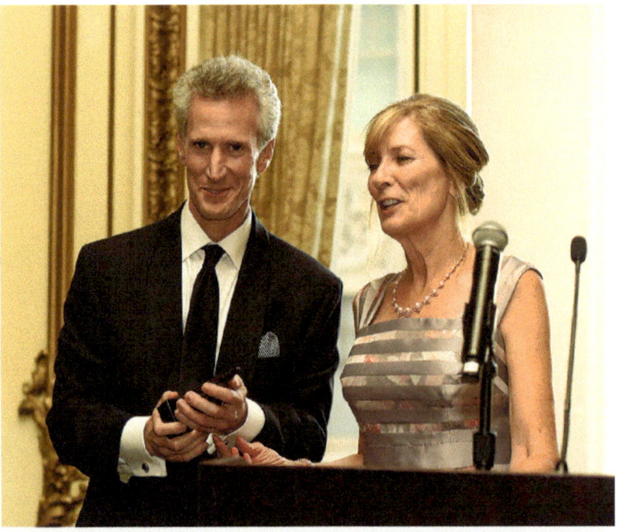

Fig. 9.10 Lisa Hannegan was my clinical nurse practitioner from the first day of my neurosurgical practice after residency to my last day at the University of California, San Francisco, 20 years later. This photograph was taken at The Aneurysm and AVM Foundation Gala in 2017, just before her retirement from nursing and my departure to Barrow Neurological Institute. Hannegan's sign is named after her. (Reproduced with permission of the family of Lisa Hannegan.)

importance of spending time thinking about your strategy (the 5-minute limit). Hannegan's sign recognizes the importance of challenging yourself to elevate your skills (trying to decide whether to operate). Hannegan's sign prioritizes the best outcome for the patient ("you probably should not"). Neurosurgeons have a big surgical appetite, but nurses are uniquely positioned to curb it. Lisa knew, as only a nurse can, that surgical selection decisions have profound consequences under the microscope and at the bedside and that we must reckon with those consequences well beyond the clinic or the operating room. We are accountable to the patients who entrust us with their lives to *do no harm*, yet go beyond, to do good.

Lisa's story has a tragic ending. She retired from nursing when I left San Francisco, and she rode off into the sunset to focus on global neurosurgery. Unfortunately, she was involved in a bicycle crash several years later and experienced a severe traumatic brain injury that took her life. That someone so caring and generous of spirit could be dealt a fate so cruel is beyond comprehension. Her story is another reminder that time is precious, that we need to pursue life with urgency, and that the journey is richer when one finds an angel who helps along the way. In addition to helping make the right selection decisions, Hannegan's sign reminds me to look for and listen to these guardian angels.

10 CARTOGRAPHY

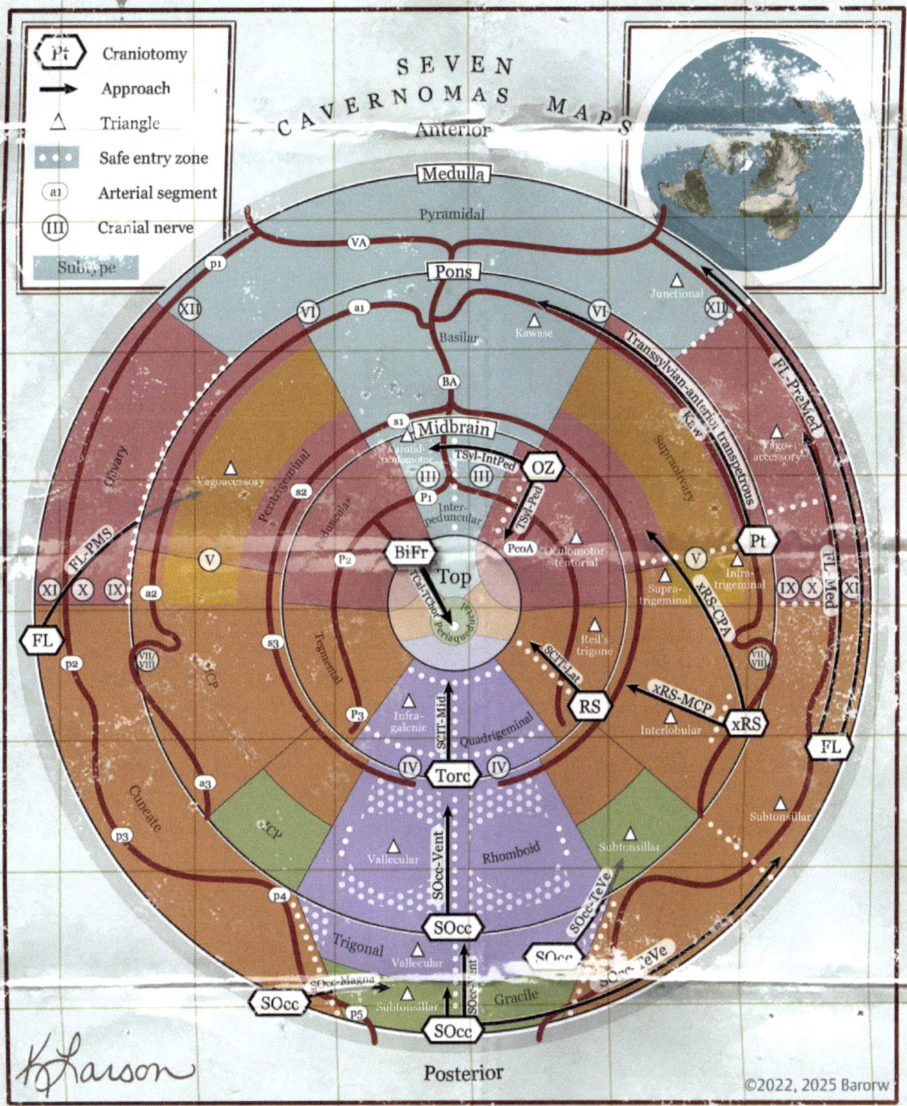

Reproduced with permission from Barrow Neurological Institute, Phoenix, AZ.

10 Neurosurgical Cartography

Summary

The Jackson Hole trail map is a classic James Niehues painting that captures the enormity of Rendezvous Mountain and Grand Teton National Park in a single folded page. That map will launch a 4,000-ft vertical drop in a single ski run of pure exhilaration. The Niehues trail map gives more than directions. It instills confidence, peace of mind, and safe passage with its symbolic representation of the wilderness. Just as Niehues provides peace of mind, Massimo Vignelli's famous New York Subway guide transforms the nightmarish and chaotic labyrinth of the subway system into a system five million people willingly brave every day. Neurosurgical cartography is built on foundational structures within the brain and skull base, the fissures and gyri, arteries and veins, peduncles and cranial nerves, and bony ridges and tubercles. How does one synthesize, condense, and clarify this vast anatomical knowledge into a comprehensive guide for a diverse array of neurosurgeons? We can look to the persistence of maps from our predecessors and contemporaries (e.g., Wilder Penfield's homunculus, Lars Leksell's Cartesian coordinates in the cranium, and Gazi Yaşargil's redefinition of the basal cistern and subarachnoid spaces) to judge the importance of neurosurgical mapping. Intracranial taxonomies of cavernous malformations map this diverse pathology to brainstem anatomy to guide the targeting of the lesion by location, approach, and nuanced execution of resection, following unmistakable landmarks. The Seven Cavernomas framework integrates quintessential clinical, anatomical, and microsurgical concepts into a comprehensive heuristic that leads neurosurgeons to achieve their best outcomes in microsurgery.

Keywords: brainstem, cavernoma, cavernous malformation, Frank Netter, Gazi Yaşargil, Harvey Cushing, Jackson Hole, map, navigation, orienteer

10.1 Jackson Hole

From my cabin window, I see falling snow accumulating on tree branches and porch railings outside in the vanishing light of the Wyoming sunset. Tomorrow will be an epic ski day, with 12 inches of fresh powder by morning. Thoughts of first tracks and soft turns set my pulse racing. A pass is purchased, the skis are tuned, and my coat pockets are stuffed with protein bars and nuts that will sustain me without stopping for lunch. My attention turns to the Jackson Hole trail map, a classic James Niehues painting that somehow captures the enormity of Rendezvous Mountain and Grand Teton National Park in a single folded page. Tomorrow, I will begin with the Aerial Tram to Corbet's Cabin on the top of the mountain and drop into Rendezvous Bowl. A left turn on Laramie Traverse will take me to Bird in the Hand and Split Rock, where there are less traveled runs that should be thick with powder. The intersection with Rendezvous Trail will take me to Sublette Lift, farthest from the hordes in Teton Village, and to the steepest terrain. If conditions are right, Sublette will position me to take Middle Hoback, which drops much of the mountain's 4,000 vertical feet in a single run that gets the adrenaline surging and the quadriceps screaming. At the bottom, the Union Pass lift will return me to the tram station, where I will plan my next descent.

The trail map catalyzes the anticipation and thrill of skiing into an action plan. Niehues' maps are known for their synthesis of information and perspective. His creative process begins with photographs of the mountain from an airplane to gain an aerial perspective. He then studies the mountain's topography from U.S. Geological Survey maps and spends time on the mountain in the snow. He combines these diverse impressions into a pencil sketch that aligns the mountain's slopes, maintains the lengths of the lifts, and captures the terrain's signature rock formations and peaks. He distorts and repositions elements of the drawing to transform three-dimensional geography into a two-dimensional map, showing skiers things that cannot be seen and giving them an understanding of the mountain. After reviewing his sketch with the resort, Niehues meticulously paints his map with a signature aesthetic that is accurate to the level of individual trees. These field guides inhabit the pockets of every ski jacket, are posted as signs at every chairlift station, and are often mounted on the chairlift harness bars. In addition to directions down the mountain, these maps offer confidence, peace of mind, and safe passage.

10.2 Cartography

What is a map? In practical terms, it is a symbolic and accurate representation of relationships between elements in a space. Road maps depict streets, buildings, and homes within a city; classroom globes depict countries, continents, and oceans on the earth; and trail maps depict mountains, rivers, and lakes in the wilderness. A map's two specific purposes are to locate where you are and find the route to where you are going. It transcends its basic representational function when it creates a novel internal language and becomes an accessible system of logic. Transcendent maps are rich with meaning and aesthetics but can be understood at a glance. Edward Tufte, a scholar of information theory, describes the successful map as the "clear portrayal of complexity ... not the complication of the simple." The cartographer gives "visual access to the subtle and the difficult—that is, the revelation of the complex."

Niehues' trail maps achieve this mark of accessible complexity, as does the modernist graphic designer Massimo Vignelli's famous 1972 edition of the *New York City Subway Guide*. Vignelli's map pairs the functional priority of wayfinding in a complicated transit system with a visual language that New York's diverse citizens and visitors can interpret quickly and easily. Alexander Tochilovsky, curator of the Herb Lubalin Study Center of Design and Typography, explained the power of Vignelli's map: "A significant part of the map's design strategy comes from withholding information that isn't necessary to make the experience of gaining the actual information that you do need much easier." Vignelli transformed the nightmare of

10

navigating the chaotic labyrinth of New York's subway into an experience that five million people willingly brave every day. Subway guides and Google maps on car dashboards emphasize the value of the cartographer in all aspects of the modern world, including neurosurgery.

Neurosurgical cartography is built on foundational structures within the brain and skull base: fissures and gyri, arteries and veins, peduncles and cranial nerves, and bony ridges and tubercles. As neuroanatomical study and cadaveric dissection continue to expand our understanding of this unique landscape, elevated cartography must edit and condense the information to preserve complexity while remaining understandable to a wide range of neurosurgeons. Operative experience helps differentiate the anatomy of interest from the anatomy of importance; in other words, the neurosurgical cartographer's hand is guided by its many experiences wielding the microsurgical knife. Many neurosurgeons with busy practices have extensively traveled these surgical corridors and acquired deep anatomical knowledge. However, few endeavor to resolve the complex into the accessible—to synthesize, condense, and clarify insights into a map. The profound challenge of this charge resonates in how persistent and insightful the maps of our early neurosurgical cartographers remain, including Wilder Penfield's homunculus for motor and sensory somatotopy, Gazi Yaşargil's microscopic redefinition of the basal cisterns and subarachnoid spaces, and Lars Leksell's application of Cartesian coordinates to the intracranial compartment.

10.3 Maps as Metaphors for the Seven Cavernomas

Dissecting through subarachnoid spaces to reach and resect a cavernoma is like downhill skiing—or hiking, if you prefer a summer mountain metaphor. The operation is an exercise in surveying the pathology and the adjacent anatomy, selecting the best approach from a menu of options, assessing your technical abilities, and embarking on the journey. Central to *Seven Cavernomas: Tenets and Techniques for Resection* is the taxonomy that categorizes a pathology that is endlessly diverse in size, shape, and location into 7 types (midbrain, pons, medulla, thalamus, basal ganglia, cerebrum, and cerebellum) and 35 subtypes. The taxonomy initiates analyses that lead to the diagnosis, surgical decision-making, and technical execution. Subtyping allows us to recognize a unique lesion in an individual patient as the manifestation of a prototypical entity with a characteristic clinical presentation, defined anatomical location, and established approach for its resection.

Elaborating on our mountain metaphor, we turn to the craniotomy as the trailhead or point of departure for the hike. The microsurgical approach is the trail coursing through the wilderness of the subarachnoid spaces. Landmarks and waypoints keep hikers on the right trail, just as the intersections of arteries, cranial nerves, and dural structures form anatomical triangles to guide the course of our dissection (▸ Table 10.1).

Table 10.1 Brainstem CM taxonomy of types and subtypes and their associated craniotomies, approaches, anatomical triangles, SEZ, and arterial segments

Type	Subtype	Craniotomy	Approach	Triangle	SEZ	Arterial target
Midbrain	Interpeduncular	Orbitozygomatic	TSyl-IntPed; cTSyl-IntPed	Carotid-oculomotor	Interpeduncular	P1
	Peduncular	Orbitozygomatic	TSyl-Ped	Oculomotor-tentorial	Anterior mesencephalic sulcus	P2A
	Tegmental	Retrosigmoid	SCIT-Lat	Supratrochlear and infratrochlear	Lateral mesencephalic sulcus	s3
	Quadrigeminal	Torcular	SCIT-Mid	Infragalenic	Intercollicular; supracollicular; infracollicular	mPChA
	Periaqueductal	Bifrontal	TCal-TChor	None	None	None
Pontine	Basilar	Orbitozygomatic	Kaw; TSyl-Cav-Pon	Kawase, infratrigeminal; carotid-oculomotor	Supratrigeminal; infratrigeminal	BA
	Peritrigeminal	Retrosigmoid	xRS-CPA	Supratrigeminal and infratrigeminal, GCT	Supratrigeminal; infratrigeminal	s2
	Middle peduncular	Retrosigmoid	xRS-MCP	Interlobular	Middle cerebellar peduncle/ lateral pontine	a3
	Inferior peduncular	Suboccipital	SOcc-TeVe	Subtonsillar	Area acustica	p4
	Rhomboid	Suboccipital	SOcc-Vent	Vallecular	Median sulcus; suprafacial collicular; superior foveal	p3
	Supraolivary	Far lateral	FL-PMS	Vagoaccessory (suprahypoglossal)	Pontomedullary sulcus	a2
Medullary	Pyramidal	Far lateral	FL-PreMed	Junctional	Anterolateral sulcus	VBJ
	Olivary	Far lateral	FL-Med	Vagoaccessory (supra- or hypoglossal-hypoglossal)	Olivary zone; posterolateral sulcus; lateral medullary zone	p2
	Trigonal	Suboccipital	SOcc-Vent	Vallecular	Median sulcus; infrafacial collicular	p3
	Gracile	Suboccipital	SOcc-Magna	Vallecular	Posterior median sulcus	p3
	Cuneate	Suboccipital	SOcc-TeVe	Subtonsillar	Posterior intermediate sulcus	PSA

Table 10.2 Brainstem CM subtypes and the presence of the arterial segments and veins associated with each subtype within the surgical field, based on the analysis of intraoperative images

Type	Subtype	Arterial target	Venous target	Total, *n* (%)	Artery observed, *n* (%)	Vein observed, *n* (%)	Dissection code[a]
All				128	117 (91)	96 (75)	
Midbrain	Interpeduncular	P1	Anterior pontomesencephalic vein	1 (1)	1 (100)	1 (100)	M3-M2-M1-C6-AChA-PCoA-P1
	Peduncular	P2A	Peduncular vein	8 (6)	8 (100)	7 (88)	M3-M2-M1-C6-AChA-PCoA-P2A
	Tegmental	s3	Lateral mesencephalic vein	12 (9)	11 (92)	7 (58)	s4-s3
	Quadrigeminal	mPChA	ICV	8 (6)	8 (100)	6 (75)	s4-s3-P3-PreCenCblV-BVR-mPChA
	Periaqueductal	None	None	0	–	–	CmaA-PcaA-ThaStrV-ICV-mPChA
Pontine	Basilar	BA	Anterior pontomesencephalic vein	3 (2)	1 (33)	2 (67)	SPS-IPS-a2-a1-BA
	Peritrigeminal	s2	Superior petrosal vein	11 (9)	10 (91)	10 (91)	s4-s3-s2
	Middle peduncular	a3	Middle cerebellar peduncle vein	28 (22)	24 (86)	21 (75)	a4-a3
	Inferior peduncular	p4	Vein of inferior cerebellar peduncle	6 (5)	5 (83)	4 (67)	p2-p3-p4
	Rhomboid	p3	Vein of cerebellomedullary fissure	14 (11)	13 (93)	10 (71)	L p3-R p3
	Supraolivary	a2	Vein of pontomedullary sulcus	13 (10)	13 (100)	12 (92)	V4-p3-p2-p1-a2
Medullary	Pyramidal	VBJ	Lateral anterior medullary vein	0	–	–	V4-p1-ASA-VBJ
	Olivary	p2	Retro-olivary vein	14 (11)	14 (100)	9 (64)	V4-p3-p2
	Trigonal	p3	Median posterior medullary vein, vein of inferior cerebellar peduncle	4 (3)	4 (100)	3 (75)	L p3-R p3
	Gracile	p3	Median posterior medullary vein, vein of inferior cerebellar peduncle	2 (2)	2 (100)	2 (100)	L p3-R p3
	Cuneate	PSA	Median posterior medullary vein	4 (3)	3 (75)	2 (50)	V4-p3-p2-PSA

[a]Dissection code is the sequence of arterial segments (and, in some cases, veins of the ventricles or deep venous system) followed through the subarachnoid corridor to reach the target lesion.

We may follow landmarks for a stretch, such as when a trail parallels a river or the dissection traces an artery (▶ Table 10.2). Ultimately, the legs of the journey connect to carry adventurous explorers to their destination, whether it is a mountain peak, campsite, or brainstem cavernoma.

10.4 Seven Cavernomas Maps

The brainstem cavernous malformation (CM) maps (▶ Fig. 10.1, ▶ Fig. 10.2, ▶ Fig. 10.3, ▶ Fig. 10.4, ▶ Fig. 10.5, ▶ Fig. 10.6, ▶ Fig. 10.7, ▶ Fig. 10.8) contain a system of logic that emphasizes clinical decision-making and surgical wayfinding. The taxonomy is the centerpiece of *Seven Cavernomas* because it defines each lesion, explains the constellation of bedside findings, and suggests the optimal surgical approach. The taxonomic framework establishes the optimal craniotomies, approaches, and triangles as the key features that guide dissection through subarachnoid spaces to reach CM targets in the brainstem. By analogy, the triangles provide the equivalent of the front sight on a marksman's rifle, which in turn is aligned with the rear sight (craniotomy) to aim the gun barrel (approach) more accurately at the target (cavernoma). The craniotomy-approach-triangle combination, or triangle concept, guides microdissection, just as the combination of rear sight–barrel–front sight increases the shooter's accuracy. The brainstem CM maps integrate taxonomy, craniotomies, approaches, triangles,

Arterial Segments: Anterior Brainstem CM Subtypes

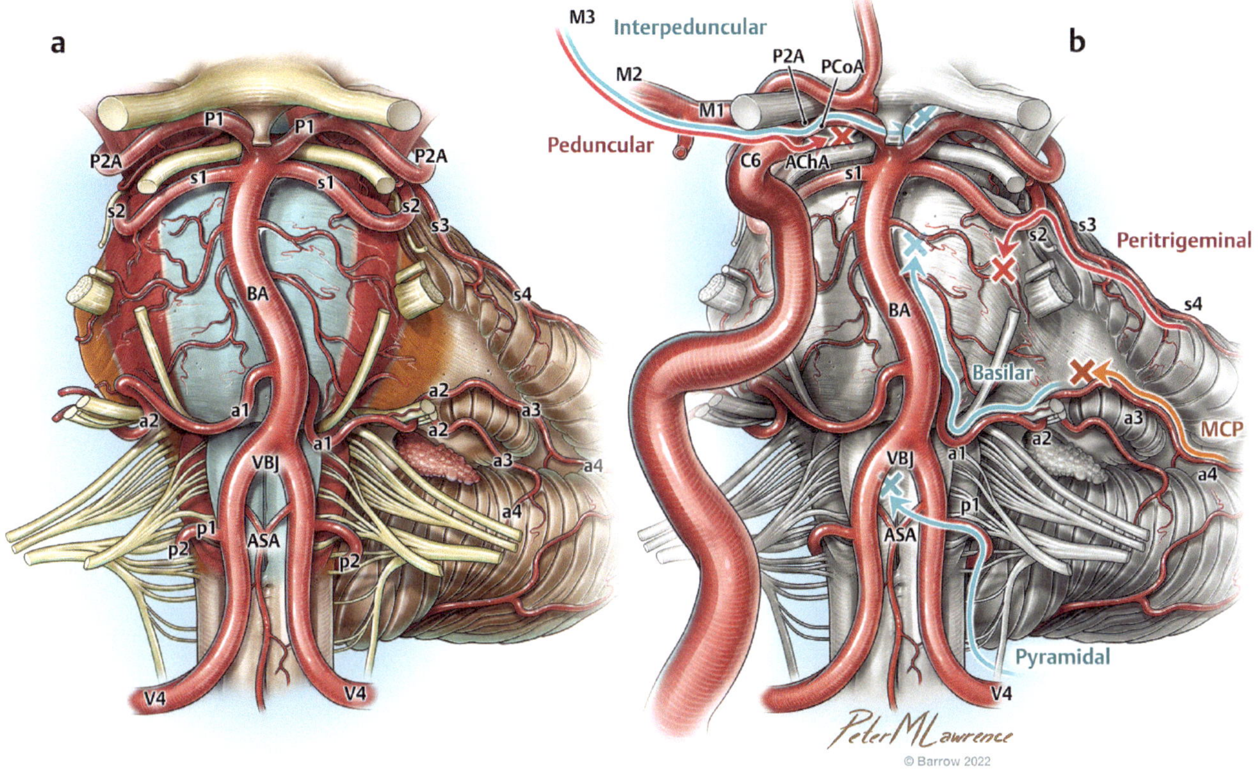

Fig. 10.1 Arterial segments associated with specific brainstem CM subtypes. **(a)** Anterior view of the brainstem shows surface locations of anterior (*teal*), anterolateral (*red*), and lateral (*orange*) subtypes. Anterior subtypes comprise interpeduncular, basilar, and pyramidal; anterolateral subtypes are peduncular, peritrigeminal, and olivary; and lateral subtypes are tegmental, middle peduncular, and cuneate. **(b)** Dissection routes to six specific brainstem CM subtypes that follow arterial waypoints are depicted with *arrows* that correspond to the colors of that CM's anatomical surface. The target CM is depicted with a matching colored X. (Reproduced with permission from Barrow Neurological Institute, Phoenix, AZ.)

arterial addresses, and safe entry zones. Each medical illustrator incorporates a range of perspectives and aesthetic choices to elevate the map to the next level of clarity.

10.5 Maps for Safe Passage

The true value of these maps is that they invest neurosurgeons with advanced tools for understanding and safely navigating the brain's corridors to reach the pathology. Good management decisions and intraoperative guidance translate to safe surgery and optimal outcomes. Brainstem CM maps help the neurosurgeon prepare and rehearse surgery before entering the operating room, just like Niehues' trail maps help plan tomorrow's ski routes. Simulation through maps helps the neurosurgeon anticipate intraoperative situations and think through contingency plans rather than confront new technical and emotional challenges unprepared or under duress. Combining preoperative map reading and imaging review fosters mental readiness, translating to clarity, calm, and confidence in the operating room. Based on good microsurgical results with our patients with brainstem CMs, I submit that the Seven Cavernomas framework integrates quintessential clinical, anatomical, and microsurgical concepts into a comprehensive heuristic that will lead neurosurgeons to achieve their best outcomes in microsurgery.

The skillful use of maps differs from intraoperative navigation. Frameless stereotactic image guidance has become the standard of care for CM surgery, especially with brainstem CMs, because surface presentation can be overestimated on preoperative magnetic resonance imaging, and confirmation of the lesion's location is reassuring before transgressing a safe entry zone. Navigation identifies one's position in the brain on cross-sectional imaging. It shows the approach trajectory to the target, which is an essential element of successful neurosurgical navigation akin to compass reading. However, orienteers need more. Orienteers interpret these readings within the context of their surroundings, relate them to checkpoints on the map, and

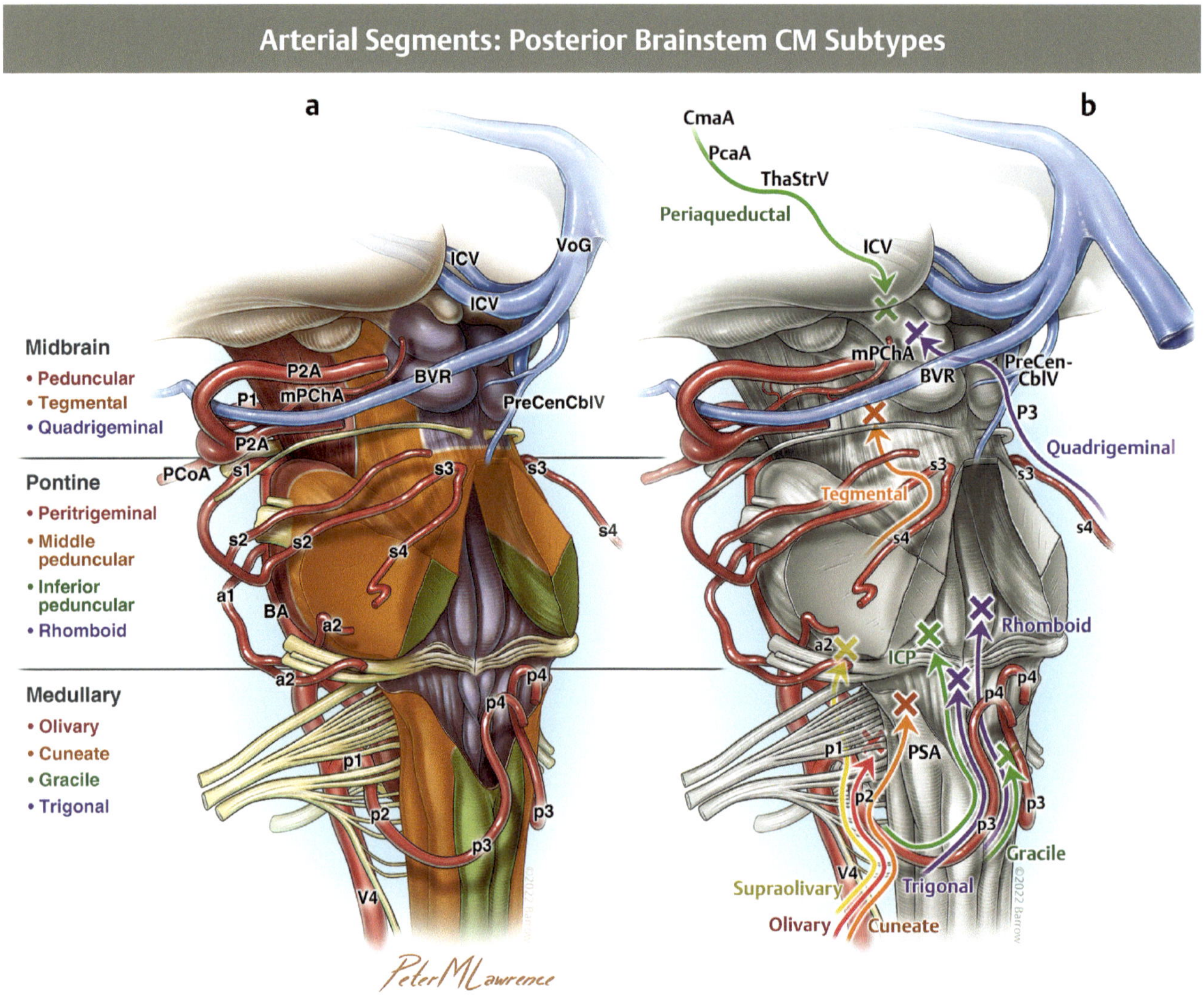

Fig. 10.2 Arterial segments associated with specific brainstem CM subtypes. **(a)** Posterolateral view of the brainstem surface locations shows posterior (*purple*), posterolateral (*green*), lateral (*orange*), and anterolateral (*red*) brainstem CM subtypes. Posterior subtypes are quadrigeminal, rhomboid, and trigonal; posterolateral subtypes are inferior peduncular and gracile; lateral subtypes are tegmental, middle peduncular, and cuneate; anterolateral subtypes comprise peduncular, peritrigeminal, and olivary; periaqueductal and supraolivary subtypes are not shown. **(b)** Dissection routes to 10 specific brainstem CM subtypes that follow vascular waypoints are depicted with *arrows* that correspond to the colors of that CM's anatomical surface. The target CM is depicted with a matching colored X. These arterial paths are summarized as dissection codes in ▶ Table 10.2. (Reproduced with permission from Barrow Neurological Institute, Phoenix, AZ).

chart a course through the territory ahead. A neurosurgeon without map-reading skills follows vectors on a computer screen like a driver shackled to his GPS (global positioning system). In contrast, the neurosurgeon-orienteer integrates anatomical knowledge, observational awareness, and navigational information to operate with a true sense of direction. These neurosurgeons know exactly where they are and do not get lost, demonstrating a keen synergy of visuospatial intelligence, three-dimensional ability, and operative intuition. Neurosurgical maps are meant to encourage neurosurgeons to become orienteers of the brain and not rely solely upon stereotactic navigation but to apply the concepts of visuospatial intelligence and information from multiple sources during active microdissection.

10.6 Maps for Education

For elementary school students, the globe provides insight into and perspective on the structure and geography of our world: Earth is a spherical planet covered with oceans and seven continents divided into nearly 200 countries. Similarly, the neurosurgical maps we have created in the Seven Cavernomas framework orient medical students and residents to the neuroanatomic terrain, ranging from overviews of superstructures

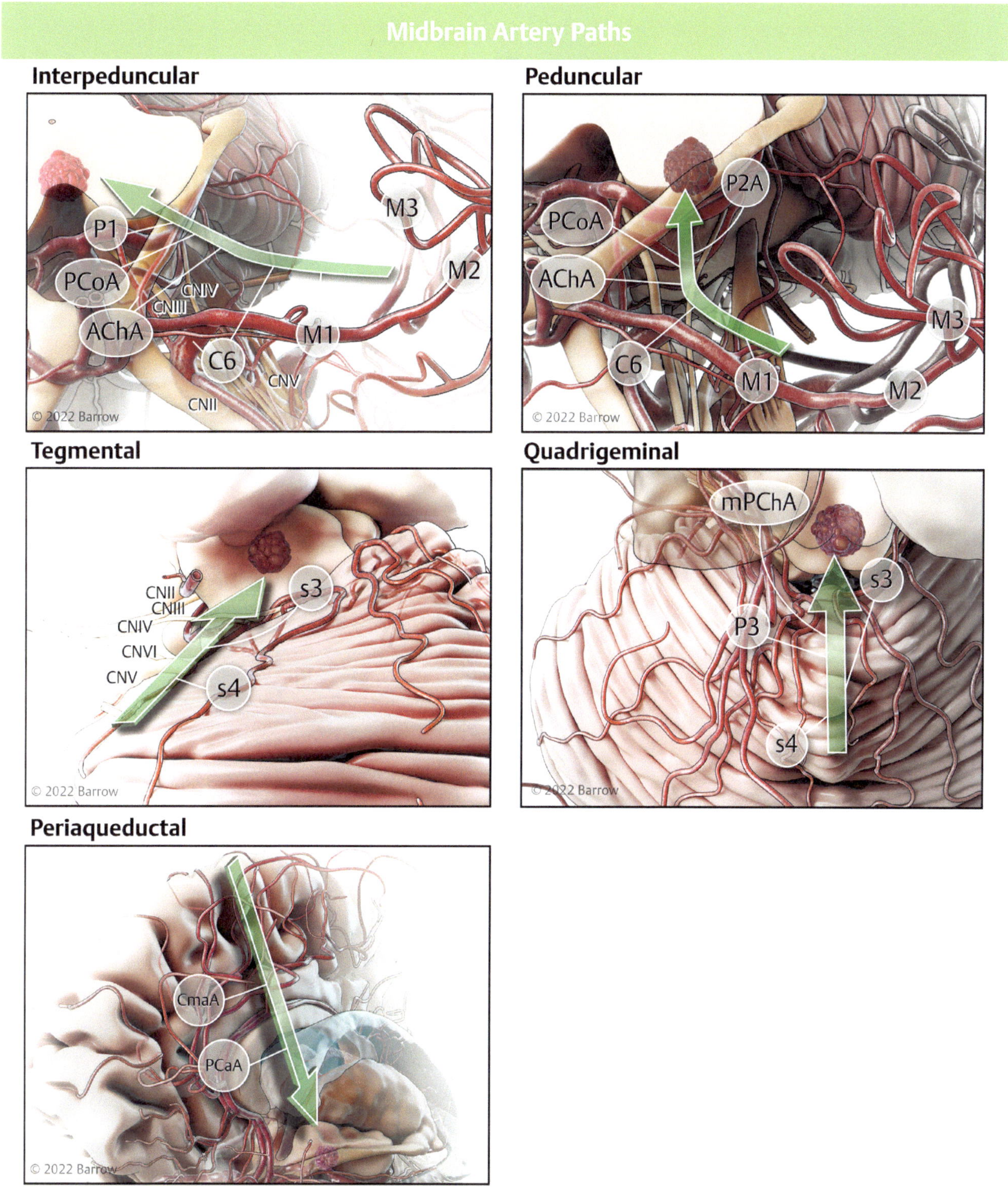

Fig. 10.3 Midbrain artery paths (*green arrows*), established by following arterial segments (*gray circles*) sequentially to reach targeted brainstem CMs (*red spheres*), are shown for interpeduncular, peduncular, tegmental, quadrigeminal, and periaqueductal CM subtypes. These arterial paths are summarized as dissection codes in ▶ Table 10.2. (Reproduced with permission from Barrow Neurological Institute, Phoenix, AZ.)

10

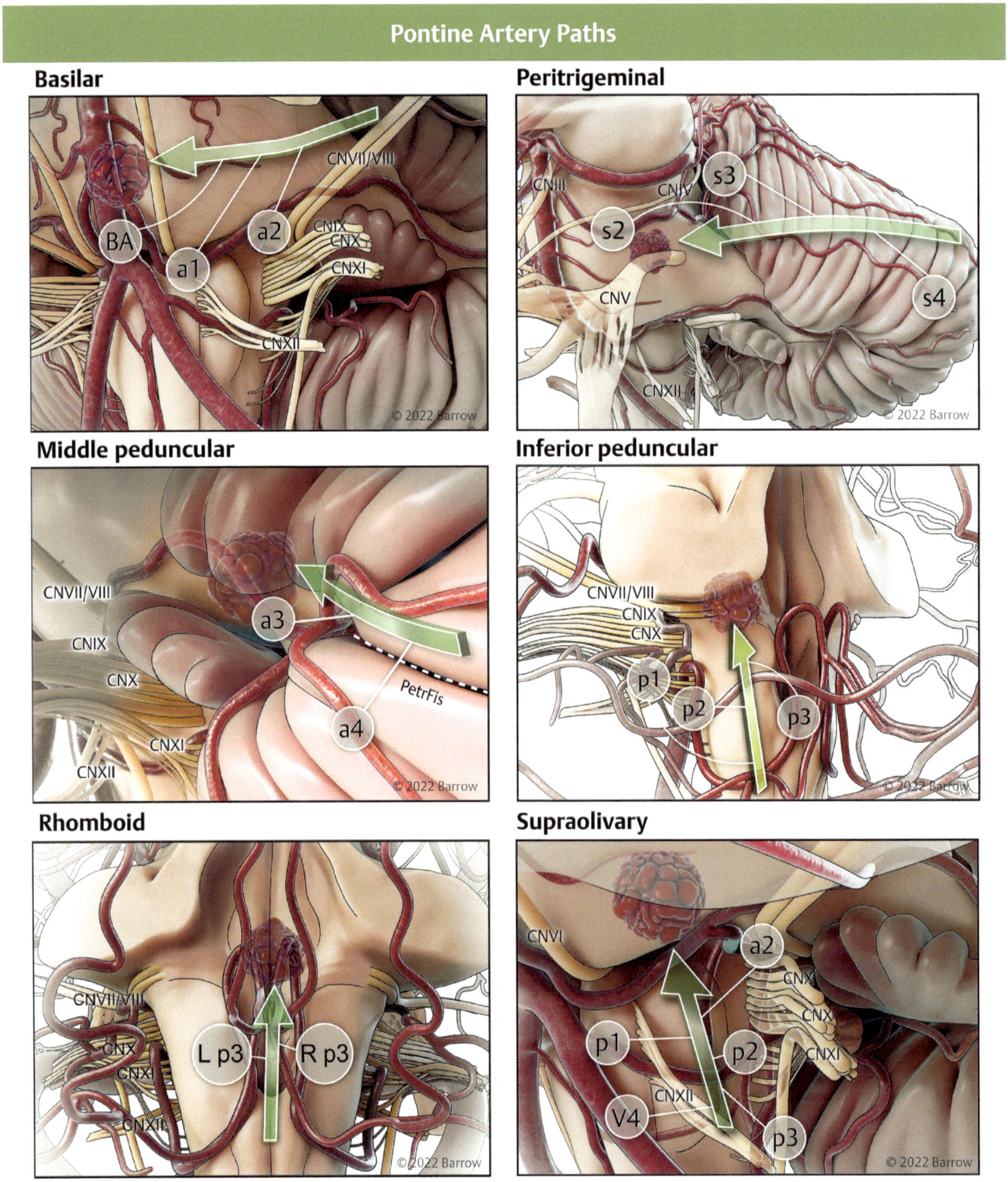

Fig. 10.4 Pontine artery paths (*green arrows*), established by following arterial segments (*gray circles*) sequentially to reach targeted CM (*red spheres*), are shown for basilar, peritrigeminal, middle peduncular, inferior peduncular, rhomboid, and supraolivary CM subtypes. These arterial paths are summarized as dissection codes in ▶ Table 10.2. (Reproduced with permission from Barrow Neurological Institute, Phoenix, AZ.)

10

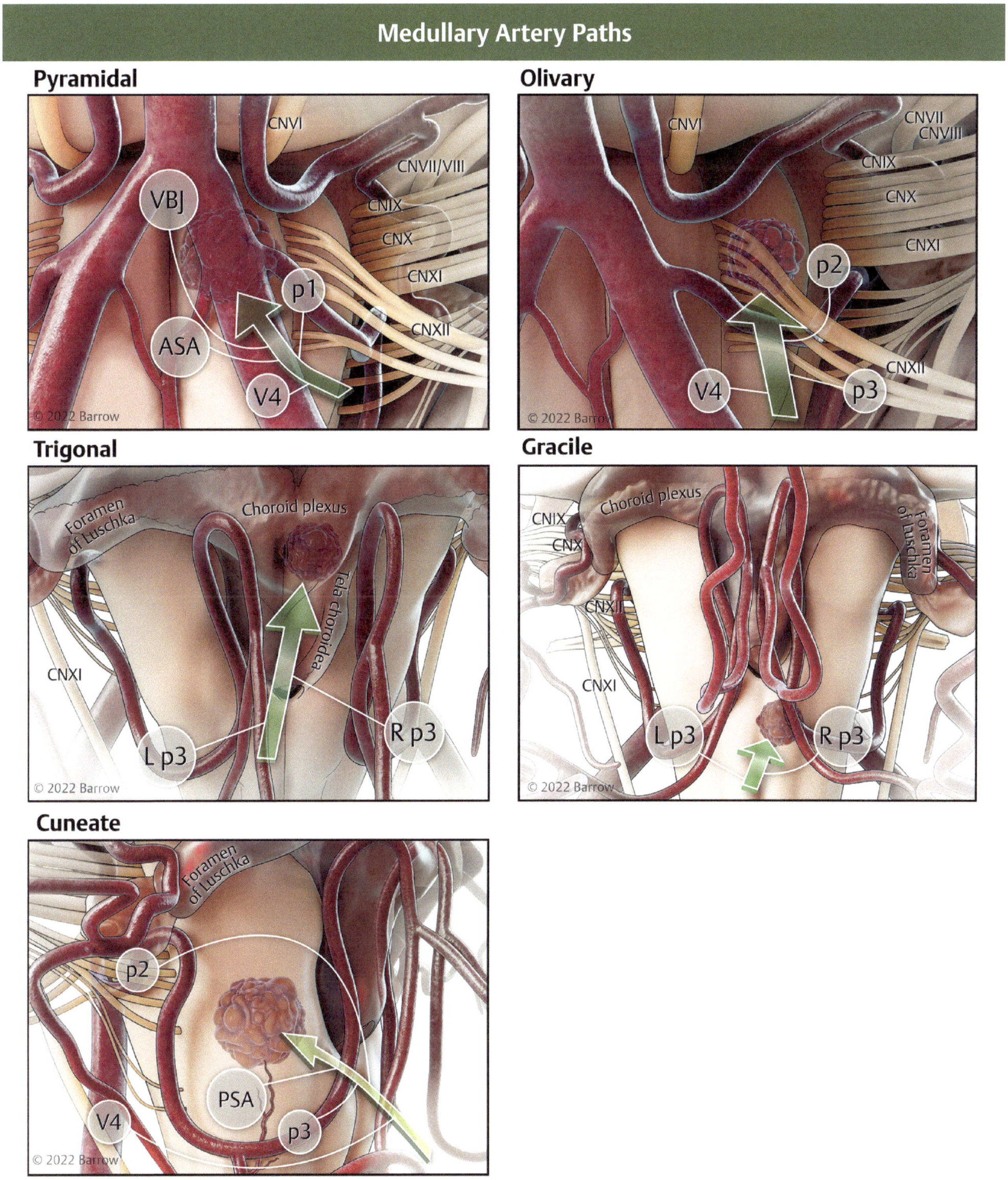

Fig. 10.5 Medullary artery paths (*green arrows*), established by following arterial segments (*gray circles*) sequentially to reach targeted CM (*red spheres*), are shown for pyramidal, olivary, trigonal, gracile, and cuneate CM subtypes. These arterial paths are summarized as dissection codes in ▸ Table 10.2. (Reproduced with permission from Barrow Neurological Institute, Phoenix, AZ.)

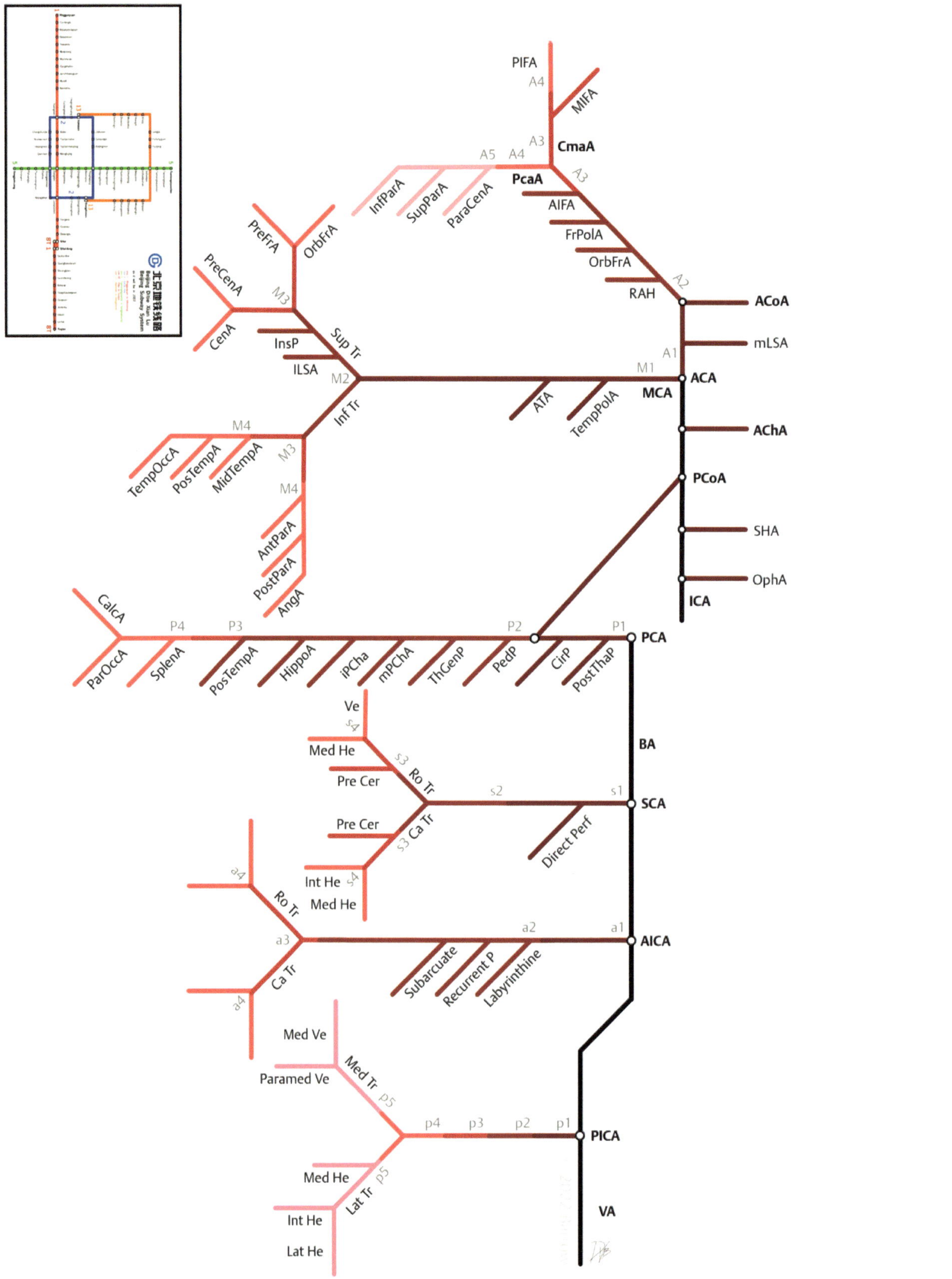

Fig. 10.6 Like Vignelli's New York City subway map or the Beijing subway map (*inset*), this arterial map captures the complexity of the cerebral circulation, portrays the arteries as tracks, and helps navigate to the brainstem CM target or arterial segment associated with that lesion's subtype. (Reproduced with permission from Lawton MT, Graffeo CS, Srinivasan VM, et al. Seven cavernomas and neurosurgical cartography, with an assessment of vascular waypoints. J Neurosurg 2022;138(4):1148–1162.)

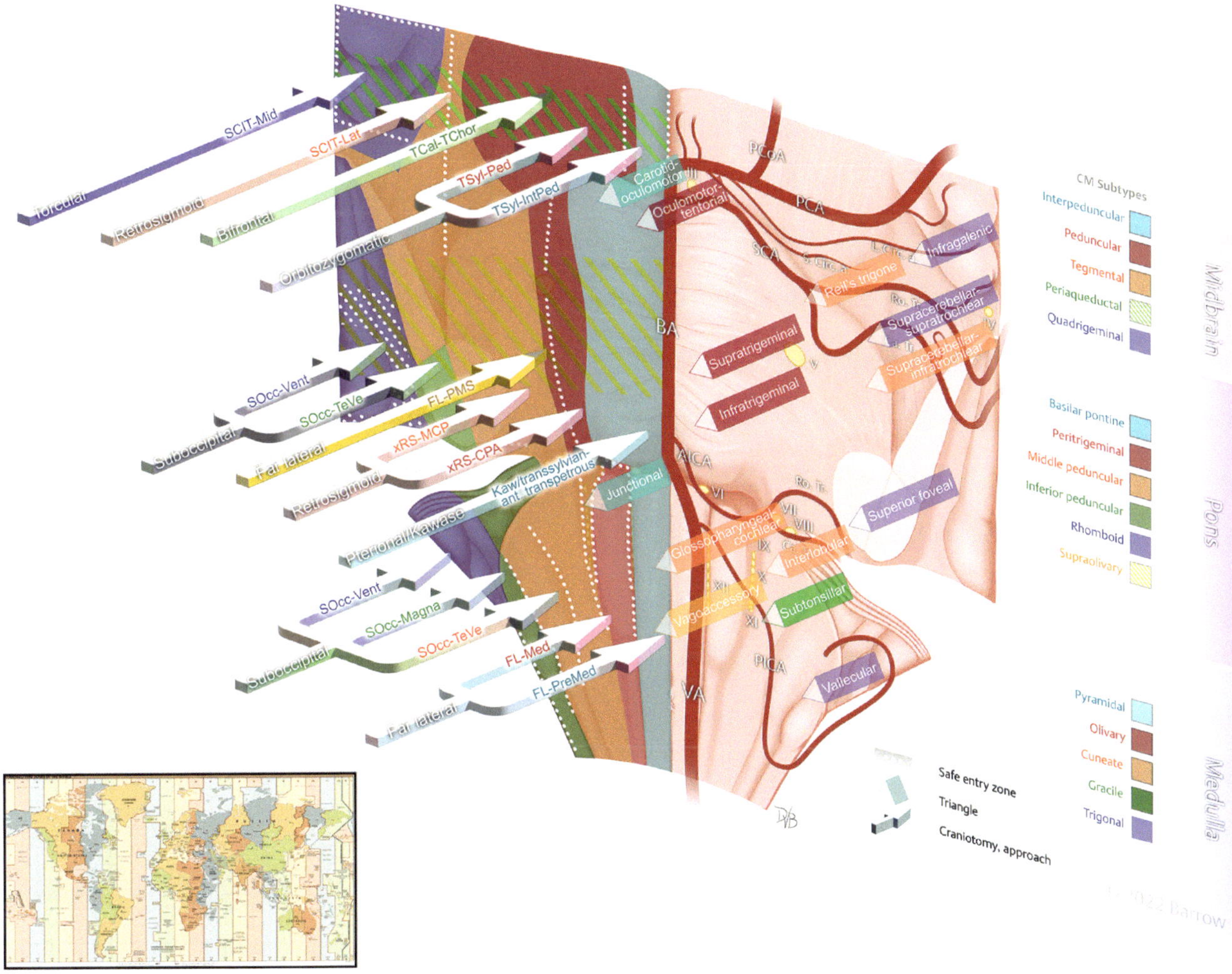

Fig. 10.7 Like the equirectangular or plate carrée map projection that converts a spherical globe into a rectangular grid of parallels and meridians (*inset*), this map projects the cylindrical brainstem and its arteries onto a flat plane. Anterior subtypes (*teal*) include interpeduncular, basilar, and pyramidal. Anterolateral subtypes (*red*) are peduncular, peritrigeminal, and olivary. Lateral subtypes (*orange*) are tegmental, middle peduncular, and cuneate. Posterolateral subtypes (*green*) include inferior peduncular and gracile, and posterior subtypes (*purple*) include quadrigeminal, rhomboid, and trigonal. Craniotomies and microsurgical approaches are depicted as *arrows* on the left side of the map, with the craniotomy labeled on the back of the *arrow* and the approach on the shaft, color coded to match the associated brainstem CM subtype. Safe entry zones (*dotted white lines*) are depicted at the *tips of the arrows*. Anatomical triangles are depicted as *triangular bars* on the right side of the map, color coded to match the associated CM subtype. Abbreviations for craniotomies and approaches are summarized in ▶ Table 10.1. Roman numerals denote cranial nerves. (Reproduced with permission from Barrow Neurological Institute, Phoenix, AZ.)

and tracts to the long menus of craniotomies, approaches, triangles, and other critical features that describe this singular landscape. In parallel, circuit diagrams of brainstem anatomy, previously developed to understand brainstem strokes, have been refined and applied to hemorrhagic presentations of brainstem CMs. These brainstem circuit maps reconnect neurosurgeons with neurology fundamentals and increase diagnostic acumen at the bedside.

The relationships between brainstem CMs, their pathoanatomy, approaches, and surgical outcomes are so complex that some researchers have proposed technology-based algorithms with computer-generated atlases and artificial intelligence to derive surgical plans. A clear conceptual framework crystallized in maps and heuristics provides a more robust strategy. Maps render the complex understandable and empower their readers to higher levels of navigational ability, whereas dependence on technology without deeper understanding often limits creativity or independent thought. Furthermore, when the younger generation of neurosurgeons is taught the principles of orienteering and shown the value of cartography, our maps will be dynamic, and we may see opportunities for a new guard to conjure a bigger vision of our microsurgical future that renders today's definitive map tomorrow's rough draft.

Neurosurgical cartographers are at once observers, reporters, archivists, and teachers. Their maps must distill countless operative forays into a simplified reconstruction of the surgical terrain, just as Niehues' time in airplanes and on skis coalesced into his trail maps. A key challenge confronting

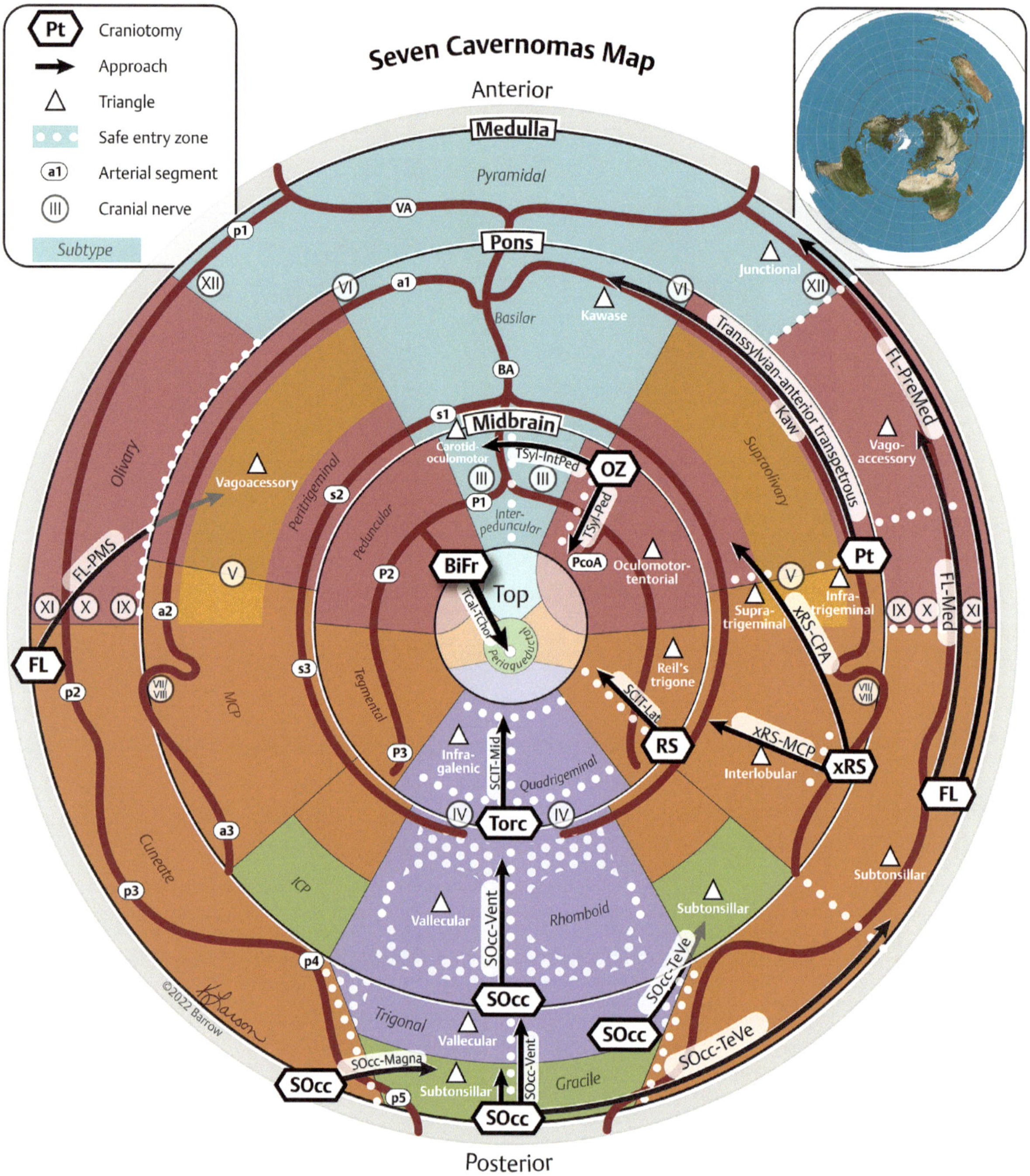

Fig. 10.8 In this azimuthal equidistant projection, where all points on the map are at proportionally correct distances from the center and in the correct direction from the center (*inset*), the brainstem is viewed from above, with brainstem CM types portrayed as concentric rings and brainstem CM subtypes distributed circumferentially, including anterior subtypes (*teal*), anterolateral (*red*), lateral (*orange*), posterolateral (*green*), posterior (*purple*), and supraolivary subtype (*yellow*). Craniotomies are abbreviated inside *white hexagons*, and microsurgical approaches are depicted as *black arrows*. Anatomical triangles are depicted as *white triangles* within the area of the associated brainstem CM subtype. Safe entry zones are depicted as *dotted white lines*. Arterial anatomy is superimposed on the map as *red lines*, with arterial segments labeled in *white ovals*. Cranial nerves are labeled with Roman numerals in *white circles* within the area of the associated brainstem CM subtype. (Reproduced with permission from Barrow Neurological Institute, Phoenix, AZ.)

10

the neurosurgical cartographer is the vital importance of artistic skill, which is a rare talent among physicians, Harvey Cushing and Frank Netter notwithstanding. Originally, Netter aspired to be an artist, studying at the National Academy of Design and the Art Students League of New York before switching to medicine in response to his family's disapproval of his art career. He completed medical school at New York University and a surgical internship at Bellevue Hospital, but he ultimately returned to visual art as a medical illustrator, producing the *Atlas of Human Anatomy*, which remains a core medical textbook even today and is Netter's personal Sistine Chapel. Pragmatically, most neurosurgeons who aspire to chart their cartography are better suited to collaborations with medical illustrators, with the neurosurgeon curating concepts and constructing the internal language of the map that the illustrators then transform into art. Transcendent maps are stripped of unnecessary information, rich in meaning and complexity, and easily interpretable. Eight such maps are presented here (▶ Fig. 10.1, ▶ Fig. 10.2, ▶ Fig. 10.3, ▶ Fig. 10.4, ▶ Fig. 10.5, ▶ Fig. 10.6, ▶ Fig. 10.7, ▶ Fig. 10.8), and although they depict the same cavernoma taxonomy and concepts, their contrasting styles emphasize the expressive nature of art and the importance of intensive collaboration and alchemy between the neurosurgeon-cartographer and the illustrators.

10.7 Maps for Exploration

Neurosurgeons are a curious lot, often compelled by a need to explore. We are driven to discover new approaches and novel surgical solutions. In addition to being everyday field guides and educational tools, maps are records of exploration at the neurosurgical frontier. Cartography can push neurosurgeons with pioneering spirits to blaze new passageways through the intracranial wilderness, offering a glimpse of how they might achieve what was once thought impossible.

Alex Honnold is one of the most accomplished rock climbers of all time. His most impressive feat was a free solo climb of the 3,000-ft granite wall known as El Capitan in Yosemite Valley, California, which he ascended without the safety of a rope or harness. Honnold's climb fused extreme difficulty, potentially deadly consequences, physical and mental challenges, and an almost unthinkable goal. It was described as one of the greatest athletic feats of any kind. His experience was captured in the Academy Award-winning documentary *Free Solo* (National Geographic Documentary Films), which highlighted the fundamentally death-defying nature of his achievement and how he came to view the nearly impossible climb as achievable and relatively low risk. For Honnold, although the free solo El Capitan climb was conceived with a go-big mentality, its execution was reducible to choreography and testing—the summation of years of preparation and self-study, detailed analysis of rock slabs, careful rehearsal of key maneuvers, and precise charting of a singular route. After an incredible career of setting routes, refining techniques, and constantly pushing beyond his limits, Honnold transcended the vertical cartographer's role as a true explorer at the frontier of possibility.

This explorer's mindset is needed more than ever in neurosurgery. New approaches require original ideas that can be tested and honed, in a stepwise fashion, first through anatomical study in the cadaver lab, then by sequencing the microsurgical steps, rehearsing the operation, waiting for the appropriate patient, and finally committing to the flawless execution, the neurosurgical free solo. Innovation, whether in climbing or in neurosurgery, is centered on freedom and exploration, with a premium placed on discovering first ascents or newer, safer surgical approaches. Both disciplines are also free from the constraints of other performance sports, where success often depends on following the rules and remaining within bounds. On the wall or under the operating microscope, the smallest movements can have tremendous consequences, and innovation occurs when training, experience, and creativity merge to empower the explorer to break from convention and deploy their new move.

In this spirit and equipped with this operating microscope, I have contributed to the development of novel approaches, including the contralateral transcallosal, contralateral transcingulate, supracarotid-infrafrontal, contralateral supracerebellar-transtentorial, trans-pontomedullary sulcus, and supratonsillar approaches. Some of these innovations represent wholly novel pathways. Others have demonstrated the value of a creative perspective by applying new concepts such as gravity retraction, contralaterality, or dural transgression to make an established approach safer, bolder, or more effective. Other frontiers center on surgical techniques, such as novel intracranial-intracranial bypasses, including double reimplantation, azygos, binder-ring, and middle communicating artery bypasses.

10.8 The Metaphor

Cartography is *Seven Cavernomas*' metaphor, and insofar as these maps reflect our best rendering of surgical neuroanatomy, they also represent a log of the collective explorations that have brought us to this frontier. Maps archive new surgical routes that comprise our neurosurgical Manifest Destiny. CMs are an ideal substrate for acts of discovery, as they are completely resectable and lack the confounding pathobiology of neoplasms, allowing us to isolate and interpret the effect of our approaches and innovations more accurately. Furthermore, their potential to precipitate major, avoidable morbidity with hemorrhage, particularly within the brainstem, motivates a trailblazing, go-big mindset, which continues to redefine our neurosurgical frontier. Neurosurgical exploration requires equal measures of insight, expertise, and boldness, and cartography charts the overarching course we have navigated as pioneers in neurosurgery. Indeed, maps have a purpose for even the foremost among us: to motivate bold feats of ingenuity that blaze new trails for neurosurgery.

Section II

The Seven Cavernomas

II

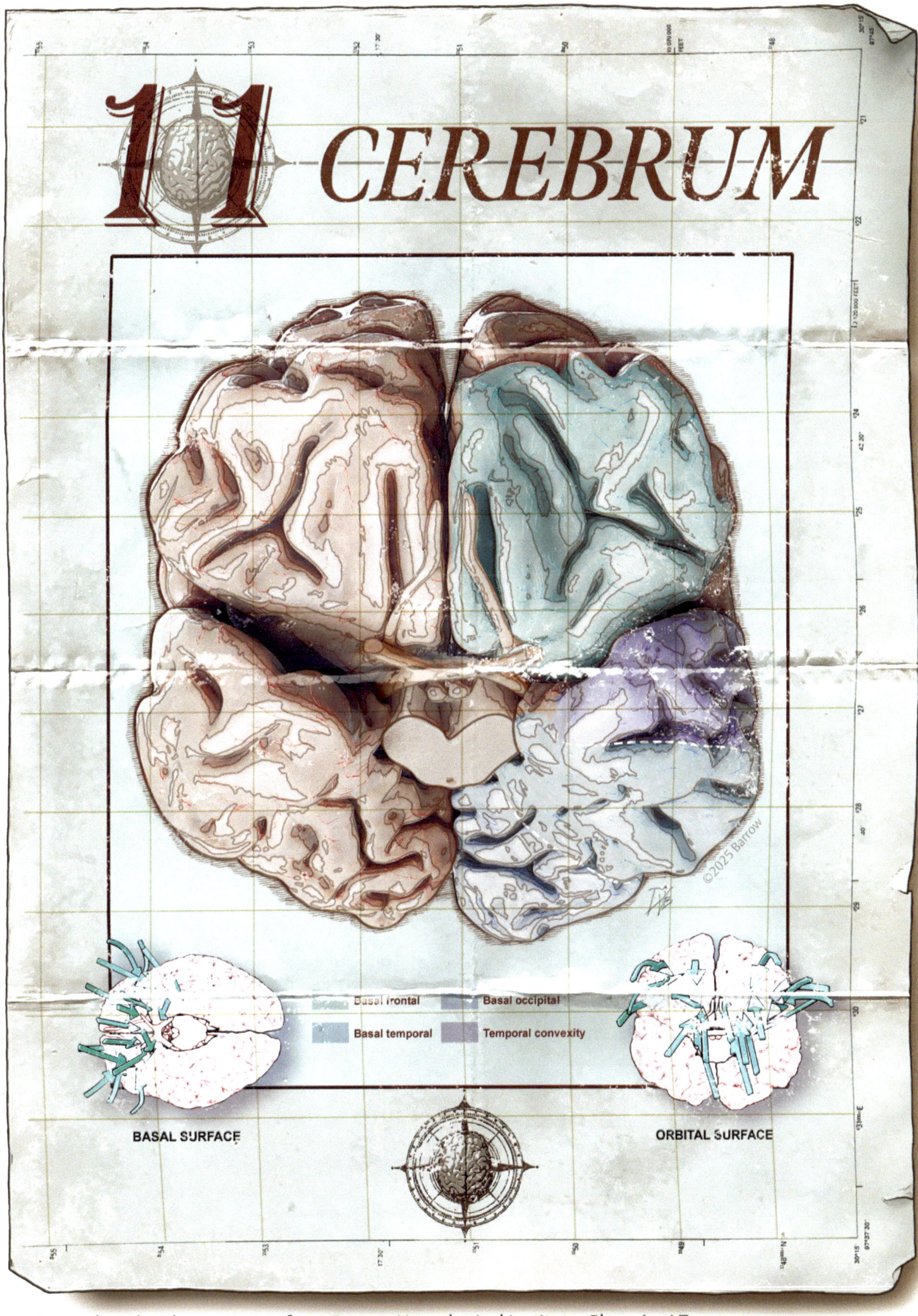

Reproduced with permission from Barrow Neurological Institute, Phoenix, AZ.

11 Superficial Cerebral Cavernous Malformations

Summary
Superficial cerebral cavernous malformations (CMs) are cortically based in gyral gray matter or subcortically based in underlying white matter, making them shallow and more accessible than deep cerebral CMs and brainstem CMs. Superficial cerebral CMs are defined on the basis of their cortical or subcortical (< 1 cm) proximity to the nearest cerebral surface. They are classified as convexity, medial, basal, and sylvian. Lobar location is also considered in subtyping, with frontal, temporal, parietal, or occipital designations. Approaches to superficial convexity CMs are transgyral (42 approaches) or transsulcal (24 approaches). Transgyral dissection is direct but transgressive. Cortical and subcortical eloquence and the possibility of brain network disruption must be considered. In contrast, transsulcal dissection minimizes or eliminates tissue transgression to preserve cortical eloquence and reduce morbidity unless the CM lies below the bottom of the sulcus. This taxonomy for superficial cerebral CMs provides valuable guidance for craniotomy planning. It was applied to a consecutive series of 346 patients with 362 CMs treated microsurgically during a 13-year period. The series included 132 (36.5%) convexity, 78 (21.5%) medial, 72 (19.9%) basal, and 80 (22.1%) sylvian CMs. Frontal CMs were most common (155, 42.8%), followed by parietal (89, 24.6%), temporal (87, 24.0%), and occipital (31, 8.6%). Of all CMs, 302 (83.4%) were cortical, and 60 (16.6%) were subcortical. Good outcomes (modified Rankin Scale [mRS] score ≤ 2) were observed in 314 patients (86.7%), and poor outcomes (mRS score > 2) were observed in 25 patients (6.9%). The Human Connectome Project and advances in cognitive neurosciences raise hope that the clinical manifestations of cortical and subcortical CMs can be understood relative to preserving the large-scale brain networks to reduce overall surgical morbidity.

Keywords: cavernoma, convexity, frontal, occipital, parietal, sylvian, taxonomy, temporal, transgyral, transsulcal

11.1 Introduction

The cerebrum comprises 85% of the brain's volume, which makes superficial cerebral cavernous malformations (CMs) the most commonly encountered CMs in clinical practice. Superficial cerebral CMs are cortically based in gyral gray matter or subcortically based in underlying white matter, making them shallow and more accessible than brainstem CMs or deep cerebral CMs. Brainstem CMs have 16 subtypes, each with a unique surgical exposure that requires nuanced approach selection and skull base techniques. Cerebral CMs have only four subtypes and are approached either transgyrally or transsulcally. Brainstem CM management is facilitated by a taxonomy that informs the selection of craniotomies, approaches, dissection triangles, and safe entry zones, whereas superficial cerebral CM management is simpler from the strategic and technical points of view. Of the seven CM types (midbrain, pons, medulla, thalamus, basal ganglia, cerebrum, and cerebellum), superficial cerebral CMs occupy the largest territory. The size and surface complexity of the cerebrum makes the taxonomy valuable for clear anatomical descriptions.

11.2 Neuroanatomy of Superficial Cerebral Cavernous Malformation Subtypes

Superficial cerebral CMs are categorized into four subtypes based on their cortical location or, if subcortical, proximity to the nearest cerebral surface: (1) convexity, (2) medial, (3) basal, and (4) sylvian. Cortical CMs are defined as lesions in the cerebrum where the closest presentation is ≤ 1 cm from the cortical surface. Subcortical CMs are defined as lesions in the cerebrum for which the closest presentation is greater than 1 cm deep to the cortical surface. Thus, subcortical CMs require transgression into the cerebral cortex, whereas cortical CMs do not.

Four lobar locations are also considered in cerebral CM subtyping: frontal, temporal, parietal, and occipital. Frontal and temporal lobes have all four cerebral surfaces (convexity, medial, basal, and sylvian), whereas the parietal lobe lacks a basal surface, and the occipital lobe lacks a sylvian surface. Convexity and medial CMs can be frontal, temporal, parietal, or occipital. Basal CMs can be frontal, temporal, or occipital. Sylvian CMs can be frontal, temporal, or parietal, depending on which side of the fissure the lesion resides. CMs in the insular cortex on the medial side of the sylvian fissure are included with deep cerebral CMs, either thalamic or basal ganglia, and are described in later chapters.

11.2.1 Convexity

Convexity CMs lie in the cerebrum adjacent to the calvarium, extending from the frontal to occipital poles in the anteroposterior plane, from the midline to the temporal squamosal bone in the mediolateral plane, and from the vertex to the skull base in the superoinferior plane (▶ Fig. 11.1). The cerebral convexity is the largest hemispheric surface. The central sulcus separates the frontal and parietal lobes. The lateral sulcus or sylvian fissure separates the frontal and parietal lobes from the temporal lobe, and the line between the parieto-occipital sulcus medially and the anterior occipital sulcus laterally is the boundary between the parietal and temporal lobes and the occipital lobe.

11.2.2 Medial

Medial CMs occur in the medial hemisphere facing the midline falx cerebri in the frontal, parietal, and occipital lobes. Medial CMs in the temporal lobe face the midbrain (▶ Fig. 11.2). These surfaces are not visible without gaining a perspective from a contralateral vantage point. Medial lesions lie just off the midline in the frontal, parietal, and occipital lobes but are paramedian in the temporal lobe. The vertical line drawn from the central sulcus is the boundary between

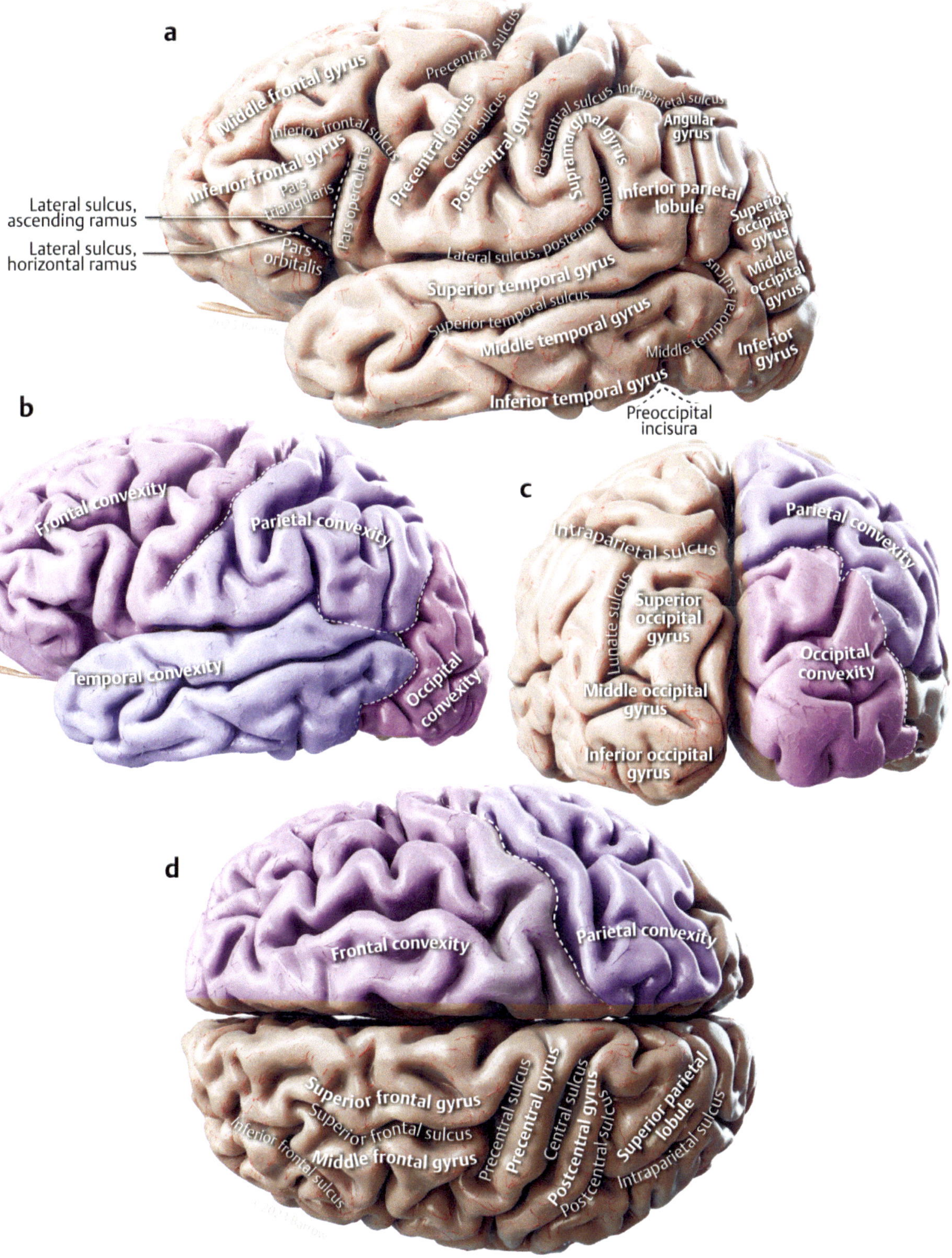

Fig. 11.1 Anatomy of the superficial cerebral convexity for subtyping cerebral CMs. **(a)** Surface anatomy of the left convexity showing gyri and sulci. **(b)** Left lateral view of the frontal, parietal, occipital, and temporal convexity subtypes shown in *shades of purple*. **(c)** Posterior view of the surface anatomy of the left posterior convexity showing gyri and sulci and right parietal and occipital convexities shown in *shades of purple*. **(d)** Superior view of the surface anatomy of the left superior convexity showing gyri and sulci and right frontal and parietal convexity subtypes shown in *shades of purple*. (Reproduced with permission from Barrow Neurological Institute, Phoenix, AZ.)

a

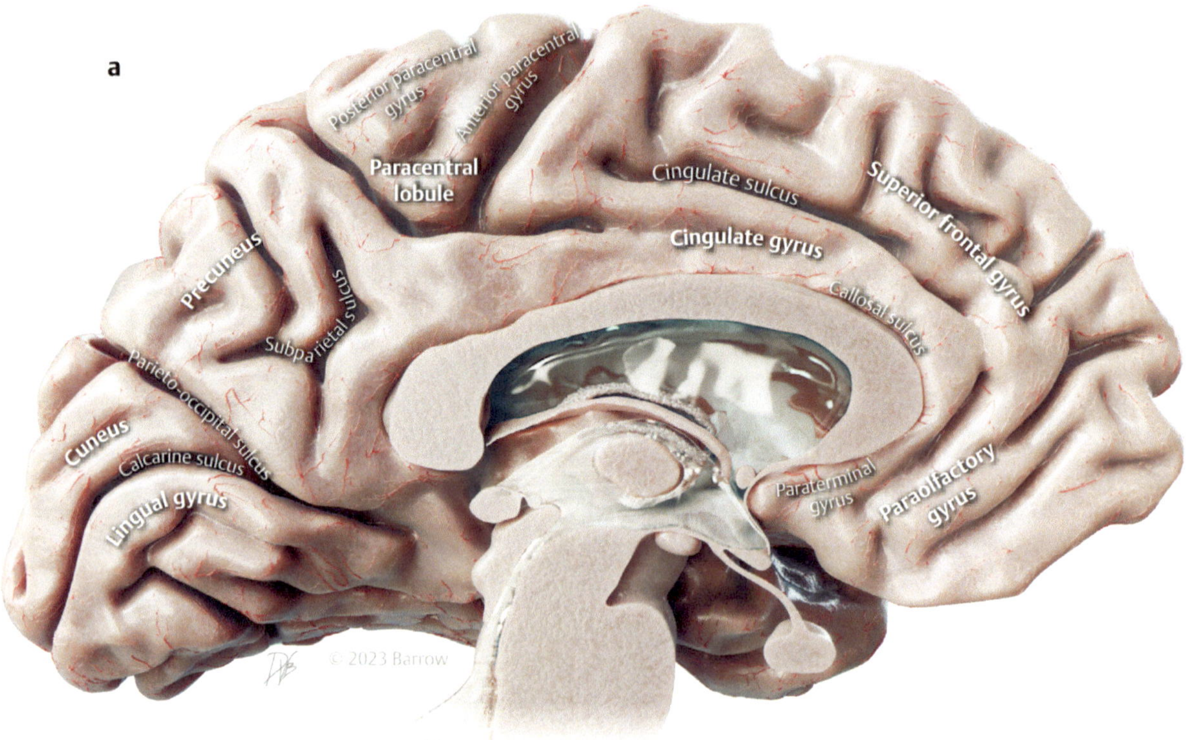

b

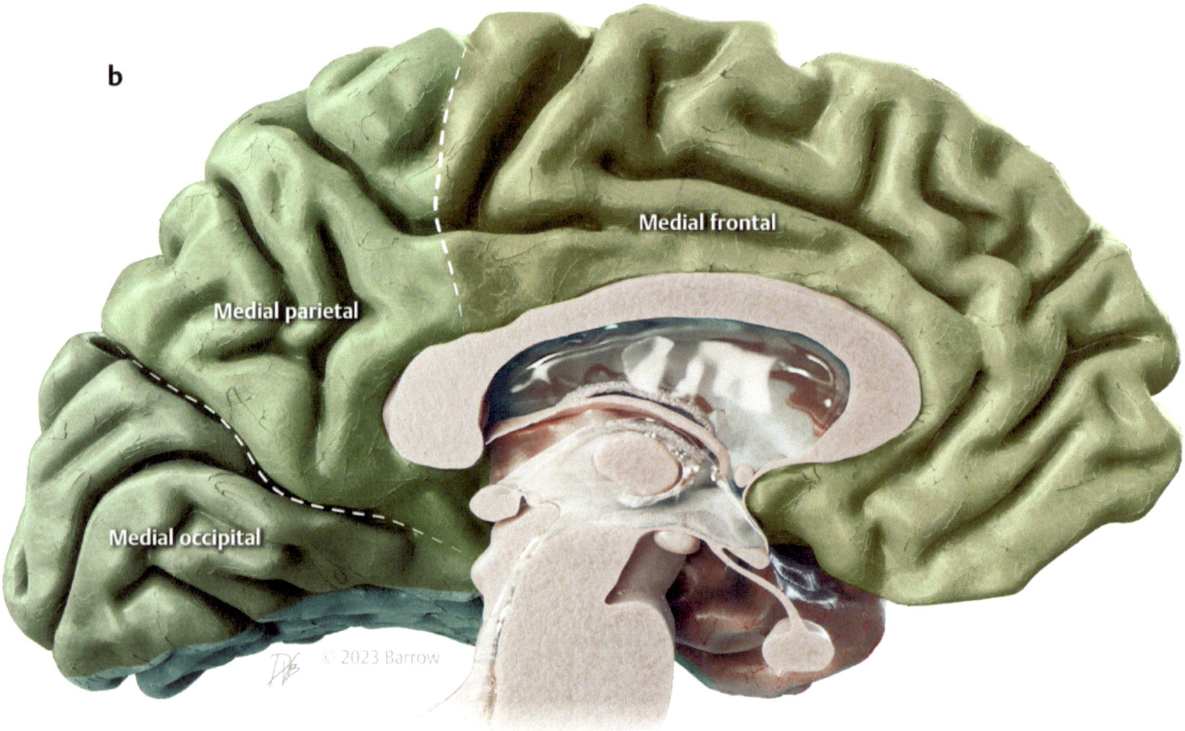

11

Fig. 11.2 Anatomy of the left medial hemisphere for subtyping superficial cerebral CMs. **(a)** Surface anatomy of the left medial hemisphere showing gyri and sulci. **(b)** Medial view of left frontal, parietal, and occipital medial subtypes shown in *shades of green*. (Reproduced with permission from Barrow Neurological Institute, Phoenix, AZ.)

the frontal and parietal lobes. The parieto-occipital sulcus is the boundary between the parietal and occipital lobes, and the preoccipital notch indicates the boundary between the temporal and occipital lobes.

11.2.3 Basal

Basal CMs lie on the inferior surfaces of the frontal, temporal, and occipital lobes (▶ Fig. 11.3). The basal frontal lobe conforms to the orbital roof and anterior cranial fossa floor, the basal temporal lobe conforms to the middle cranial fossa floor, and the basal occipital lobe conforms to the upper surface of the tentorium cerebelli. These surfaces are invisible without brain retraction or transtentorial exposure in the posterior temporal and occipital lobes. The basal surfaces of the frontal and temporal lobes are well demarcated from one another, unlike the basal surfaces of the temporal and occipital lobes. The boundary between the temporal and occipital lobes is a line extending from the preoccipital notch to the anterior end of the calcarine sulcus.

11.2.4 Sylvian

The sylvian surfaces are those portions of the frontal, temporal, and parietal lobes that face the sylvian fissure (▶ Fig. 11.4). They comprise the operculum of the sylvian cistern, and they are the smallest of the four subtype surfaces. They are visible only after widely splitting the sylvian fissure. The central sulcus is the boundary between the frontal and parietal sylvian subtype locations. The short and long gyri of the insula are not included in the sylvian subtype for superficial cerebral CMs. Given their deep location and proximity to the basal ganglia and thalamus, they are included in the subtypes for deep cerebral CMs. Specifically, CMs in the short gyri are included in the putaminal subtype of basal ganglial CMs, and CMs in the long gyri are included in the lateral thalamic subtype.

11.3 Clinical Evidence

The taxonomy for superficial cerebral CMs based cortically in gyral gray matter or subcortically in underlying white matter was applied to a consecutive series of 346 patients with 362 CMs that Robert M. Spetzler or I treated microsurgically during a 13-year period. The CMs included 132 (36.5%) convexity, 78 (21.5%) medial, 72 (19.9%) basal, and 80 (22.1%) sylvian subtypes. Frontal CMs were the most common (155, 42.8%), followed by parietal (89, 24.6%), temporal (87, 24.0%), and occipital (31, 8.6%). Of all CMs, 302 (83.4%) were cortical, and 60 (16.6%) were subcortical. The mean (standard deviation [SD]) subcortical lesion depth was 2.97 (1.09) cm, and the mean lesion volume was 4.68 (9.03) cm^3.

Overall, 228 lesions (63.0%) were resected through a transgyral approach, and 134 (37.0%) were resected through a transsulcal approach (▶ Table 11.1). Good outcomes (modified Rankin Scale [mRS] score ≤ 2) were observed in 314 patients (86.7%), poor outcomes (mRS score > 2) in 25 patients (6.9%), and 23 patients (6.4%) were lost to late follow-up (mean [SD] follow-up duration, 11.5 [22.8] months). Relative outcomes were good (unchanged or improved mRS) in 327 patients (90.3%) and poor (worse or died) in 35 patients (9.7%; ▶ Table 11.2). Good outcomes were more likely in patients with cortical CMs (85.3%) than in those with subcortical CMs (80%; $p = 0.003$). Patients with outcomes that deteriorated after surgery had a mean (SD) lesion volume of 7.9 (18.5) cm^3, whereas those whose outcomes did not deteriorate had a mean (SD) lesion volume of 4.3 (7.2) cm^3.

11.4 Resection Strategies for Superficial Cerebral Cavernous Malformations

Approaches to superficial cerebral CMs are either transgyral (42 possible routes) or transsulcal (24 possible routes; ▶ Table 11.1 and ▶ Table 11.3 detail all routes). In general, transgyral approaches are used twice as often as transsulcal approaches. Transgyral and transsulcal approaches are used with similar frequency for convexity lesions, partly because sulci are accessible and easily entered on this surface. Transgyral approaches outnumber transsulcal approaches with medial and basal subtypes, but transsulcal approaches outnumber transgyral approaches with sylvian lesions.

11.4.1 Convexity Subtype

The two most common transgyral approaches to frontal convexity subtype CMs were through the middle (41%, 11/27) and superior (26%, 7/27) frontal gyri. Parietal convexity CMs were approached through the inferior (35%, 6/17) and superior (29%, 5/17) parietal lobules, whereas all occipital convexity CMs were approached through the middle occipital gyrus (100%, 11/11). Temporal convexity CMs were approached through the middle temporal gyrus in 64% of cases (14/22) (▶ Fig. 11.5; ▶ Video 11.1, ▶ Video 11.2, ▶ Video 11.3).

Transsulcal approaches to convexity CMs traversed the superior frontal sulcus (52%, 15/29) in the frontal lobe, the superior temporal sulcus (63%, 5/8) and the inferior temporal sulcus (38%, 3/8) in the temporal lobe, the postcentral sulcus (73%, 11/15) in the parietal lobe, and the intraoccipital sulcus (100%, 3/3) in the occipital lobe (▶ Table 11.1).

11.4.2 Medial Subtype

The most common transgyral approach to medial CM subtypes in the frontal lobe transgressed the cingulate gyrus (58%, 21/36; ▶ Table 11.1). Approaches to the medial temporal CM subtypes transgressed the middle temporal gyrus in 40% (2/5), using a lateral trajectory to a medial lesion. In the parietal lobe, approaches to medial CM subtypes transgressed the precuneus in

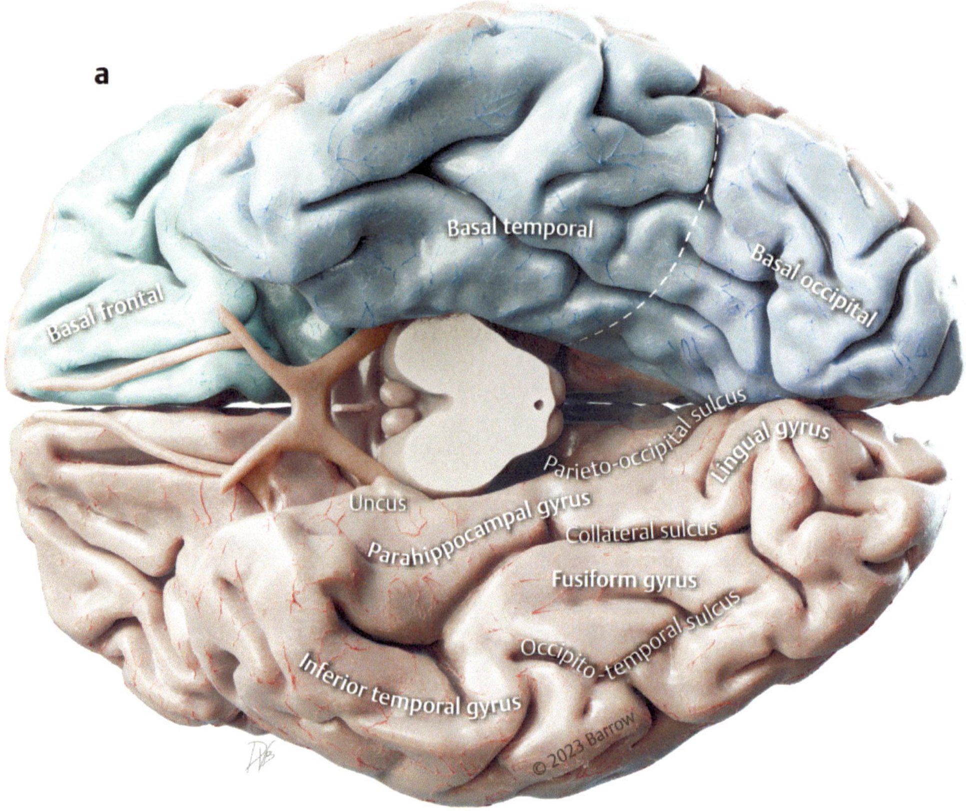

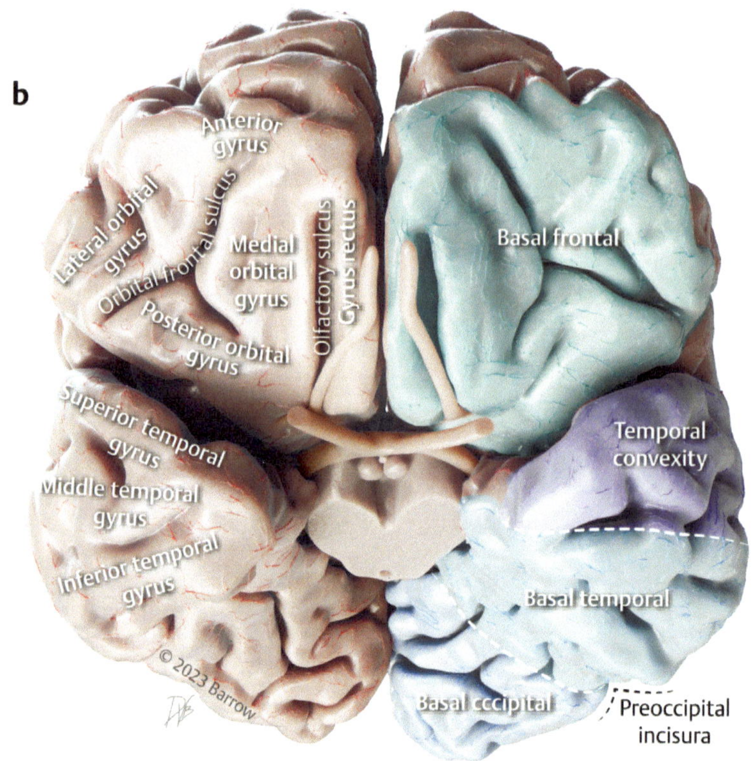

Fig. 11.3 Anatomy of basal surfaces for subtyping superficial cerebral CMs. **(a)** Inferior view of the surface anatomy of the right basal temporal and occipital surfaces showing gyri and sulci and left basal frontal, temporal, and occipital subtypes shown in *shades of blue*. **(b)** Anteroinferior view of the surface anatomy of the right basal frontal and temporal surfaces showing gyri and sulci and left basal frontal, temporal, and occipital subtypes shown in *shades of blue*. (Reproduced with permission from Barrow Neurological Institute, Phoenix, AZ.)

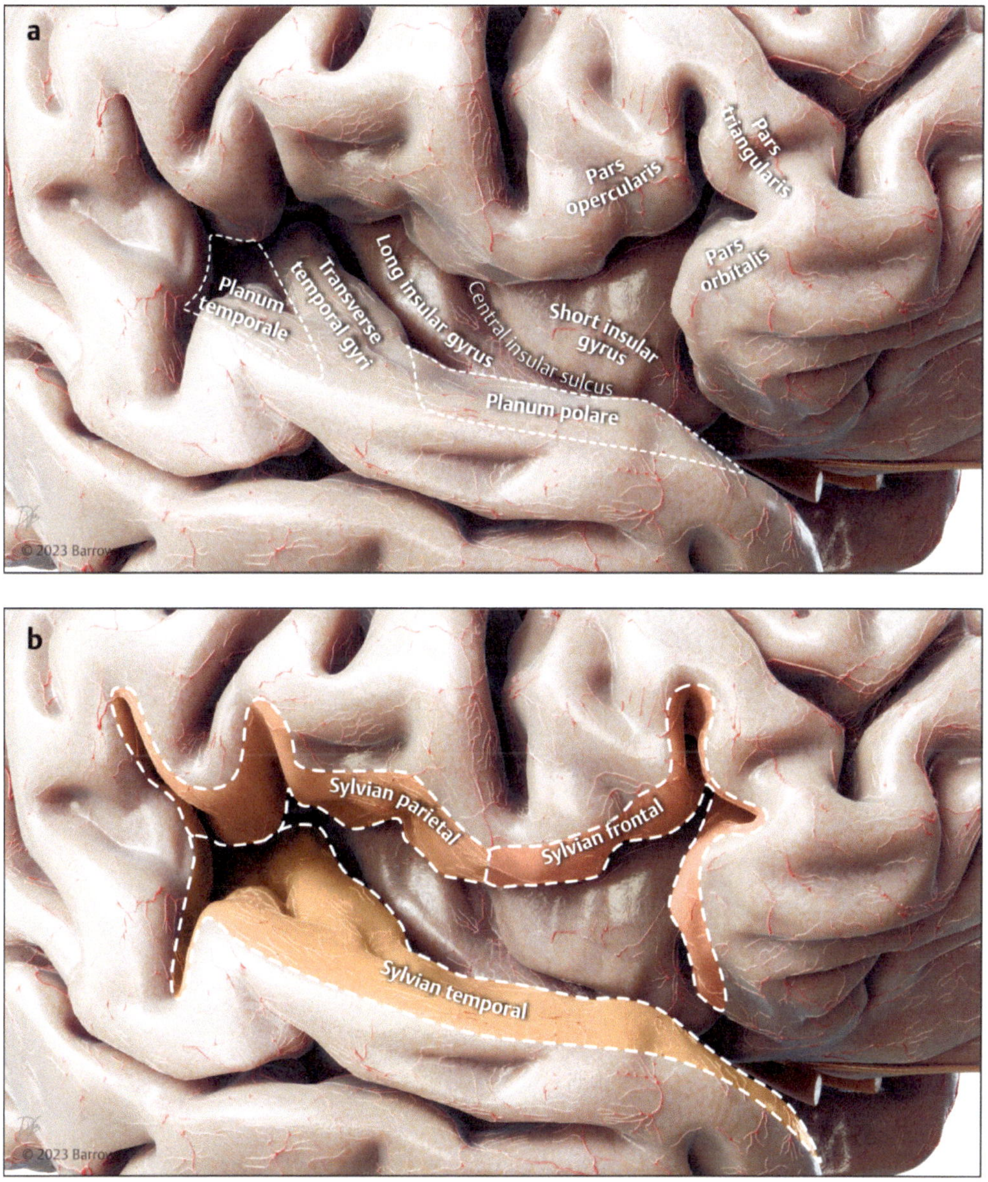

Fig. 11.4 Anatomy of sylvian surfaces for subtyping superficial cerebral CMs. **(a)** Lateral view of the anatomy of the right sylvian surfaces showing gyri and sulci. **(b)** Lateral view of the right sylvian frontal, parietal, and temporal subtypes shown in *shades of orange*. Note that the insular cortex is not included in the superficial cerebral CM subtype. Instead, it is included in the deep cerebral basal ganglia and thalamus subtypes. (Reproduced with permission from Barrow Neurological Institute, Phoenix, AZ.)

50% (7/14), and in the occipital lobe, they transgressed the cuneus (33%, 1/3), lingual gyrus (33%, 1/3), and superior occipital gyrus (33%, 1/3) (▶ Fig. 11.6; ▶ Video 11.4, ▶ Video 11.5).

The most common transsulcal approaches to medial CMs were from a lateral direction through the superior frontal sulcus in the frontal lobe (50%, 3/6), postcentral sulcus in the parietal lobe (50%, 5/10), and the superior temporal sulcus (50%, 1/2) and inferior temporal sulcus (50%, 1/2) in the temporal lobe.

11.4.3 Basal Subtype

The two most frequent transgyral approaches to basal subtype CMs in the frontal lobe transgressed the gyrus rectus (17%, 4/24) and posterior orbital gyrus (17%, 4/24). Approaches in the temporal lobe transgressed the inferior temporal gyrus (38%, 9/24), and approaches in the occipital lobe transgressed the inferior occipital gyrus (70%, 7/10) (▶ Fig. 11.7; ▶ Video 11.6, ▶ Video 11.7).

Transsulcal approaches to basal CMs were used infrequently.

11.4.4 Sylvian Subtype

The most common transgyral approaches to sylvian subtype CMs in the frontal lobe transgressed the pars opercularis (43%, 3/7) and inferior frontal gyrus (43%, 3/7). Approaches to sylvian CMs in the temporal lobe transgressed the superior temporal gyrus (65%, 13/20). Approaches to sylvian CMs in the parietal lobe transgressed the postcentral gyrus (50%, 4/8) (▶ Fig. 11.8; ▶ Video 11.8).

Table 11.1 Summary of microsurgical approaches to superficial cerebral CMs

Approach	Number (%) of CMs, by subtype				
	Convexity (n = 132)	Medial (n = 78)	Basal (n = 72)	Sylvian (n = 80)	Total (N = 362)
Frontal transgyral					
Overall	27/132 (20)	36/78 (46)	24/72 (33)	7/80 (9)	94/362 (26)
Superior frontal gyrus	7/27 (26)	12/36 (33)	1/24 (4)	0 (0)	20/94 (21)
Middle frontal gyrus	11/27 (41)	0 (0)	3/24 (13)	0 (0)	14/94 (15)
Inferior frontal gyrus	1/27 (4)	2/36 (6)	3/24 (13)	3/7 (43)	9/94 (10)
Precentral gyrus	4/27 (15)	0 (0)	0 (0)	0 (0)	4/94 (4)
Pars opercularis	0 (0)	0 (0)	0 (0)	3/7 (43)	3/94 (3)
Pars triangularis	1/27 (4)	0 (0)	1/24 (4)	0 (0)	2/94 (2)
Pars orbitalis	0 (0)	0 (0)	3/24 (13)	0 (0)	3/94 (3)
Gyrus rectus	0 (0)	0 (0)	4/24 (17)	0 (0)	4/94 (4)
Medial orbital gyrus	0 (0)	0 (0)	0 (0)	0 (0)	0 (0)
Lateral orbital gyrus	0 (0)	0 (0)	1/24 (4)	0 (0)	1/94 (1)
Anterior orbital gyrus	0 (0)	0 (0)	1/24 (4)	0 (0)	1/94 (1)
Posterior orbital gyrus	0 (0)	0 (0)	4/24 (17)	0 (0)	4/94 (4)
Anterior paracentral gyrus	2/27 (7)	0 (0)	0 (0)	0 (0)	2/94 (2)
Paracentral lobule	0 (0)	0 (0)	0 (0)	0 (0)	0 (0)
Cingulate gyrus	1/27 (4)	21/36 (58)	3/24 (13)	1/7 (14)	26/94 (28)
Paraolfactory gyrus	0 (0)	0 (0)	0 (0)	0 (0)	0 (0)
Subcallosal area/paraterminal gyrus	0 (0)	1/36 (3)	0 (0)	0 (0)	1/94 (1)
Frontal transsulcal					
Overall	29/132 (22)	6/78 (8)	10/72 (14)	16/80 (20)	61/362 (17)
Superior frontal sulcus	15/29 (52)	3/6 (50)	0 (0)	0 (0)	18/61 (30)
Inferior frontal sulcus	2/29 (7)	0 (0)	2/10 (20)	2/16 (13)	6/61 (10)
Lateral sulcus, ascending ramus	0 (0)	1/6 (17)	3/10 (30)	6/16 (38)	10/61 (16)
Lateral sulcus, anterior ramus	0 (0)	1/6 (17)	5/10 (50)	6/16 (38)	12/61 (20)
Olfactory sulcus	0 (0)	0 (0)	0 (0)	0 (0)	0 (0)
Orbital sulcus (lateral, medial, transverse)	0 (0)	0 (0)	0 (0)	0 (0)	0 (0)
Cingulate sulcus	0 (0)	0 (0)	0 (0)	0 (0)	0 (0)
Callosal sulcus	0 (0)	1/6 (17)	0 (0)	0 (0)	1/61 (2)
Precentral sulcus	9/29 (31)	0 (0)	0 (0)	1/16 (6)	10/61 (16)
Central sulcus	3/29 (10)	0 (0)	0 (0)	1/16 (6)	4/61 (7)
Parietal transgyral					
Overall	17/132 (13)	14/78 (18)	0 (0)	8/80 (10)	39/362 (11)
Postcentral gyrus	2/17 (12)	2/14 (14)	0 (0)	4/8 (50)	8/39 (21)
Superior parietal lobule	5/17 (29)	1/14 (7)	0 (0)	0 (0)	6/39 (15)
Inferior parietal lobule	6/17 (35)	0 (0)	0 (0)	1/8 (13)	7/39 (18)
Supramarginal gyrus	2/17 (12)	0 (0)	0 (0)	3/8 (38)	5/39 (13)
Angular gyrus	0 (0)	0 (0)	0 (0)	0 (0)	0 (0)
Posterior paracentral gyrus	1/17 (6)	4/14 (29)	0 (0)	0 (0)	5/39 (13)
Precuneus	1/17 (6)	7/14 (50)	0 (0)	0 (0)	8/39 (21)
Parietal transsulcal					
Overall	15/132 (11)	10/78 (13)	0 (0)	25/80 (31)	50/362 (14)
Postcentral sulcus	11/15 (73)	5/10 (50)	0 (0)	10/25 (40)	26/50 (52)
Intraparietal sulcus	2/15 (13)	2/10 (20)	0 (0)	0 (0)	4/50 (8)

(Continued)

11

Table 11.1 (*Continued*) Summary of microsurgical approaches to superficial cerebral CMs

Approach	Number (%) of CMs, by subtype				
	Convexity (*n* = 132)	Medial (*n* = 78)	Basal (*n* = 72)	Sylvian (*n* = 80)	Total (*N* = 362)
Parieto-occipital sulcus	2/15 (13)	3/10 (30)	0 (0)	0 (0)	5/50 (10)
Lateral sulcus, posterior ramus	0 (0)	0 (0)	0 (0)	15/25 (60)	15/50 (30)
Subparietal sulcus	0 (0)	0 (0)	0 (0)	0 (0)	0 (0)
Occipital transgyral					
Overall	11/132 (8)	3/78 (4)	10/72 (14)	0 (0)	24/362 (7)
Superior occipital gyrus	0 (0)	1/3 (33)	0 (0)	0 (0)	1/24 (4)
Middle occipital gyrus	11/11 (100)	0 (0)	0 (0)	0 (0)	11/24 (46)
Inferior occipital gyrus	0 (0)	0 (0)	7/10 (70)	0 (0)	7/24 (29)
Cuneus	0 (0)	1/3 (33)	0 (0)	0 (0)	1/24 (4)
Lingual gyrus (medial occipito-temporal)	0 (0)	1/3 (33)	3/10 (30)	0 (0)	4/24 (17)
Occipital transsulcal					
Overall	3/132 (2)	2/78 (3)	2/72 (3)	0 (0)	7/362 (2)
Calcarine sulcus	0 (0)	0 (0)	0 (0)	0 (0)	0 (0)
Lunate sulcus	0 (0)	0 (0)	0 (0)	0 (0)	0 (0)
Intraoccipital sulcus	3/3 (100)	2/2 (100)	1/2 (50)	0 (0)	6/7 (86)
Inferior occipital sulcus	0 (0)	0 (0)	1/2 (50)	0 (0)	1/7 (14)
Preoccipital incisura	0 (0)	0 (0)	0 (0)	0 (0)	0 (0)
Temporal transgyral					
Overall	22/132 (17)	5/78 (6)	24/72 (33)	20/80 (25)	71/362 (20)
Superior temporal gyrus	2/22 (9)	1/5 (20)	0 (0)	13/20 (65)	16/71 (23)
Middle temporal gyrus	14/22 (64)	2/5 (40)	4/24 (17)	5/20 (25)	25/71 (35)
Inferior temporal gyrus	5/22 (23)	1/5 (20)	9/24 (38)	1/20 (5)	16/71 (23)
Fusiform gyrus	1/22 (5)	1/5 (20)	4/24 (17)	0 (0)	6/71 (8)
Parahippocampal gyrus	0 (0)	0 (0)	5/24 (21)	1/20 (5)	6/71 (8)
Hippocampus, head	0 (0)	0 (0)	0 (0)	0 (0)	0 (0)
Hippocampus, body	0 (0)	0 (0)	1/24 (4)	0 (0)	1/71 (1)
Hippocampus, tail	0 (0)	0 (0)	0 (0)	0 (0)	0 (0)
Uncus	0 (0)	0 (0)	1/24 (4)	0 (0)	1/71 (1)
Transverse temporal gyrus (Heschl gyrus)	0 (0)	0 (0)	0 (0)	0 (0)	0 (0)
Planum polare	0 (0)	0 (0)	0 (0)	0 (0)	0 (0)
Planum temporale	0 (0)	0 (0)	0 (0)	0 (0)	0 (0)
Temporal transsulcal					
Overall	8/132 (6)	2/78 (3)	2/72 (3)	4/80 (5)	16/362 (4)
Superior temporal sulcus	5/8 (63)	1/2 (50)	0 (0)	3/4 (75)	9/16 (56)
Inferior temporal sulcus	3/8 (38)	1/2 (50)	1/2 (50)	1/4 (25)	6/16 (38)
Occipitotemporal sulcus	0 (0)	0 (0)	0 (0)	0 (0)	0 (0)
Collateral sulcus	0 (0)	0 (0)	1/2 (50)	0 (0)	1/16 (6)
Transgyral overall	77/132 (58)	58/78 (74)	58/72 (81)	35/80 (44)	228/362 (63)
Transsulcal overall	55/132 (42)	20/78 (26)	14/72 (19)	45/80 (56)	134/362 (37)

Note: Data are presented as proportion (%).

11

Table 11.2 Cerebral CMs by patient outcome status

Lobe, subtype	All CMs (*N* = 362)	Number (%) of CMs, by patient outcome				
		Improved or unchanged	Worsened	Additional decline	Unfavorable	Favorable
Frontal						
All	155/362 (42.8)	140/327 (42.8)	15/35 (42.9)	18/47 (38.3)	33/82 (40.2)	122/280 (43.6)
Medial	42/155 (27.1)	38/140 (27.1)	4/15 (26.7)	6/18 (33.3)	10/33 (30.3)	32/122 (26.2)
Convexity	56/155 (36.1)	52/140 (37.1)	4/15 (26.7)	7/18 (38.9)	11/33 (36.7)	45/122 (36.9)
Basal	34/155 (21.9)	29/140 (20.7)	5/15 (33.3)	2/18 (11.1)	7/33 (21.2)	27/122 (22.1)
Sylvian	23/155 (14.8)	21/140 (15.0)	2/15 (13.3)	3/18 (16.7)	5/33 (15.2)	18/122 (14.8)
Parietal						
All	89/362 (24.6)	76/327 (23.2)	13/35 (37.1)	10/47 (21.3)	23/82 (28.0)	66/280 (23.6)
Medial	24/89 (27.0)	22/76 (28.9)	2/13 (15.4)	2/10 (20.0)	4/23 (17.4)	20/66 (30.3)
Convexity	32/89 (36.0)	27/76 (35.5)	5/13 (38.5)	5/10 (50.0)	10/23 (43.5)	22/66 (33.3)
Sylvian	33/89 (37.1)	27/76 (35.5)	6/13 (46.2)	3/10 (30.0)	9/23 (39.1)	24/66 (36.4)
Occipital						
All	31/362 (8.6)	29/327 (8.9)	2/35 (5.7)	2/47 (4.3)	4/82 (4.9)	27/280 (9.6)
Medial	5/31 (16.1)	5/29 (17.2)	0/2 (0)	0/2 (0)	0/4 (0)	5/27 (18.5)
Convexity	14/31 (45.2)	13/29 (44.8)	1/2 (50)	1/2 (50.0)	2/4 (50)	12/27 (44.4)
Basal	12/31 (38.7)	11/29 (37.9)	1/2 (50)	1/2 (50.0)	2/4 (50)	10/27 (37.0)
Temporal						
All	87/362 (24.0)	82/327 (25.1)	5/35 (14.3)	17/47 (36.2)	22/82 (26.8)	65/280 (23.2)
Medial	7/87 (8.0)	6/82 (7.3)	1/5 (20.0)	2/17 (11.8)	3/22 (13.6)	4/65 (6.2)
Convexity	30/87 (34.5)	28/82 (34.1)	2/5 (40.0)	2/17 (11.8)	4/22 (18.2)	26/65 (40.0)
Basal	26/87 (29.9)	26/82 (31.7)	0/5 (0)	9/17 (52.9)	9/22 (40.9)	17/65 (26.2)
Sylvian	24/87 (27.6)	22/82 (26.8)	2/5 (40.0)	4/17 (23.5)	6/22 (27.3)	18/65 (27.7)
All locations	362/362 (100)	327/362 (90.3)	35/362 (9.7)	47/362 (13.0)	82/362 (22.7)	280/362 (77.3)

Note: All data are presented as proportion (%).

Table 11.3 Summary of cerebral gyri, sulci, and abbreviations of transgyral and transsulcal approaches

Lobe	Gyrus	Transgyral approach	Sulcus	Transsulcal approach
Frontal	Superior frontal gyrus	TGyr-SFG	Superior frontal sulcus	TSul-sfs
	Middle frontal gyrus	TGyr-MFG	Inferior frontal sulcus	TSul-ifs
	Inferior frontal gyrus	TGyr-IFG	Lateral sulcus, ascending ramus	TSul-las
	Precentral gyrus	TGyr-PRG	Lateral sulcus, anterior ramus	TSul-lat
	Pars opercularis	TGyr-IFGOp	Olfactory sulcus	TSul-ols
	Pars triangularis	TGyr-IFGTr	Orbital sulcus (lateral, medial, transverse)	TSul-ors
	Pars orbitalis	TGyr-IFGOr	Cingulate sulcus	TSul-cgs
	Gyrus rectus	TGyr-GR	Callosal sulcus	TSul-scc
	Orbital gyri (medial, lateral, anterior, posterior)	TGyr-MOrG, LOrG, AOrG, POrG	Precentral sulcus	TSul-pces
	Paracentral lobule	TGyr-PCL	Central sulcus	TSul-ces
	Cingulate gyrus	TGyr-CG	–	–
	Paraolfactory gyrus	TGyr-PaOG	–	–
	Subcallosal area/paraterminal gyrus	TGyr-SCA	–	–
Parietal	Postcentral gyrus	TGyr-POG	Postcentral sulcus	TSul-pcs
	Superior parietal lobule	TGyr-SPL	Intraparietal sulcus	TSul-ips
	Inferior parietal lobule	TGyr-IPL	Parieto-occipital sulcus	TSul-pos
	Supramarginal gyrus	TGyr-SMG	Lateral sulcus, posterior ramus	TSul-lpor

(Continued)

Table 11.3 (*Continued*) Summary of cerebral gyri, sulci, and abbreviations of transgyral and transsulcal approaches

Lobe	Gyrus	Transgyral approach	Sulcus	Transsulcal approach
	Angular gyrus	TGyr-AG	Subparietal sulcus	TSul-sps
	Anterior paracentral gyrus	TGyr-APaG	–	–
	Posterior paracentral gyrus	TGyr-PPaG	–	–
	Precuneus	TGyr-PCun	–	–
Occipital	Superior occipital gyrus	TGyr-SOG	Calcarine sulcus	TSul-cas
	Middle occipital gyrus	TGyr-MOG	Lunate sulcus	TSul-ls
	Inferior occipital gyrus	TGyr-IOG	Intraoccipital sulcus	TSul-ios
	Cuneus	TGyr-Cun	Inferior occipital sulcus	TSul-ifos
	Lingual gyrus (medial occipitotemporal)	TGyr-LG	Preoccipital incisura	TSul-poi
Temporal	Superior temporal gyrus	TGyr-STG	Superior temporal sulcus	TSul-sts
	Middle temporal gyrus	TGyr-MTG	Inferior temporal sulcus	TSul-its
	Inferior temporal gyrus	TGyr-ITG	Occipitotemporal sulcus	TSul-ots
	Fusiform gyrus (lateral occipitotemporal)	TGyr-FG	Collateral sulcus	TSyl-cos
	Parahippocampal gyrus	TGyr-PHG	–	–
	Hippocampus, head	TGyr-HiH	–	–
	Hippocampus, body	TGyr-HiB	–	–
	Hippocampus, tail	TGyr-HiT	–	–
	Uncus (gyrus intralimbicus, uncinate gyrus, limbus Giacomini)	TGyr-Un	–	–
	Transverse temporal gyrus (Heschl gyrus)	TGyr-TTG (anterior, posterior)	–	–
	Planum polare	TGyr-PPo	–	–
	Planum temporale	TGyr-PTe	–	–

Sylvian subtype CMs were approached through the sylvian fissure and its anterior and ascending rami of the lateral sulcus for lesions in the frontal, temporal, and parietal lobes.

11.5 Superficial Cerebral Cavernous Malformations and Approach Selection

The taxonomy for superficial cerebral CMs initiates a comprehensive system that characterizes all the CMs encountered in the brain. With this taxonomy, a particular CM's anatomical location is uniquely defined, can be correlated with radiographic anatomy on MRI, may be associated with a constellation of symptoms and signs that help localize the lesion with bedside examination findings, and is described precisely for clearer clinical communication and publication. Perhaps even more importantly, the taxonomy informs microsurgical management by associating each subtype with a specific craniotomy and approach, and in the case of brainstem CMs, a dissection triangle and safe entry zone. These deep and complex CMs may be exposed in many ways, and the taxonomy adds clarity and guidance to surgical decision-making. In contrast, the taxonomy for superficial cerebral CMs may be less informative than the taxonomy for deeper lesions because the selection of a craniotomy and an approach reduces to a choice between transgyral and transsulcal approaches. There are no cranial nerves or skull base anatomy in the cerebral hemispheres, which eliminates the use of dissection triangles, and similarly, there are no safe entry zones for cortical and subcortical CMs.

In our experience, most superficial cerebral CMs (83%) were within 1 cm of the cortical surface, and most (63%) were resected using a transgyral approach. The depth of the overlying tissue transgression with transgyral approaches varied from 0 to 3 cm for subcortical CMs. We minimize tissue transgression by whatever means possible, including maximizing subarachnoid dissection, opening corridors like the sylvian and interhemispheric fissures, and traversing the full extent of sulci to deepen the approach. Notably, 74 of 362 cases of cortical CMs (20%) had transsulcal rather than transgyral resections, attesting to the practice of minimizing tissue transgression to preserve associated eloquence and reduce neurological morbidity.

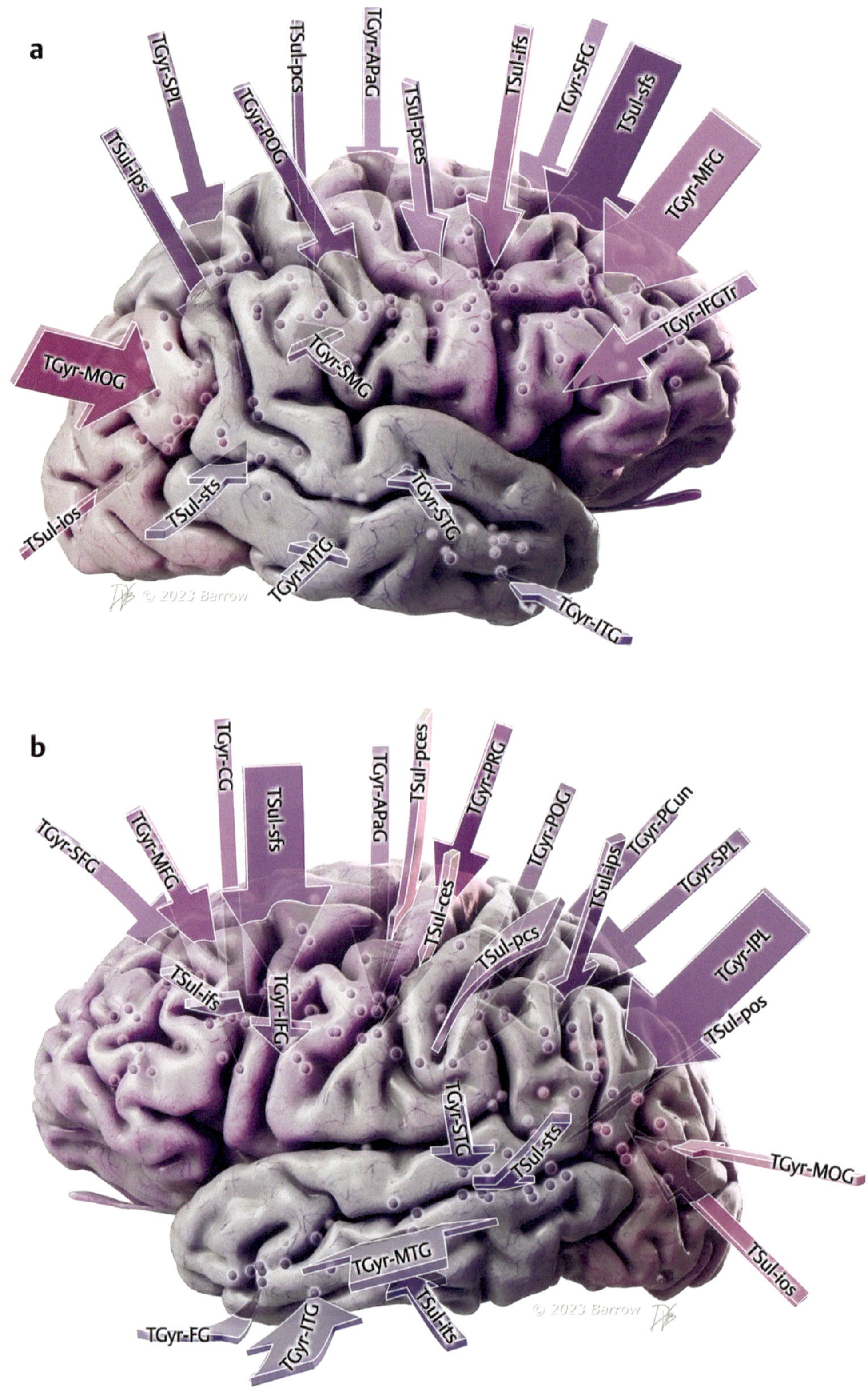

Fig. 11.5 Summary of approaches to convexity CMs. TGyr and TSul approaches to **(a)** right-sided and **(b)** left-sided convexity CMs. Approaches are shown as *arrows* in which the size or width is proportional to the number of patients. CMs are depicted as spheres of uniform size placed at the approximate center of each lesion. *Shading of the arrows* corresponds to the lobar locations (surgical cases; ▶ Video 11.1, ▶ Video 11.2, ▶ Video 11.3; QR codes). ▶ Table 11.3 lists approach abbreviations. (Reproduced with permission from Barrow Neurological Institute, Phoenix, AZ.)

Surgical Case 11.1

CEREBRAL

Cavernoma Subtype: Convexity (Frontal)

Position: Supine, nose up
Craniotomy: Frontoparietal
Approach: Transsulcal (TSul)
Triangle: None
SEZ: None
Artery: M4 MCA

Video: Resection of a left frontal convexity superficial cerebral cavernoma

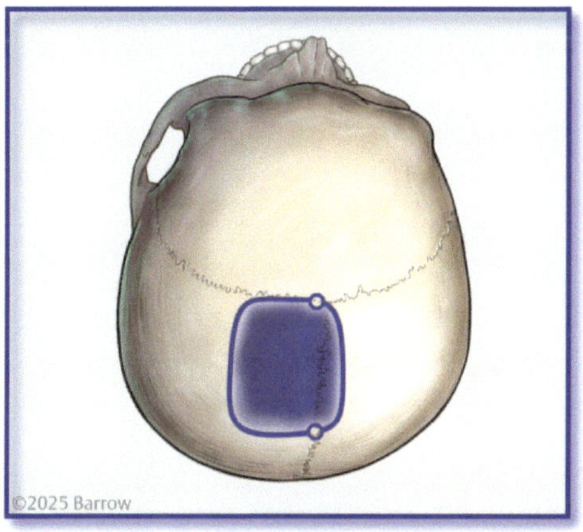

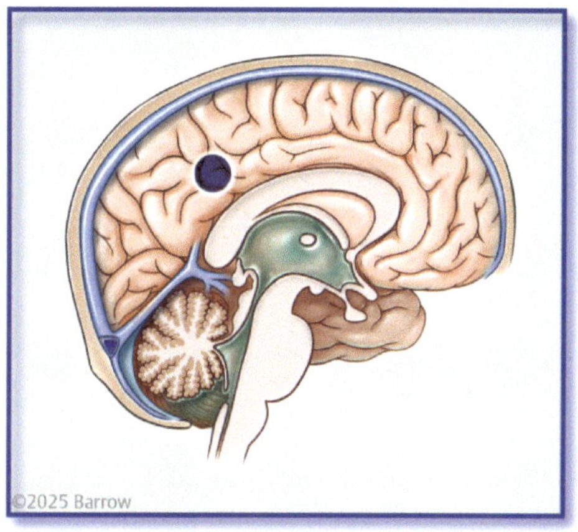

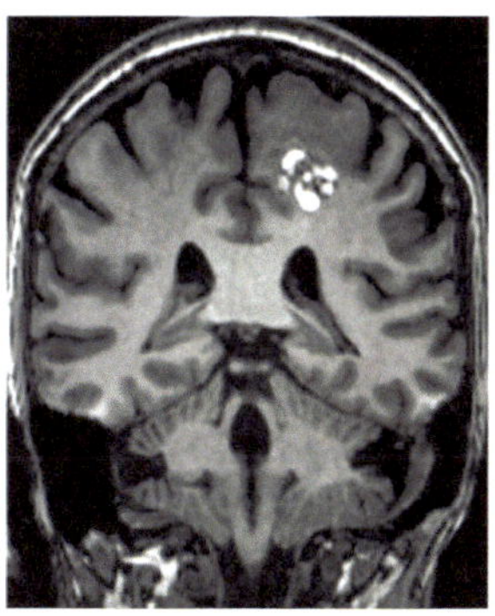

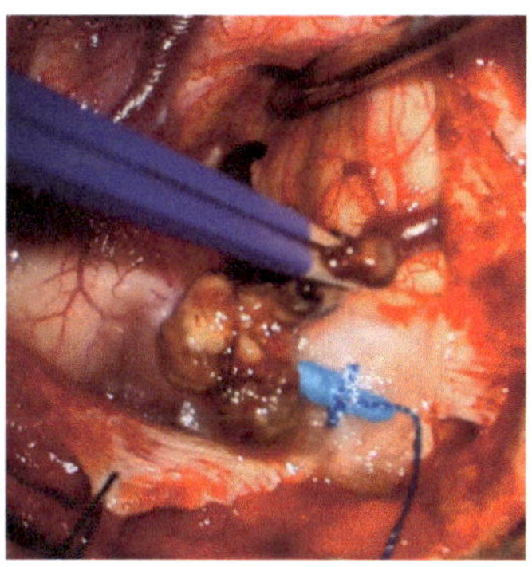

Video 11.1
Transsulcal Approach for Motor Strip Cavernous Malformation Resection (Reproduced with permission from Barrow Neurological Institute, Phoenix, AZ.)

Surgical Case 11.2

CEREBRAL

Cavernoma Subtype: Convexity (Parietal)

Position: Lateral
Craniotomy: Parietal
Approach: Transsulcal (TSul)
Triangle: None
SEZ: None
Artery: M4 MCA

Video: Resection of a cluster of left parietal convexity superficial cerebral cavernomas

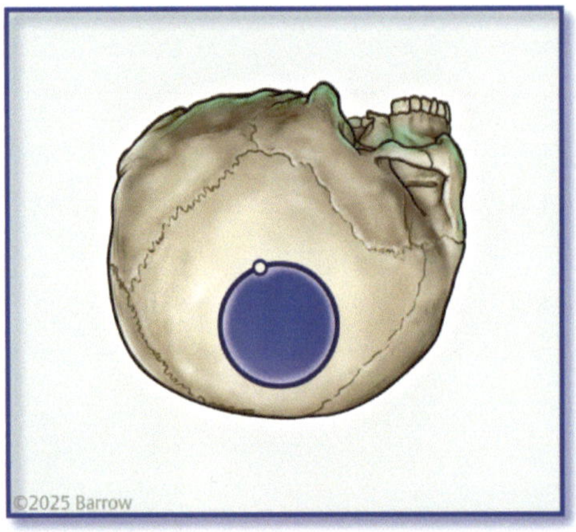

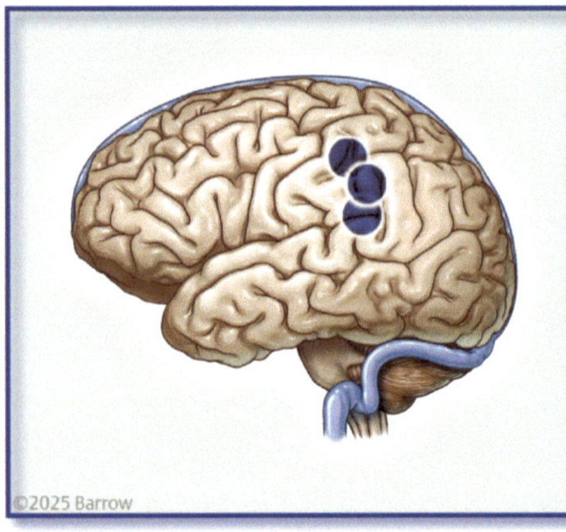

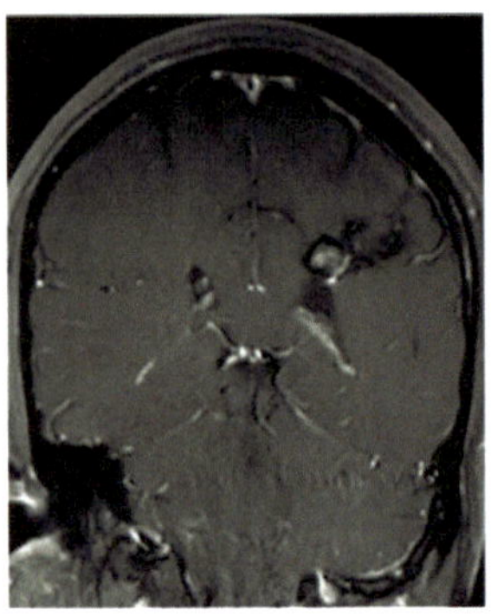

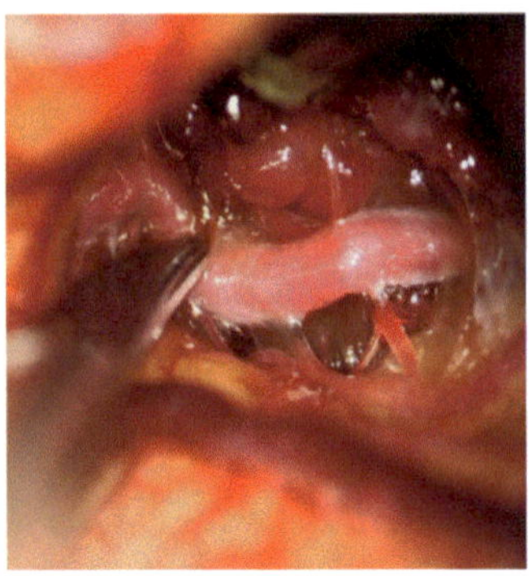

Video 11.2
Transsulcal Approach for Multiple Parietal Convexity Cavernous Malformation Resections (Reproduced with permission from Barrow Neurological Institute, Phoenix, AZ.)

11

Surgical Case 11.3

CEREBRAL

Cavernoma Subtype: Convexity (Frontoparietal, Giant)

Position: Supine
Craniotomy: Frontoparietal
Approach: Transsulcal (TSul)
Triangle: None
SEZ: None
Artery: M4 MCA

Video: Resection of a giant left frontoparietal convexity superficial cerebral cavernoma

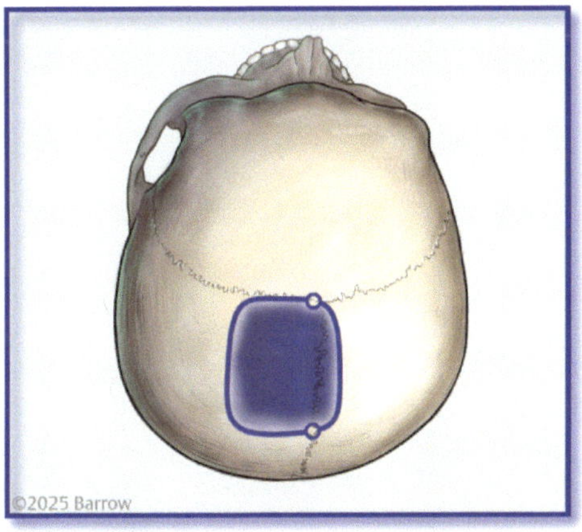

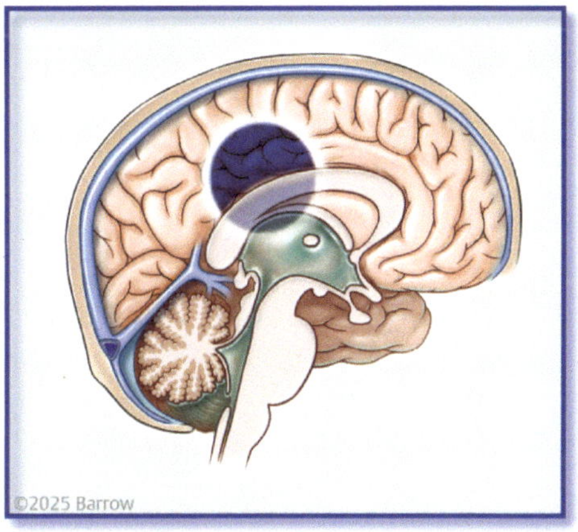

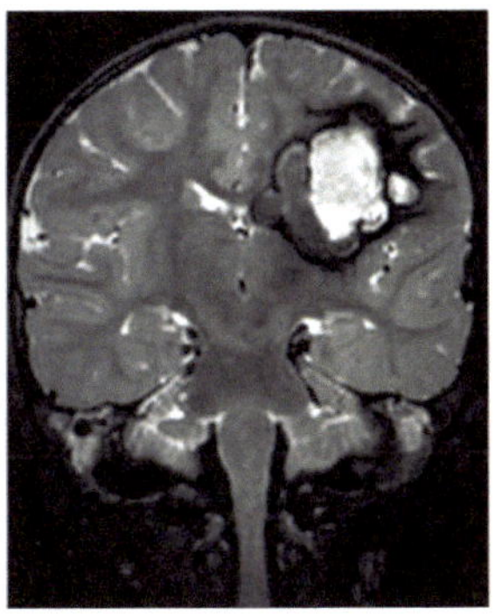

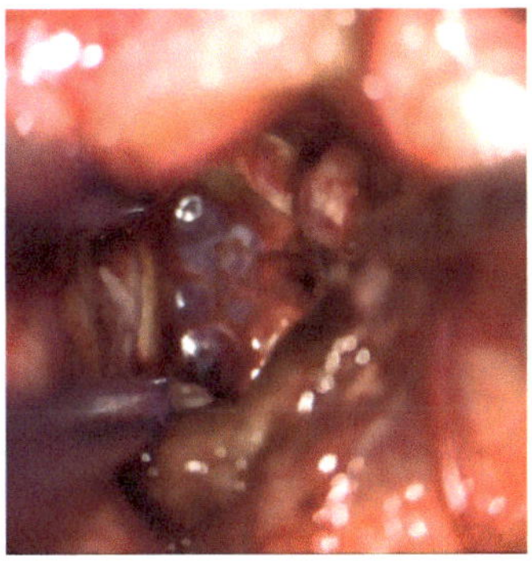

Video 11.3
Transsulcal Approach for Giant Rolandic Cavernous Malformation Resection (Reproduced with permission from Barrow Neurological Institute, Phoenix, AZ.)

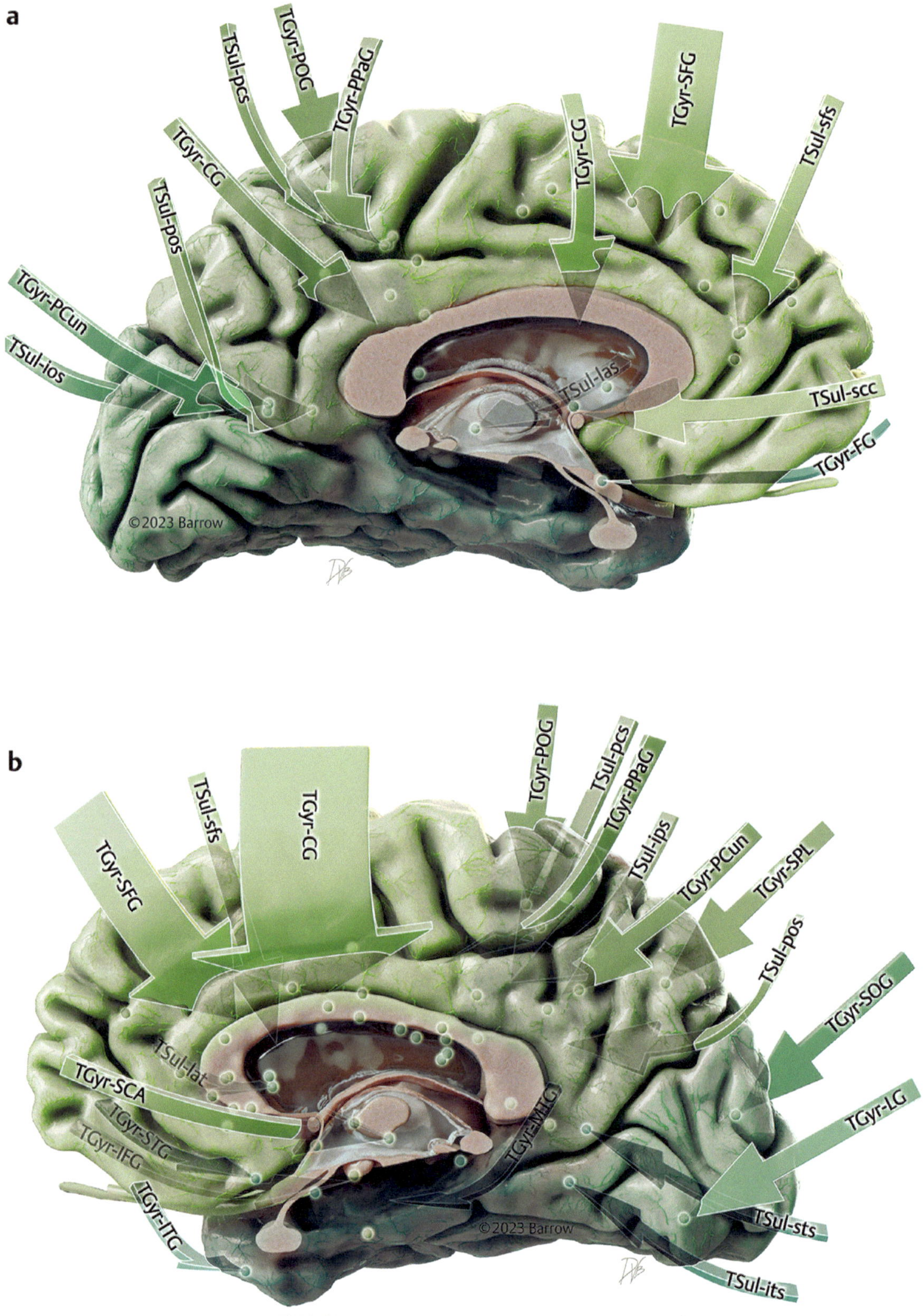

Fig. 11.6 Summary of approaches to medial CMs. TGyr and TSul approaches to **(a)** left-sided and **(b)** right-sided medial CMs. Approaches are shown as *arrows* in which the size or width is proportional to the number of patients. CMs are depicted as spheres of uniform size placed at the approximate center of each lesion. *Shading of the arrows* corresponds to the lobar locations (surgical cases; ▸ Video 11.4, ▸ Video 11.5; QR codes). ▸ Table 11.3 lists approach abbreviations. (Reproduced with permission from Barrow Neurological Institute, Phoenix, AZ.)

Surgical Case 11.4

CEREBRAL

Cavernoma Subtype: Medial (Frontal)

Position: Supine, head turned to the right
Craniotomy: Bifrontal
Approach: Anterior interhemispheric, ipsilateral transcingulate (TGyr)
Triangle: None
SEZ: None
Artery: CmaA and PcaA

Video: Resection of a right frontal medial superficial cerebral cavernoma

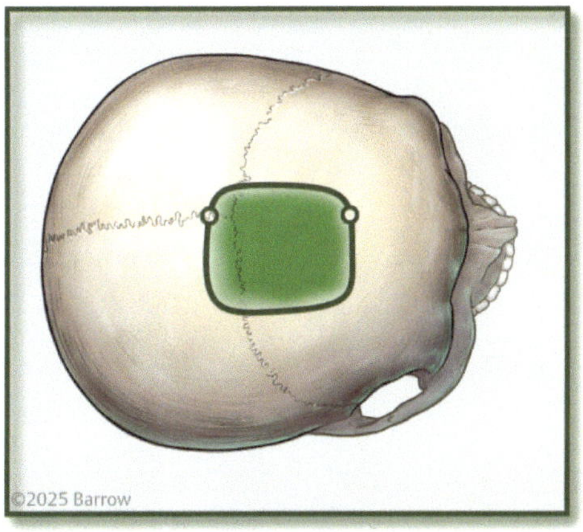

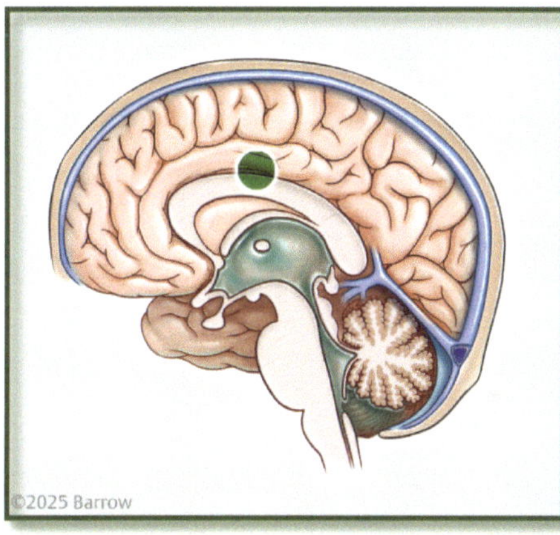

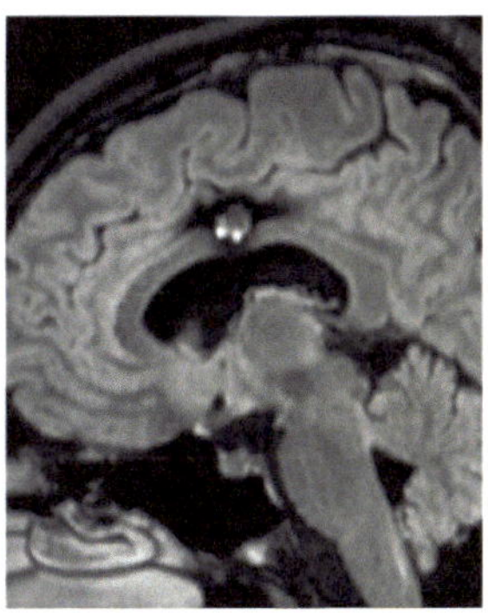

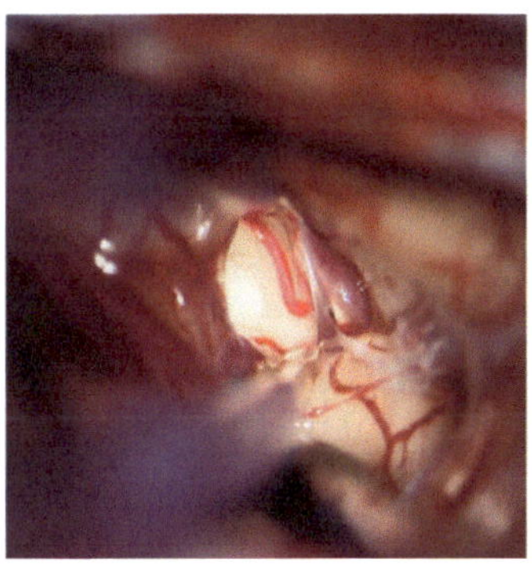

Video 11.4
Anterior Interhemispheric Ipsilateral Transcingulate Approach for Cingulate and Corpus Callosum Cavernous Malformation Resection (Reproduced with permission from Barrow Neurological Institute, Phoenix, AZ.)

11

Surgical Case 11.5

CEREBRAL

Cavernoma Subtype: Medial (Temporal)

Position: 3/4 prone, head turned toward floor
Craniotomy: Torcular
Approach: Supratentorial-infraoccipital transgyral (STIO-TGyr)
Triangle: None
SEZ: None
Artery: P3 PCA

Video: Resection of a right temporal medial superficial cerebral cavernoma

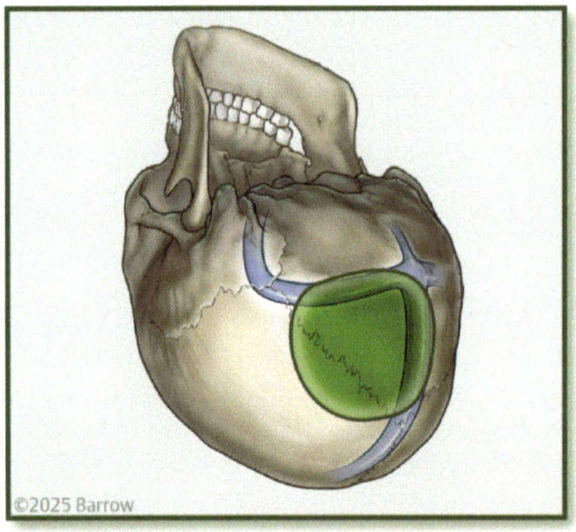

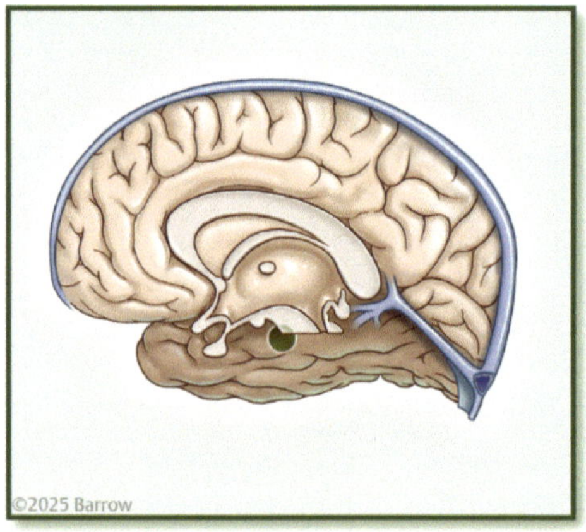

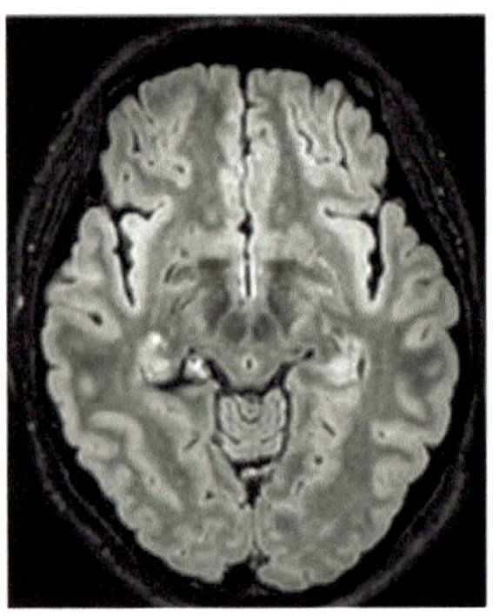

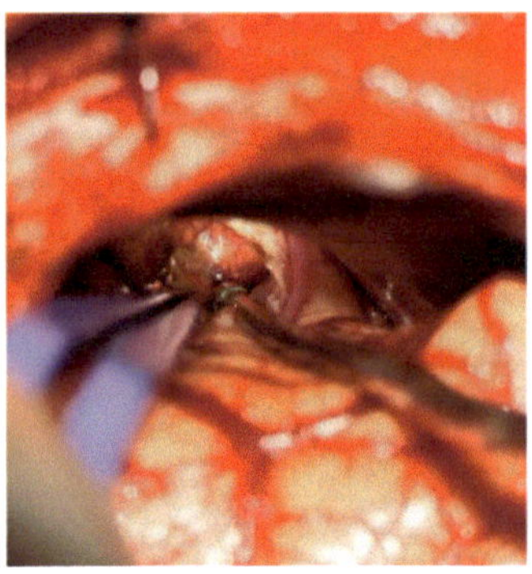

Video 11.5
Supratentorial-Infraoccipital Transgyral Approach for Medial Temporal Cavernous Malformation Resection (Reproduced with permission from Barrow Neurological Institute, Phoenix, AZ.)

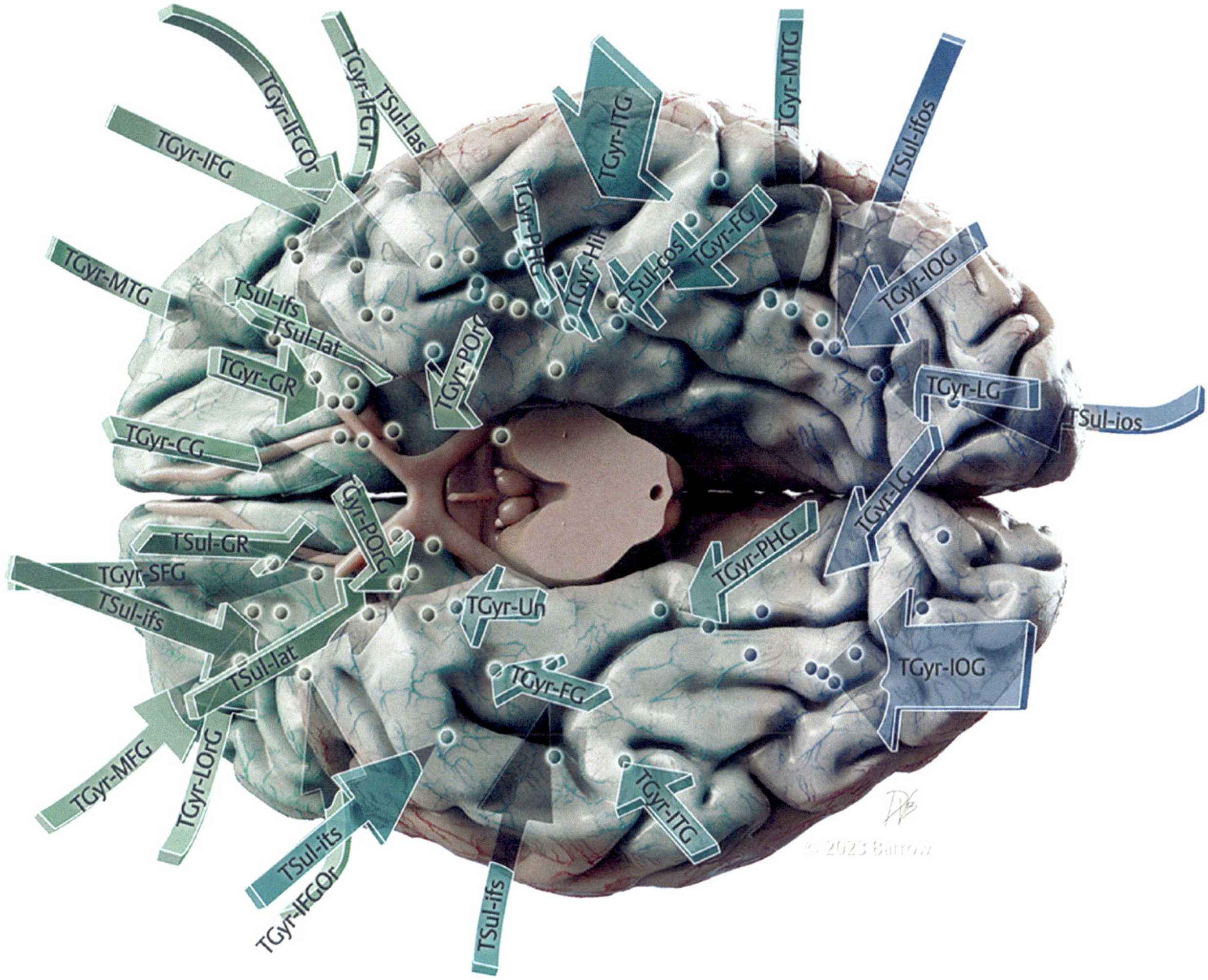

Fig. 11.7 Summary of approaches to basal CMs. TGyr and TSul approaches are shown as *arrows* in which the size or width is proportional to the number of patients. CMs are depicted as spheres of uniform size placed at the approximate center of each lesion. *Shading of the arrows* corresponds to the lobar locations (surgical cases; ▶ Video 11.6, ▶ Video 11.7; QR codes). ▶ Table 11.3 lists approach abbreviations. (Reproduced with permission from Barrow Neurological Institute, Phoenix, AZ.)

11.6 Approach Technique

Taxonomic subtyping provides valuable guidance for craniotomy planning. Small or miniature craniotomies are used with convexity subtype CMs because distances to these lesions are short and direct. Neuronavigation helps localize the CM and center the craniotomy around it. In contrast, medial subtype CMs are approached through the interhemispheric fissure, which requires larger bilateral frontal, parietal, or occipital craniotomies for direct access to the midline. Positioning the patient's head with the midline turned horizontally induces gravity retraction of the dependent hemisphere and widens the surgical corridor. Crossing trajectories to the contralateral side extend the lateral reach to the target lesion. Medial temporal subtype CMs reside in the carotid and ambient cisterns and often require pterional or orbitozygomatic craniotomies. Similarly, basal subtype CMs are frequently approached with skull base craniotomies: pterional, orbitopterional, and supraorbital craniotomies for frontal subtype CMs; pterional and subtemporal craniotomies for temporal subtype CMs; and torcular craniotomies for supratentorial-infraoccipital and supracerebellar-transtentorial approaches to occipital CMs. Sylvian subtype CMs are approached through pterional craniotomies.

Transgyral and transsulcal dissections are diametrically opposite techniques. Transgyral dissection is direct but inherently transgressive, which introduces the issue of cortical and subcortical eloquence. Dissecting through parenchyma circumvents the subarachnoid space, which removes any contact with cortical arteries and veins but might disrupt brain networks and increase surgical morbidity. In contrast, transsulcal dissection minimizes and sometimes eliminates tissue transgression, thereby preserving cortical eloquence and reducing morbidity. However, sulcal arteries are deliberately followed to open the route, which can induce hemorrhage or vascular compromise. The added proximity to the target lesion gained by sulcal

Surgical Case 11.6

CEREBRAL

Cavernoma Subtype: Basal (Occipital)

Position: Sitting
Craniotomy: Torcular
Approach: Supracerebellar-transtentorial transsulcal (SCTT-TSul)
Triangle: None
SEZ: None
Artery: P4 PCA (posterior temporal artery)

Video: Resection of a right occipital basal superficial cerebral occipital cavernoma

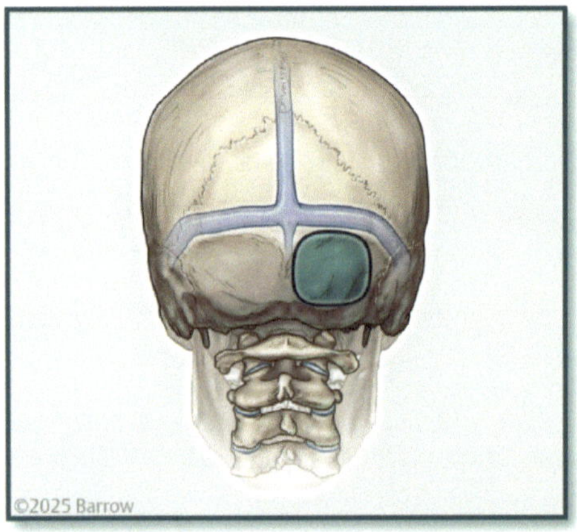

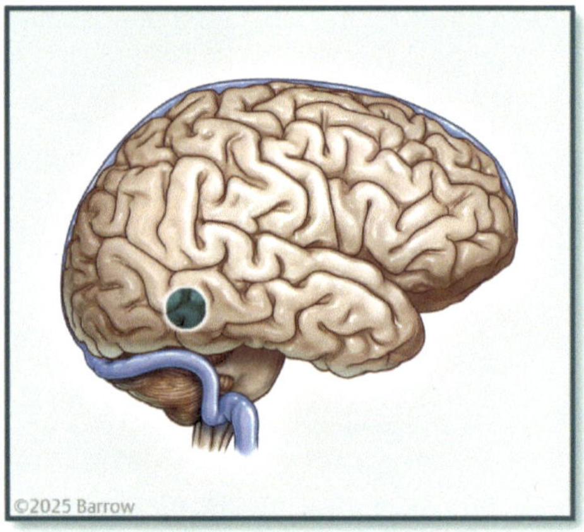

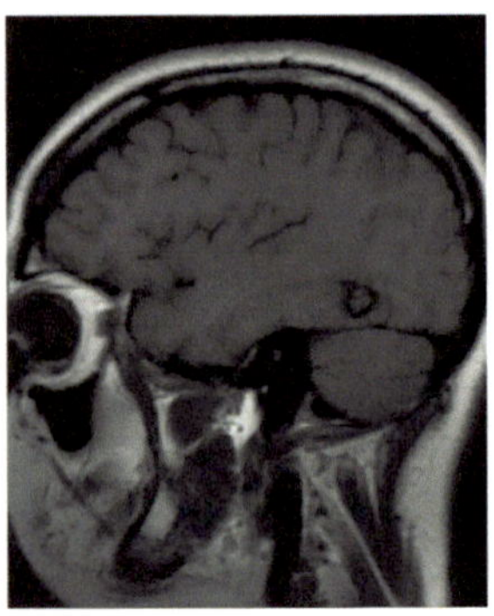

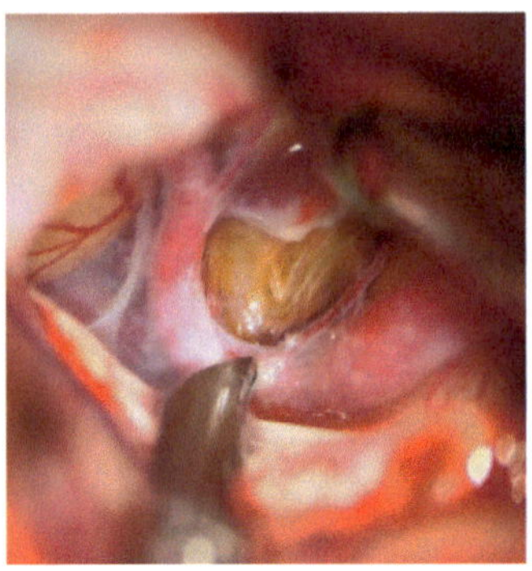

Video 11.6
Supracerebellar-Transtentorial Transsulcal Approach for Basal Occipital Cavernous Malformation Resection (Reproduced with permission from Barrow Neurological Institute, Phoenix, AZ.)

11

Surgical Case 11.7

CEREBRAL

Cavernoma Subtype: Basal (Occipital)

Position: Sitting
Craniotomy: Torcular
Approach: Supracerebellar-transtentorial transsulcal (SCTT-TSul)
Triangle: None
SEZ: None
Artery: P4 PCA (posterior temporal artery)

Video: Resection of a left occipital basal superficial cerebral cavernoma

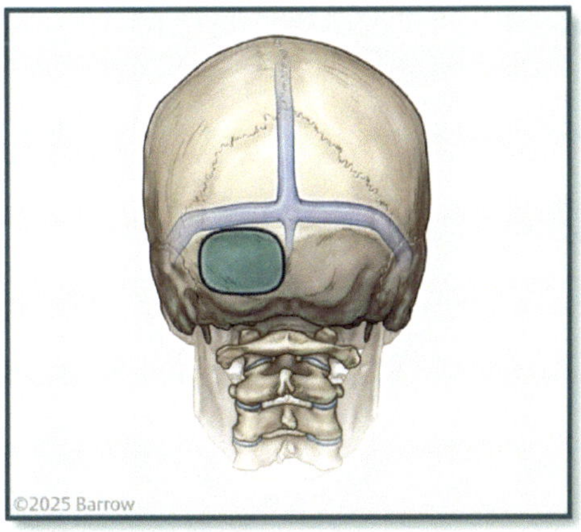

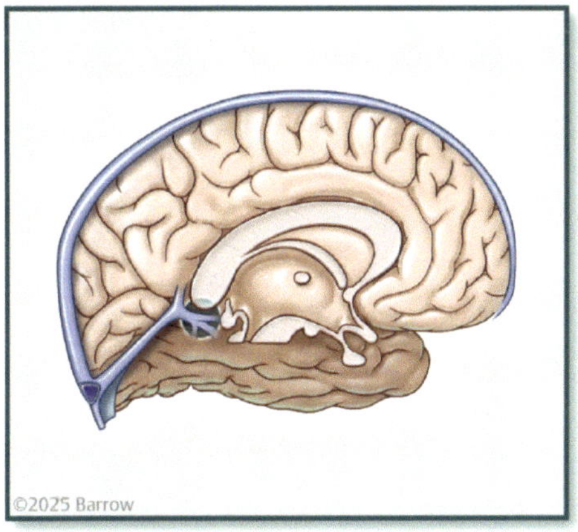

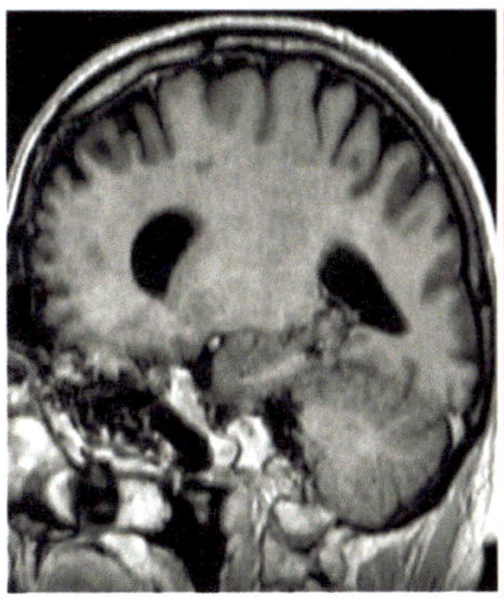

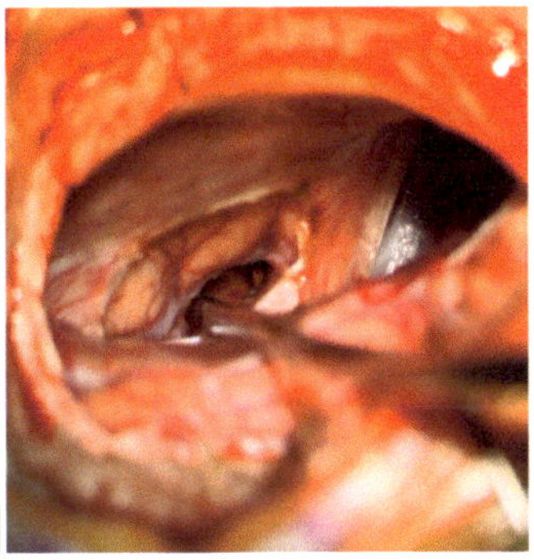

Video 11.7
Supracerebellar-Transtentorial Transsulcal Approach for Basal Occipital Cavernous Malformation Resection (Reproduced with permission from Barrow Neurological Institute, Phoenix, AZ.)

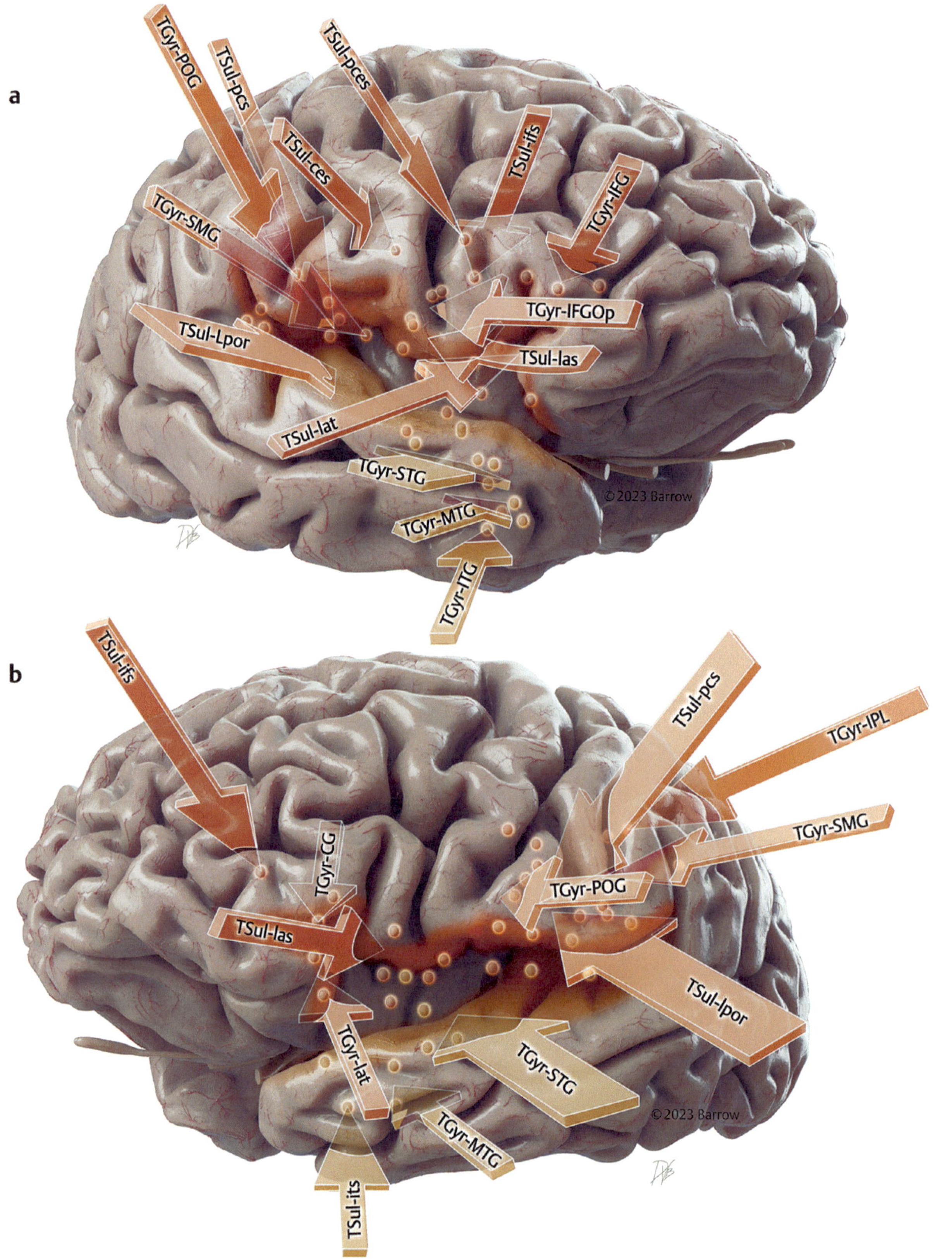

Fig. 11.8 Summary of approaches to sylvian CMs. TGyr and TSul approaches to **(a)** right-sided and **(b)** left-sided sylvian CMs. Approaches are shown as *arrows* in which the size or width is proportional to the number of patients. CMs are depicted as spheres of uniform size placed at the approximate center of each lesion. *Shading of the arrows* corresponds to the lobar locations (surgical case; ▶ Video 11.8; QR code). ▶ Table 11.3 lists approach abbreviations. (Reproduced with permission from Barrow Neurological Institute, Phoenix, AZ.)

Surgical Case 11.8

CEREBRAL

Cavernoma Subtype: Sylvian (Temporal)

Position: Supine, head turned left
Craniotomy: Temporoparietal
Approach: Posterior transsylvian-transgyral (TSyl-TGyr)
Triangle: None
SEZ: None
Artery: M3 MCA

Video: Resection of a right temporal sylvian superficial cerebral cavernoma

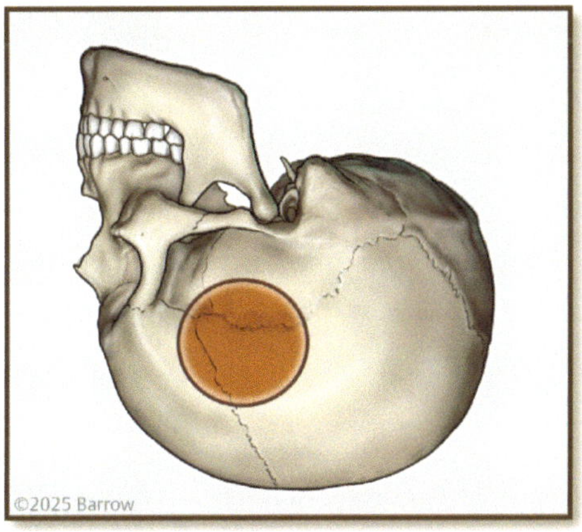

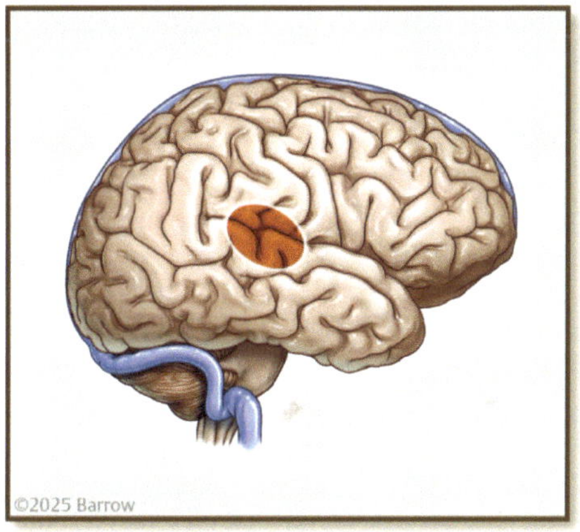

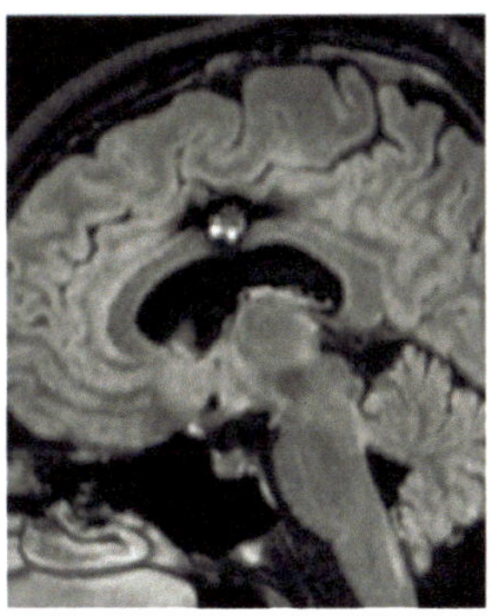

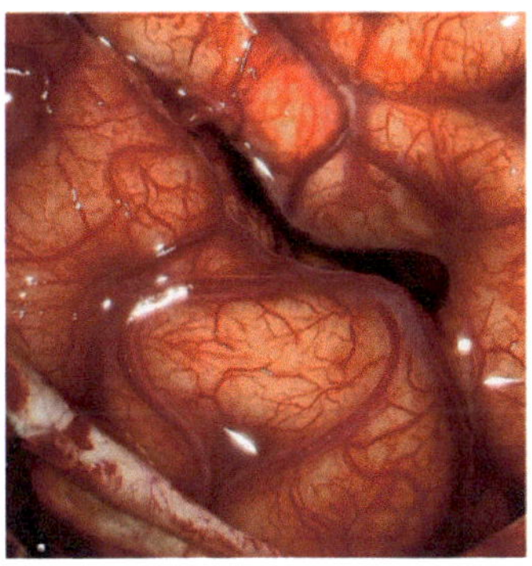

Video 11.8
Posterior Transylvian-Transgyral Approach for Temporal Sylvian Cavernous Malformation Resection (Reproduced with permission from Barrow Neurological Institute, Phoenix, AZ.)

dissection is a significant advantage with minimal risk in the hands of microvascular neurosurgeons.

Even with transsulcal dissection, the lesion may lie beneath the bottom of the sulcus, and tissue transgression may still be necessary. Neuronavigation is essential to guide parenchymal dissection, and hemosiderin staining is equally important. Subtle hemosiderin staining of the white matter increases as the distance to the target CM decreases. This visual gradient illuminates the neurosurgeon's approach like lights on a runway. Following this hemosiderin trail requires bloodless dissection, high illumination, magnification from the microscope, and meticulous stepwise dissection advances. The transgressive path should be narrow and direct, combining visual clues with neuronavigation to reach the target. In addition, dynamic retraction with bipolar forceps and a suction device, rather than a fixed retractor, facilitates more agile dissection along the hemosiderin trail.

11.7 Presenting Symptom

Seizures were the most common presenting symptom of superficial cerebral CMs, and many patients in the cohort presented with refractory epilepsy rather than neurological deficits. The surgical indications among these patients were seizure intractability and the prevention of morbidity from future hemorrhage. Seizure freedom after microsurgical CM resection has been studied in a meta-analysis of the literature and in my experience (73% Engel class 1), and predictors include gross total resection, early surgery within 1 year of seizure onset, CM size, single lesion, and absence of secondarily generalized seizures. Extended resection of the hemosiderin-stained ring was not correlated with seizure freedom, and my practice in these patients is to treat with lesion resection alone.

11.8 Clinical Syndromes

We attempted to identify unique neurological syndromes associated with each superficial cerebral CM subtype, as with our analysis of patients with brainstem CMs, but this objective was difficult. Some CMs, like frontal convexity, medial occipital, and medial temporal CMs, can have distinguishing symptoms and signs like hemiparesis, visual field deficits, and intractable seizures, respectively. However, many others do not, like basal temporal and sylvian parietal CMs. Unique neurological syndromes probably exist for many of these superficial cerebral CMs. However, their definitions require extensive neurological examinations in the form of cognitive and neuropsychological testing, which were limited for most patients in our series. Our understanding of human cognition has evolved from a modular paradigm in which the brain is composed of areas acting as independent processors of specific functions, such as Wernicke's and Broca's areas for language, to a network paradigm in which cognition arises from interactions between distributed cortical systems and areas connected by fasciculi in subcortical white matter. The Human Connectome Project and advances in cognitive neurosciences raise hope that clinical manifestations of cortical and subcortical CMs can be understood in relation to the large-scale brain networks that they influence in the same way that brainstem CMs can be understood in relation to the brainstem nuclei and tracts they affect. Obtaining the data needed to achieve this goal would require a transformation in our practices and methodologies for evaluating patients and their outcomes after surgery.

11.9 Conclusion

The proposed taxonomy defines superficial cerebral CMs on the basis of their surface presentation (convexity, medial, basal, and sylvian) and lobar location (frontal, temporal, parietal, and occipital). Superficial cerebral CMs were resected through a gyrus or sulcus to minimize tissue transgression by opening subarachnoid corridors and traversing the full extent of the sulci to deepen the approach. Transgyral dissection avoids associated arteries but is inherently transgressive, whereas transsulcal dissection preserves cortical tissue and may reduce morbidity. Superficial cerebral CMs occupy the largest territory of the seven types, and the size and surface complexity of the cerebrum makes taxonomic subtyping valuable for clear anatomical descriptions.

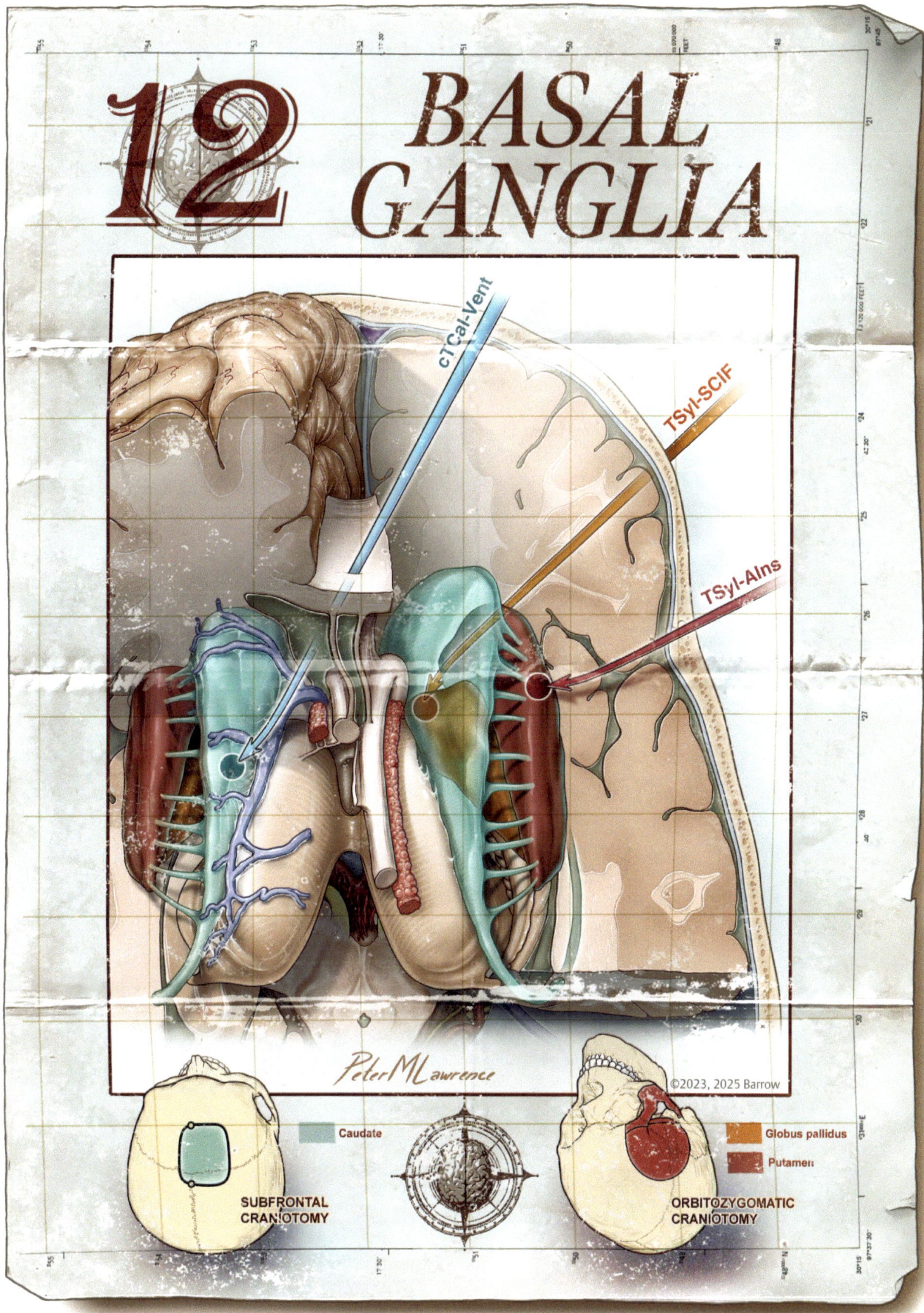

Reproduced with permission from Barrow Neurological Institute, Phoenix, AZ.

12 Basal Ganglia Cavernous Malformations

Summary

Deep in the geographical core of the cerebral hemisphere sit four structures composed of gray matter: the caudate nucleus, putamen, globus pallidus, and thalamus. The first three compose the basal ganglia and are the focus of this chapter. They are separated from the thalamus by the internal capsule. Basal ganglia cavernous malformation (CM) subtypes are named after these three components. The subtype taxonomy guides the approach and defines the key symptoms, signs, and clinical syndromes associated with each to improve patient outcomes. This taxonomy was applied to 54 patients with basal ganglia CMs resected microsurgically over an approximate 20-year period and identified 31 caudate (57%), 16 putaminal (30%), and 7 pallidal (13%) CMs. Twenty-five patients presented with severe or worsening headaches (43%), 13 had mild hemiparesis (24%), 7 had seizures (13%), and 6 had dysmetria or ataxia or both (11%). A single surgical approach was preferred for each basal ganglia subtype in greater than 80% of cases. Most caudate CMs were resected via contralateral transcallosal-transventricular approaches (90%, 28/31). Putaminal CMs were resected via the transsylvian-anterior transinsular (TSyl-AIns) approach (81%, 13/16). Pallidal CMs were resected via the transsylvian-supracarotid-infrafrontal (transperforate) (TSyl-SCIF) approach (100%, 7/7). Most patients had favorable outcomes (modified Rankin Scale score ≤ 2) after resection (94%, 44/47). Symptoms and signs were caused by the mass effects of lesional hemorrhages on the internal capsule rather than by specific circuit disruptions. Despite the basal ganglia's functional involvement with movement, cognition, executive function, and emotion, well-defined clinical syndromes were not associated with the basal ganglia CM subtypes.

Keywords: caudate nucleus, cavernoma, globus pallidus, putamen, taxonomy, thalamus, transgression

12

12.1 Introduction

The central core of the cerebral hemisphere comprises four large gray matter masses: the caudate nucleus, putamen, globus pallidus, and thalamus. The first three structures compose the basal ganglia and are separated from the thalamus by the internal capsule. Cavernous malformations (CMs) located in the central core are collectively considered deep CMs because they are located at the geographic center of the brain, are difficult to access microsurgically, and have no cortical surfaces and few subarachnoid surfaces. Unlike the thalamus, in which the inferior pulvinar presents to the quadrigeminal cistern and the geniculate bodies present to the ambient cistern, the basal ganglia have no cisternal point of access and can only be reached transventricularly or via strategic transgressions through noneloquent parenchyma. The basal ganglia CM subtypes are presented with their clinical symptoms and signs and the optimal surgical approaches for resection. This taxonomy is designed to (1) help neurosurgeons select the best surgical approach and ultimately improve patient outcomes; (2) increase diagnostic acumen at the bedside by defining key symptoms, signs, and clinical syndromes associated with each subtype; and (3) standardize discourse in the clinical setting and the literature.

12.2 Neuroanatomy of Three Basal Ganglia Cavernous Malformation Subtypes

Basal ganglia CMs are classified into subtypes based on lesion location (▶ Fig. 12.1): caudate, putaminal, and pallidal.

12.2.1 Caudate

Caudate CMs are located within this arched C-shaped structure that wraps around the lateral part of the thalamus. The caudate nucleus forms the lateral wall of the lateral ventricle, with the caudate head walling the frontal horn and the caudate body walling the body of the lateral ventricle. The slender tail courses around the pulvinar and forms the lateral wall of the atrium and roof of the temporal horn. The largest caudate surface is in the frontal horn anterior and lateral to the foramen of Monro along the prominent medial aspect of the caudate head. Posterior to the foramen of Monro, the stria terminalis and thalamostriate vein define the inferior border of the caudate body. This caudate surface extends superiorly to the undersurface of the corpus callosum, which forms the roof of the lateral ventricle. Caudate CMs are found medial to the anterior limb of the internal capsule, which forms the lateral border of the caudate nucleus.

12.2.2 Putaminal

The largest of the basal ganglia structures, the putamen, lies between the insula and external capsule laterally, the anterior limb of the internal capsule anteromedially, and the globus pallidus posteromedially. Its lateral surface is slightly smaller than the insular surface area. The claustrum, a thin gray matter layer, and the extreme capsule, a thin white matter layer, are lateral to the putamen beneath the insular cortex. The putamen faces the caudate head across the anterior limb of the internal capsule, and they fuse anteroinferiorly below the anterior limb. The lateral medullary lamina is a thin layer of white matter that separates the putamen and globus pallidus and acts as a dividing line between these two subtypes.

12.2.3 Pallidal

The globus pallidus lies between the putamen laterally, the anterior limb of the internal capsule anteromedially, and the posterior limb of the internal capsule posteromedially. The globus pallidus is smaller and medial to the putamen and faces the thalamus across the posterior limb of the internal capsule. The globus

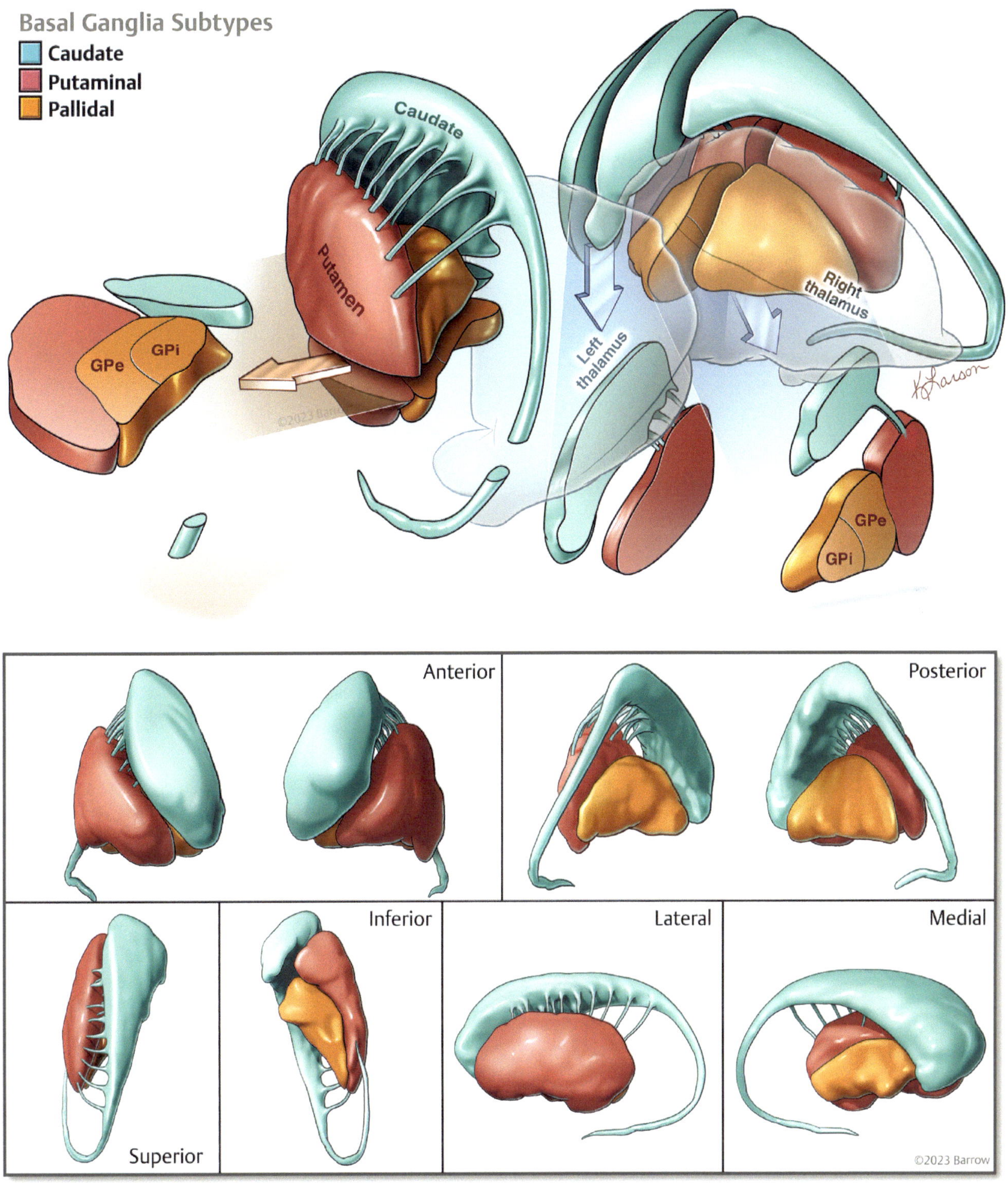

Fig. 12.1 Overview of basal ganglia anatomy and the three CM subtypes, seen from a left posterior oblique view. Subtypes are shown in the left and right basal ganglia: caudate (*teal*), putaminal (*red*), and pallidal (*orange*). An axial slice is shown through the left basal ganglia (*orange arrow*), and anterior and middle coronal slices are shown through the right basal ganglia (*blue arrows*). Surface locations of basal ganglial subtypes are shown in different perspectives (*insets*): anterior and posterior, superior, inferior, lateral, and medial. (Reproduced with permission from Barrow Neurological Institute, Phoenix, AZ.)

pallidus is subdivided into medial (pars interna) and lateral (pars externa) parts by the medial medullary lamina. The lateral medullary lamina separates the putamen and the globus pallidus. Anteroinferiorly, the globus pallidus lies below the anterior limb of the internal capsule and above the anterior perforated substance, immediately above the carotid terminus.

12.3 Clinical Evidence

The taxonomy was applied to Robert F. Spetzler's and my experience with CM management; 54 patients with basal ganglia CMs resected microsurgically over an approximately 20-year period were studied (▸ Table 12.1). CMs involving the basal ganglia were subtyped on the basis of their predominant presentation identified on preoperative magnetic resonance imaging (MRI) and included the caudate (57%, 31/54), putaminal (30%, 16/54), and pallidal (13%, 7/54) subtypes. Each basal ganglia CM subtype was associated with a recognizable constellation of neurological symptoms (▸ Table 12.2). The most common symptoms at presentation were severe or worsening headaches (43%, 25/54), mild hemiparesis (24%, 13/54), seizures (13%, 7/54), and dysmetria, ataxia, or both (11%, 6/54). Patients

Table 12.1 Clinical presenting symptoms and signs by basal ganglia CM subtype

Symptom or sign	Number (%) of patients, by basal ganglia CM subtype			
	All (*N* = 54)	Caudate (*n* = 31)	Putaminal (*n* = 16)	Pallidal (*n* = 7)
Severe headache	25 (46)	14 (45)	8 (50)	3 (43)
Mild hemiparesis[a]	13 (24)	5 (16)	5 (31)	3 (43)
Hemianesthesia deficit	7 (13)	3 (10)	3 (19)	1 (14)
Dysmetria or dyscoordination	6 (11)	2 (7)	3 (19)	1 (14)
Seizure	7 (13)	4 (13)	2 (13)	1 (14)
Visual field deficit	4 (7)	0 (0)	3 (13)	2 (29)
Diplopia	2 (4)	1 (6)	1 (9)	0 (0)
Blurry vision	1 (2)	1 (3)	0 (0)	0 (0)
CN III palsy	1 (2)	0 (0)	0 (0)	1 (14)
Dysarthria or dysphagia	3 (6)	1 (3)	0 (0)	2 (29)
Memory or cognitive	3 (6)	2 (7)	0 (0)	1 (14)
Facial weakness	2 (4)	1 (3)	0 (0)	1 (14)
Hydrocephalus	1 (2)	1 (3)	0 (0)	0 (0)

[a]Mild hemiparesis (4/5) strength for the worst muscle group.

Table 12.2 Surgical approaches and preoperative and postoperative outcome measures for patients who underwent resection of basal ganglia CMs, by subtype

Variable	All subtypes (*N* = 54)	Caudate (*n* = 31)	Putaminal (*n* = 16)	Pallidal (*n* = 7)	*p*-value[a]
Surgical approach	54	28 (90) cTCal-Vent; 3 (10) Fro-Sul-Vent	13 (81) TSyl-AIns, 3 (19) Fro-Sul-Vent	7 (100) TSyl-SCIF	
Preoperative mRS score					
> 2	13/53 (24)	3/30 (10)	6/16 (38)	4/7 (57)	**0.01**
≤ 2	40/53 (75)	27/30 (90)	10/16 (62)	3/7 (43)	**0.01**
Postoperative mRS score					
> 2	8/53 (15)	2/30 (7)	3/16 (19)	3/7 (43)	**0.049**
≤ 2	45/53 (85)	28/30 (93)	13/16 (81)	4/7 (57)	**0.049**
Follow-up (mo), mean (SD)	32 (44)	30 (39)	24 (36)	68 (78)	0.11
Final mRS score					
> 2	3/47 (6)	1/26 (4)	1/15 (7)	1/6 (17)	0.51
≤ 2	44/47 (94)	25/26 (96)	14/15 (93)	5/6 (83)	0.51
Worsened	3/47 (6)	2/26 (8)	1/15 (7)	0/6 (0)	0.79
Stable or improved	44/47 (94)	24/26 (92)	14/15 (93)	6/6 (100)	0.79

Note: Data are reported as proportion (%) of patients with available data unless otherwise specified. **Bold** p-values indicate statistical significance ($p < 0.05$).
[a]Pearson chi-squared test.

12

with caudate CMs were the most likely to present with headaches and constitutional symptoms. Patients with putaminal CMs were the most likely to present with hemibody sensory deficits and dysmetria, ataxia, or both. Patients with pallidal CMs were the most likely to present with mild hemiparesis and visual field deficits.

A single surgical approach was preferred for each basal ganglia subtype in more than 80% of cases (▶ Fig. 12.2, ▶ Fig. 12.3). Most caudate CMs were resected through a contralateral transcallosal-transventricular (cTCal-Vent) approach (90%, 28/31). Putaminal CMs were primarily resected through a TSyl-AIns approach (81%, 13/16). Pallidal CMs were resected via the TSyl-SCIF approach (100%, 7/7). Most patients with follow-up had favorable outcomes (modified Rankin Scale [mRS] score ≤ 2) after microsurgical resection (94%, 44/47), as well as stable or improved mRS scores postoperatively (94%, 44/47). Absolute and relative outcomes at the final follow-up did not differ among the three basal ganglia subtypes.

12.4 Basal Ganglia Cavernous Malformation Subtypes

The basal ganglia nuclei are involved with movement, cognition, executive function, and emotions. Despite the functional importance of the basal ganglia, well-defined clinical syndromes were not observed with basal ganglia CMs, in contrast with brainstem CMs. Symptoms and signs were caused by the mass effect of a lesional hemorrhage on the internal capsule rather than by specific circuit disruptions.

12.4.1 Caudate

The caudate nucleus is involved with learning, memory, motivation, reward, emotion, and movement planning. It receives input from the ipsilateral frontal cortex about planned movements via the corticostriatal pathway (▶ Fig. 12.4). The caudate nucleus acts as the main input nucleus for the basal ganglia and initiates movement, especially eye movement. Patients with caudate lesions often present with behavioral disorders. Deficits in spatial memory, goal-directed action, sleep, and language that might be associated with caudate CMs are difficult to detect, and these patients were often intact on neurological examination at presentation. In our study, patients with caudate CMs most often presented with severe headaches (45%).

Most of the tissue in the C-shaped caudate nucleus is in its anterior portion, forming the lateral wall of the frontal horn and body of the lateral ventricle. Therefore, caudate CMs are exposed through the cTCal-Vent approach to create a steep crossing trajectory to the lateral wall (▶ Fig. 12.5; ▶ Video 12.1). Gravity retraction drops the dependent hemisphere, extends the reach off the midline, and pulls the lesion downward into the line of sight. The CM is placed on the upside with the midline oriented horizontally and the head and neck angled 30 degrees upward from the floor. A bifrontal craniotomy exposes the superior sagittal sinus to eliminate any calvarial ledge over the anterior interhemispheric fissure and visually directly along the falx. Meticulous dissection of the anterior interhemispheric fissure below the falx releases the dependent hemisphere and protects the callosomarginal and pericallosal arteries. A transcallosal incision made beneath the upside pericallosal artery, ipsilateral to the CM, ensures entry into the correct ventricle. Low-lying CMs may be visible through this standard cTCal-Vent corridor. However, high-riding lesions may require resection of the lateral callosum, incision of the falx, and retraction or resection of the cingulate gyrus to extend the view laterally. The transition from a contralateral transcallosal to a transcingulate approach may require a corridor above the pericallosal artery beneath the callosomarginal artery. The anterior caudate vein is a landmark that confirms the identity of the caudate head. The thalamostriate vein runs between the thalamus and caudate nucleus atop the stria terminalis and identifies the inferior border of the caudate subtype and the lateral border of the choroidal thalamic subtype (caudate-thalamostriate triangle). The territory between the anterior caudate and septal veins belongs to the anterior thalamic subtype (septocaudate triangle). The columns of the fornix diverge laterally as they descend beyond the foramen of Monro. These columns must be avoided when entering the caudate head anteroinferiorly.

12.4.2 Putaminal

The putamen regulates movements, influences learning, and drives goal-directed behaviors, acting as the basal ganglia's input area for cortical information about desired movements. Exiting neurons connect to the substantia nigra, globus pallidus, subthalamic nucleus, and thalamus to inhibit or facilitate movement (▶ Fig. 12.6). Contemporary studies suggest a possible cerebellar component to basal ganglia function. Patients with putaminal lesions most often present with extrapyramidal motor symptoms. In our study, dysmetria and dyscoordination were differentiating findings in 19% of patients with putaminal CMs. These patients were the most likely to present with severe headaches (50%), followed by hemiparesis (31%). Some of the classic symptoms associated with other diseases of putaminal dysfunction, namely, Parkinson's disease, Huntington's disease, Alzheimer's disease, and various psychiatric disorders, were not observed in these patients.

Putaminal CMs are exposed through a standard pterional craniotomy and TSyl-AIns approach (▶ Fig. 12.7; ▶ Video 12.2, ▶ Video 12.3). The putamen is the largest of the basal ganglia structures. It runs nearly the length of the insula beneath the short and long gyri. Transinsular dissection and transgression through the claustrum and extreme capsule are neurologically well tolerated. The critically eloquent internal capsule lies safely deeper than the putamen. A TSyl-AIns approach to CMs located in front of the foramen of Monro reaches lesions in the anterior putamen and those lying low and lateral in the caudate head. This dissection is performed through a pterional craniotomy with wide splitting of the sylvian fissure. Exposure of the M1 and M2 segments in the sylvian cistern leads to the limen insula at or near the middle cerebral artery (MCA) bi-trifurcation, and M2 stem arteries are followed distally across the insula. A transsylvian-posterior transinsular (TSyl-PIns) approach may be needed for lesions in the posterior putamen lateral to the globus

12

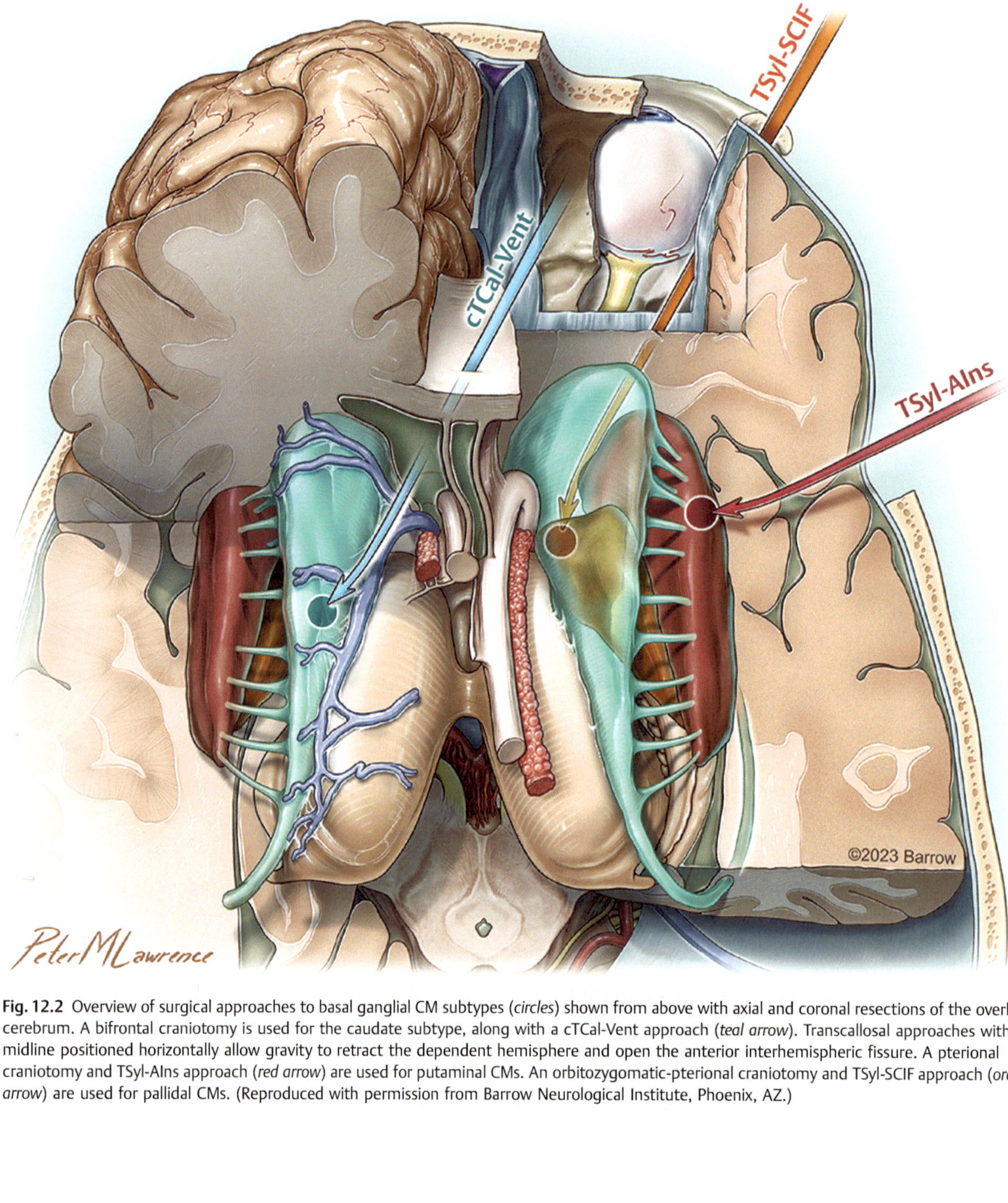

Fig. 12.2 Overview of surgical approaches to basal ganglial CM subtypes (*circles*) shown from above with axial and coronal resections of the overlying cerebrum. A bifrontal craniotomy is used for the caudate subtype, along with a cTCal-Vent approach (*teal arrow*). Transcallosal approaches with the midline positioned horizontally allow gravity to retract the dependent hemisphere and open the anterior interhemispheric fissure. A pterional craniotomy and TSyl-AIns approach (*red arrow*) are used for putaminal CMs. An orbitozygomatic-pterional craniotomy and TSyl-SCIF approach (*orange arrow*) are used for pallidal CMs. (Reproduced with permission from Barrow Neurological Institute, Phoenix, AZ.)

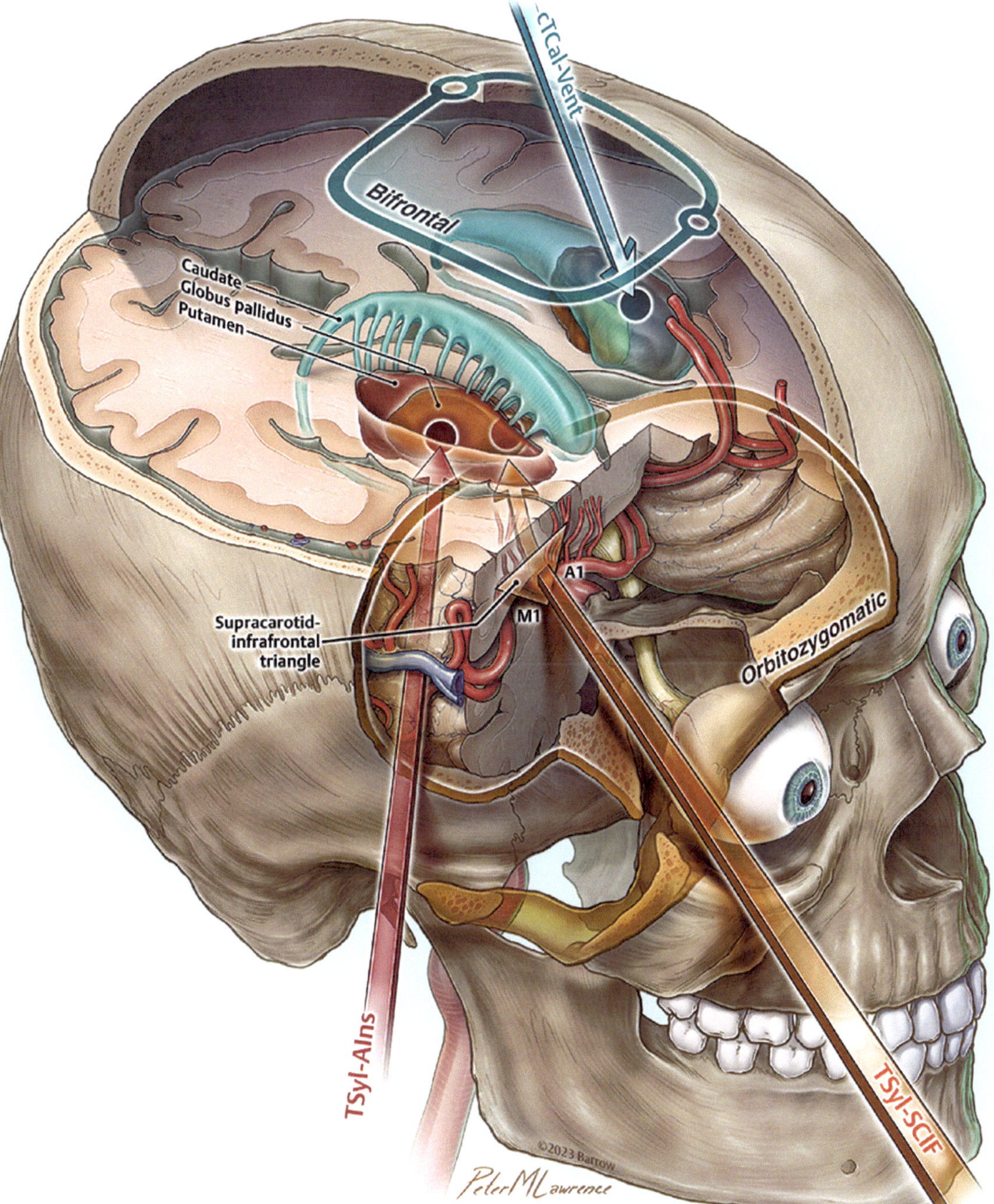

Fig. 12.3 Overview of surgical approaches to basal ganglial CM subtypes shown from a right anterior oblique view with axial and coronal resections of the overlying cerebrum. This illustration highlights the bifrontal craniotomy and cTCal-Vent approach (*teal arrow*) used for the caudate subtype (*teal circle*), the pterional craniotomy and TSyl-AIns approach (*red arrow*) used for the putaminal subtype (*red circle*), and the orbitozygomatic-pterional craniotomy and TSyl-SCIF approach (*orange arrow*) used for the pallidal subtype (*orange circle*). The relationships between these approaches and intracranial arteries are shown. Note the supracarotid-infrafrontal triangle formed by the A1 ACA medially, the M1 MCA laterally, and the anterior perforated substance superiorly. (Reproduced with permission from Barrow Neurological Institute, Phoenix, AZ.)

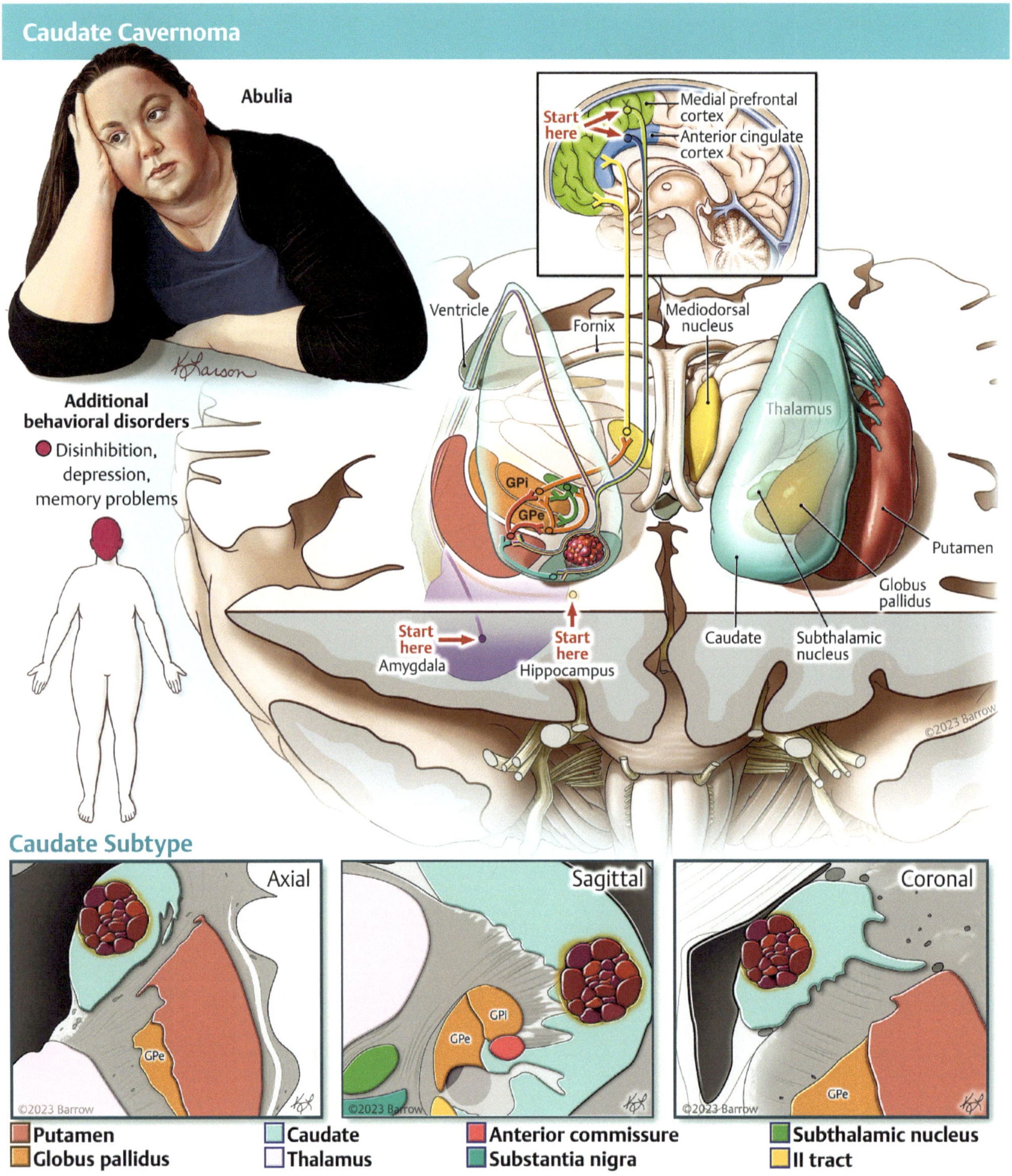

12

Fig. 12.4 Patients with caudate lesions can present with behavioral disorders, including abulia, disinhibition, depression, and memory deficits. The anterior caudate nucleus receives input from the amygdala, hippocampus, and medial prefrontal and anterior cingulate cortices (*upper right inset*). Caudate lesions disrupt the normally balanced physiology of the excitatory and inhibitory connections between the striatum, globus pallidus, subthalamic nucleus, and mediodorsal nucleus of the thalamus. The relationships between this left-sided caudate CM, the ventricles, and the surrounding anatomy are shown in axial, sagittal, and coronal views (*lower insets*). (Reproduced with permission from Barrow Neurological Institute, Phoenix, AZ.)

Surgical Approach

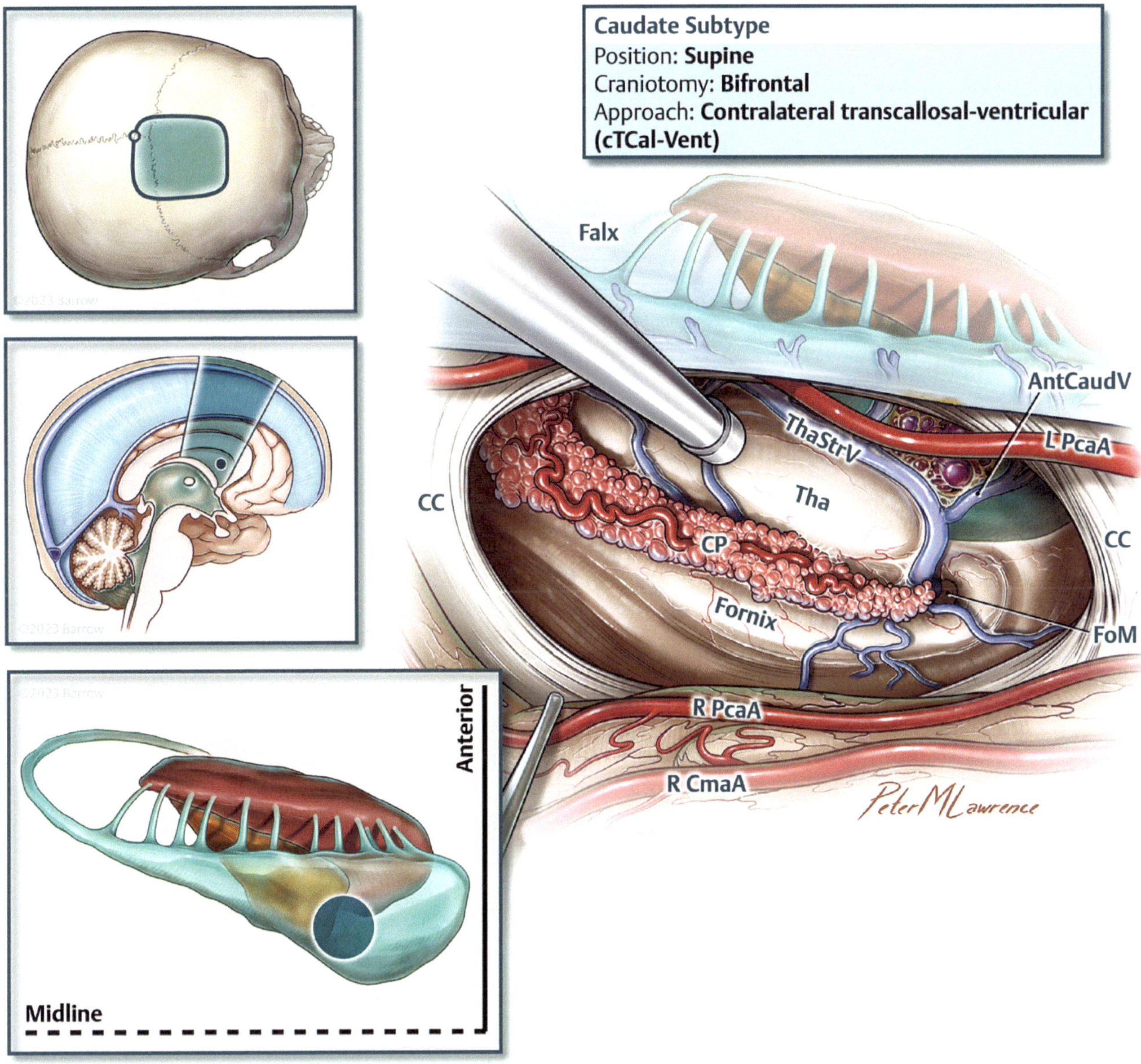

Fig. 12.5 Caudate CMs are exposed through the cTCal-Vent approach to create a steep crossing trajectory to the lateral wall of the frontal horn and body of the lateral ventricle. The lesion is placed on the upside with the midline oriented horizontally to allow gravity to retract the dependent hemisphere. A bifrontal craniotomy exposes the superior sagittal sinus (*upper left inset*). Dissection of the anterior interhemispheric fissure and a transcallosal incision made beneath the upside pericallosal artery ipsilateral to the CM leads to the correct ventricle (*middle left inset, teal circle*). Most caudate CMs are located in the head or body (*lower left inset, teal circle*). The AntCaudV identifies the caudate head, and the ThaStrV identifies the inferior border of the caudate subtype and lateral border of the choroidal thalamic subtype (caudate-thalamostriate triangle). The territory between the AntCaudV and SepV belong to the anterior thalamic subtype (septocaudate triangle) (surgical case; ▶ Video 12.1; QR code). (Reproduced with permission from Barrow Neurological Institute, Phoenix, AZ.)

12

Surgical Case 12.1

BASAL GANGLIAL

Cavernoma Subtype: Caudate

Position: Supine, head turned 90°
Craniotomy: Bifrontal
Approach: Anterior interhemispheric, contralateral transcallosal-transventricular (cTCal-Vent)
Triangle: Septocaudate
SEZ: None
Artery: PcaA

Video: Resection of a left caudate cavernoma

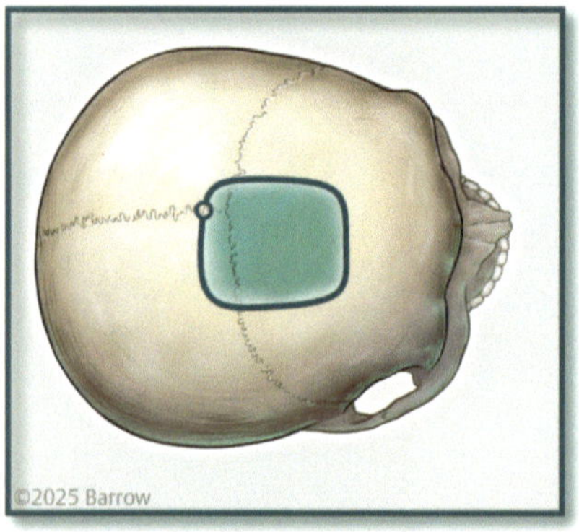

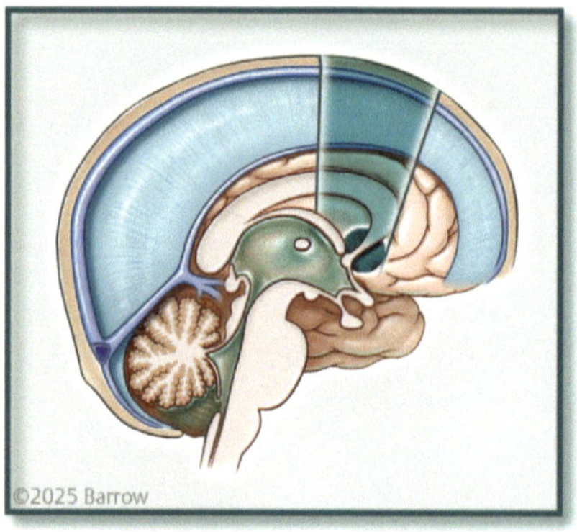

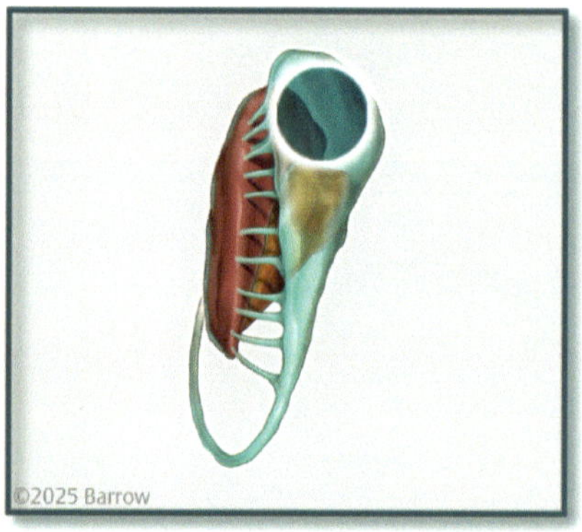

12

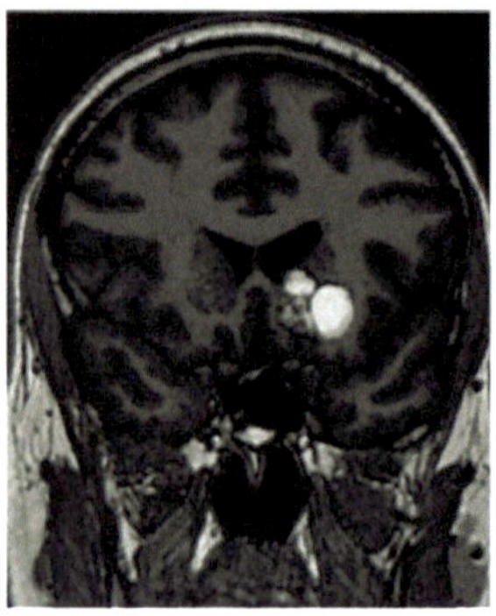

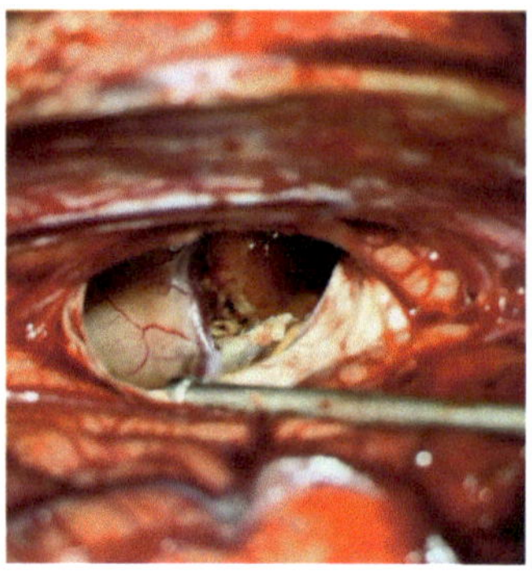

Video 12.1
Anterior Interhemispheric Contralateral Transcallosal Approach for Caudate Basal Ganglia Cavernous Malformation Resection (Reproduced with permission from Barrow Neurological Institute, Phoenix, AZ.)

Putaminal Cavernoma

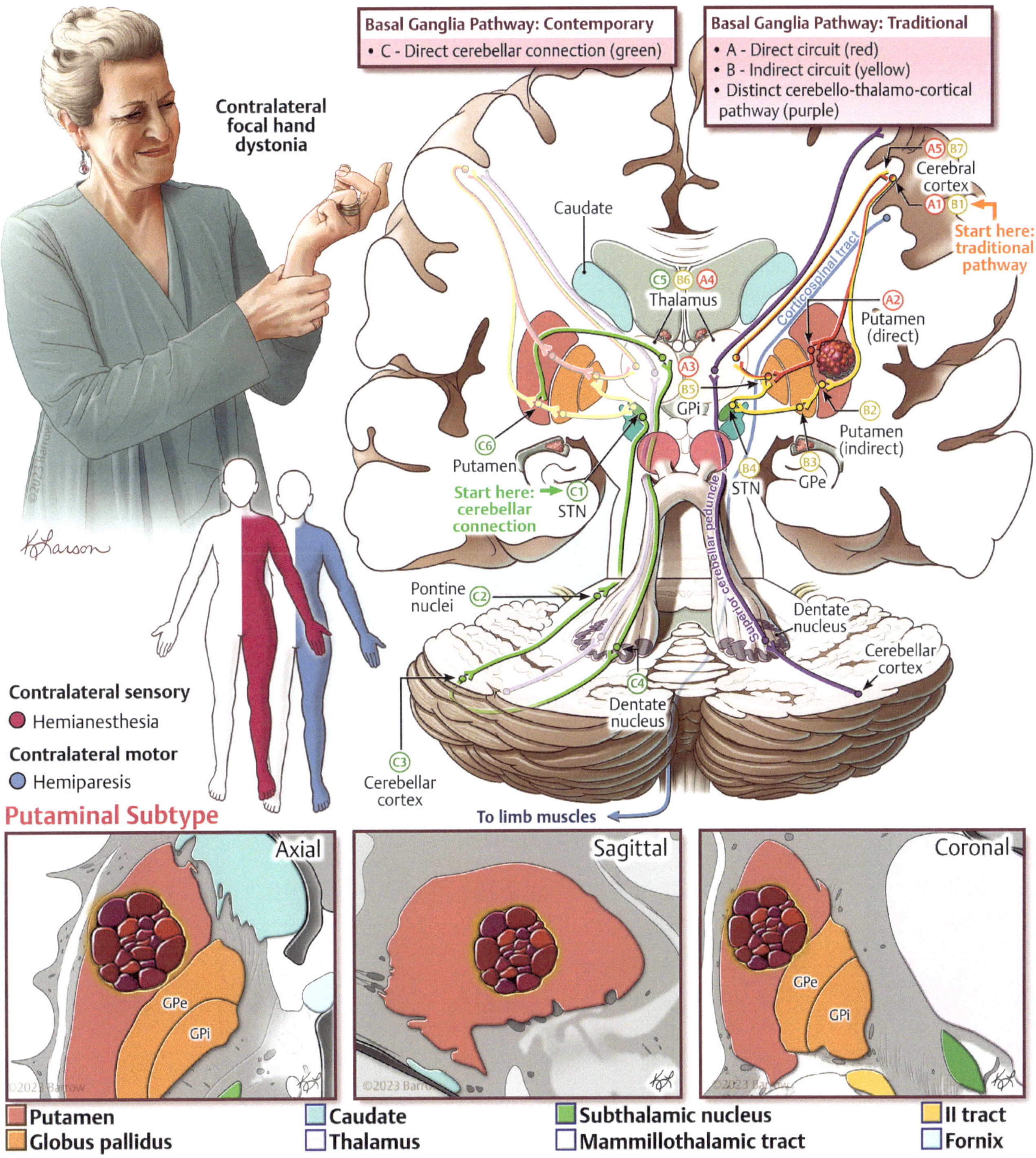

Fig. 12.6 Patients with putaminal lesions often present with motor symptoms, including contralateral focal hand dystonia and hemiparesis. The middle and dorsal regions of the putamen receive input from the motor cortex. These afferent connections may follow the direct pathway (direct circuit A [*red*]: putamen, GPi, thalamus, cortex) or the indirect pathway (indirect circuit B [*yellow*]: putamen, GPe, STN, GPi, thalamus, cortex) to complete the circuit. Recent studies also suggest a direct basal ganglia connection to the cerebellum via the STN with a reciprocal cerebellar connection to the striatum via the dentate nucleus and thalamus (contemporary circuit C [*green*]). Patients with putaminal CMs can also present with headaches and hemianesthesia. The relationships between this right-sided putaminal CM and the surrounding anatomy are shown in axial, sagittal, and coronal views (*lower insets*). (Reproduced with permission from Barrow Neurological Institute, Phoenix, AZ.)

12

Surgical Approach

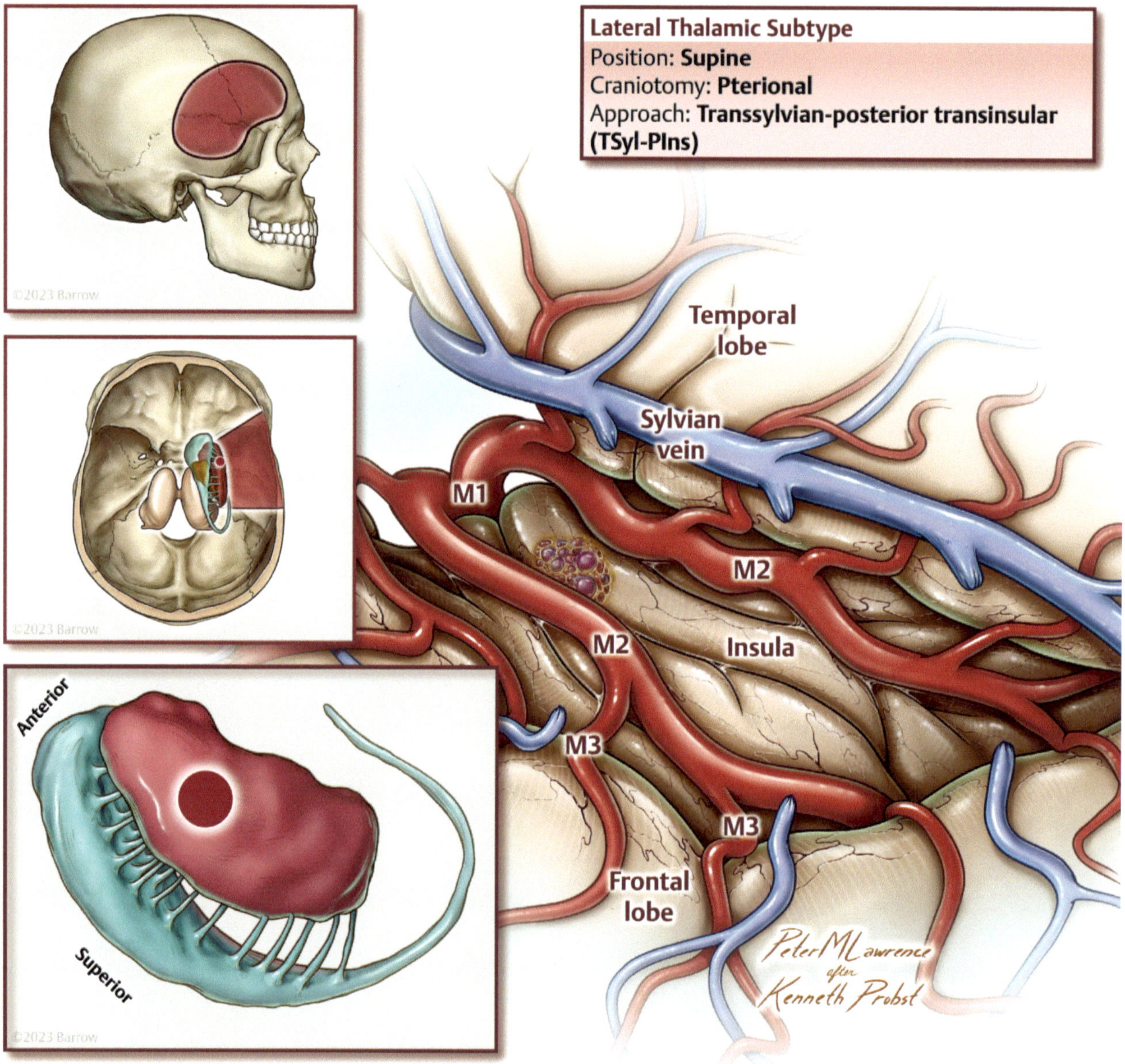

Fig. 12.7 Putaminal CMs are exposed through a pterional craniotomy and TSyl-AIns approach. Pterional craniotomy (*upper left inset*) and superior view showing CM (*middle left inset, red circle*). Wide splitting of the sylvian fissure exposes the short and long gyri of the insula overlying the putamen (*lower left inset, red circle*). Exposure of M1 and M2 segments in the sylvian cistern identifies the limen insula at or near the MCA bi-trifurcation, and M2 stem arteries are followed distally across the insula. A TSyl-PIns approach may be needed for lesions in the posterior putamen lateral to the globus pallidus and the posterior limb of the internal capsule. The transinsular dissection route depends on the lesion location. Anterior putaminal CMs are reached through the short gyri, posterior putaminal CMs are reached through the long gyri, and inferior putaminal CMs are reached through the limen insulae. The pathway to the target passes close by the eloquent pre-, post-, and subcentral gyri and above the Wernicke area in the dominant hemisphere. It passes through the candelabra below, above, or between the M2 stem arteries (surgical cases, ▶ Video 12.2 and ▶ Video 12.3; QR codes). (Reproduced with permission from Barrow Neurological Institute, Phoenix, AZ.)

Surgical Case 12.2

BASAL GANGLIAL

Cavernoma Subtype: Putamen

Position: Supine
Craniotomy: Pterional
Approach: Transsylvian-anterior transinsular (TSyl-AIns)
Triangle: None
SEZ: None
Artery: M2 MCA

Video: Resection of a right putaminal cavernoma

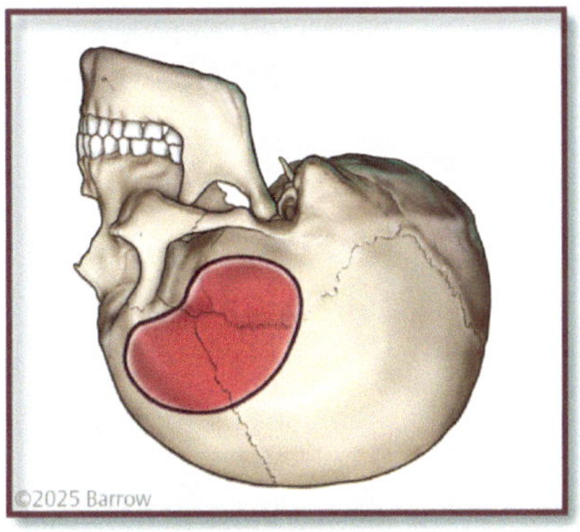

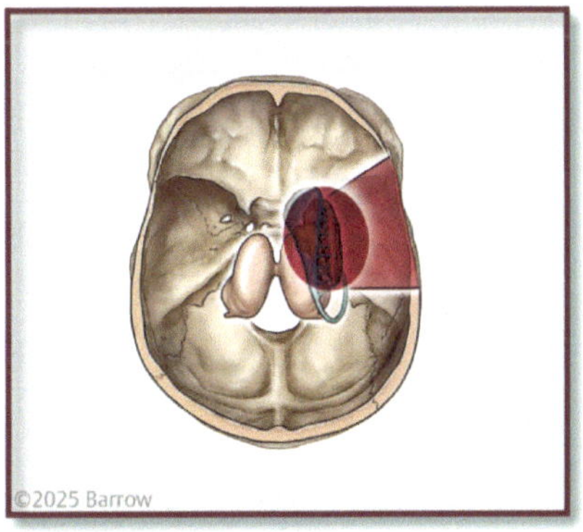

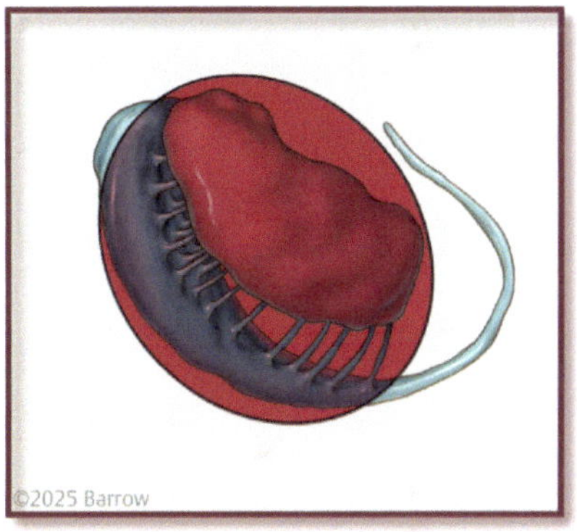

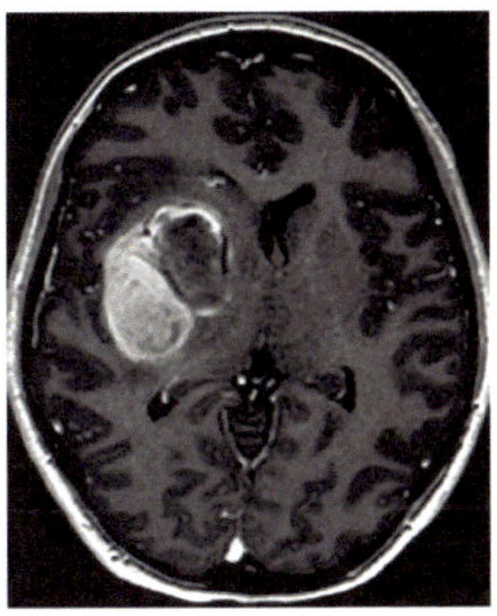

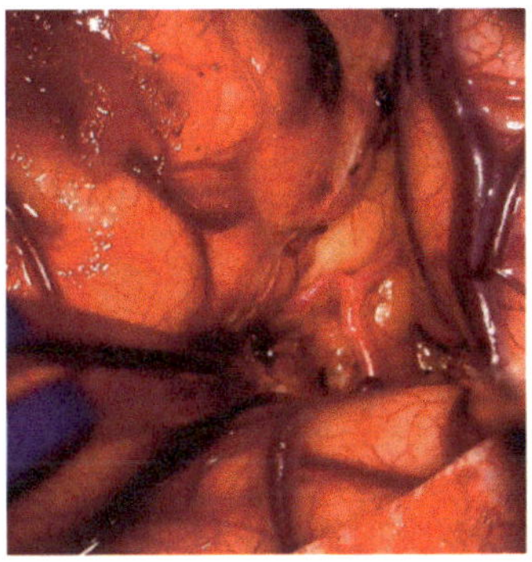

Video 12.2
Transsylvian-Anterior Transinsular Approach for Putaminal Basal Ganglia Cavernous Malformation Resection (Reproduced with permission from Barrow Neurological Institute, Phoenix, AZ.)

Surgical Case 12.3

BASAL GANGLIAL

Cavernoma Subtype: Putamen

Position: Supine
Craniotomy: Pterional
Approach: Transsylvian-anterior transinsular (TSyl-AIns)
Triangle: None
SEZ: None
Artery: M2 MCA

Video: Resection of a right putaminal cavernoma

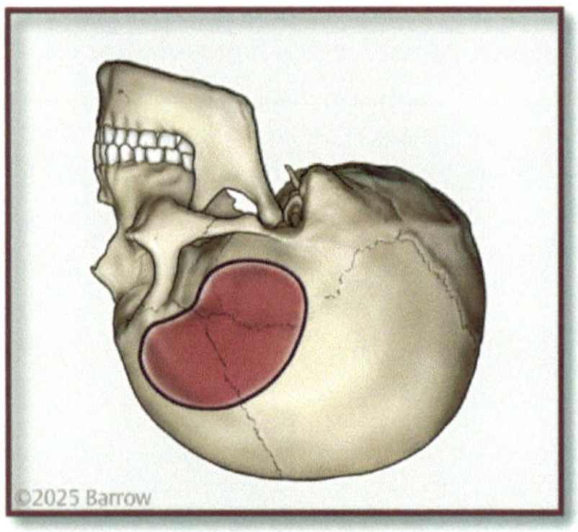

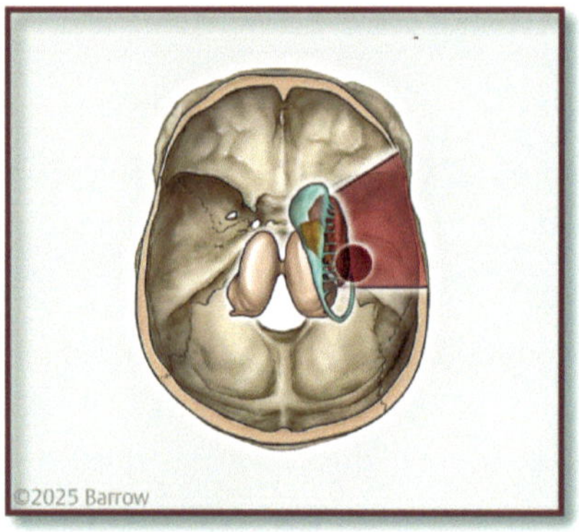

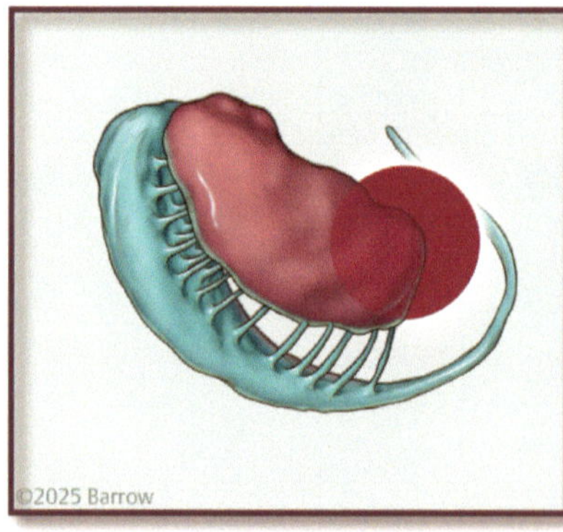

12

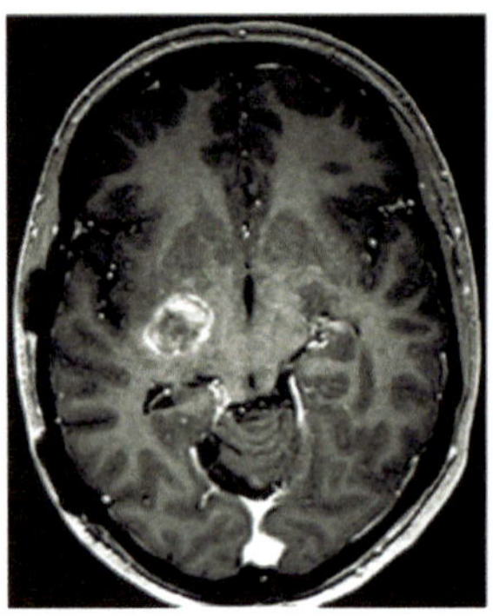

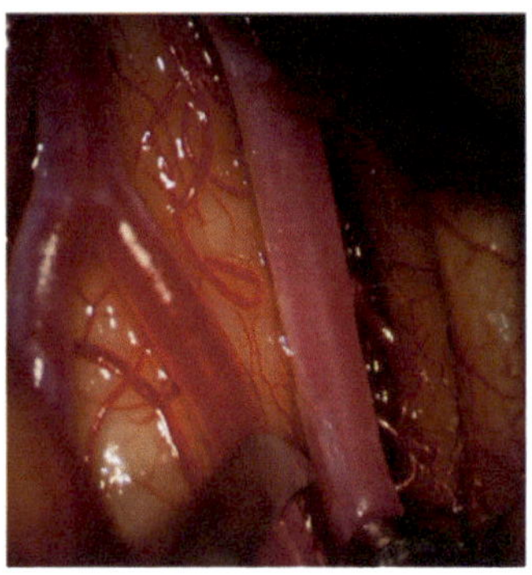

Video 12.3
Transsylvian-Anterior Transinsular Approach for Putaminal Basal Ganglia Cavernous Malformation Resection (Reproduced with permission from Barrow Neurological Institute, Phoenix, AZ.)

pallidus and the posterior limb of the internal capsule. As seen on an axial brain image, a transverse line through the foramen of Monro bisects the insula into anterior and posterior parts. The craniotomy for the TSyl-PIns approach extends further posteriorly than the standard pterional craniotomy through a question mark skin incision and fronto-temporo-parietal craniotomy. The more posterior the CM, the more the opercular dissection is required. Apposition or interdigitation of the frontal and temporal lobes and overlying venous complexes can make the operculum difficult to open. A smaller temporoparietal craniotomy with direct entry into the distal sylvian fissure is ideal for patients with open or atrophic fissures. The dissection route through the insular cortex depends on the location of the lesion. Anterior putaminal CMs are reached through the short gyri; posterior putaminal CMs are reached through the long gyri, and inferior putaminal CMs are reached through the limen insulae. Hemosiderin staining on the overlying insula is a helpful clue for insular entry, but neuronavigation remains essential for subcortical lesions. The MCA vessels in the sylvian cistern lie between the neurosurgeon and the CM, and the pathway to this target must course through the candelabra below, above, or between the M2 stem arteries. Anterior putaminal CMs are close to ascending lateral lenticulostriate arteries (LSAs) arising from M1 and must be protected on the deep separation plane. Large CMs may reach medially through the globus pallidus to the posterior limb of the internal capsule, where motor and sensory tracts must be protected. Transsylvian-transinsular approaches pass eloquent pre-, post-, and subcentral gyri and above the Wernicke area in the dominant hemisphere, requiring meticulous dissection in the sylvian fissure.

12.4.3 Pallidal

The globus pallidus, or *pale globe* in Latin, is part of the extrapyramidal motor system. It consists of internal and external parts, has inputs from the striatum, and has outputs to the thalamus (medial dorsal nucleus), subthalamic nucleus, and substantia nigra (▶ Fig. 12.8). The globus pallidus serves as a limbic–motor interface involved in planning and inhibiting voluntary movement as well as regulating movements that occur on the subconscious level. Dysarthria and dysphagia observed in patients with pallidal CMs reflect this relationship with the cerebellum; visual field deficits (29%) reflect CM proximity to the optic tract.

The globus pallidus is surrounded by the putamen laterally, the anterior limb of the internal capsule anteromedially, and the posterior limb of the internal capsule posteromedially. Proximity to the internal capsule and increased deficits resulting from hemorrhage explain the higher mRS scores observed in these patients pre- and postoperatively relative to others with basal ganglia lesions. This anatomy makes pallidal CMs accessible only through anteroinferior routes below the anterior limb of the internal capsule (▶ Fig. 12.9; ▶ Video 12.4). The anterior perforated substance or substantia innominata above the carotid terminus is the gateway to lesions at or near this surface. Candidate CMs are recognized on coronal MRIs showing the lesion sitting on the carotid terminus like a golf ball on its tee. The TSyl-SCIF approach is a variation of the transsylvian approach that is worked transfrontally through the supracarotid triangle to access these lesions from below. This triangle is formed by the initial portions of the A1 segment medially and the M1 segment laterally as they originate from the carotid terminus. The base of this triangle is the anterior perforated substance superiorly. Pallidal CMs are directly accessed when they come to the surface of the anterior perforated substance. More superiorly located lesions require parenchymal transgression through the posterior part of the medial orbital gyrus and lateral olfactory stria to climb up into the substantia innominate and reach the globus pallidus. The orbitozygomatic or orbitopterional craniotomy lowers the floor of this approach over the orbit and is necessary to create this climbing trajectory. The supracarotid triangle contains lenticulostriate perforators originating from the A1 (medial LSA) and M1 (lateral LSA) segments and perforators from the terminal internal carotid artery and anterior choroidal artery. The recurrent artery of Heubner originates from the A2 segment of the anterior cerebral artery (ACA) just distal to the anterior communicating artery (ACoA) and courses through the supracarotid triangle parallel to its base, in contrast to other perforators that run perpendicular to its base. This dense collection of perforators in the supracarotid triangle supplies the caudate nucleus, globus pallidus, putamen, internal capsule, and anterior thalamus and is the critical obstacle with the approach. Parenchymal transgression must proceed between these ascending perforators. Deep sylvian veins draining the insula and contributing to the basal vein of Rosenthal are also found in the supracarotid triangle but have little functional significance. The transorbital exposure enables the microscope to angle low and medial over the globe and gives this infrafrontal approach its upward reach into the globus pallidus.

Compared to the standard transsylvian approach, the head is rotated less (only 15 degrees off midline) and extended more. Microsurgical steps include wide splitting of the sylvian fissure to expose the entire M1 and A1 segments, occasional use of a retractor on the medial orbital gyrus, generous release of cerebrospinal fluid in the carotid cisterns and third ventricle, identification and protection of the ascending perforators and recurrent artery of Heubner, and entry into the parenchyma at the site of parenchymal hemosiderin staining. The entry points into the frontal lobe vary from the A1 side of the triangle medially to the M1 side laterally to underneath the triangle below the M1 segment after mobilizing it superiorly. Parting of perforators opens a perpendicular corridor to their course and allows the dissection to deepen beyond them. Cottonoids or hemostatic agents are used to cover and protect perforators immediately adjacent to the corridor. The blind spot with this approach is its superior pole, which is closest to the internal capsule. Preservation of the CM capsule and pulling it inferiorly help deliver it into the surgical corridor. The lateral margin can also be a blind spot that requires meticulous inspection for residual tissue. The advantage of this approach over the TSyl-AIns approach in the dominant hemisphere is that it avoids the Broca area on the lateral convexity.

Pallidal Cavernoma

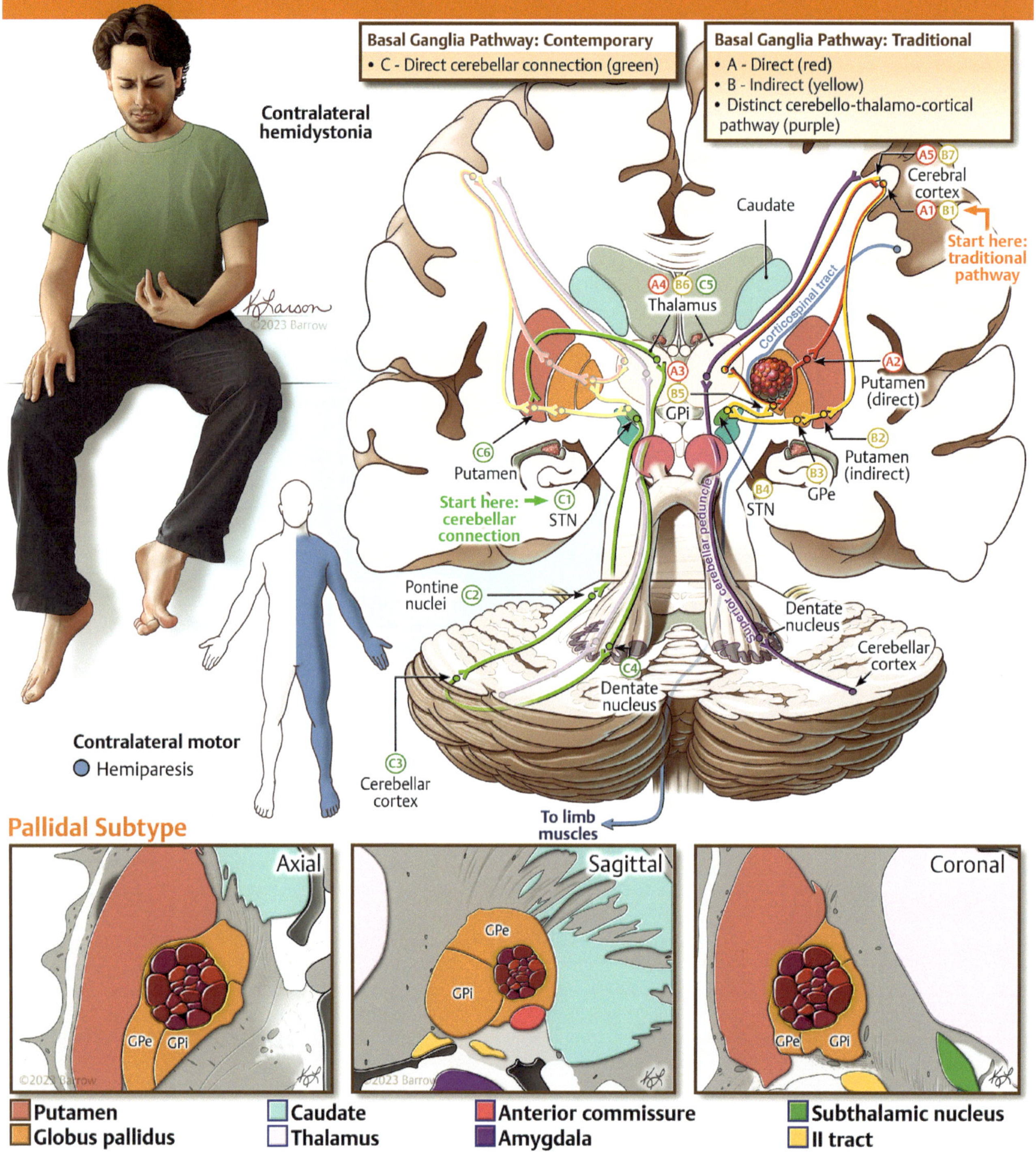

Fig. 12.8 Patients with pallidal lesions often present with motor symptoms, including contralateral hemidystonia. The globus pallidus is integral to the direct and indirect basal ganglia pathways (direct circuit A [*red*]: putamen, GPi, thalamus, cortex; and indirect circuit B [*yellow*]: putamen, GPe, STN, GPi, thalamus, cortex). Recent studies also suggest a reciprocal basal ganglia connection to the cerebellum via the STN, dentate nucleus, and thalamus (contemporary circuit C [*green*]). The inhibitory action of the globus pallidus counters the excitatory action of the cerebellum to smooth movements. Patients with pallidal CMs can also present with symptoms of headache and hemiparesis. The relationships between this right-sided CM and the surrounding anatomy are shown in axial, sagittal, and coronal views (*lower insets*). (Reproduced with permission from Barrow Neurological Institute, Phoenix, AZ.)

Surgical Approach

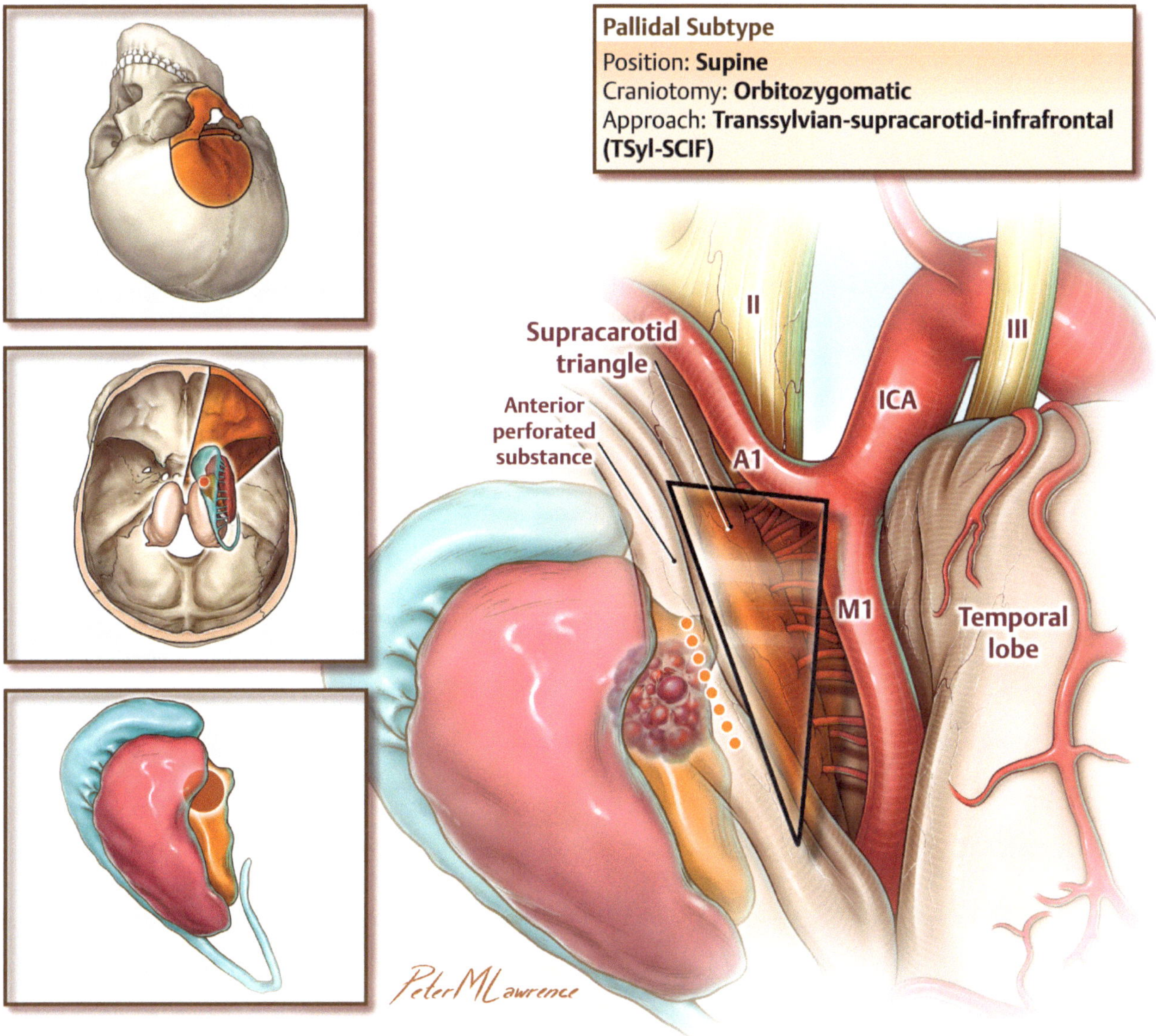

Fig. 12.9 The TSyl-SCIF approach is a variation of the transsylvian approach that works through the supracarotid triangle to access pallidal CMs from below. This triangle is formed by the initial portions of the A1 segment medially and the M1 segment laterally as they originate from the carotid terminus (*orange triangle*). The base of this triangle is the anterior perforated substance superiorly. Pallidal CMs (*lower left inset, orange circle*) are directly accessed when they come to the surface of the anterior perforated substance. In contrast, more superiorly located lesions require parenchymal transgression through the posterior part of the medial orbital gyrus and lateral olfactory stria (*orange dotted line*). The orbitozygomatic or orbital-pterional craniotomy (*upper left inset*) and superior view showing CM (*middle left inset, orange circle*) lowers the floor of this approach over the orbit to create this climbing trajectory. The supracarotid triangle contains lenticulostriate perforators originating from the A1 (mLSA) and M1 (lLSA) segments and perforators from the terminal ICA and AChA. The recurrent artery of Heubner originates from A2 of the ACA just distal to the ACoA and courses through the supracarotid triangle parallel to its base, in contrast to other perforators that run perpendicular to its base. Parenchymal transgression must proceed between these ascending perforators (surgical case, ▶ Video 12.4; QR code). Roman numerals denote cranial nerves. (Reproduced with permission from Barrow Neurological Institute, Phoenix, AZ.)

Surgical Case 12.4

BASAL GANGLIAL

Cavernoma Subtype: Pallidal

Position: Supine
Craniotomy: Pterional
Approach: Transsylvian-anterior transinsular (TSyl-AIns)
Triangle: None
SEZ: None
Artery: M2 MCA

Video: Resection of a right pallidal cavernoma

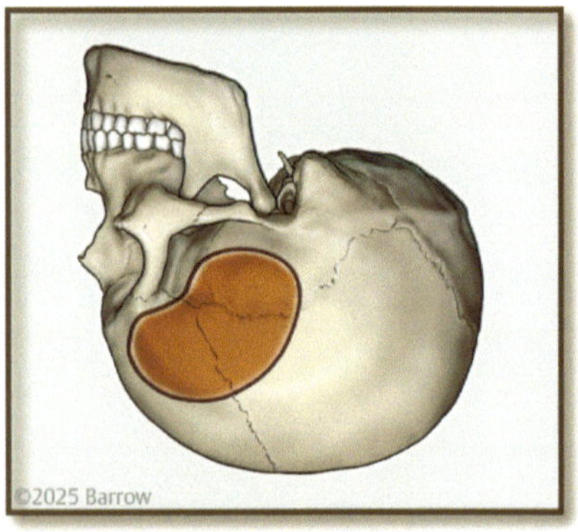

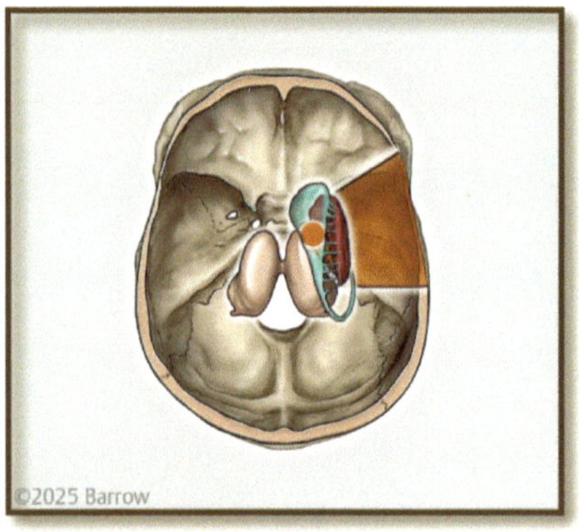

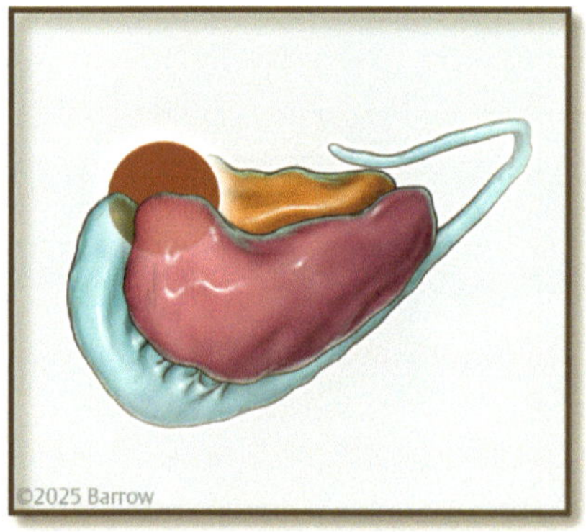

12

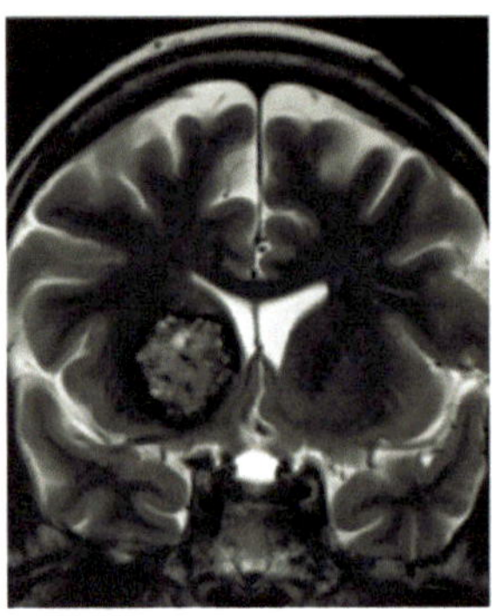

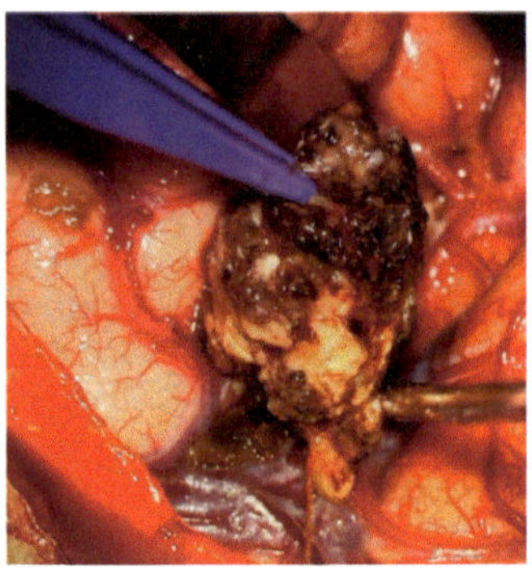

Video 12.4
Transsylvian-Anterior Transinsular Approach for Pallidal Basal Ganglia Cavernous Malformation Resection (Reproduced with permission from Barrow Neurological Institute, Phoenix, AZ.)

12.5 Conclusion

The basal ganglia nuclei are involved with movement, cognition, executive function, and emotion. Despite the functional importance of the basal ganglia, well-defined clinical syndromes were not observed with basal ganglia CMs, unlike with brainstem CMs. Symptoms and signs were caused by the effects of lesional hemorrhage on the internal capsule rather than by specific circuit disruptions. Nonetheless, the classification of basal ganglia CMs into subtypes guides surgical decision-making for selecting the appropriate craniotomy and approach. The taxonomy simplifies the choice between the three different and nuanced approaches used with basal ganglia CMs: the cTCal-Vent approach for caudate lesions, the TSyl-AIns approach for putaminal lesions, and the TSyl-SCIF approach for pallidal lesions.

13 THALAMUS

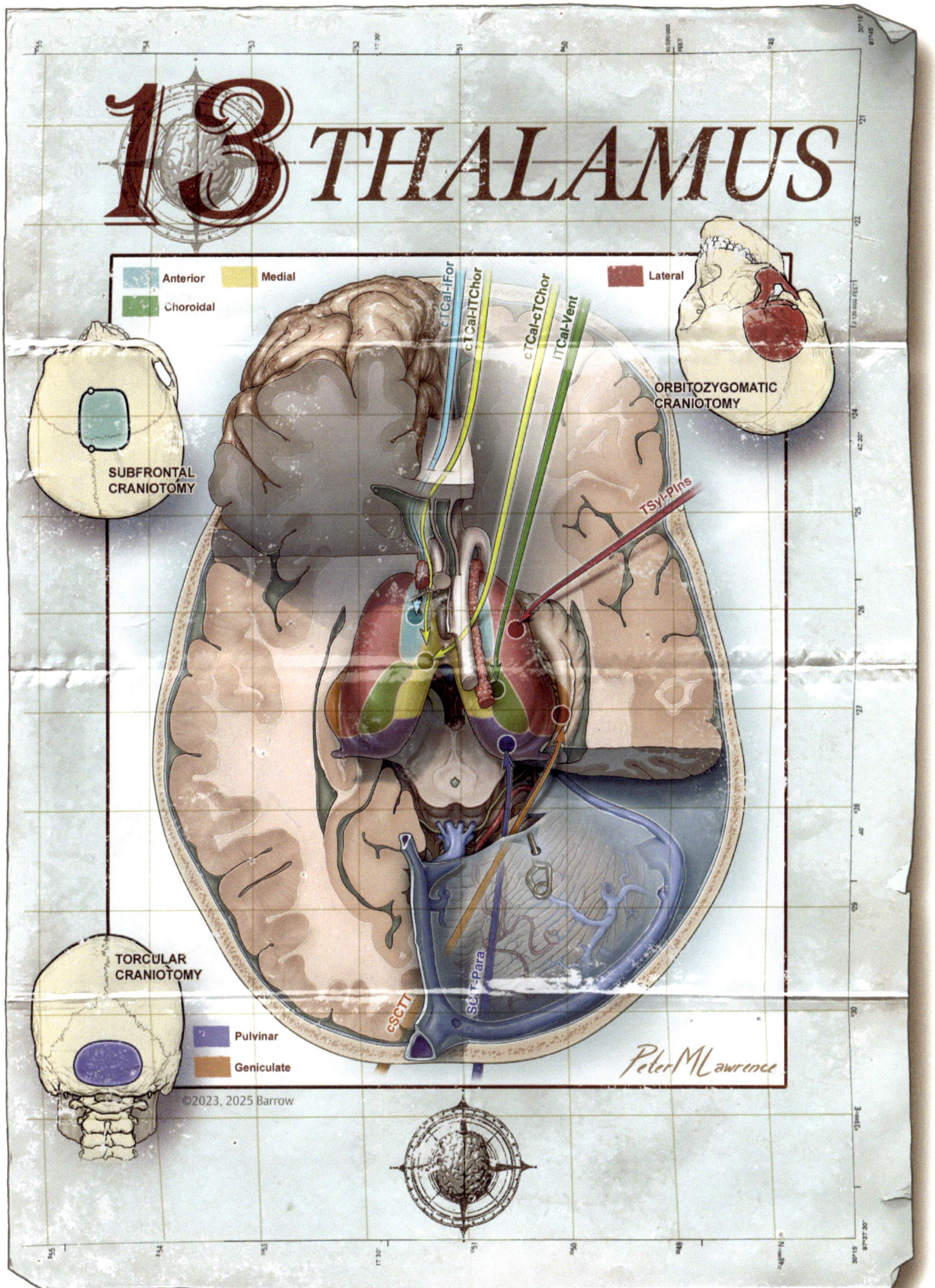

Reproduced with permission from Barrow Neurological Institute, Phoenix, AZ.

13 Thalamic Cavernous Malformations

Summary

The thalamus comprises paired gray matter structures located in the center of the brain that serve as the brain's information gateway. The deep central location of the thalamus makes access to targeted thalamic cavernous malformations (CMs) difficult. The thalamic taxonomy is based on the lesion's intrathalamic location and presentation to an ependymal surface, resulting in six CM subtypes. The thalamic taxonomy was applied to 75 patients that Dr. Robert F. Spetzler and I treated over an approximately 20-year period. The CM subtypes included anterior (7/75, 9%), medial (22/75, 29%), lateral (10/75, 13%), choroidal (9/75, 12%), pulvinar (19/75, 25%), and geniculate (8/75, 11%). The most common presentations were severe or worsening headaches and hemiparesis. Each thalamic CM subtype was associated with a recognizable constellation of neurologic symptoms. Favorable outcomes (modified Rankin Scale [mRS] score ≤ 2) after microsurgical resection were observed in 80% (53/66) of patients with follow-up. Relative outcomes assessed by mRS scores were unchanged or improved in most patients (61/66, 92%). The CM subtype guides the selection of the surgical approach. Anterior CMs are resected through contralateral transcallosal-ipsilateral transforaminal (cTCal-iFor) approaches. Medial CMs are resected through contralateral transcallosal-transchoroidal fissure (cTCal-TChor) approaches, and lateral CMs are resected through transsylvian-posterior transinsular (TSyl-PIns) approaches. Choroidal CMs are resected through ipsilateral transcallosal-transventricular (iTCal-Vent) approaches, with anterior (ATCal-Vent) or posterior (PTCal-Vent) approaches. Pulvinar CMs are resected through paramedian supracerebellar-infratentorial (SCIT-Para) approaches, with occasional use of superior parietal lobule-transatrial (SPL-Atr) approaches. Although some medial geniculate CMs are resected using SCIT-Para approaches, most are located more laterally and require contralateral supracerebellar-transtentorial (cSCTT) approaches. The CM taxonomy improves diagnostic acumen at the patient's bedside, guides surgical approach selection, and helps improve patient outcomes.

Keywords: cavernoma, choroidal, ependymal, geniculate, neural pathway, pial, pulvinar, relay nucleus, supracerebellar, thalamic nucleus

13.1 Introduction

The thalamus is a paired gray matter structure occupying the center of the brain that serves as the brain's information gateway, relaying and modulating information coming from the periphery to the cerebral cortex. In almost all neural pathways, including motor, limbic, somatosensory, visual, auditory, and taste, the first synapse within a thalamic nucleus is where information is sorted, analyzed, and integrated. Relay nuclei, like the ventral posterolateral (VPL) nucleus, ventral posteromedial (VPM) nucleus, or lateral geniculate nucleus (LGN), transmit these signals to cortical centers, whereas association nuclei, like the anterior nucleus and pulvinar, receive cortical information and project it back to association areas that interpret sensory information. These processing functions make the thalamus one of the brain's most critical and eloquent areas.

The central location of the thalamus makes it difficult to access. It has no cortical surface, and its pial surfaces are limited to a small piece of the inferior pulvinar in the quadrigeminal cistern and the geniculate bodies in the ambient cistern. However, its location within the ventricular system gives it multiple points of transependymal access, albeit at the end of long surgical corridors that are technically challenging to reach, anatomically complex, and associated with surgical risks. Therefore, cavernous malformations (CMs) in the thalamus have long been considered inoperable and best managed conservatively, like CMs in the brainstem. This perception has changed with the continued refinement of microsurgical approaches that capitalize on natural subarachnoid and intraventricular pathways to deep targets. For example, traditional midline supracerebellar approaches have advanced to contralateral supracerebellar-transtentorial (cSCTT) approaches that use gravity retraction of the cerebellum, a tentorial incision to access the ambient cistern, and a crossing trajectory to extend the lateral reach to the geniculate nuclei.

As with brainstem CMs, select thalamic CMs are now considered for microsurgical resection as the treatment of choice in patients with symptomatic hemorrhage and surgically accessible pathology. Judicious surgical selection depends on a critical analysis of the patient's unique pathoanatomy and a pairing with a surgical approach to provide optimal exposure for complete and safe resection.

13.2 Neuroanatomy of Thalamic Cavernous Malformation Subtypes

The thalamic CM taxonomy is based on intrathalamic location or presentation to a pial or ependymal surface. CM subtyping based on nuclear groups and ventricular or cisternal presentations results in six thalamic subtypes: (1) anterior, (2) medial, (3) lateral, (4) choroidal, (5) pulvinar, and (6) geniculate subtypes (▸ Fig. 13.1). This taxonomy is intended to guide the selection of the optimal surgical approach and to improve neurosurgical decision-making and outcomes.

13.2.1 Anterior

The anterior thalamic nuclei (anteroventral, anterodorsal, and anteromedial) are situated between the limbs of the Y-shaped internal medullary lamina. Anterior thalamic CMs are lateral and inferior to the foramen of Monro and the venous angle formed by the confluence of the thalamostriate vein (ThaStrV), caudate vein, and septal vein (septocaudate triangle). These lesions are situated posterior to the descending columns of the fornix and medial to the genu of the internal capsule, within

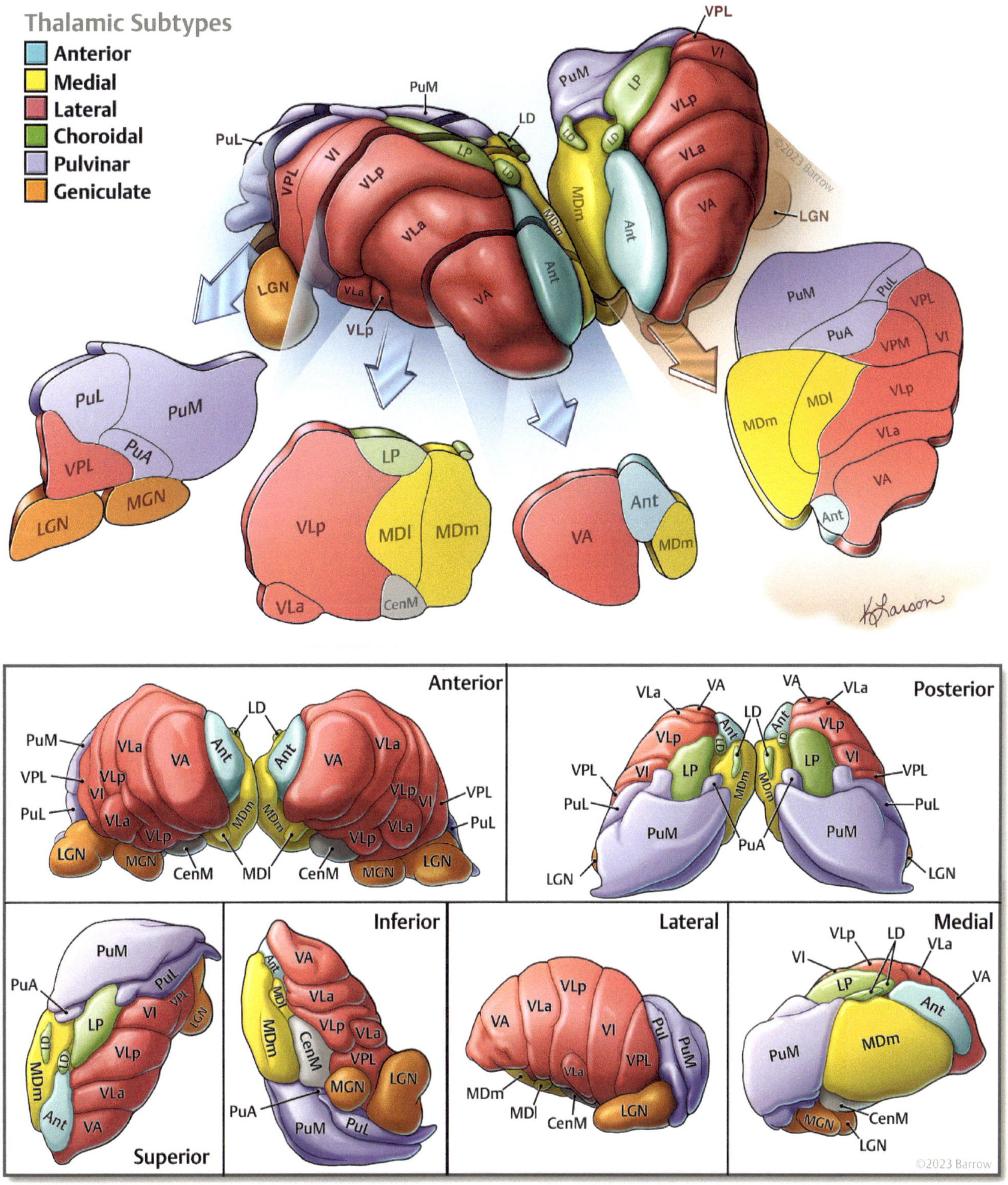

Fig. 13.1 Overview of thalamic anatomy and the six CM subtypes, as seen from an anterior oblique view. Subtypes are shown in the right and left thalami, with anterior in *teal*, medial in *yellow*, lateral in *red*, choroidal in *green*, pulvinar in *blue*, and geniculate in *orange*. Thalamic nuclei within each subtype are labeled with their abbreviations. Anterior, middle, and posterior coronal slices are shown through the right thalamus (*blue arrows*), and an axial slice is shown through the left thalamus (*orange arrow*). Surface locations of thalamic subtypes are shown in different perspectives (*insets*): anterior and posterior views of both thalami (*upper row*) and superior, inferior, lateral, and medial views of the left thalamus (*lower row*). (Reproduced with permission from Barrow Neurological Institute, Phoenix, AZ.)

millimeters of these critical structures. The anterior thalamic tubercle is a prominent landmark overlying these CMs at the posterior edge of the foramen of Monro.

13.2.2 Medial

Medial thalamic CMs are located in the medial nuclear group (medial dorsal magnocellular [MDm], medial dorsal parvocellular [MDl], and median nuclei) that forms the third ventricle's lateral wall. Lesions on this surface lie between the tenia thalami superiorly and the hypothalamic sulcus inferiorly, delineating the border between the thalamus and hypothalamus. Stria medullaris is a fiber bundle in the epithalamus that parallels the tenia thalami on this upper medial surface. The massa intermedia or interthalamic adhesion is a prominent bridge between the two thalami found at the center of this medial surface in most patients.

13.2.3 Lateral

Lateral thalamic CMs can occur in the ventral group of thalamic nuclei and include the ventral anterior (VA) nucleus, ventral lateral anterior (VLa) subnucleus, ventral lateral posterior (VLp) subnucleus, ventral intermediate (VI) nucleus, VPM, and VPL in the lateral portion of the thalamus, deep to the posterior half of the insula. They have no surface presentation in the lateral ventricle, lying underneath the body of the caudate nucleus. They have no subarachnoid presentation, lying beneath the insula's long gyri. Lateral thalamic lesions are located medial to the posterior limb of the internal capsule. Although the lateral dorsal (LD) nucleus and lateral posterior (LP) nucleus are part of the lateral nuclear group, they are considered choroidal thalamic CMs, not lateral thalamic CMs.

13.2.4 Choroidal

Choroidal thalamic CMs are located in the superior thalamus. The superior thalamus comprises the LD and LP nuclei and forms the floor of the body of the lateral ventricle. This subtype is named for the choroid plexus that covers it. The superior surface lies between the anterior thalamic nucleus and the pulvinar and lacks clear surface landmarks. Instead, the superior thalamic surface is delineated anteriorly by a transverse line drawn through the point where the choroid plexus exits the foramen of Monro at its posterior aspect. Posteriorly, this superior surface is delineated by a transverse line drawn through the point where the body of the fornix ends and the crus bends laterally toward the atrium. The pulvinar curves steeply downward at this line to form the posterior thalamic surface. This superior surface extends medially from the tenia thalami in the choroidal fissure to the stria terminalis and ThaStrV laterally in the groove between the body of the caudate nucleus and thalamus. The medial posterior choroidal artery (mPChA) courses in the choroid plexus along this surface.

13

13.2.5 Pulvinar

Pulvinar thalamic CMs are located within the posterior thalamus. This singular nucleus has three parts: the anterior pulvinar, medial pulvinar, and lateral pulvinar. The pulvinar presents to three compartments: the anterior wall of the atrium inside the lateral ventricle (posterolateral part), the anterior wall of the quadrigeminal cistern under the crus of the fornix (posteromedial part), and the roof of the ambient cistern near the geniculate bodies (inferolateral part). The pulvinar is draped superiorly in the ventricle by the crus of the fornix and the choroid plexus of the atrium, between which the tenia fornicea and tenia thalami anchor the choroid plexus and the choroidal fissure. The pulvinar is draped inferiorly in the quadrigeminal and ambient cisterns by the basal vein of Rosenthal (BVR), a loop of the P3 (quadrigeminal) segment of the posterior cerebral artery (PCA), and the mPChA.

13.2.6 Geniculate

Geniculate thalamic CMs are situated in the posteroinferior aspect of the thalamus, where the medial geniculate nucleus (MGN) and LGN attach to the pulvinar. They occupy the inferolateral part of the pulvinar that forms the roof of the ambient cistern. Although small lesions can reside in the MGN or LGN, these nuclei provide a gateway to access larger lesions extending into the ventral posterior nuclei. Geniculate CMs are associated with the vascular anatomy of the ambient cistern, specifically the BVR, the P3 segment of the PCA, and the mPChA.

13.3 Clinical Evidence

The thalamic taxonomy was applied to an extensive microsurgical experience of 75 patients that Robert F. Spetzler and I treated over an approximately 20-year period (2001–2019) (▶ Table 13.1). CMs involving the thalamus were subtyped based on the predominant surface presentation identified on preoperative magnetic resonance imaging. Six subtypes of thalamic CMs were defined: anterior (7/75, 9%), medial (22/75, 29%), lateral (10/75, 13%), choroidal (9/75, 12%), pulvinar (19/75, 25%), and geniculate (8/75, 11%). Each thalamic CM subtype was associated with a recognizable constellation of neurologic symptoms. The most common symptoms were severe or worsening headaches (30/75, 40%), hemiparesis (27/75, 37%), hemianesthesia (21/75, 28%), blurred vision (14/75, 19%), and hydrocephalus (9/75, 12%) (▶ Fig. 13.2). Patients with anterior and lateral CMs presented with hemiparesis and hemisensory deficits related to the involvement of or proximity to the internal capsule (▶ Fig. 13.3). Hemisensory deficits in patients with lateral CMs may also have been due to involvement of the sensory relay nuclei (VPM and VPL). Patients with medial CMs were the most likely to present with hydrocephalus (23%). Patients with anterior and choroidal CMs were the most likely to present with memory or cognitive deficits due to proximity of the fornix (43 and 29%, respectively). Patients with pulvinar CMs were the most likely to present with contralateral hemisensory deficits (58%) and blurred vision (38%). Patients with geniculate CMs were the most likely to present with visual field deficits (25%). Favorable outcomes (mRS ≤ 2) after microsurgical resection were observed in 80% (53/66) of patients with follow-up. Relative outcomes by mRS scores were unchanged or improved in most patients (61/66, 92%).

Table 13.1 Preoperative and postoperative outcome measures for patients who underwent resection of thalamic CMs by subtype

Variable	All subtypes (*N* = 75)	Anterior (*n* = 7)	Medial (*n* = 22)	Lateral (*n* = 10)	Choroidal (*n* = 9)	Pulvinar (*n* = 19)	Geniculate (*n* = 8)
Preoperative mRS score							
> 2	18 (24)	3 (43)	7 (32)	3 (30)	0 (0)	3 (16)	2 (25)
≤ 2	57 (76)	4 (57)	15 (68)	7 (70)	9 (100)	16 (84)	6 (75)
Postoperative mRS score							
> 2	18/72 (25)	2/7 (29)	4/21 (19)	4/10 (40)	0/9 (0)	5/18 (28)	3/7 (43)
≤ 2	54/72 (75)	5/7 (71)	17/21 (81)	6/10 (60)	9/9 (100)	13/18 (72)	4/7 (57)
Follow-up (mo), mean (SD)	23 (30)	27 (31)	16 (20)	26 (35)	41 (45)	27 (33)	6 (10)
Final mRS score							
> 2	13/66 (20)	1/6 (17)	4/20 (20)	4/10 (40)	0/8 (0)	5/16 (31)	1/6 (17)
≤ 2	53/66 (80)	5/6 (83)	16/20 (80)	6/ (60)	8/8 (100)	11/16 (69)	5/6 (83)
Worse	5/66 (8)	0/6 (0)	2/20 (10)	0/10 (0)	0/8 (0)	3/16 (19)	0/6 (0)
Stable or improved	61/66 (92)	6/6 (100)	18/20 (90)	10/10 (100)	8/8 (100)	13/16 (81)	6/6 (100)

Note: All data are reported as proportion (%) unless otherwise specified.

	Subtype					
Symptom	Anterior (n=7)	Medial (n=22)	Lateral (n=10)	Choroidal (n=9)	Pulvinar (n=19)	Geniculate (n=8)
Hemianesthesia	2 (29)	0 (0)	5 (50)	1 (11)	11 (58)	2 (25)
Pain syndrome	1 (14)	0 (0)	0 (0)	1 (11)	2 (11)	0 (0)
Hemiparesis	4 (57)	6 (27)	7 (70)	1 (11)	8 (42)	1 (13)
Facial weakness	0 (0)	1 (5)	0 (0)	1 (11)	3 (16)	0 (0)
Blurry vision	0 (0)	3 (14)	0 (0)	2 (22)	6 (32)	3 (38)
CN III	0 (0)	0 (0)	0 (0)	0 (0)	2 (11)	0 (0)
Visual field	0 (0)	0 (0)	0 (0)	0 (0)	0 (0)	2 (25)
Memory, cognitive	3 (43)	2 (9)	0 (0)	2 (22)	2 (11)	1 (13)
Hydrocephalus	0 (0)	5 (23)	0 (0)	1 (11)	3 (16)	0 (0)

Fig. 13.2 Heat map showing symptoms of patients with thalamic CMs according to subtype. Percentages were calculated as the frequency of a particular symptom within a given thalamic subtype. Conditional formatting was applied on a scale of least common (*red*) to most common (*green*). The symptoms associated with each subtype are most closely aligned with cells with green formatting. (Reproduced with permission from Catapano JS, Rumalla K, Srinivasan VM, et al. A taxonomy for deep cerebral cavernous malformations: subtypes of thalamic lesions. J Neurosurg 2023;139(6):1681–1696.).

13.4 Resection Strategies for Thalamic Cavernous Malformation Subtypes

The thalamic CM subtype determined the selection of the surgical approach (▶ Fig. 13.4). Anterior CMs are resected through a contralateral transcallosal-transforaminal (TCal-For) approach. Medial CMs are resected through a contralateral transcallosal-transchoroidal fissure (TCal-TChor) approach, and lateral CMs are resected through a transsylvian-posterior transinsular (TSyl-PIns) approach. Choroidal CMs are resected through a transcallosal-transventricular (TCal-Vent) approach, with occasional use of anterior (ATCal-Vent) or posterior (PTCal-Vent) approaches. Pulvinar CMs are resected through a paramedian supracerebellar-infratentorial (SCIT-Para) approach, with occasional use of the superior parietal lobule-transatrial (SPL-Atr) approach. Although some medial geniculate CMs are resected using a SCIT-Para

Clinical Presentation of Thalamic Subtypes

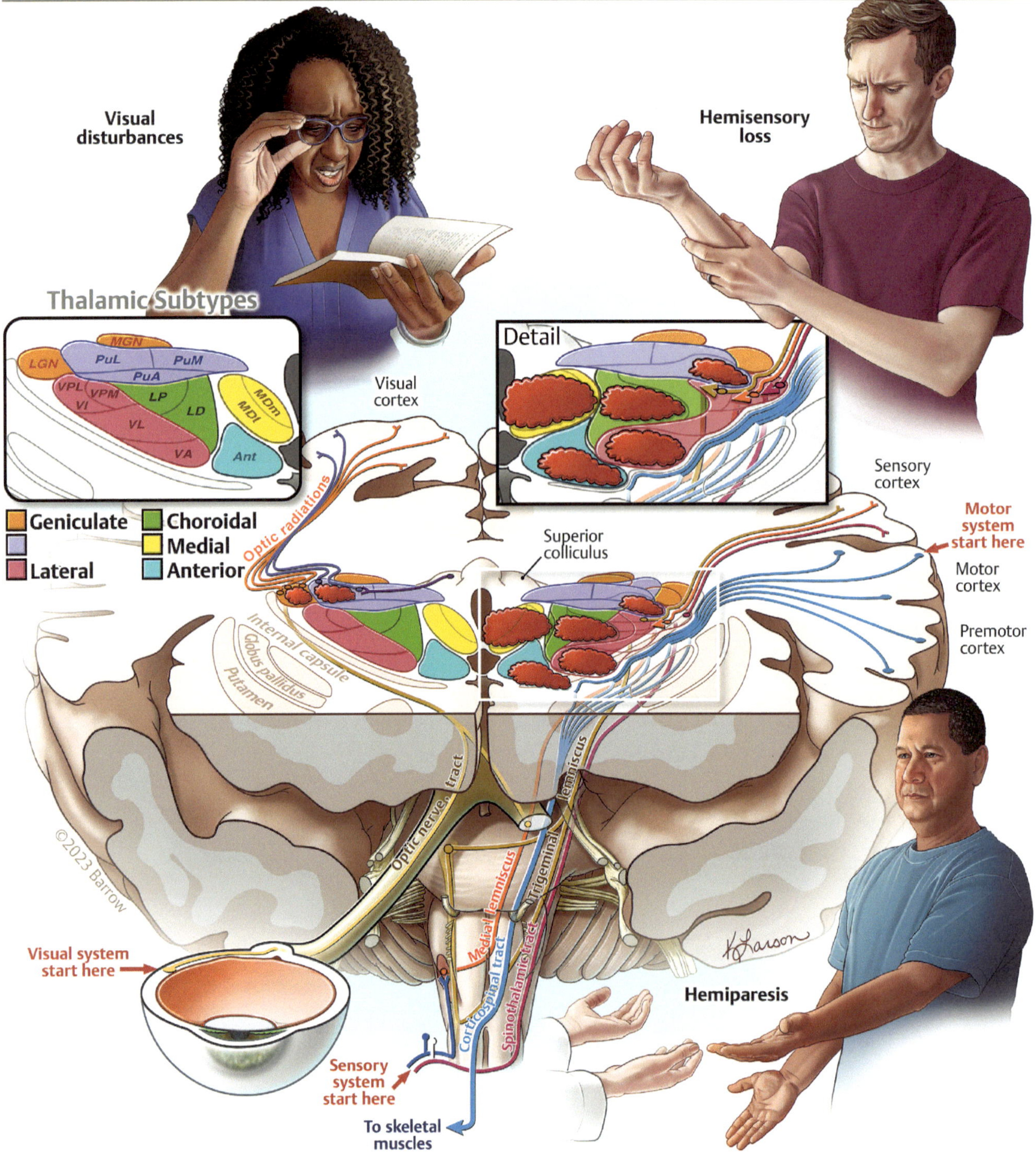

Fig. 13.3 Overview of clinical symptoms and signs associated with thalamic CMs. Patients with anterior and lateral CMs presented with hemiparesis or hemisensory deficits related to the involvement of or proximity to the internal capsule (*right inset*). Hemisensory deficits in patients with lateral CMs may also have been due to the involvement of the sensory relay nuclei (*left inset*; VPM and VPL). Visual disturbances were observed in patients with pulvinar and geniculate CMs, with blurred vision in the former and visual field deficits in the latter (optic tract and radiations). Patients with anterior and choroidal CMs were the most likely to present with memory or cognitive deficits due to proximity of the fornix. Patients with medial CMs were the most likely to present with hydrocephalus. (Reproduced with permission from Barrow Neurological Institute, Phoenix, AZ.)

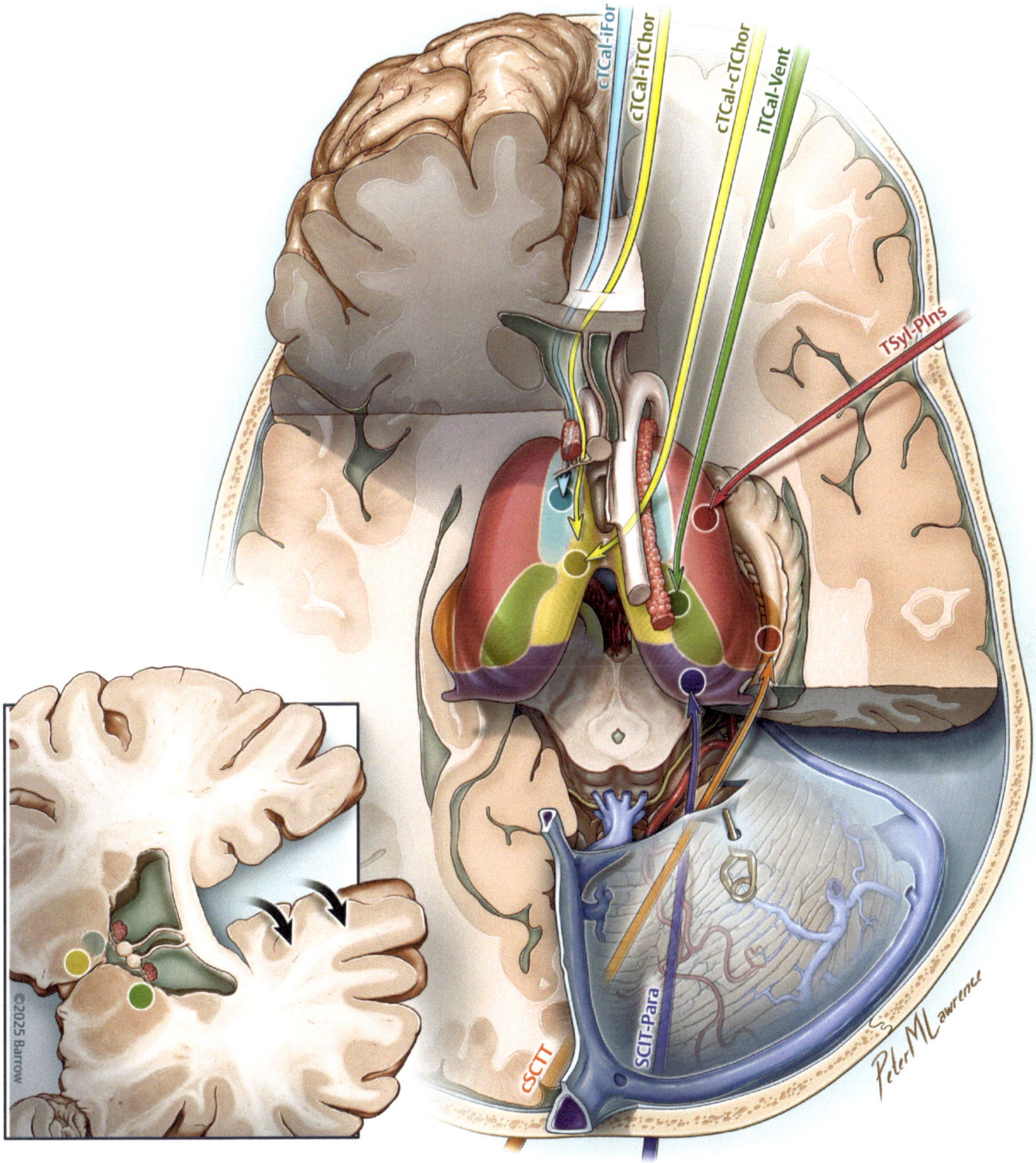

Fig. 13.4 Overview of surgical approaches to thalamic CM subtypes (*circles*) shown from above with axial and coronal resections of the overlying cerebrum. Bifrontal craniotomies are used for anterior, medial, and choroidal subtypes. A cTCal-iFor approach is taken for anterior CMs (*teal arrow*); a contralateral transcallosal-transchoroidal approach is taken for medial CMs through the ipsilateral choroidal fissure (cTCal-iTChor) or contralateral choroidal fissure (cTCal-cTChor; *yellow arrows*), and an iTCal-Vent approach is taken for choroidal CMs (*green arrow*). Transcallosal approaches were performed with the midline horizontal to allow gravity to retract the dependent hemisphere (*inset*; *black arrows*) and open the anterior interhemispheric fissure. A pterional craniotomy and TSyl-PIns approach are taken for lateral CMs (*red arrow*). Torcular craniotomies are used for pulvinar and geniculate subtypes. A SCIT-Para approach is taken for pulvinar CMs (*purple arrow*), and a cSCTT approach is taken for geniculate CMs (*orange arrow*). (Reproduced with permission from Barrow Neurological Institute, Phoenix, AZ.)

approach, most geniculate CMs are located more laterally and require a cSCTT approach.

13.4.1 Anterior

Anterior CMs were the least common, making their clinical constellation of symptoms and signs difficult to characterize. Anterior thalamic nuclei influence emotions, alertness, attention, and memory function, receiving inputs from the mamillary bodies via the mammillothalamic tract and projecting to the cingulate gyrus, anterior limbic area, parahippocampal gyrus, and prefrontal cortex. These patients were symptomatic from hemorrhages that affected the internal capsule. Anatomically, this small portion of the thalamus is adjacent to the foramen of Monro, posterior to the descending columns of the fornix, and only millimeters medial to the genu of the internal capsule. Hemiparesis and hemisensory loss were recorded among these patients, whereas memory disturbance was not.

Anterior CMs were approached through a contralateral transcallosal-ipsilateral transforaminal (cTCal-iFor) approach with gravity retraction (▶ Fig. 13.5; ▶ Video 13.1). In this approach, the head is turned laterally 90 degrees to align the midline horizontally with the lesion on the upside. A bifrontal craniotomy exposes the interhemispheric fissure, and the dependent frontal lobe falls away from the falx to separate the frontal lobes and widen the fissure. The interhemispheric fissure is traversed contralateral to the lesion, and the midline is crossed at the level of the corpus callosum. By performing the callosotomy under the pericallosal artery ipsilateral to the CM, the ipsilateral ventricle is entered, and the crossing trajectory optimizes the view of the anterior thalamus through the foramen of Monro. In addition, the fornix lies medially in the foramen, away from the dissection path and protected from manipulation. The internal medullary lamina that defines this subtype is an internal structure that is not visible microsurgically, but the tributaries of the internal cerebral vein (ICV) are surrogate landmarks. Anterior CMs occur anterior to the ThaStrV as it arcs into the venous angle in the septocaudate triangle between the septal vein and anterior caudate vein. Although the presence and caliber of these venous landmarks vary, the choroid plexus reliably courses over the venous angle and U-turns through the foramen of Monro. The anterior thalamus is entered at or anterior to the intersection of the ThaStrV and choroid plexus. A transforaminal descent is needed to access anteroventral CMs, but opening the choroidal fissure was not typically needed. Resection is performed within the transforaminal window with the column of the fornix anteriorly, pre- and supraoptic nuclei of the hypothalamus inferiorly, and the genu of the internal capsule laterally. The regions of two other subtypes adjoin this spot: choroidal CMs, located posterior to the venous angle or ThaStrV and lateral to the tenia thalami, and medial CMs, located posterior to the venous angle or ThaStrV and medial to the tenia thalami.

13.4.2 Medial

Medial CMs accounted for nearly one-third of thalamic lesions and were the most common subtype. Medial nuclei consist of the median (or midline) and medial dorsal nuclei, which are association nuclei between the limbic system and the prefrontal association cortex. The larger MDm is composed of an anteromedial magnocellular part that receives olfactory inputs from the piriform cortex, adjacent olfactory cortex, ventral pallidum, and amygdala. The posterolateral parvocellular part (MDl) receives inputs from the prefrontal cortex, anterior cingulate cortex, anterior insula, and inferior parietal cortex. The specific functions of medial thalamic nuclei are unclear, but they influence emotions. The location of this CM subtype on the third ventricular wall made hydrocephalus a common finding. However, these patients presented more frequently with hemiparesis due to the proximity of the CM to the genu of the internal capsule.

The medial thalamic surface between the tenia thalami superiorly and the hypothalamic sulcus inferiorly provides transventricular access to CMs using a contralateral TCal-TChor approach with gravity retraction (▶ Fig. 13.6; ▶ Video 13.2, ▶ Video 13.3). Like anterior CMs, the midline is oriented horizontally with the lesion on the upside. After bifrontal craniotomy and dissection through the interhemispheric fissure, callosotomy is performed under the pericallosal artery contralateral to the CM to enter the contralateral ventricle. The midline is crossed later below the level of the choroidal fissure, not at the level of the corpus callosum as it is with anterior CMs. The approach remains contralateral through the corpus callosum, into the lateral ventricle, and through the choroidal fissure, crossing ipsilaterally in the third ventricle to reach targeted medial CMs in the opposite thalamus. This deeper midline crossing offers a more favorable reach under the fornix and a trajectory across and into the medial thalamus. Careful opening of the choroidal fissure consists of incising tenia fornicea along the lateral border of the fornix, entering the velum interpositum, and dissecting the confluence of the ThaStrV, caudate vein, and ICV. These transchoroidal maneuvers open the third ventricular roof posteriorly and double the size of the foramen of Monro. A 2-cm oval window is created with the fornix medially, caudate vein anterolaterally, and ICV posterolaterally. The massa intermedia or interthalamic adhesion may be divided if it blocks access to the CM. The entry site into the thalamus is selected at the exophytic portion of the lesion or through its hemosiderin stain, taking care to stay above the hypothalamic sulcus inferiorly. This cTCal-cTChor trajectory into the medial thalamus targets inferomedial CMs on or immediately below the ependymal surface. Larger CMs extending centrally into the thalamus to the internal medullary lamina create a blind spot in the superolateral corner that requires the lesion to be mobilized inferomedially into the surgical corridor. The more superior and lateral the reach, the greater the deflection of the fornix. To minimize fornix manipulation, the neurosurgeon can consider a cTCal-iTChor approach that crosses the midline at the corpus callosum and opens the ipsilateral choroidal fissure by dropping the fornix below the dissection pathway.

13.4.3 Lateral

The largest group of thalamic nuclei are the lateral nuclei, consisting of the ventral group (VA, VLa and VLp, VI, VPM, and VPL), dorsal group (LD, LP, and pulvinar), and geniculate group (MGN and LGN). The ventral group forms the lateral surface of the thalamus and is the defining group of this lateral subtype. The

Surgical Approach

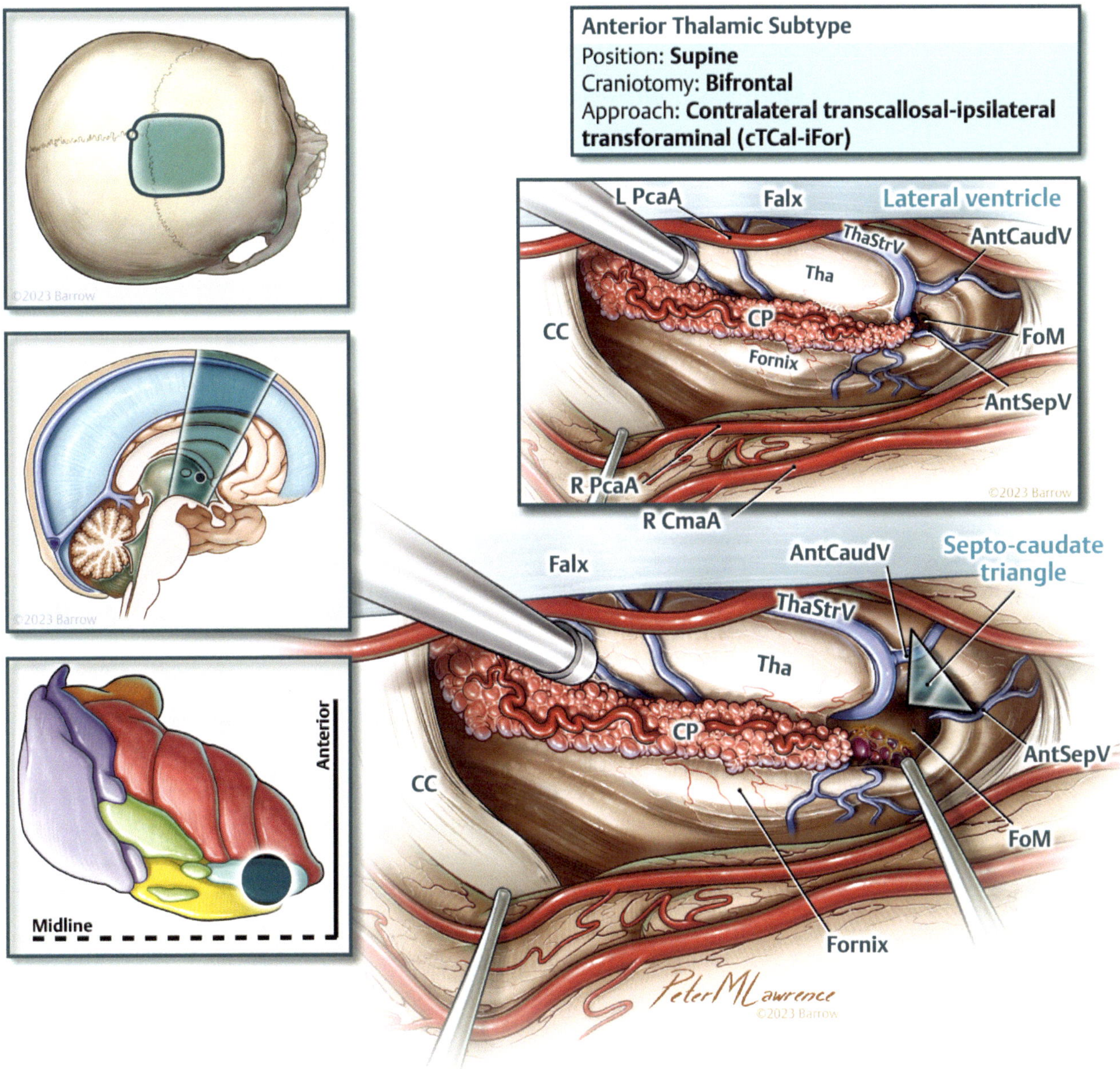

Fig. 13.5 Anterior thalamic CMs are accessed through a bifrontal craniotomy and cTCal-iFor approach. Gravity opens the interhemispheric fissure by turning the head 90 degrees laterally with the lesion on the upside (*upper left inset*). The interhemispheric fissure is traversed contralateral to the lesion (*middle left inset*; *teal circle*), the midline is crossed at the level of the corpus callosum, and the ipsilateral ventricle is entered with a view of the anterior thalamus through the foramen of Monro (*lower left and upper right insets*). Anterior CMs (*lower left inset*; *teal circle*) lie anterior to the ThaStrV as it arcs into the venous angle in the septocaudate triangle between the AntSepV and the AntCaudV (*teal triangle*). Resection is performed within the transforaminal window with a column of fornix anteriorly, pre- and supraoptic nuclei of the hypothalamus inferiorly, and the knee of the internal capsule laterally (surgical case; ▶ Video 13.1; QR code). (Reproduced with permission from Barrow Neurological Institute, Phoenix, AZ.)

Surgical Case 13.1

THALAMIC

Cavernoma Subtype: Anterior

Position: Lateral position, midline horizontal
Craniotomy: Bifrontal
Approach: Contralateral transcallosal-contralateral transchoroidal (cTCal-cTChor)
Triangle: Septocaudate
SEZ: None
Artery: mPChA

Video: Resection of a left anterior thalamic cavernoma

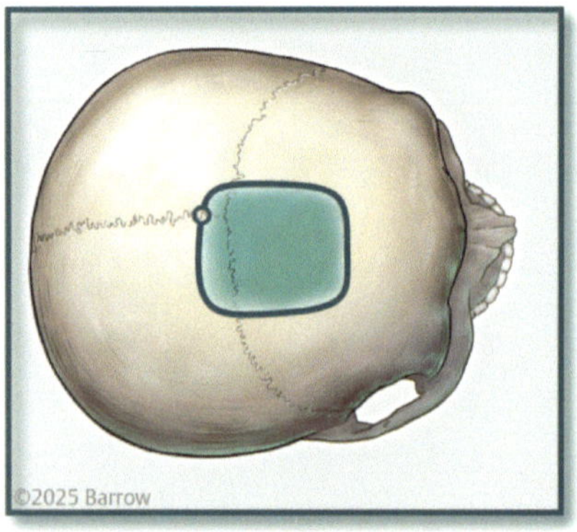

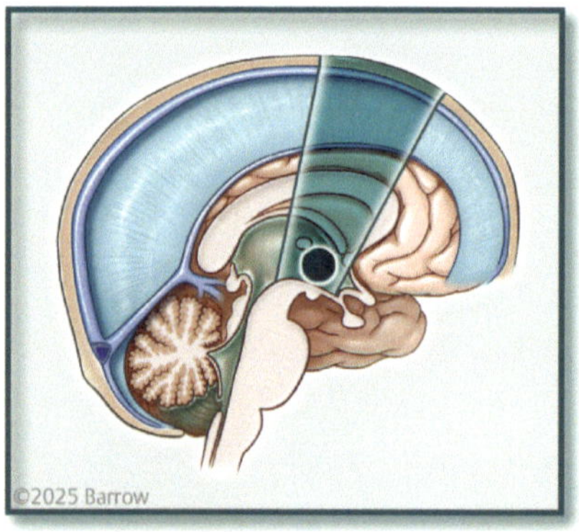

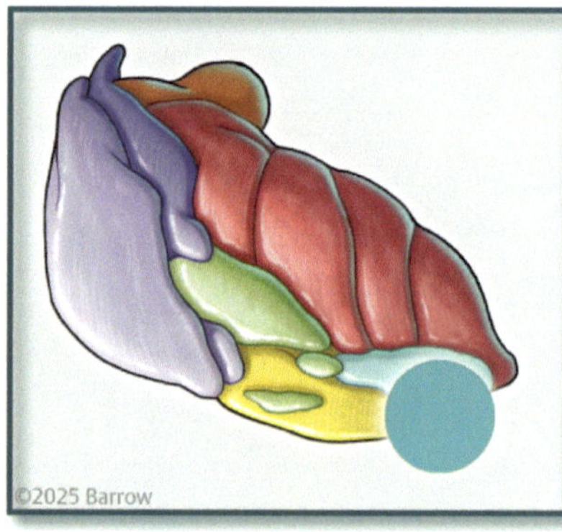

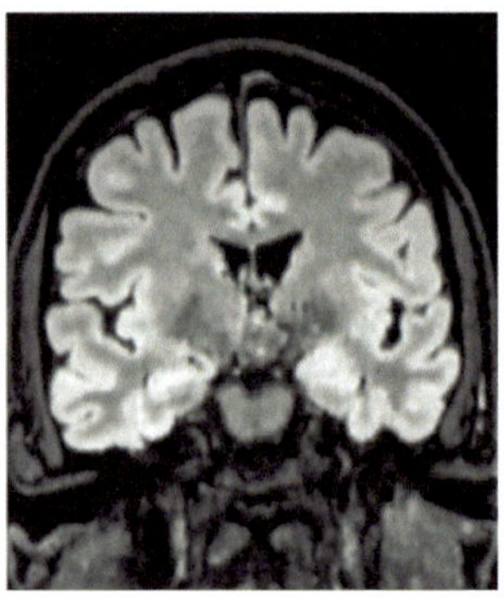

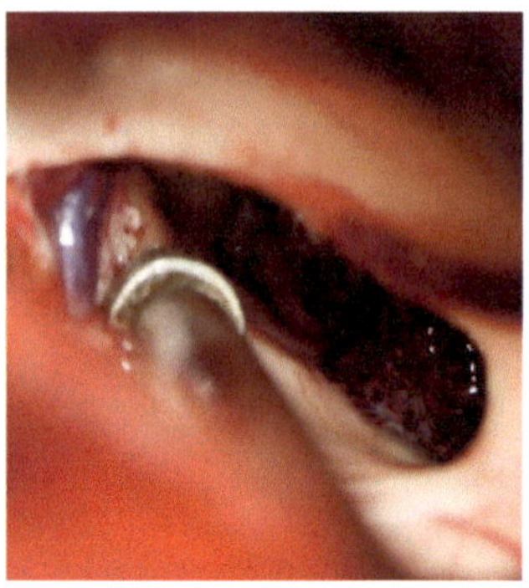

Video 13.1
Contralateral Transcallosal–Contralateral Transchoroidal Approach for Anterior Thalamic Cavernous Malformation Resection (Reproduced with permission from Barrow Neurological Institute, Phoenix, AZ.)

13

Surgical Approach

Medial Thalamic Subtype

Position: **Supine**
Craniotomy: **Bifrontal**
Approach: **Contralateral transcallosal-contralateral transchoroidal (cTCal-cTChor)**

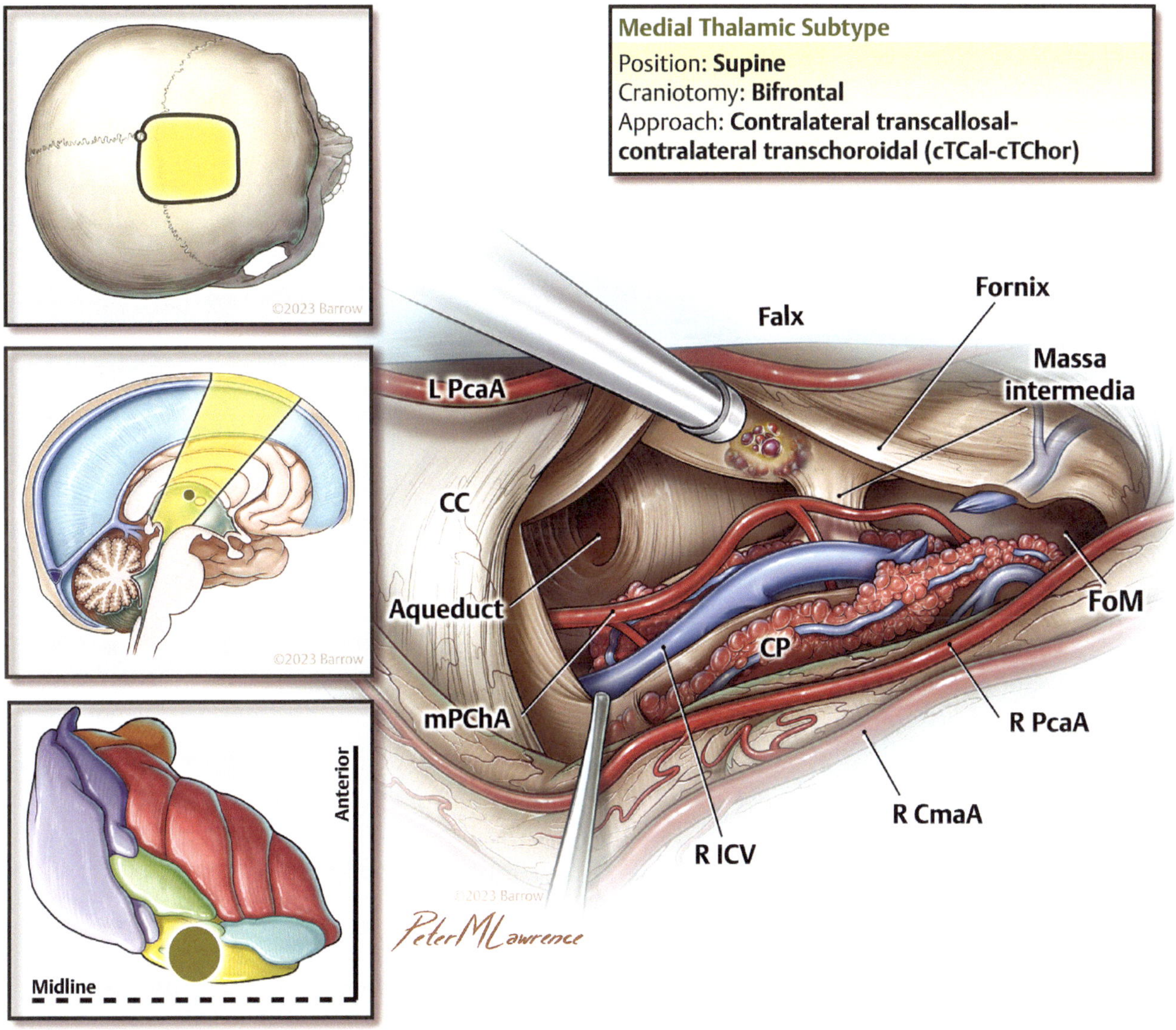

Fig. 13.6 Medial thalamic CMs are accessed through a bifrontal craniotomy and cTCal-cTChor approach. Gravity opens the interhemispheric fissure by turning the head 90 degrees laterally with the lesion on the upside (*upper left inset*). The interhemispheric fissure is navigated contralateral to the lesion (*middle left inset*; *yellow circle*), as is the corpus callosum and the choroidal fissure. The midline is crossed in the third ventricle to reach the medial CM in the opposite thalamus (*lower left inset*; *yellow circle*). The choroidal fissure is opened by incising the tenia fornicea along the lateral border of the fornix, entering the velum interpositum, and dissecting the confluence of the ThaStrV, caudate vein, and ICV. This opening of the third ventricular roof enlarges the foramen of Monro and positions the fornix medially, caudate vein anterolaterally, and ICV posterolaterally. This cTCal-cTChor trajectory under the fornix and across the midline reaches medial CMs on or immediately below the thalamus's ependymal surface (surgical cases; ▶ Video 13.2, ▶ Video 13.3; QR codes). (Reproduced with permission from Barrow Neurological Institute, Phoenix, AZ).

Surgical Case 13.2

THALAMIC

Cavernoma Subtype: Medial

Position: Lateral position, midline horizontal
Craniotomy: Bifrontal
Approach: Contralateral transcallosal-contralateral transchoroidal (cTCal-cTChor)
Triangle: None
SEZ: None
Artery: mPChA

Video: Resection of a left medial thalamic cavernoma

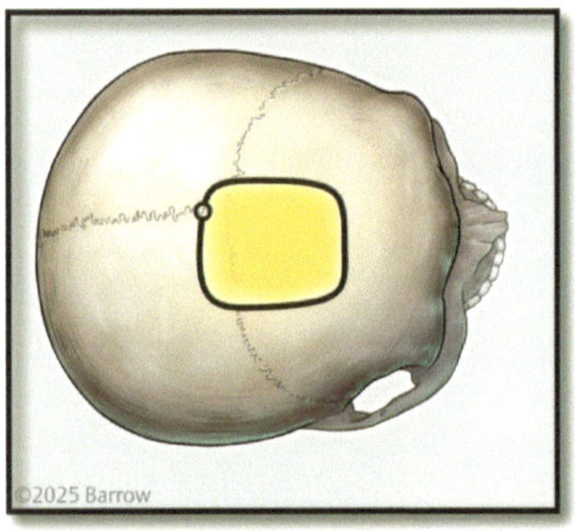

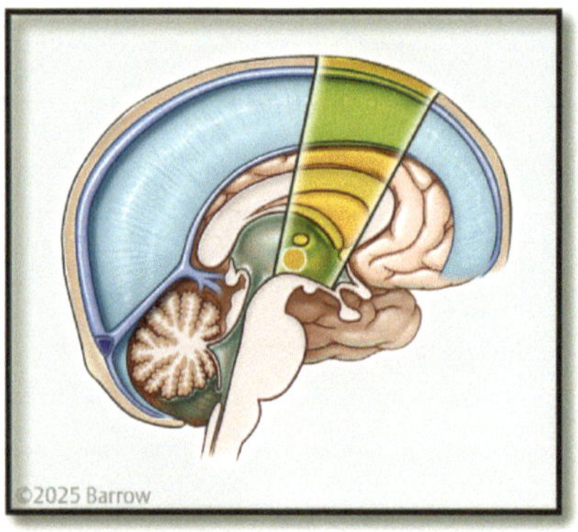

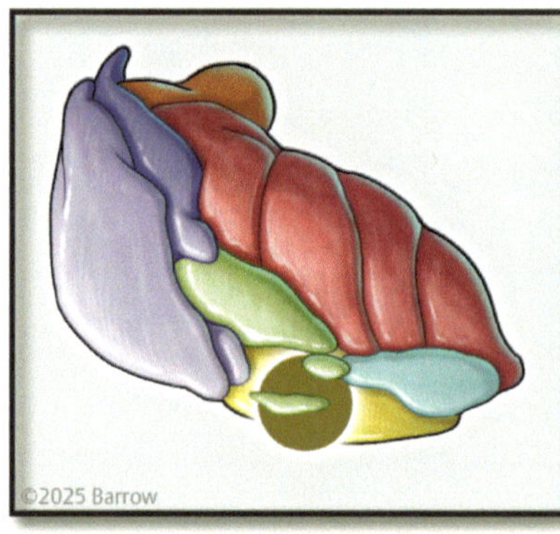

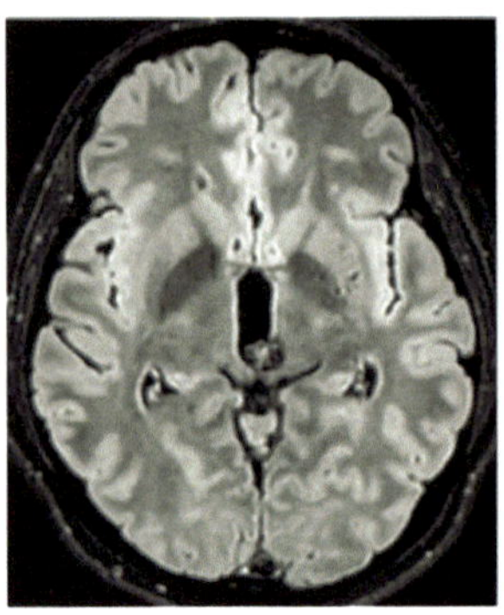

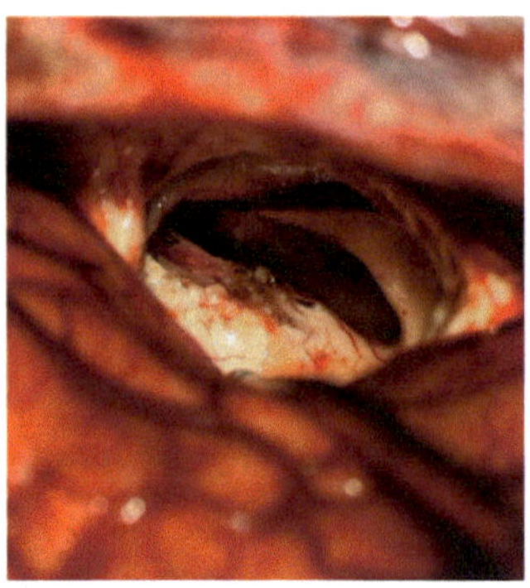

Video 13.2
Contralateral Transcallosal–Contralateral Transchoroidal Approach for Medial Thalamic Cavernous Malformation Resection (Reproduced with permission from Barrow Neurological Institute, Phoenix, AZ.)

13

Surgical Case 13.3

THALAMIC

Cavernoma Subtype: Medial

Position: Lateral position, midline horizontal
Craniotomy: Bifrontal
Approach: Contralateral transcallosal-ipsilateral transchoroidal (cTCal-iTChor)
Triangle: None
SEZ: None
Artery: mPChA

Video: Resection of a right medial thalamic cavernoma

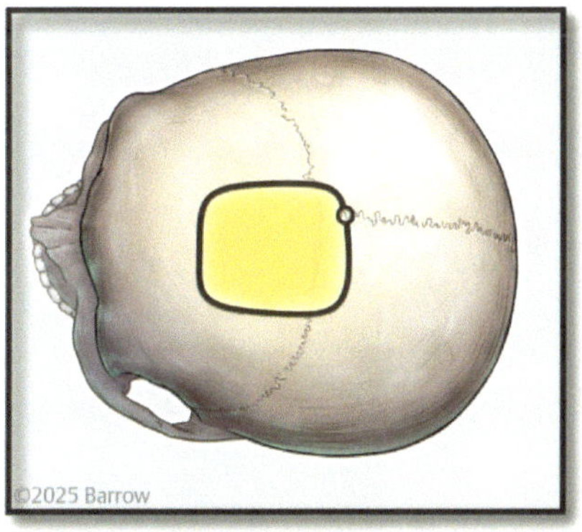

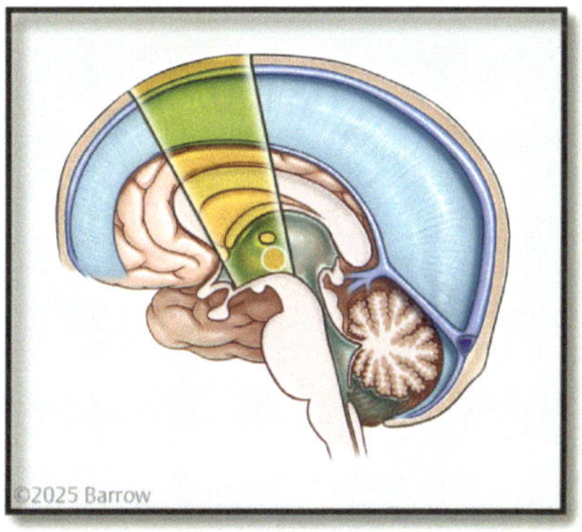

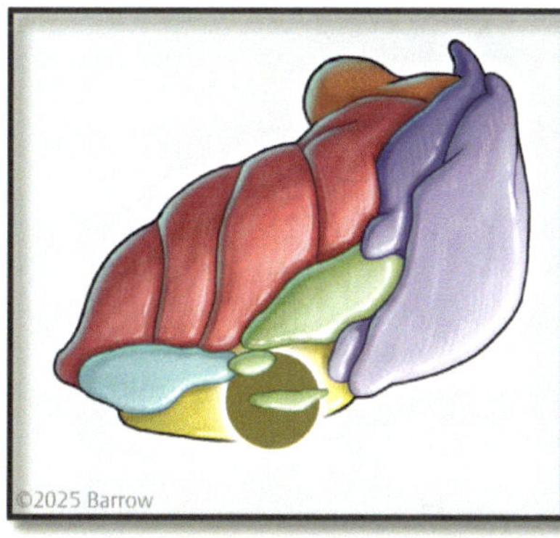

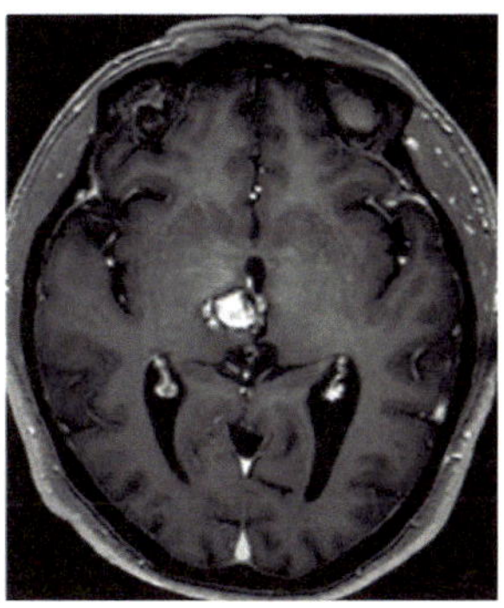

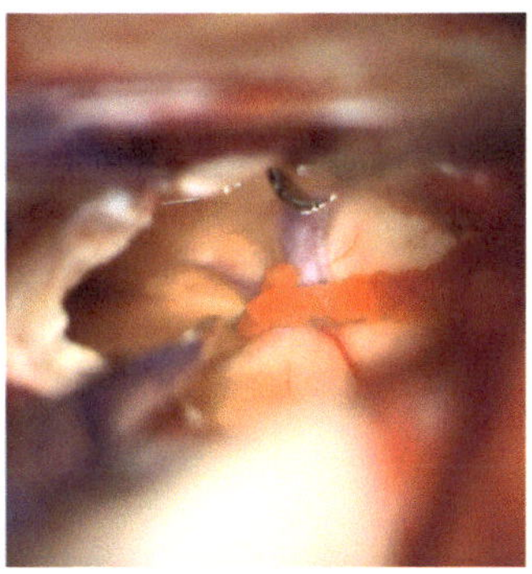

Video 13.3
Contralateral Transcallosal–Ipsilateral Transchoroidal Approach for Medial Thalamic Cavernous Malformation Resection (Reproduced with permission from Barrow Neurological Institute, Phoenix, AZ.)

pulvinar and geniculate nuclei are separate subtypes, and the dorsal nuclei form the lateral ventricular surface of the thalamus and are part of the choroidal subtype. Ventral nuclei relay sensory signals from the body to the sensory cortex, which makes hemisensory deficits the characteristic presentation of patients with this CM subtype. The medial lemniscus and spinothalamic tract relay to the VPL, the trigeminothalamic tract relays to the VPM, and their efferent fibers project to the primary somatosensory cortex. Ventral nuclei also help plan and initiate movements, which makes hemiparesis the other characteristic presentation of these patients. The VA nucleus receives afferent signals from the globus pallidus and substantia nigra and sends efferent signals to the premotor cortex. The VLa and VLp nuclei process motor feedback from the cerebellum, receiving afferent signals from deep cerebellar nuclei and the globus pallidus and sending efferent signals to the supplementary motor area, premotor, and motor cortex.

Lateral thalamic CMs are exposed through a TSyl-PIns approach that skirts the posterior limb of the internal capsule (▶ Fig. 13.7; ▶ Video 13.4, ▶ Video 13.5). On an axial brain section, a transverse line through the foramen of Monro bisects the insula into anterior and posterior parts. A transsylvian-anterior transinsular (TSyl-AIns) approach in front of the foramen of Monro reaches the basal ganglia structures, including the caudate head, putamen, and globus pallidus, as well as the anterior limb of the internal capsule. In contrast, a TSyl-PIns approach behind the foramen of Monro reaches the posterior limb of the internal capsule and lateral thalamus. Lateral CMs in the VA, VLa, and VLp lie just inside the descending motor tracts and are inaccessible, while those in the VPL and VPM nuclei are more accessible. A pterional craniotomy with the wide splitting of the sylvian fissure exposes the M2 (insular) segments of the middle cerebral artery (MCA) in the sylvian cistern at the limen insulae and follows them distally across the insula. Apposition or interdigitation of the frontal and temporal lobes or overlying venous complexes makes the operculum difficult to open. Dissection through the sylvian sulcus follows multiple M3 (opercular) segments to reach the circular sulcus, separates the pia-to-pia adhesions of the intervening operculum, and opens widely into the circular sulcus to access the insular cortex. A smaller parietotemporal craniotomy and more direct entry into the distal sylvian fissure can be used in patients with open or atrophic fissures. Access to lateral CMs requires dissection through one of the long gyri of the insula, typically inferior to the M2 segments. This entry zone is deepened through the external capsule, putamen, and posterior limb to reach the thalamus, taking great care to stay in the posterior third of the posterior limb to avoid sensorimotor tracts. This eloquent dissection proceeds below the pre- and postcentral gyri and above Wernicke's area in the dominant hemisphere.

13.4.4 Choroidal

Although the choroid plexus is not part of the thalamus, it is an adherent intraventricular landmark on the thalamus's superior surface that approximates the location of the otherwise invisible internal medullary lamina. Choroidal CMs surfacing on this floor of the lateral ventricle are lateral to the choroid plexus in the LD and LP nuclei or under the choroid plexus in the medial dorsal nucleus. This distribution of nuclei in the choroidal subtype demonstrates that although the internal medullary lamina neatly subdivides the thalamic nuclei into anterior, medial, and lateral groups, it offers no visible landmarks to locate targeted CMs. The taxonomy relies on visible anatomy apparent intraoperatively and on microsurgically accessible thalamic surfaces.

Choroidal CMs are accessed through a transcallosal-transventricular approach with gravity retraction to open the anterior interhemispheric fissure, as discussed with anterior and medial CMs (▶ Fig. 13.8; ▶ Video 13.6). The superior thalamic surface is at the center of the lateral ventricle. Ipsilateral approaches are usually adequate to reach the targeted CM. Nonetheless, contralateral approaches were occasionally chosen to reach laterally or to approach left-sided lesions from the right and avoid the bridging veins to the superior sagittal sinus in the dominant hemisphere. Choroidal CMs located underneath the choroid plexus were exposed by dissecting through the tenia thalami and mobilizing the choroid plexus medially (subchoroidal approach). Once the exophytic CM or its hemosiderin stain is reached, the exposure provides a working window within the venous angle between the ThaStrV and the stria terminalis laterally and the choroid plexus and the fornix medially. CMs located medial to the choroid plexus belong to the medial subtype and require a contralateral TCal-TChor approach. Similarly, CMs located posterior to the bend of the fornix where the crus begins belong to the pulvinar subtype and require an SPL-Atr approach.

13.4.5 Pulvinar

The pulvinar, which Rhoton calls the *buttock* of the thalamus, is its largest nucleus (accounting for ~40% of its volume). It receives information about eye movements from the superior colliculi and movements of the visual image from the LGN. The pulvinar connects with the visual cortex and helps the secondary visual cortex detect rapid motion, stabilizes perception during saccadic eye movements, and subtracts eye movements from movements of the retinal image. Despite the pulvinar's involvement in visual processing and attention, visual symptoms and signs were recorded in less than half of the patients in our cohort. They were less common than the hemisensory deficits and hemiparesis related to the adjacent posterior limb of the internal capsule.

Pulvinar CMs that presented posterolaterally to the anterior wall of the atrium inside the lateral ventricle were accessed through an SPL-Atr approach. Those that presented posteromedially to the anterior wall of the quadrigeminal cistern were accessed through a SCIT-Para approach (▶ Fig. 13.9; ▶ Video 13.7, ▶ Video 13.8). An anatomical dividing line formed by the crus of the fornix guides the selection of approach, with the SPL-Atr approach chosen for superolateral lesions at the atrial ependyma underneath the choroid plexus and the SCIT-Para approach chosen for inferomedial lesions below the crus of the fornix. It should be noted that CMs presenting to the inferolateral pulvinar on the roof of the ambient cistern in the region of the MGN and LGN are classified as geniculate CMs and accessed through the cSCTT approach. The SPL-Atr approach is performed through a parietal craniotomy, with the patient positioned laterally and the head turned toward the floor to bring the parietal convexity uppermost in the field. A trajectory through the superior parietal lobe is selected using frameless stereotactic

Surgical Approach

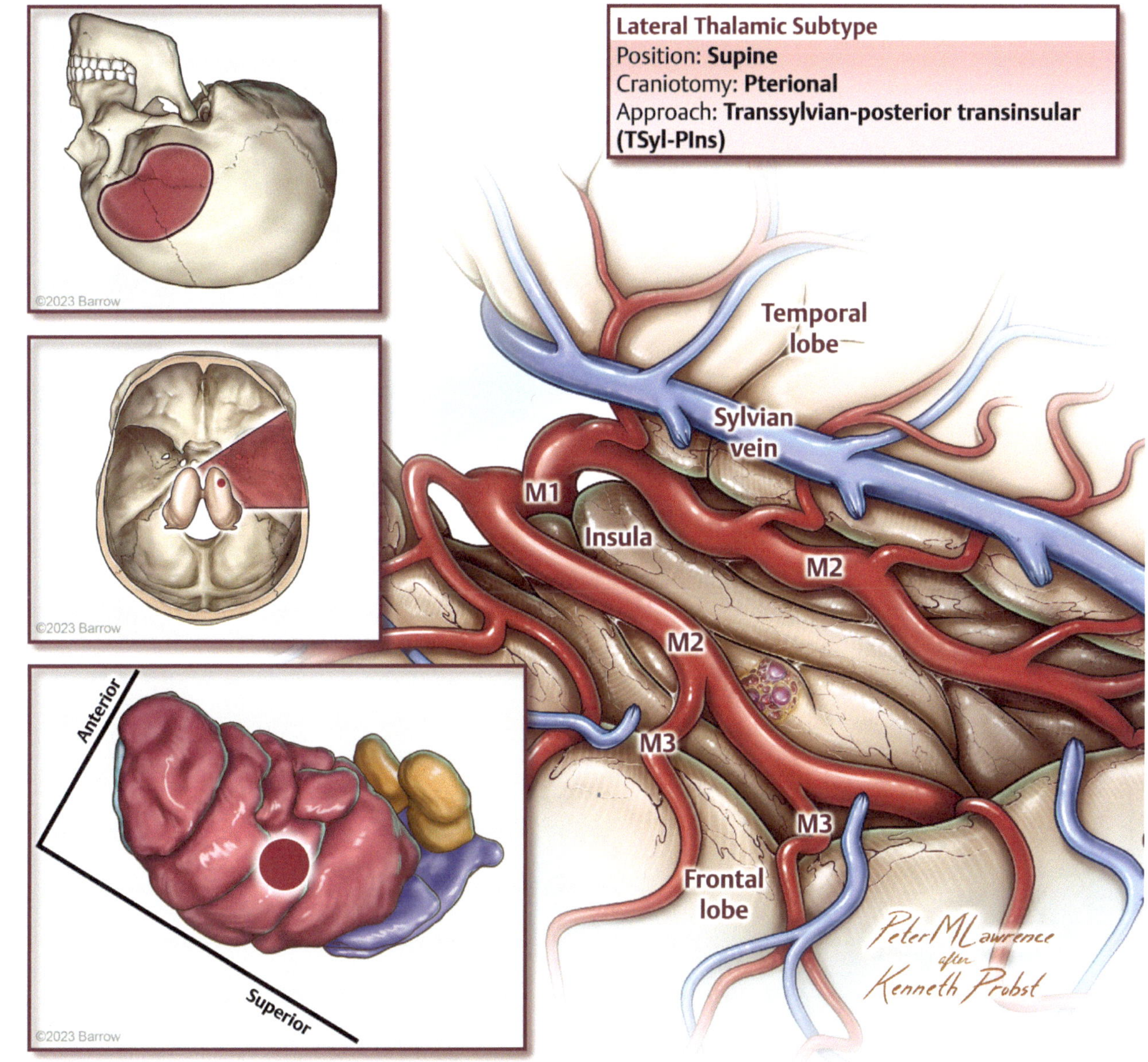

Fig. 13.7 Lateral thalamic CMs are accessed through a pterional craniotomy (*upper left inset*). Superior view shows CM (*middle left inset*; *red circle*) and TSyl-PIns approach. Wide splitting of the sylvian fissure exposes the M2 segments in the sylvian cistern at the limen insulae and follows them distally across the insula. A smaller parietotemporal craniotomy and more direct entry into the distal sylvian fissure can be used in patients with open or atrophic fissures. Access to lateral thalamic CMs requires dissection through one of the long gyri of the insula, typically inferior to the M2 segments. This entry zone is deepened through the external capsule, putamen, and posterior limb to reach the thalamus (*lower left inset*; *red circle*), staying in the posterior third of the posterior limb to avoid sensorimotor tracts (surgical cases; ▸ Video 13.4, ▸ Video 13.5; QR codes). (Reproduced with permission from Barrow Neurological Institute, Phoenix, AZ.)

Surgical Case 13.4

THALAMIC

Cavernoma Subtype: Lateral

Position: Supine
Craniotomy: Frontotemporal
Approach: Transsylvian–posterior transinsular (TSyl-PIns)
Triangle: None
SEZ: None
Artery: M2 MCA

Video: Resection of a right lateral thalamic cavernoma

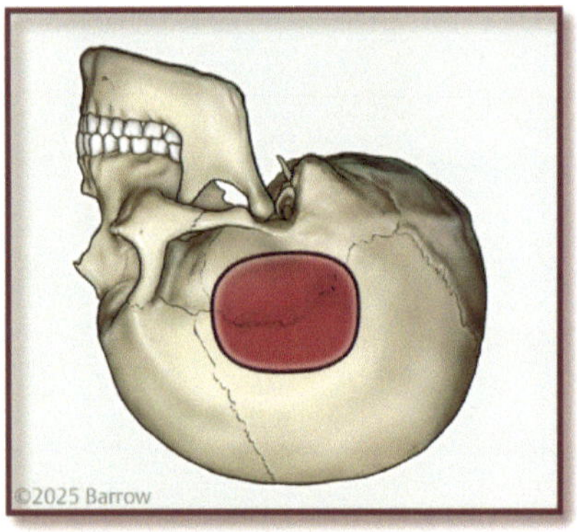

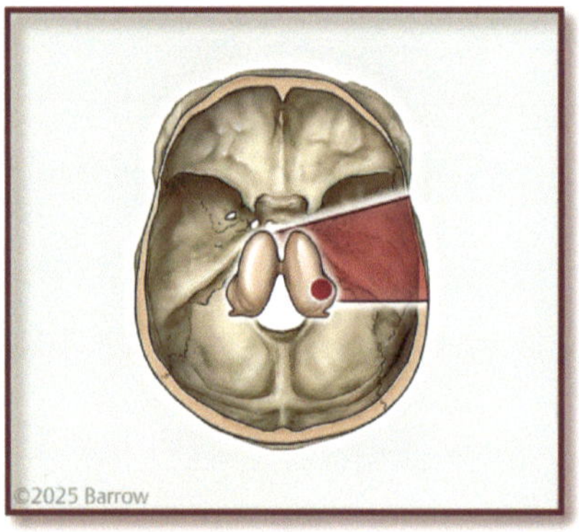

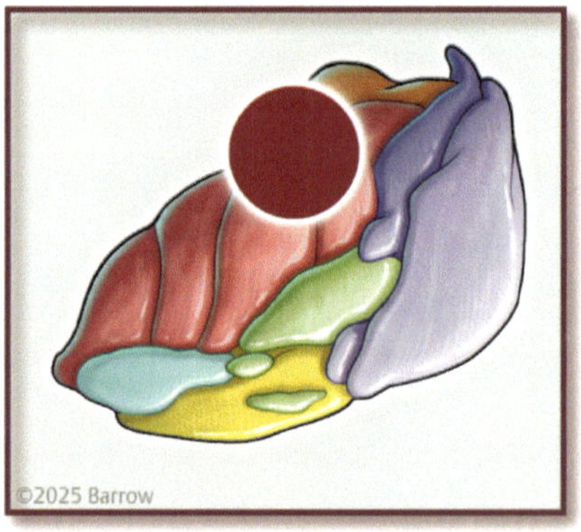

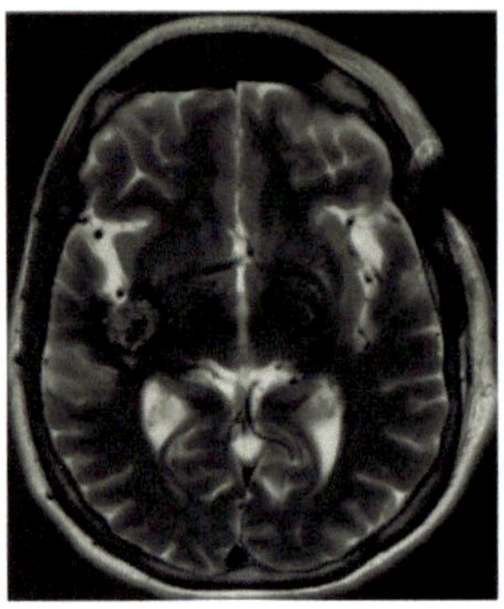

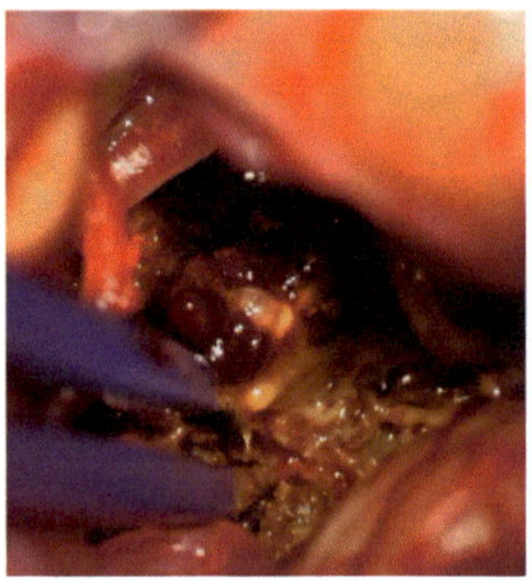

Video 13.4
Transsylvian–Posterior Transinsular Approach for Insular and Lateral Thalamic Cavernous Malformation Resection (Reproduced with permission from Barrow Neurological Institute, Phoenix, AZ.)

13

Surgical Case 13.5

THALAMIC & BASAL GANGLIAL

Cavernoma Subtype: Lateral

Position: Supine
Craniotomy: Pterional
Approach: Transsylvian–posterior transinsular (TSyl-PIns)
Triangle: None
SEZ: None
Artery: M2 MCA

Video: Resection of a right putaminal thalamic cavernoma

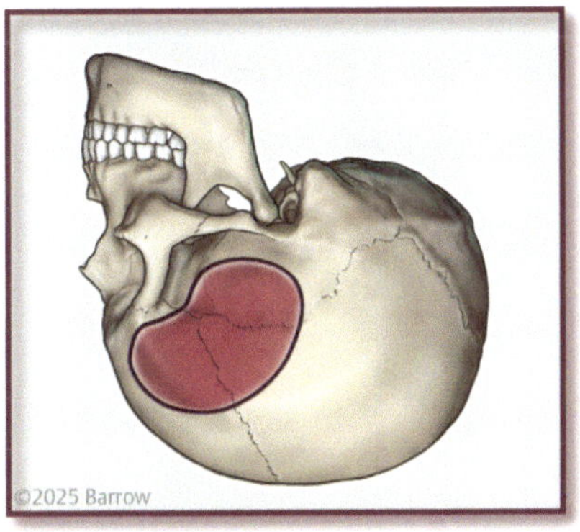

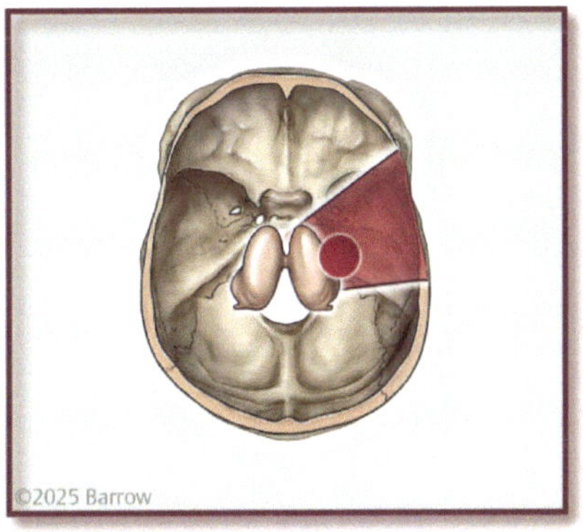

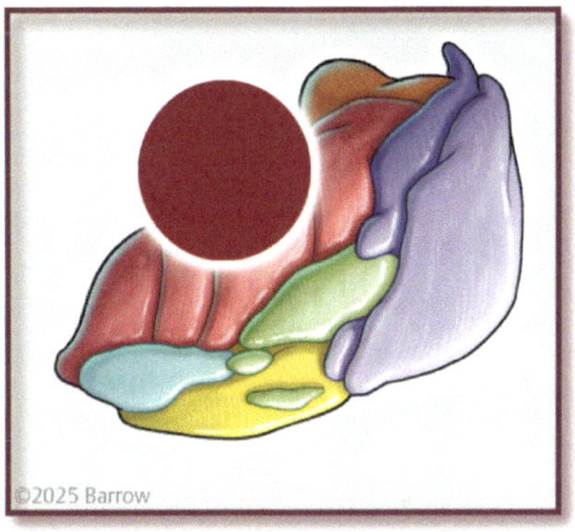

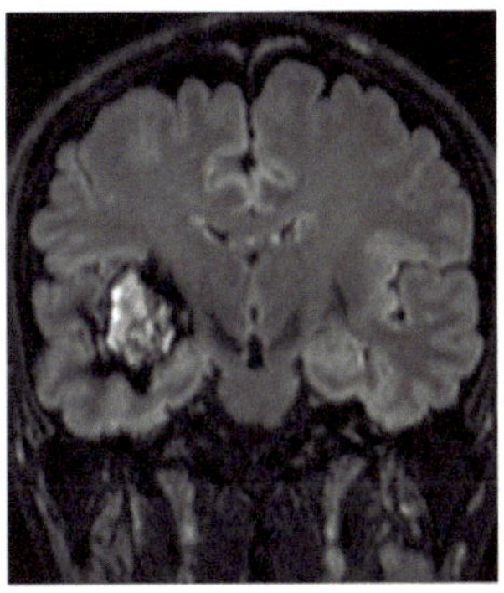

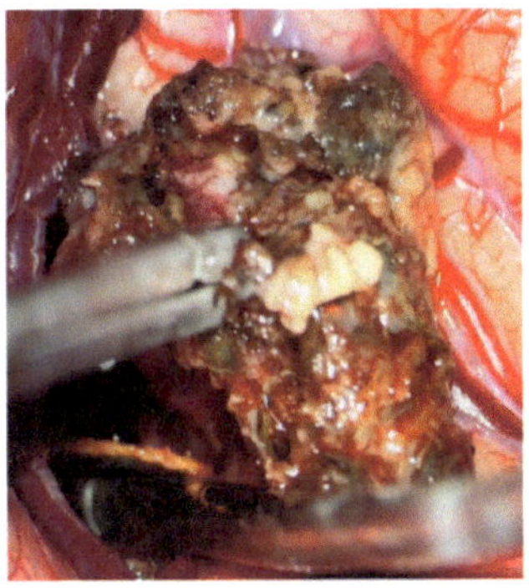

Video 13.5
Transsylvian–Posterior Transinsular Approach for Putaminal Basal Ganglia and Lateral Thalamic Cavernous Malformation Resection (Reproduced with permission from Barrow Neurological Institute, Phoenix, AZ.)

13

Surgical Approach

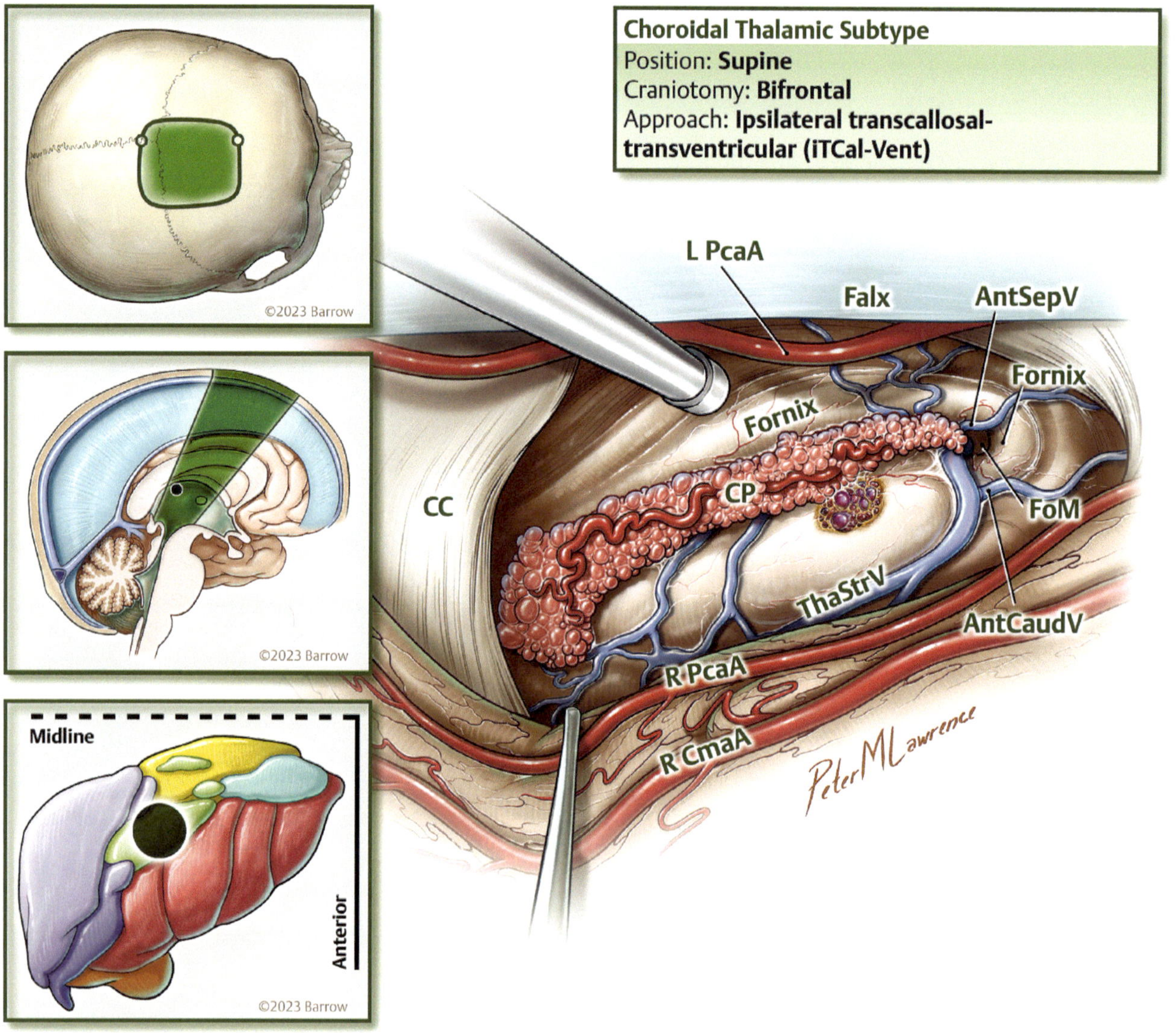

Fig. 13.8 Choroidal thalamic CMs are accessed through a bifrontal craniotomy and iTCal-Vent approach with gravity retraction of the ipsilateral hemisphere (*upper left inset*). An anterior interhemispheric approach was used for most choroidal subtype CMs (*middle left inset*; *green circle*), but a posterior trajectory was used occasionally. The *light green oval* represents the interthalamic adhesion. The superior thalamic surface is exposed in the body of the lateral ventricle (*lower left inset*; *green circle*). Choroidal CMs were exposed by dissecting through the tenia thalami and mobilizing the choroid plexus medially (subchoroidal approach). Once the exophytic CM or its hemosiderin stain is reached, the exposure provides a working window inside the venous angle, between the ThaStrV and stria terminalis laterally and the choroid plexus and fornix medially (surgical case; ▶ Video 13.6; QR code). (Reproduced with permission from Barrow Neurological Institute, Phoenix, AZ.)

navigation; alternatively, an entry point may be selected between 6 and 9 cm above the inion and between 3 and 5 cm lateral to the midline. A C-shaped scalp incision is centered over this entry point, a parietal craniotomy flap is elevated, and a transcortical corridor is opened to the atrium. The atrial portion of the choroidal fissure lies anteriorly between the pulvinar and the crus of the fornix posteriorly. The medial and lateral atrial veins, superior and inferior choroidal veins, and posterior caudate vein often obscure the pulvinar. These veins converge in the choroidal fissure and collect in the ICV and BVR en route to the vein of Galen (VoG). Choroidal arteries (anterior, medial posterior, and lateral posterior) also converge on the atrial

Surgical Case 13.6

THALAMIC

Cavernoma Subtype: Choroidal

Position: Lateral position, midline horizontal
Craniotomy: Bifrontal
Approach: Contralateral transcallosal-transventricular (cTCal-Vent)
Triangle: None
SEZ: None
Artery: mPChA

Video: Resection of a right choroidal thalamic cavernoma

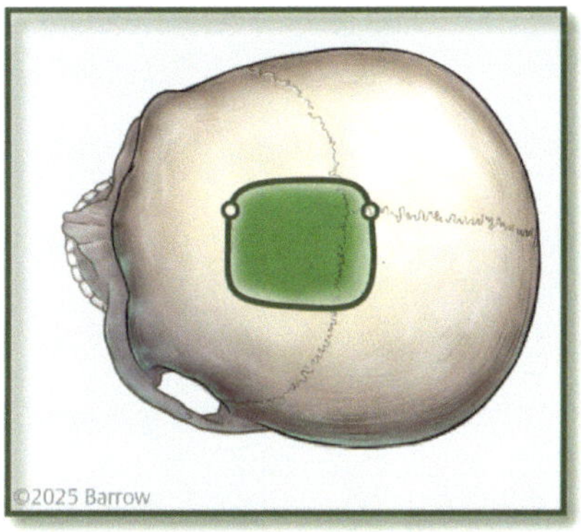

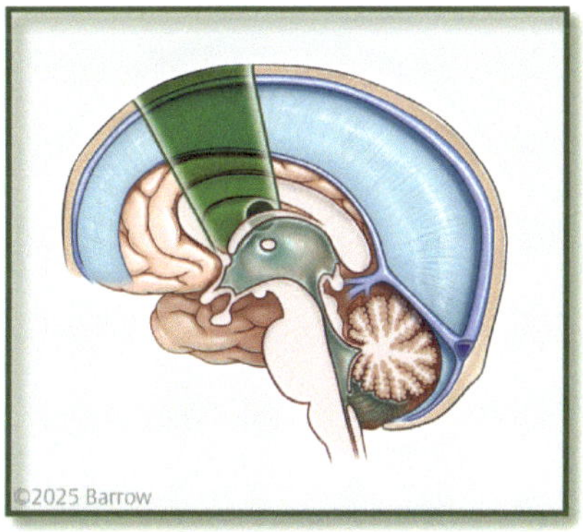

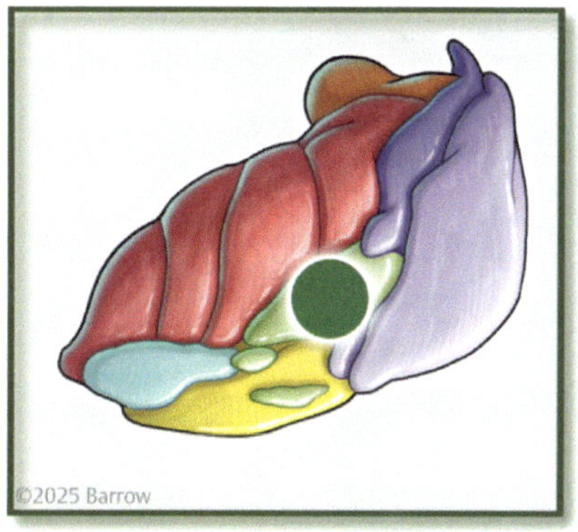

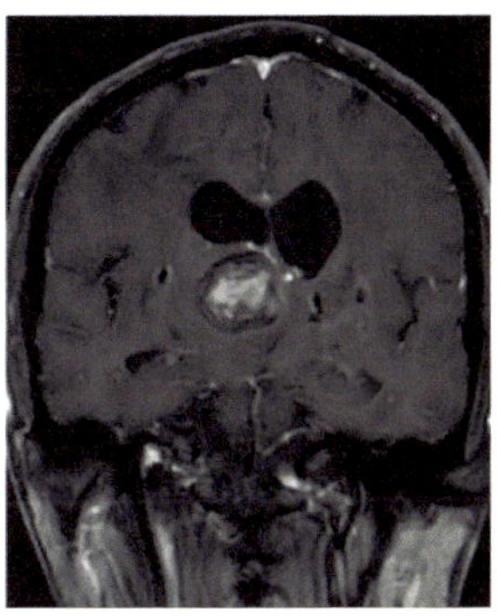

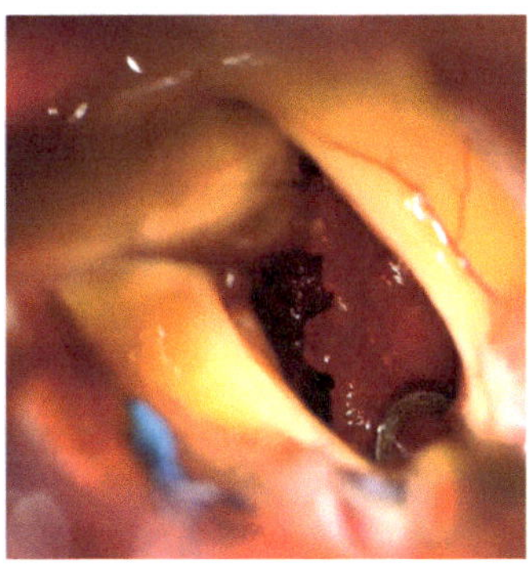

Video 13.6
Contralateral Transcallosal-Transventricular Approach for Choroidal Thalamic Cavernous Malformation Resection (Reproduced with permission from Barrow Neurological Institute, Phoenix, AZ.)

Surgical Approach

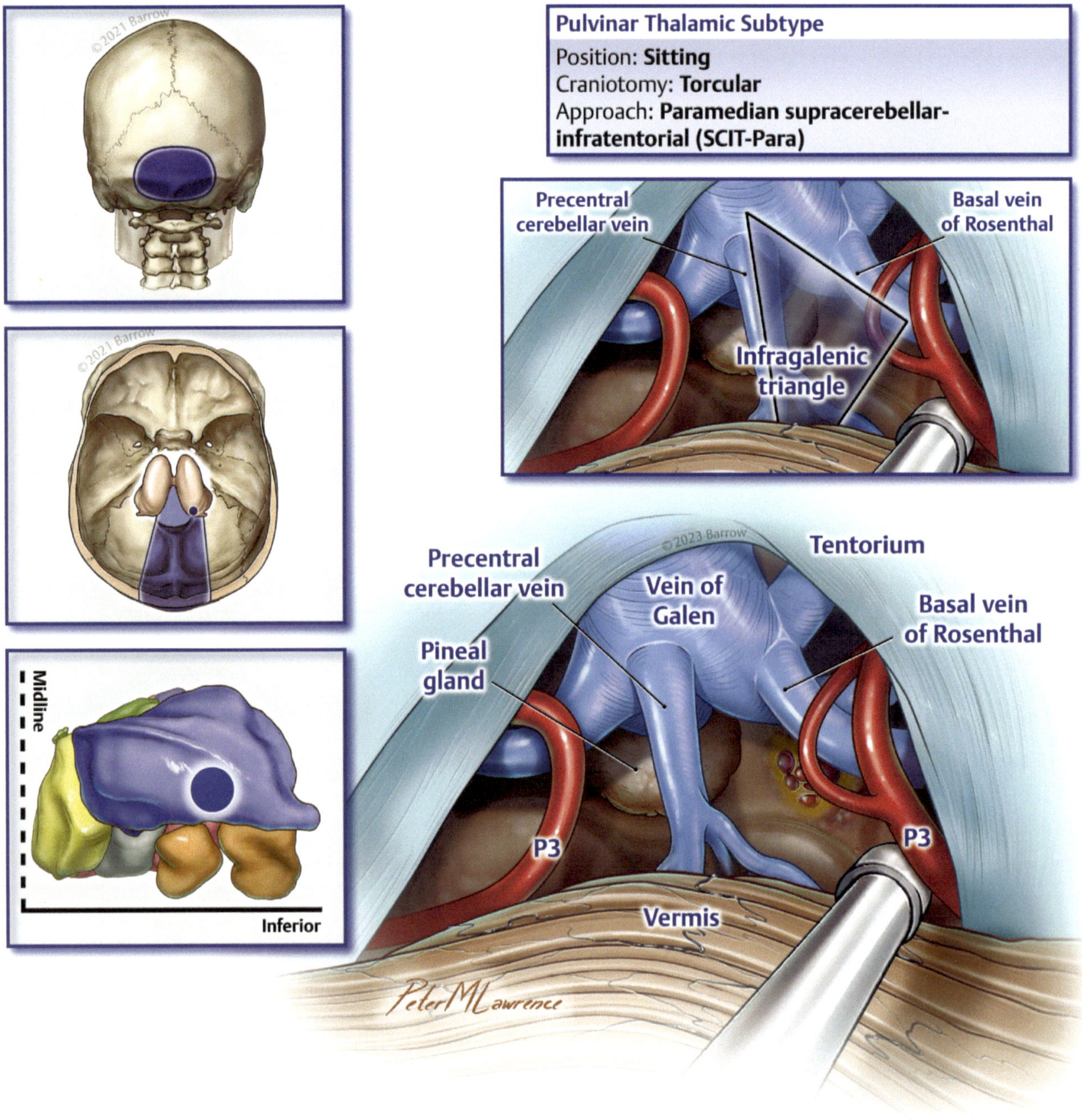

Fig. 13.9 Pulvinar thalamic CMs that present posteromedial to the anterior wall of the quadrigeminal cistern are accessed through a torcular craniotomy (*upper left inset*) and SCIT-Para approach. The torcular craniotomy exposes the transverse sinuses and torcula to remove bony obstructions in the supracerebellar corridor to reach the CM (*middle left inset*; *purple circle*). The sitting position and release of cerebrospinal fluid allow the cerebellum to sag with gravity and the corridor to widen, bringing the tectum and inferolateral thalamus into view (*lower left inset*; *purple circle*). The paramedian trajectory exposes the infragalenic triangle (*upper right inset*) through which the CM can be reached without needing an incision in the tentorium or a contralateral trajectory. Pulvinar CMs that present posterolaterally to the anterior wall of the atrium inside the lateral ventricle are accessed through a SPL-Atr approach (not shown). An anatomical dividing line formed by the crus of the fornix guides the selection of approach, with the SPL-Atr approach chosen for superolateral lesions at the atrial ependyma underneath the choroid plexus and the SCIT-Para approach chosen for inferomedial lesions below the crus of the fornix (surgical cases; ▸ Video 13.7, ▸ Video 13.8; QR codes). (Reproduced with permission from Barrow Neurological Institute, Phoenix, AZ.)

Surgical Case 13.7

THALAMIC

Cavernoma Subtype: Pulvinar

Position: Sitting
Craniotomy: Torcular
Approach: Midline supracerebellar-infratentorial (SCIT-Mid)
Triangle: Infragalenic
SEZ: None
Artery: mPChA

Video: Resection of a left pulvinar thalamic cavernoma

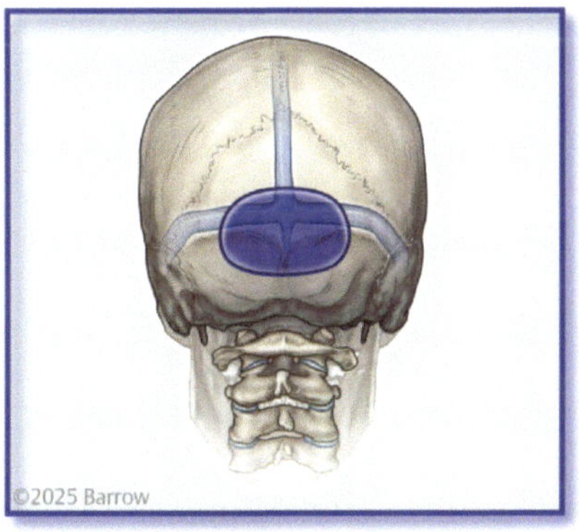

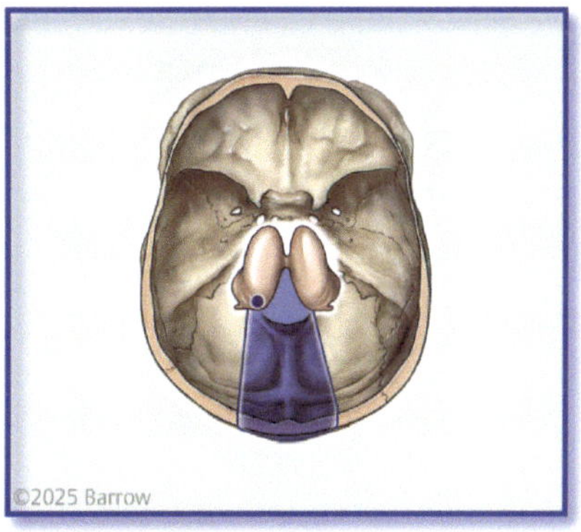

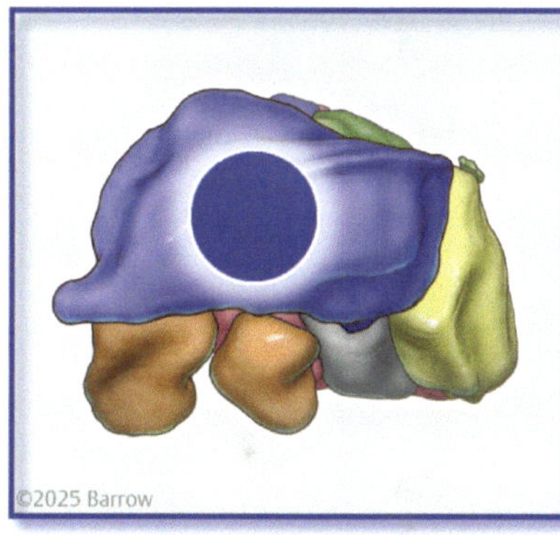

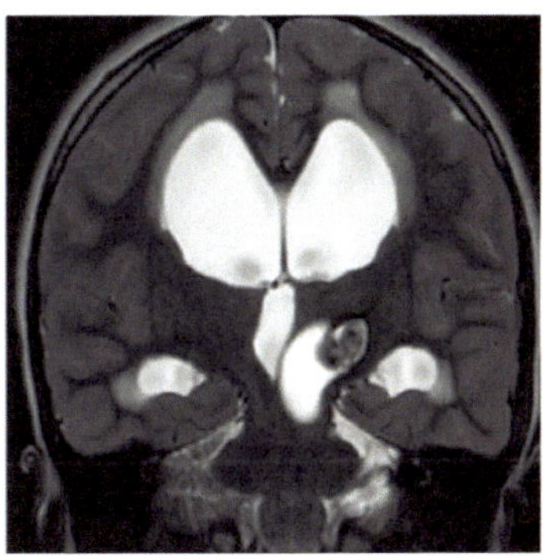

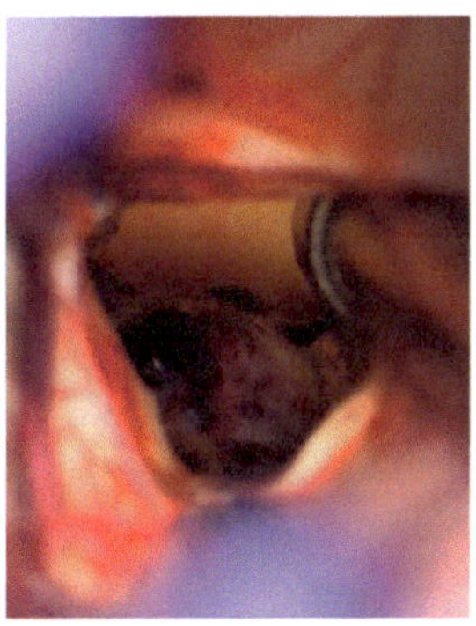

Video 13.7
Midline Supracerebellar-Infratentorial Approach for Pulvinar Thalamic Cavernous Malformation Resection (Reproduced with permission from Barrow Neurological Institute, Phoenix, AZ.)

Surgical Case 13.8

THALAMIC

Cavernoma Subtype: Pulvinar

Position: Sitting
Craniotomy: Torcular
Approach: Midline supracerebellar-infratentorial (SCIT-Mid)
Triangle: Infragalenic
SEZ: None
Artery: mPChA

Video: Resection of a right pulvinar thalamic cavernoma

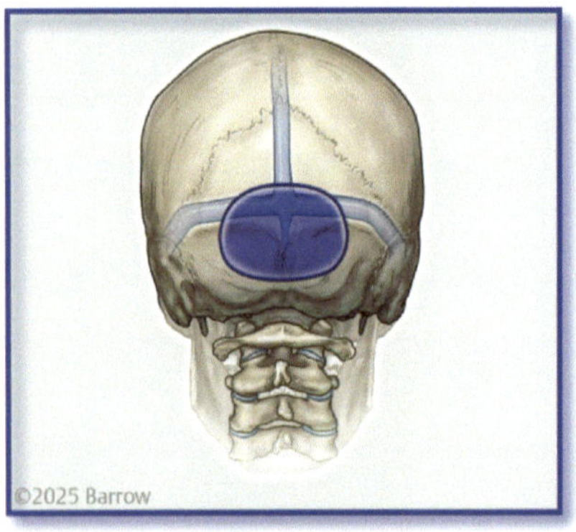

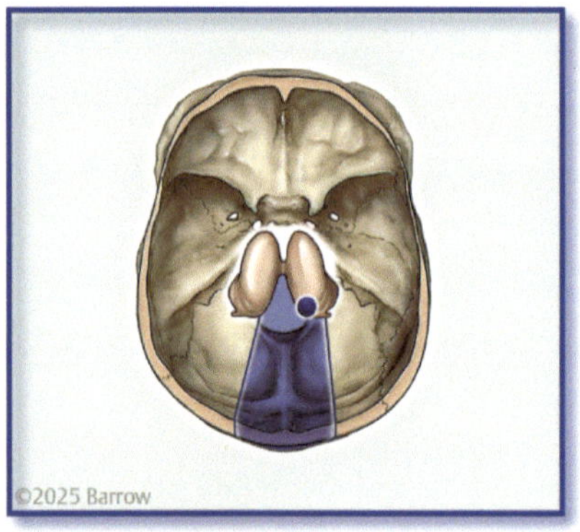

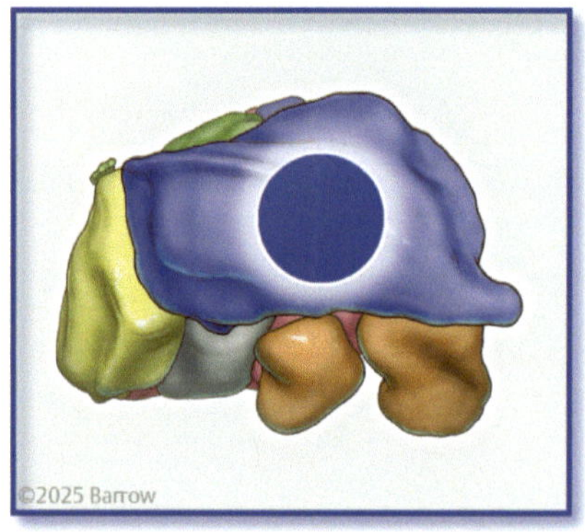

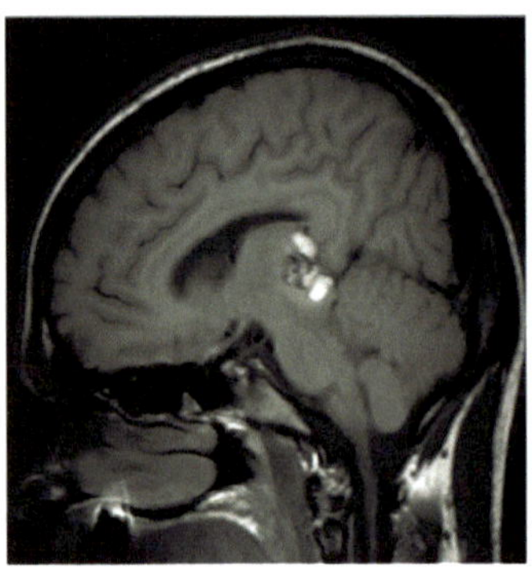

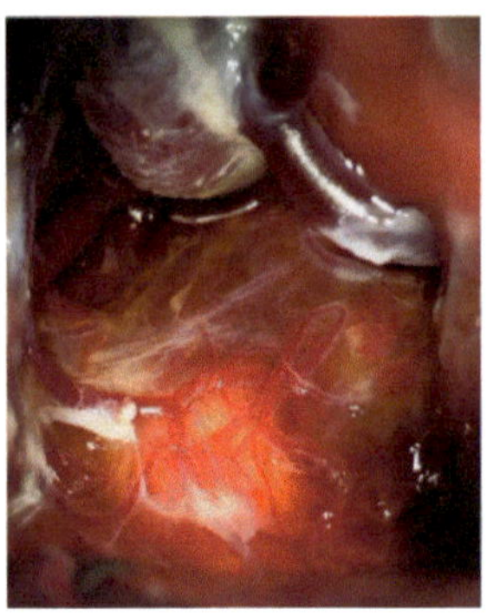

Video 13.8
Midline Supracerebellar-Infratentorial Approach for Pulvinar Thalamic Cavernous Malformation Resection (Reproduced with permission from Barrow Neurological Institute, Phoenix, AZ.)

choroid plexus, sometimes forming a prominent tuft or glomus. This vascular anatomy is mobilized off the CM by opening the choroidal fissure. However, unlike in transchoroidal dissection of medial CMs, the tela choroidea is opened on the thalamic side of the choroid plexus (tenia thalami) to access the pathology directly.

The SCIT-Para approach is performed in the sitting position to allow gravity to retract the cerebellum and steepen the trajectory upward to the pulvinar, as described below for geniculate CMs. The paramedian trajectory lines up nicely with the medial pulvinar and reaches the MGN laterally without needing an incision in the tentorium or a contralateral trajectory. Patients with a patent foramen ovale on echocardiography (with positive bubble test) have an increased surgical risk of air embolism in the sitting position, and the approach must be performed in the prone position instead.

13.4.6 Geniculate

The LGN is the visual relay center of the thalamus. It receives input from the ascending retinal ganglion via the optic nerve and tract and sends axons to the visual cortex via the optic radiations. Therefore, patients with geniculate CMs commonly present with blurred vision and visual field deficits. The MGN is the thalamus's auditory nucleus, directing auditory attention and responses to sound. Hearing deficits were documented infrequently in patients with geniculate CMs.

Geniculate CMs are uniquely surgically accessible because their location in the roof of the ambient cistern is one of the few subarachnoid surfaces of the thalamus. The preferred route is a torcular craniotomy in the sitting position and a cSCTT approach (▸ Fig. 13.10; ▸ Video 13.9, ▸ Video 13.10). The torcular craniotomy exposes the transverse sinuses and torcula to remove any bony obstruction into the supracerebellar corridor. The dural flap lifts the torcula further. The sitting position and release of cerebrospinal fluid allow the cerebellum to sag with gravity and lower the inferior limit of the corridor. These maneuvers open the quadrigeminal and ambient cisterns, bringing the tectum and inferolateral thalamus into view. The conventional SCIT-Para approach may be sufficient to visualize small CMs located in the MGN, and the cSCTT approach increases access laterally. Incising the tentorium removes the lateral constraints of the incisura, and the approach from the side opposite the lesion steepens the crossing trajectory to enter the ambient cistern for lesions located in the LGN. Working in the infragalenic triangle formed by the confluence of the precentral cerebellar vein (PreCenCblV), BVR, and VoG steers the approach to the LGN. Excursions over the shoulder of the BVR lead to the lateral pulvinar. The P3 segments of the PCA course supratentorially and vanish behind the tentorium. Similarly, the supratentorial location of the medial occipital vein differentiates it from the BVR. Immediately deep to geniculate CM targets along this cSCTT trajectory lies the VPL, the posterior limb of the internal capsule, and the optic radiations, which can cause hemisensory and visual field deficits. Therefore, the deep margin of geniculate CMs must be carefully monitored and protected during resection.

13.5 Iterative Advances

Classification of thalamic CMs into anterior, medial, lateral, choroidal, pulvinar, or geniculate subtypes meaningfully guides the selection of surgical approach from many possible options. Variations of the transcallosal approach were used for three subtypes (anterior, medial, and choroidal), including ipsi- and contralateral trajectories that adjust the laterality of approach or maneuver above or below the fornix. Variations through the foramen of Monro or choroidal fissure drop deeper into the ventricular system to access anterior and medial target CMs. Variations of the supracerebellar approach that use paramedian, transtentorial, or contralateral trajectories were used for two subtypes. Favorable functional outcomes were observed in most of these patients, validating the use of these modifications.

This taxonomy is not the first attempt at classifying thalamic CMs. Rangel-Castilla and Spetzler proposed a classification with anteroinferior, medial, lateral, posterosuperior, lateral posteroinferior, and medial posteroinferior regions. These six thalamic regions had different allocations of thalamic nuclei than our taxonomy. For example, some anterior nuclei are included in their medial region (region 2), and others are included in their anteroinferior region (region 1). In contrast, all the anterior nuclei were included together in the anterior subtype. Similarly, the previous classification partitioned the pulvinar into three regions (posterosuperior, region 4; lateral posteroinferior, region 5; and medial posteroinferior, region 6), which reside in a singular subtype in our taxonomy. Differences between regions and subtypes did not significantly change the surgical approach used, except in region 1. Region 1 lesions appeared to be predominantly in the basal ganglia, and we describe such lesions as pallidal CMs in the previous chapter and recommend the orbitozygomatic transsylvian supracarotid-infrafrontal (TSyl-SCIF) approach for these lesions. However, the intervening internal capsule makes the TSyl-SCIF approach unsafe for pure thalamic lesions and was not used for our patients. Therefore, our proposed taxonomy can be viewed as an iterative advance to clarify previous territorial definitions of the thalamic CMs and make them more practical and memorable.

Surgical Approach

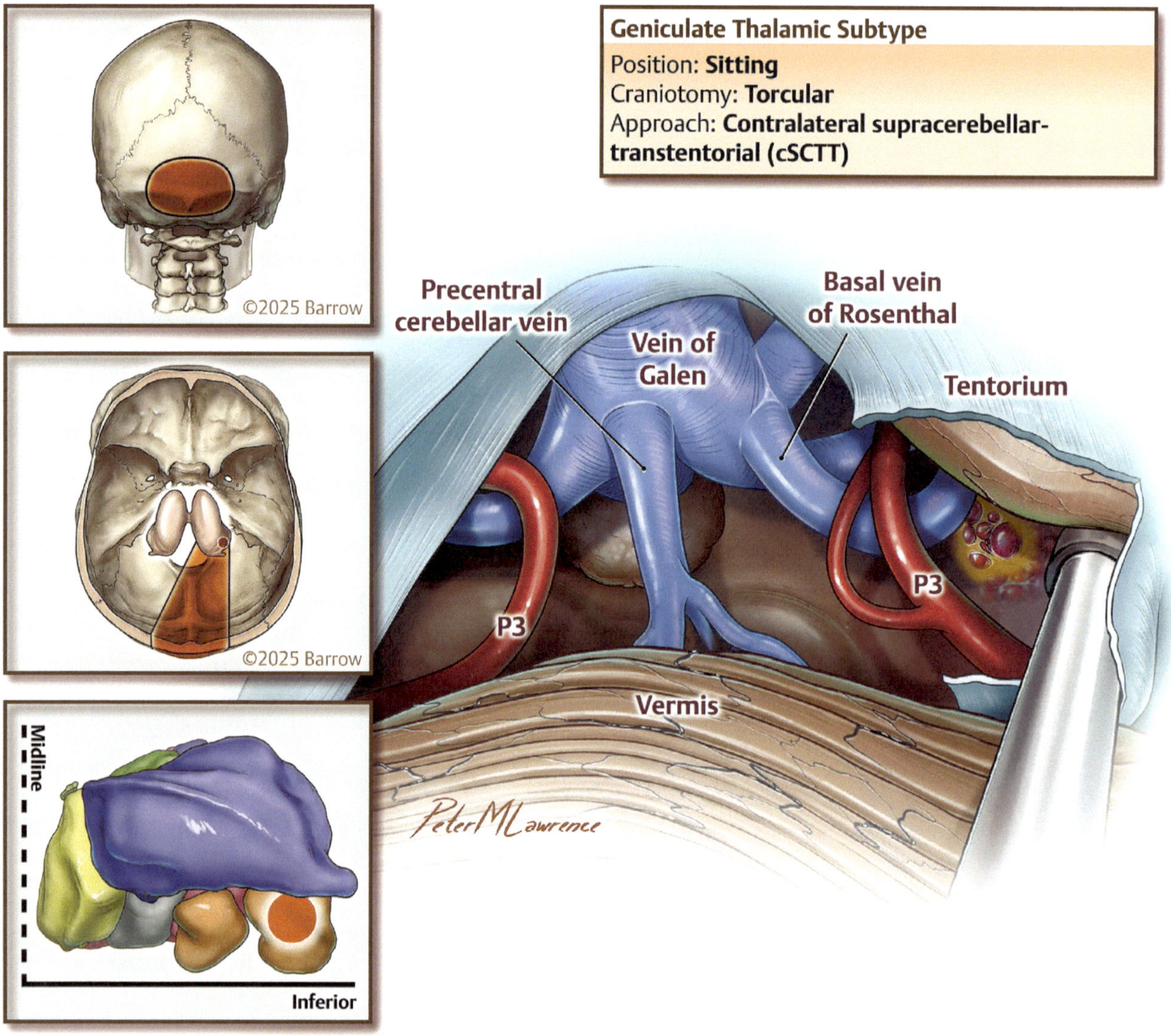

Fig. 13.10 Geniculate thalamic CMs, shown as *orange dots*, are accessed through a torcular craniotomy (*upper left inset*) and cSCTT approach. The conventional SCIT-Para approach may be sufficient to visualize small CMs located in the MGN, but the cSCTT approach increases access to reach more laterally located CMs (*middle left inset*; *orange circle*). Incising the tentorium removes the lateral constraints of the incisura, and the approach from the side opposite the lesion steepens the crossing trajectory to enter the ambient cistern for lesions located in the LGN (*lower left inset*; *orange circle*). Working in the infragalenic triangle formed by the confluence of the PreCenCblV, BVR, and VoG steers the approach to the region of the LGN, whereas excursions over the shoulder of the BVR lead to the lateral pulvinar. The P3 segment of the PCA courses supratentorially and vanishes behind the tentorium, as does the medial occipital vein (surgical cases; ▶ Video 13.9, ▶ Video 13.10; QR codes). (Reproduced with permission from Barrow Neurological Institute, Phoenix, AZ.)

Surgical Case 13.9

THALAMIC

Cavernoma Subtype: Geniculate

Position: Sitting
Craniotomy: Torcular
Approach: Contralateral supracerebellar-transtentorial (cSCTT)
Triangle: Infragalenic
SEZ: None
Artery: mPChA

Video: Resection of a right geniculate thalamic cavernoma

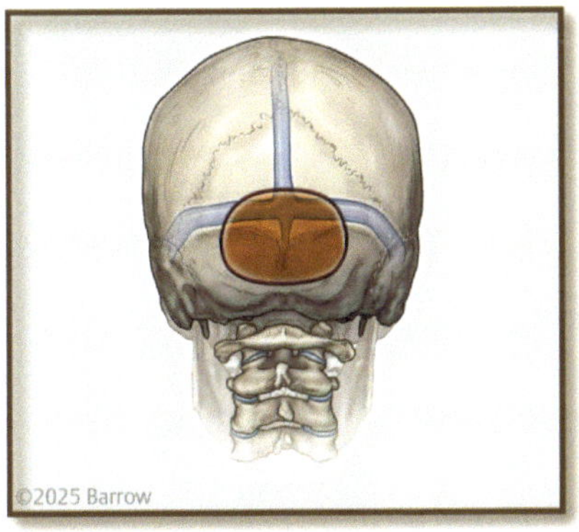

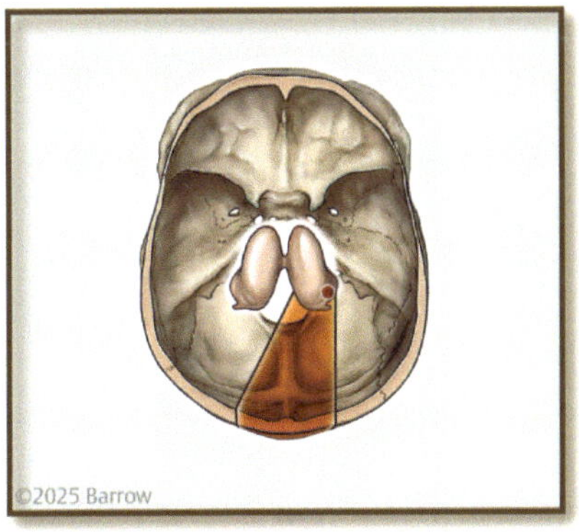

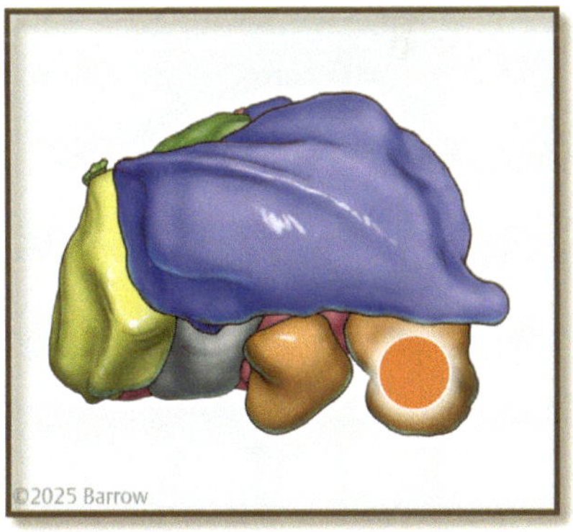

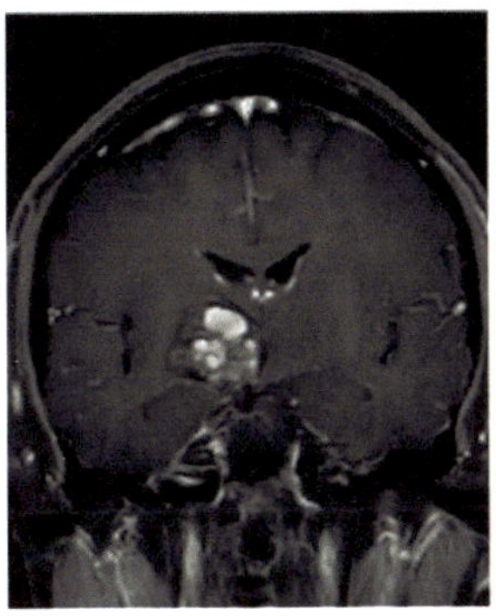

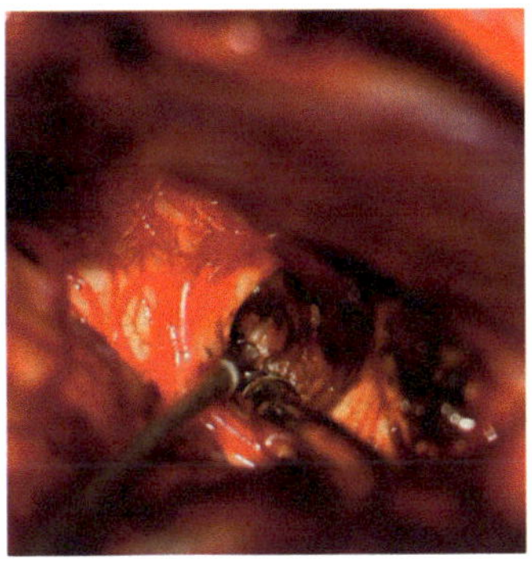

Video 13.9
Contralateral Supracerebellar-Transtentorial Approach for Geniculate Thalamic Cavernous Malformation Resection (Reproduced with permission from Barrow Neurological Institute, Phoenix, AZ.)

13

Surgical Case 13.10

THALAMIC

Cavernoma Subtype: Geniculate

Position: Sitting
Craniotomy: Torcular
Approach: Contralateral supracerebellar-transtentorial (cSCTT)
Triangle: Infragalenic
SEZ: None
Artery: mPChA

Video: Resection of a right geniculate thalamic cavernoma

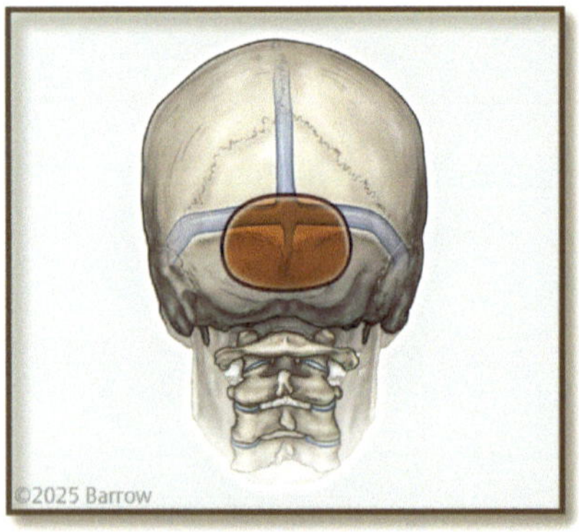

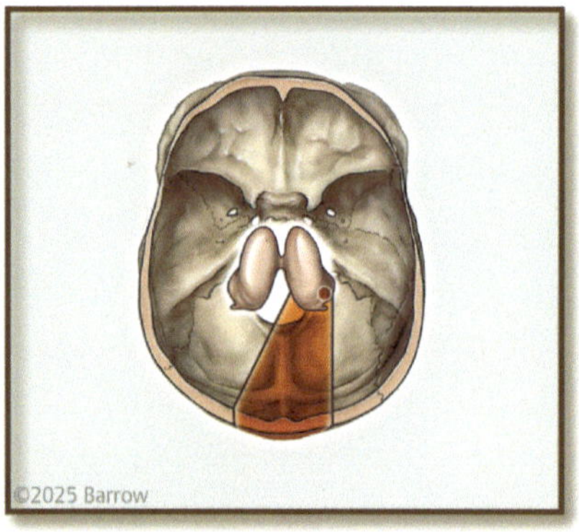

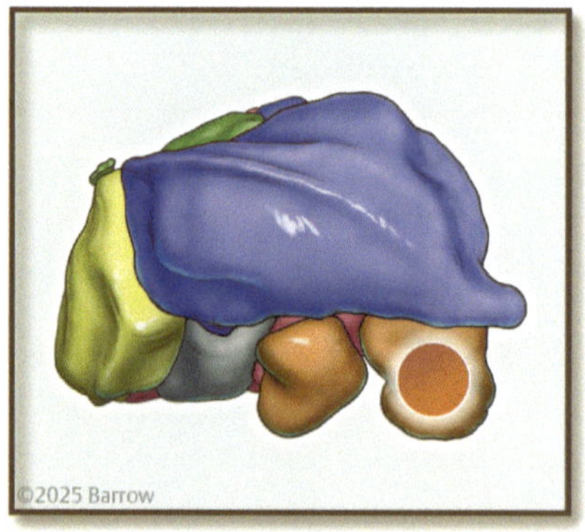

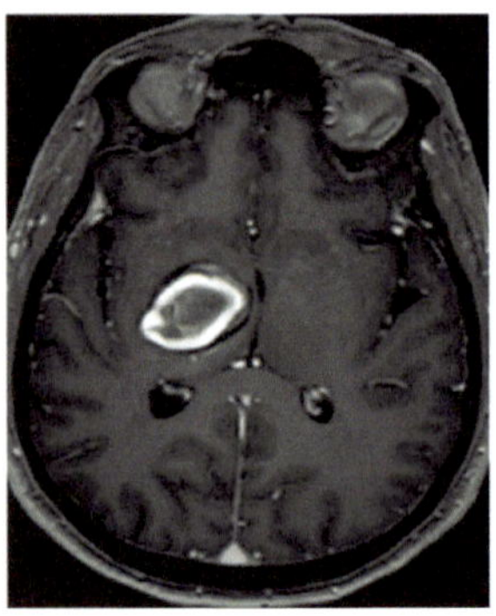

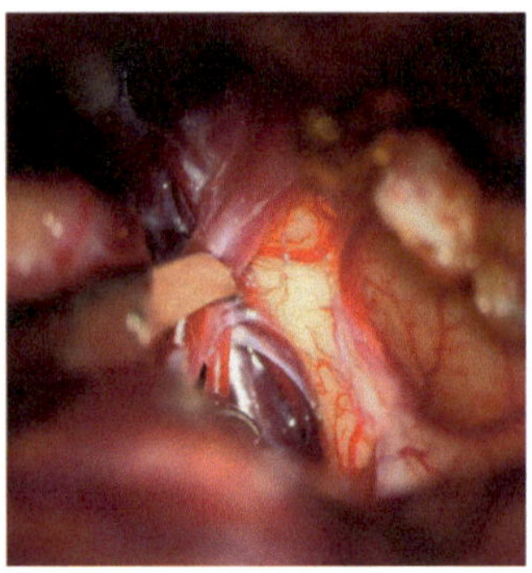

Video 13.10
Contralateral Supracerebellar-Transtentorial Approach for Geniculate Thalamic Cavernous Malformation Resection (Reproduced with permission from Barrow Neurological Institute, Phoenix, AZ.)

13

13.6 Conclusion

The proposed taxonomy can increase diagnostic acumen at the patient's bedside by recognizing the symptoms and signs associated with each subtype. However, unique clinical syndromes were not observed with thalamic CMs as they were with brainstem CMs, which reflects the higher density of cranial nerve nuclei and tracts in the brainstem, as we will see in the next chapters.

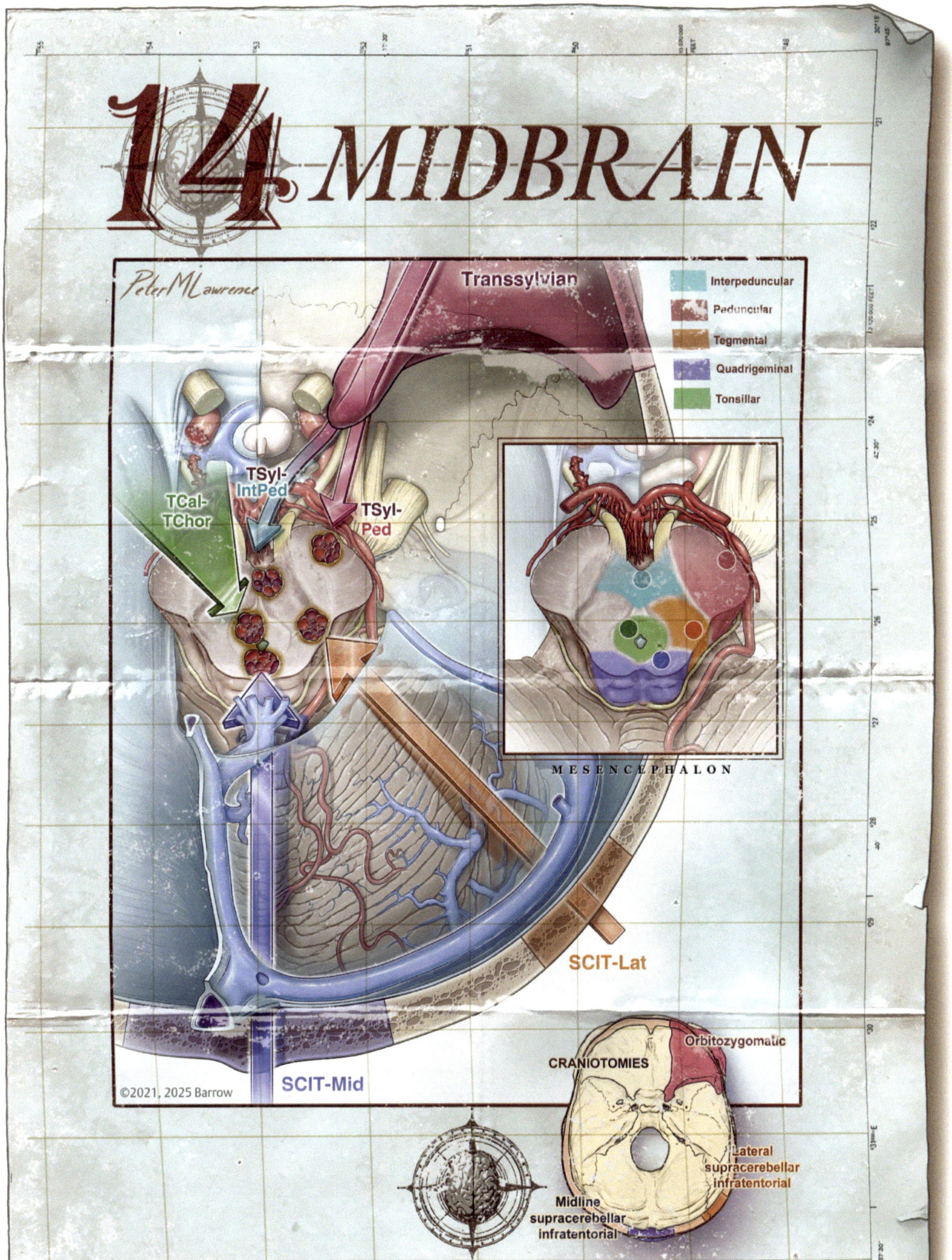

Reproduced with permission from Barrow Neurological Institute, Phoenix, AZ.

14 Midbrain Cavernous Malformations

Summary
Cavernous malformations (CMs) in the midbrain, pons, and medulla were once considered inoperable because of their eloquent location. Managing midbrain CMs is the focus of this chapter. Heuristic grading accounts for lesion size, location, venous anomalies, patient age, and hemorrhage. Traditionally, the surgical approach has been selected on the basis of where the CM presented to a pial or ependymal surface, the optimal approach to that location, and the optimal surgical trajectory. The midbrain CM taxonomy guides the approach selection and resection strategy. Five subtypes of midbrain CMs are defined by surface presentation: interpeduncular, peduncular, tegmental, quadrigeminal, and periaqueductal. This taxonomy was applied to 151 cases of midbrain CMs microsurgically resected over a 30-year period. Seven of 151 midbrain CMs (5%) were the interpeduncular subtype, 37 (24%) were peduncular, 73 (48%) were tegmental, 27 (18%) were quadrigeminal, and 7 (5%) were periaqueductal. Each midbrain CM subtype was associated with a recognizable constellation of neurologic symptoms. A single surgical approach was preferred for each midbrain CM subtype in over 90% of cases. Transsylvian-interpeduncular approaches were preferred for interpeduncular CMs, transsylvian-transpeduncular approaches were preferred for peduncular CMs, and lateral supracerebellar-infratentorial approaches were preferred for tegmental CMs. Midline supracerebellar-infratentorial or paramedian supracerebellar-infratentorial approaches were preferred for quadrigeminal CMs, and transcallosal-transchoroidal fissure approaches were preferred for periaqueductal CMs. The taxonomy for midbrain CMs meaningfully guided the selection of surgical approaches and resection strategies. It increased diagnostic acumen at the bedside and offered an interventional alternative to manage the difficult and destructive natural history of midbrain CMs and improve patient outcomes.

Keywords: brainstem, cavernoma, constellation, hemorrhage, interpeduncular, peduncular, periaqueductal, quadrigeminal, surgical approach, tegmental

14.1 Introduction

Listen to your patient; he is telling you the diagnosis.

—Sir William Osler; *Books and Men;* remarks made at the opening of the new building of the Boston Medical Library, January 12, 1901

Brainstem cavernous malformations (CMs), once considered inoperable because of their eloquent location, are now routinely resected in patients with symptomatic hemorrhage and surgically accessible lesions. Managing brainstem CMs requires answering two critical questions. First, should the lesion be observed or resected microsurgically? Heuristic grading (e.g., Lawton brainstem CM grading) accounts for lesion size, location, venous anomalies, patient age, and hemorrhage and helps answer this question (see Chapter 9). Surgery is recommended for patients with low-grade (0–II) or intermediate-grade (III–V) CMs and not recommended for patients with high-grade (VI–VII) CMs. However, few guidelines exist for the second question: How should brainstem CMs be approached for resection? The surgical approach has traditionally been selected on the basis of where the CM presented to a pial or ependymal surface, the approach that exposed that location, and the optimal surgical trajectory ascertained by simple concepts like the two-point method. This critical question can now be answered by the midbrain CM taxonomy.

We hypothesized that the Seven Cavernomas taxonomy would guide the surgical approach and resection strategies for brainstem CMs more meaningfully than current heuristics. The taxonomy holds particular value for brainstem CMs relative to other superficial CMs because of the many approach options for the former. In addition, we hypothesized that, with the dense packing of tracts and cranial nerve nuclei in the brainstem, the constellation of neurologic symptoms and signs associated with a hemorrhagic brainstem CM subtype would define it clinically just as its location would define it anatomically. Therefore, any patient with a brainstem CM would have a recognizable neurologic syndrome at the bedside and characteristic radiographic anatomy on magnetic resonance imaging (MRI). Notably, nowhere would Osler's words about clinical presentation and physician acumen ring truer than in the midbrain, pons, and medulla.

14.2 Neuroanatomy of the Five Midbrain Cavernous Malformation Subtypes

Five subtypes of midbrain CMs are defined by surface presentation (▸ Fig. 14.1): interpeduncular, peduncular, tegmental, quadrigeminal, and periaqueductal.

14.2.1 Interpeduncular

Interpeduncular midbrain CMs are located anteriorly in the interpeduncular fossa between the cerebral peduncles, below the mammillary bodies, and above the pontomesencephalic sulcus. This small space, located posterior to the basilar quadrifurcation and the P1 (precommunicating) segment of the posterior cerebral artery (PCA), contains the exit zone of the oculomotor nerves and the entry zone of posterior thalamoperforating arteries in the posterior perforated substance. The interpeduncular midline contains the ventral and dorsal tegmental decussations anteriorly and the oculomotor nerve nuclei, Edinger–Westphal nuclei, and medial longitudinal fasciculi posteriorly. The red nuclei are the largest parenchymal structures and lie at the lateral edges of this region.

14.2.2 Peduncular

Peduncular midbrain CMs occur in the cerebral peduncles on the anterolateral surfaces of the midbrain. Lesions are located at the lateral edge of the oculomotor nerve medially to the lateral mesencephalic sulcus laterally and from the optic tracts superiorly to the pontomesencephalic sulcus inferiorly. Peduncular brainstem CMs are located beneath the distal P1 and P2A (crural) segments of the PCA. Critical motor fibers in the corticospinal tracts occupy the middle third of the peduncle, with frontopontine tracts medially and temporoparieto-occipitopontine fibers laterally. The substantia nigra lies below these tracts, with its reticular and compact parts with pallidonigral, nigrostriatal, and corticonigral fibers between them. Peduncular lesions are lateral to oculomotor nerve fibers and the red nuclei.

14.2.3 Tegmental

Tegmental midbrain CMs occur on the posterolateral midbrain surface between the lateral mesencephalic sulcus and the tectal plate. They lie below the thalamic medial geniculate body and overhanging pulvinar and lie above the pontomesencephalic sulcus. The brachia of the inferior and superior colliculi coursing to the medial and lateral geniculate bodies, respectively, define the upper portion of this tegmental surface. The lemniscal trigone between the brachium of the inferior colliculus and the trochlear nerve defines the lower portion of this surface. These lesions are deep to the s3 (cerebellomesencephalic) segments of the superior cerebellar arteries (SCAs) and their rostral and caudal trunks. Tegmental lesions occur posterior to the cerebral peduncle and red nucleus, lateral to the periaqueductal gray matter, and anterolateral to the tectum. The midbrain tegmentum contains eloquent structures, including the spinothalamic tract, ventral trigeminothalamic tract, medial lemniscus, reticular formation, central tegmental tracts, and brachium and external nucleus of the inferior colliculus.

14.2.4 Quadrigeminal

Quadrigeminal midbrain CMs occur on the posterior surface and present to the tectum or collicular plate. They lie inferior to the pineal gland and superior to the trochlear nerves. These CMs may involve the superior colliculus, inferior colliculus, or both and may be in the midline or eccentric to one side. They lie inside the vertical lines formed by the lateral margins of the colliculi and the exit zone of the trochlear nerves. They are anteroinferior to the vein of Galen complex and are draped by circumflex perforating arteries and the medial posterior choroidal artery. Quadrigeminal CMs involve the colliculi and may extend into the midbrain parenchyma up to the periaqueductal gray matter.

14.2.5 Periaqueductal

The periaqueductal gray matter encircles the aqueduct and is the locus of periaqueductal midbrain CMs. These lesions occur superiorly in the midbrain and centrally around the cerebral (sylvian) aqueduct. They come to an ependymal rather than a pial surface along the aqueduct near the third ventricle. Periaqueductal midbrain CMs are located in the midline or are slightly eccentric and surrounded by the tectum posteriorly, red nuclei and oculomotor nuclei anteriorly, and tegmentum laterally. The mesencephalic nucleus and tract of the trigeminal nerve and dorsal trigeminothalamic tract lie on the lateral periphery of targeted periaqueductal lesions.

14.3 Clinical Evidence

The taxonomy was applied to a two-surgeon experience (M.T.L. and Robert F. Spetzler) of 151 midbrain CMs resected microsurgically over a 30-year period (1990–2019) (▸ Table 14.1). These midbrain CMs were subtyped on the basis of their predominant surface presentation identified on preoperative MRI: interpeduncular (7/151, 5%), peduncular (37/151, 24%), tegmental (73/151, 48%), quadrigeminal (27/151, 18%), and periaqueductal (7/151, 5%). Each midbrain CM subtype was associated with a recognizable constellation of neurologic symptoms (▸ Fig. 14.2). Patients with interpeduncular lesions commonly presented with ipsilateral oculomotor nerve palsy and contralateral cerebellar ataxia or dyscoordination. Peduncular lesions were associated with contralateral hemiparesis and ipsilateral oculomotor nerve palsy. Patients with tegmental lesions were the most likely to present with contralateral sensory deficits, whereas those with quadrigeminal lesions commonly presented with features of Parinaud syndrome. Periaqueductal lesions were the most likely to cause obstructive hydrocephalus.

The Lawton brainstem CM grades were determined for 87 patients: 28 (32%) had low-grade CMs (grades 0–II), 45 (52%) had intermediate-grade CMs (grades III–V), and 14 (16%) had high-grade CMs (grades VI and VII). A single surgical approach was preferred in more than 90% of cases for each midbrain subtype: transsylvian-interpeduncular (TSyl-IntPed) for interpeduncular (7/7), peduncular transsylvian-transpeduncular (TSyl-Ped) for peduncular (24/37), lateral supracerebellar-infratentorial (SCIT-Lat) for tegmental (73/73), midline supracerebellar-infratentorial (SCIT-Mid) or paramedian supracerebellar-infratentorial (SCIT-Para) for quadrigeminal (27/27), and

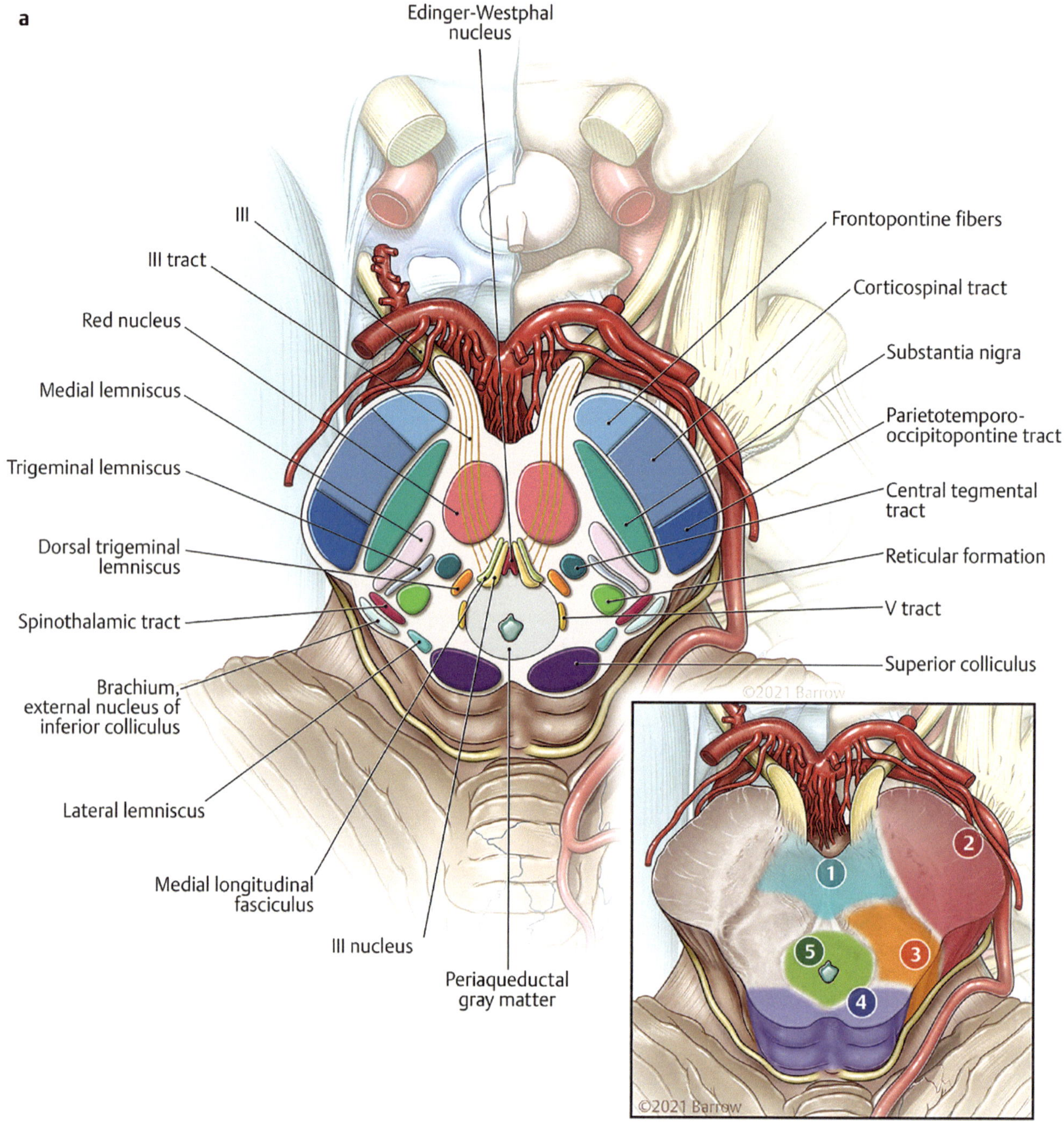

Fig. 14.1 Overview of midbrain anatomy and CM subtypes. **(a)** The anatomy of midbrain nuclei and tracts is shown in axial cross-section. The locations of the five subtypes are shown (*inset with numbered*; *colored circles*) with interpeduncular in *teal*, peduncular in *red*, tegmental in *orange*, quadrigeminal in *purple*, and periaqueductal in *green*.

(Continued)

b

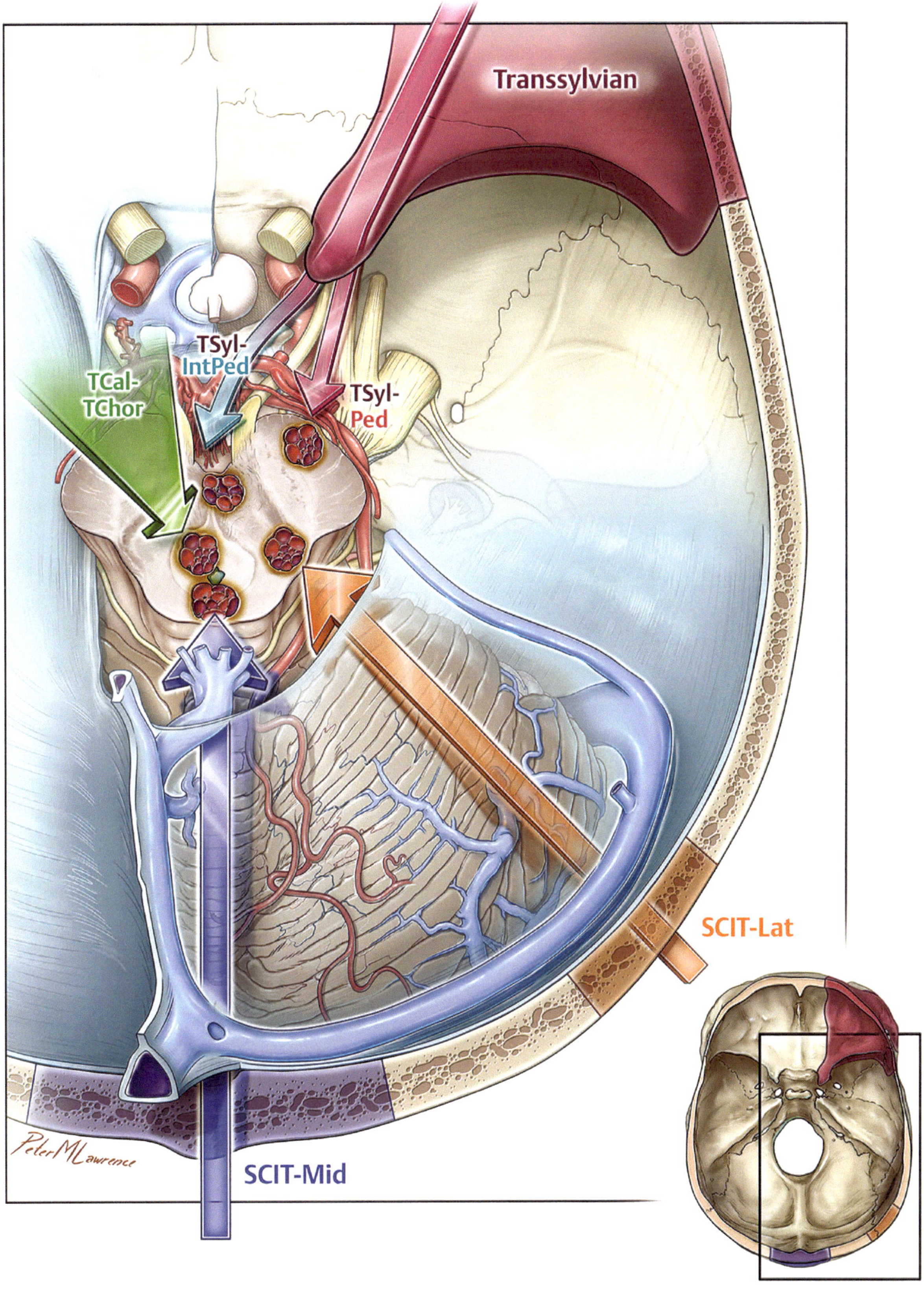

Fig. 14.1 *(Continued)* **(b)** Overview of surgical approaches to midbrain CMs shown in axial cross-section viewed from above. The TSyl-IntPed approach is used for interpeduncular CMs, the TSyl-Ped approach for peduncular CMs, and the SCIT-Lat approach for tegmental CMs. The SCIT-Mid approach is used for quadrigeminal CMs, and the TCal-TChor approach is used for periaqueductal CMs. An orbitozygomatic craniotomy is used for the TSyl-IntPed (*teal arrow*) and TSyl-Ped approaches (*red arrow*), a retrosigmoid craniotomy for the SCIT-Lat approaches (*orange arrow*), a torcular craniotomy for SCIT-Mid approaches (*purple arrow*), and a bifrontal craniotomy for TCal-TChor approaches (*green arrow*). *Inset* shows the skull base view. Roman numerals denote cranial nerves. (Reproduced with permission from Barrow Neurological Institute, Phoenix, AZ.)

Table 14.1 Preoperative and postoperative outcome measures for patients with resection of midbrain CMs by subtype

Variable	All (*N* = 151)	Interpedun-cular (*n* = 7)	Peduncular (*n* = 37)	Tegmental (*n* = 73)	Quadrigeminal (*n* = 27)	Periaqueductal (*n* = 7)	*p*-value
Brainstem CM grade							0.36
Patients with data available	87	0	20	51	14	2	
Low	26 (30)	0 (0)	8 (62)	15 (33)	2 (17)	1 (50)	
Intermediate	35 (40)	0 (0)	3 (23)	22 (48)	9 (75)	1 (50)	
High	12 (14)	0 (0)	2 (15)	9 (20)	1 (8)	0 (0)	
Follow-up							
Mean (SD), mo	25.8 (33.3)	41.1 (45.1)	29.5 (40.0)	23.3 (30.2)	28.4 (30.8)	7.3 (5.3)	0.30
> 30 d	130 (86)	7 (100)	31 (84)	61 (84)	24 (89)	7 (100)	0.49
Preop mRS score							
Median (IQR)	2 (1–2)	2 (1–2)	2 (1–2)	1 (1–2)	2 (1–2)	2 (1–2)	0.37
> 2	20 (13)	1 (14)	7 (19)	7 (10)	4 (15)	1 (14)	0.76
Postop mRS score							
Median (IQR)	2 (1–3)	1 (1–2)	2 (1–3)	2 (1–3)	2 (1–3)	2 (1–3)	0.85
> 2	46 (30)	1 (14)	14 (38)	20 (28)	8 (30)	3 (43)	0.63
Final mRS score							
Patients with data available	136	7	30	67	25	7	
Median (IQR)	1 (1–2)	1 (1–2)	1 (1–2)	1 (1–2)	2 (1–2)	1 (0–2)	0.59
> 2	26 (19)	1 (14)	5 (17)	15 (22)	4 (16)	1 (14)	0.92
≤ 2	110 (81)	6 (86)	25 (83)	52 (78)	21 (84)	6 (86)	0.92
Worsened vs. preop mRS score	31 (23)	0 (0)	5 (17)	17 (25)	7 (28)	2 (29)	0.48

Note: Data are presented as n (%) unless otherwise indicated. Percentages might not total 100% due to rounding.

	Subtype				
Symptom	Interpeduncular (n=7)	Peduncular (n=37)	Tegmental (n=73)	Quadrigeminal (n=27)	Periaqueductal (n=7)
Hemisensory loss	3 (43%)	15 (41%)	45 (62%)	12 (44%)	2 (29%)
Hemiparesis	3 (43%)	24 (65%)	21 (29%)	7 (26%)	5 (71%)
Diplopia	3 (43%)	17 (46%)	26 (36%)	16 (59%)	4 (57%)
Ataxia, dysmetria	5 (71%)	9 (24%)	21 (29%)	5 (19%)	1 (14%)
Oculomotor nerve palsy	3 (43%)	11 (30%)	8 (11%)	3 (11%)	1 (14%)
Trochlear nerve palsy	0 (0%)	0 (0%)	0 (0%)	4 (15%)	0 (0%)
Hemifacial numbness	3 (43%)	5 (14%)	16 (22%)	5 (19%)	0 (0%)
Facial weakness	2 (29%)	8 (22%)	10 (14%)	3 (11%)	2 (29%)
Hydrocephalus	0 (0%)	0 (0%)	3 (4%)	5 (19%)	2 (29%)

Fig. 14.2 Heat map showing symptoms of patients with midbrain CMs by midbrain CM subtype. Percentages were calculated as the frequency of a particular symptom within a given midbrain subtype. The sensitivity and specificity of neurologic examination findings vary substantially. For example, hemiparesis is more likely to be accurately documented in the medical record than trochlear nerve palsy. Thus, rates were sorted for each symptom or sign according to their relative frequency across the five subtypes. Conditional formatting was applied on a scale of least common (*red*) to most common (*green*). Symptoms associated with each subtype are most closely aligned with cells with *green formatting*. (Reproduced with permission from Catapano JS, Rumalla K, Srinivasan VM, Lawrence PM, Larson Keil K, Lawton MT. A taxonomy for brainstem cavernous malformations: subtypes of midbrain lesions. J Neurosurg 2021;136(6):1667–1686).

transcallosal-transchoroidal fissure (TCal-TChor) for periaqueductal (6/7). Favorable outcomes (modified Rankin Scale [mRS] score ≤ 2) were observed in most patients with follow-up (110/136, 81%). Relative outcomes according to mRS scores were improved or unchanged postoperatively in most patients (105/136, 77%). No significant differences in outcomes were observed between subtypes ($p = 0.92$).

14.4 Resection Strategies for Midbrain Cavernous Malformations

A single surgical approach was preferred for each midbrain subtype in over 90% of cases. TSyl-IntPed approaches were preferred for interpeduncular CMs, TSyl-Ped approaches were preferred for peduncular CMs, and SCIT-Lat approaches were preferred for tegmental CMs. SCIT-Mid or SCIT-Para approaches were preferred for quadrigeminal CMs, and TCal-TChor approaches were preferred for periaqueductal CMs.

14.4.1 Interpeduncular

The interpeduncular fossa is a small space traversed by incoming posterior thalamoperforating arteries and outgoing oculomotor nerve fibers, with the red nucleus deep to the posterior perforated substance. Interpeduncular CMs were the least common midbrain subtype (7 of 151, 5%). These patients present with Claude syndrome, characterized by ipsilateral oculomotor nerve palsy, contralateral cerebellar ataxia, and dyscoordination, with or without tremors (▶ Fig. 14.3a). The oculomotor nerve palsy reflects the involvement of fibers coursing through the midbrain from the nerve's nucleus. In contrast, ataxia reflects the involvement of the red nucleus, which receives the cerebellum's major output from the dentate nuclei and decussated superior cerebellar peduncle before projecting to the ventrolateral and anterior nuclei of the thalamus and motor and premotor cortex. Patients with large lesions present with Benedikt syndrome encompassing Claude syndrome and contralateral hemiparesis or hemiplegia due to corticospinal tract involvement in the adjacent peduncle.

Interpeduncular midbrain CMs are accessed through an orbitozygomatic craniotomy and TSyl-IntPed approach (▶ Fig. 14.3b; ▶ Video 14.1, ▶ Video 14.2, ▶ Video 14.3, ▶ Video 14.4). As with basilar bifurcation aneurysms, the orbitozygomatic craniotomy provides an upward panoramic view into the interpeduncular fossa. The keys to accessing these CMs include (1) a wide sylvian fissure split, (2) dissection of the anterior choroidal artery into the crural cistern, (3) posterolateral mobilization of the temporal pole, and (4) the wide opening of the carotid-oculomotor triangle with the possible division of the posterior communicating artery, posterior clinoidectomy, or transcavernous dissection to mobilize the oculomotor nerve laterally. The working space is through the carotid-oculomotor triangle, above the basilar terminus and P1 segments of the PCA, and through intervening thalamoperforators. The interpeduncular fossa extends below the basilar terminus and oculomotor nerves. However, the working space between the P1 and s1 (anterior pontomesencephalic segment of the SCA) segments medial to the oculomotor nerve is small and contains perforating arteries. The interpeduncular safe entry zone (SEZ) lies in the posterior perforate substance off the midline because of the midline interpeduncular nucleus. Paramedian interpeduncular CMs extending behind the cerebral peduncle align favorably with a contralateral TSyl-IntPed approach. A contralateral TSyl-IntPed approach for the treatment of patients with ipsilateral oculomotor nerve palsy can result in debilitating bilateral palsies. This approach should be considered only when the ipsilateral oculomotor nerve is functional.

14.4.2 Peduncular

The cerebral peduncle contains the corticospinal, corticopontine, and corticobulbar tracts that refine movements, learn motor skills, and convert proprioceptive information into balance and posture. The most eloquent of these tracts is the corticospinal tract, occupying the peduncle's central one-third, with somatotopic fibers for the face organized medially, the arm in the middle, and the leg laterally. Patients with midbrain peduncular CMs present with Weber syndrome, combining contralateral hemiparesis or hemiplegia of the limbs and face with ipsilateral oculomotor nerve palsy (▶ Fig. 14.4a). Among the 37 patients with peduncular CMs, hemiparesis (24 of 37, 65%) was more common than oculomotor paresis (11 of 37, 30%) because the motor tract is inside the peduncle, and the oculomotor circuit is in the interpeduncular region.

The orbitozygomatic craniotomy and TSyl-Ped approach are preferred for peduncular CMs (▶ Fig. 14.4b; ▶ Video 14.5, ▶ Video 14.6, ▶ Video 14.7). The approach is centered on the sylvian fissure and oculomotor nerve but is lateral to the nerve, unlike the approach to interpeduncular CMs. The TSyl-Ped approach requires greater mobilization of the temporal pole than the TSyl-IntPed approach for interpeduncular lesions. This requirement can indicate transposition of the sphenoparietal sinus, which preserves critical temporal bridging veins. The dissection transitions from the carotid-oculomotor triangle during the approach to the oculomotor-tentorial triangle for the resection. Peduncular lesions present to the surface of the upper peduncle above the P2A segment of the PCA or in the lower peduncle between the P2A segment of the PCA and s2 (lateral pontomesencephalic) segment of the SCA. The s2 segment parallels the pontomesencephalic sulcus, with lesions below this artery located in the pons. The anterior mesencephalic SEZ entails a vertical incision in the medial one-third of the peduncle, lateral to the oculomotor nerve in the anterior corner. Entry through

Interpeduncular Midbrain Cavernoma

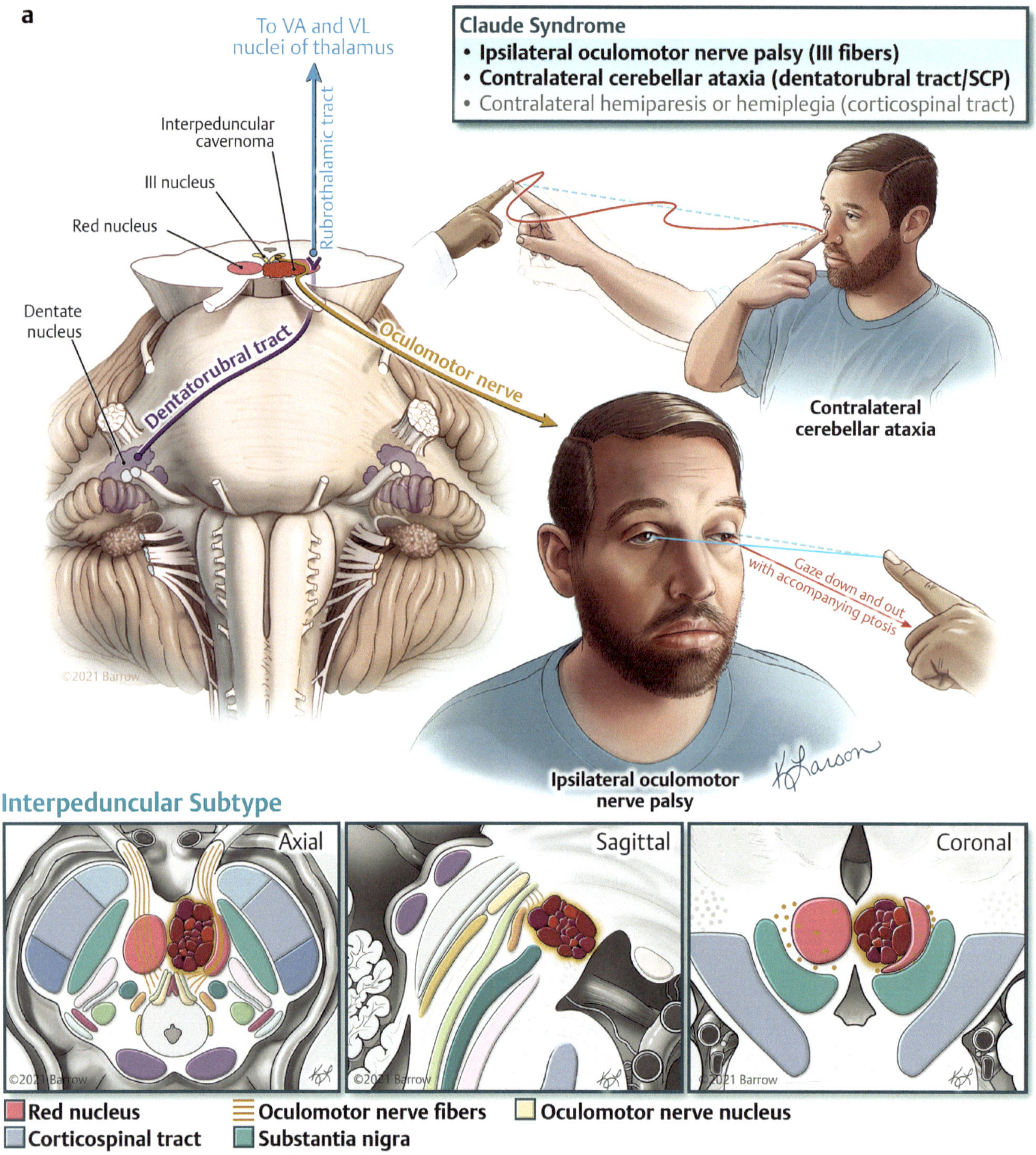

Fig. 14.3 Interpeduncular midbrain CMs. **(a)** Patients with interpeduncular midbrain CMs present with Claude syndrome (ipsilateral oculomotor nerve palsy, contralateral cerebellar ataxia, and dyscoordination). Patients with larger lesions present with Benedikt syndrome, which includes Claude syndrome symptoms and contralateral hemiparesis or hemiplegia due to corticospinal tract involvement in the adjacent cerebral peduncle. The relationships between this left-sided interpeduncular CM and the oculomotor nerve nucleus, red nucleus, and superior cerebellar peduncle are shown in axial, sagittal, and coronal views (*lower insets*).

(Continued)

Surgical Approach

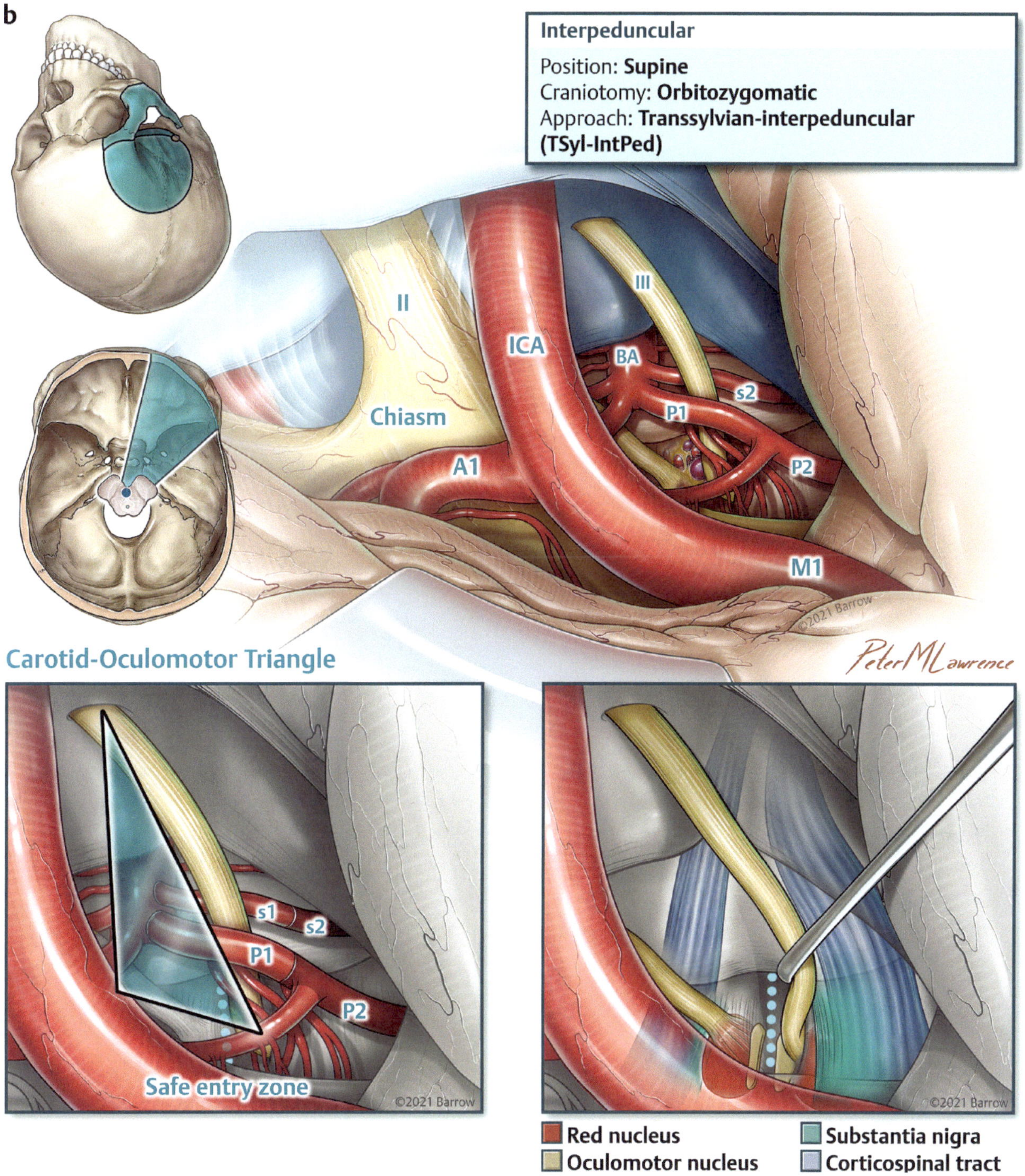

Fig. 14.3 *(Continued)* **(b)** Interpeduncular CMs are accessed through an orbitozygomatic craniotomy (*upper left inset*). Superior view shows TSyl-IntPed approach and CM (*middle left inset; teal circle*). The dissection route is through the carotid-oculomotor triangle (*teal, lower left inset*) above the basilar terminus and P1 segments of the PCA and through intervening thalamoperforators. The interpeduncular SEZ lies in the posterior perforate substance off the midline (*lower left and right insets; teal dotted line*). Safe entry requires dissection medial to the oculomotor nerve, red nucleus, and corticospinal tract and anterior to the oculomotor nucleus (*lower right inset; ghosted structures*) (surgical cases; ▶ Video 14.1, ▶ Video 14.2, ▶ Video 14.3, ▶ Video 14.4, QR codes). Roman numerals denote CNs. (Reproduced with permission from Barrow Neurological Institute, Phoenix, AZ).

14

Surgical Case 14.1

MIDBRAIN

Cavernoma Subtype: Interpeduncular

Position: Supine
Craniotomy: Right orbitozygomatic-pterional
Approach: Transsylvian-interpeduncular (TSyl-IntPed)
Triangle: Carotid-oculomotor
SEZ: Interpeduncular
Artery: P1 PCA

Video: Resection of a midline interpeduncular midbrain cavernoma

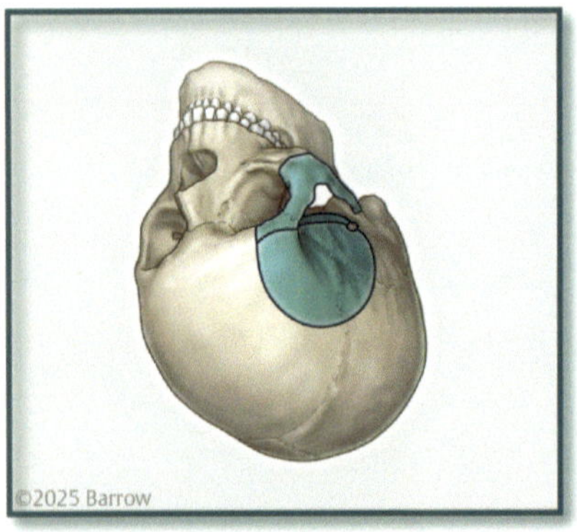

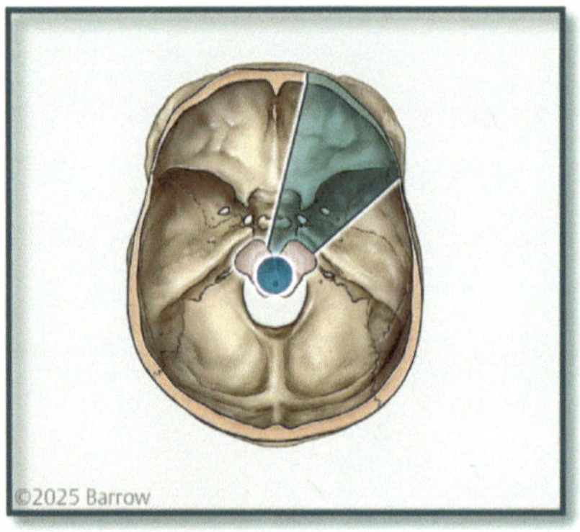

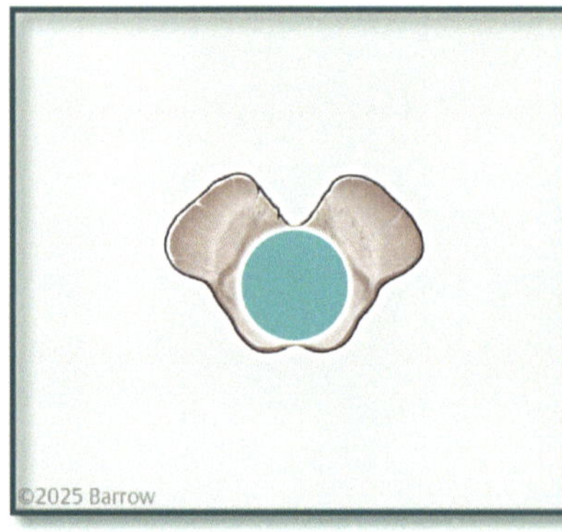

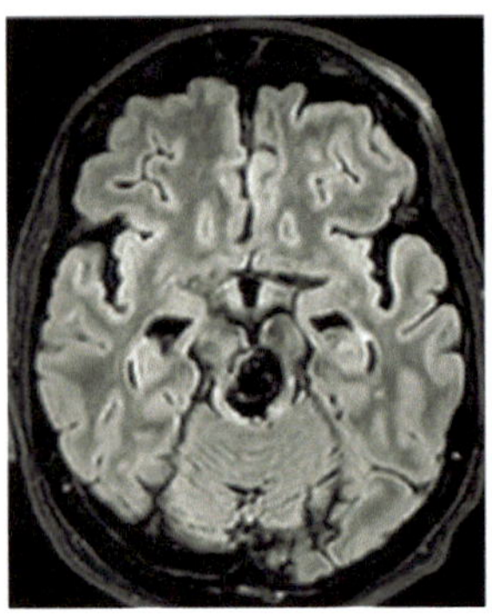

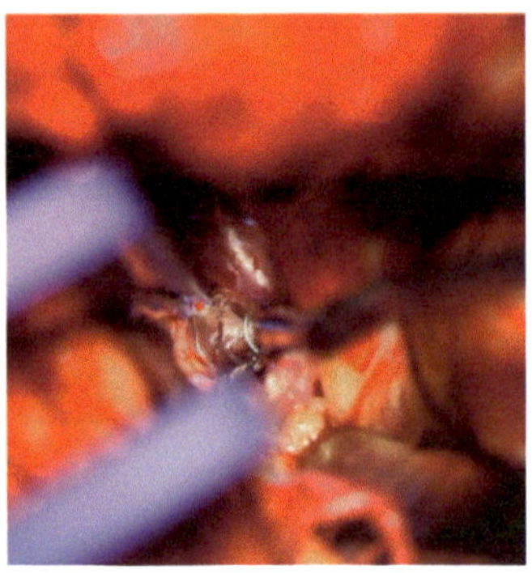

Video 14.1
Transsylvian-Interpeduncular Approach for Interpeduncular Midbrain Cavernous Malformation Resection (Reproduced with permission from Barrow Neurological Institute, Phoenix, AZ.)

14

Surgical Case 14.2

MIDBRAIN

Cavernoma Subtype: Interpeduncular

Position: Supine
Craniotomy: Left orbitozygomatic-pterional
Approach: Transsylvian-interpeduncular (TSyl-IntPed)
Triangle: Carotid-oculomotor
SEZ: Interpeduncular
Artery: P1 PCA

Video: Resection of a right interpeduncular midbrain cavernoma

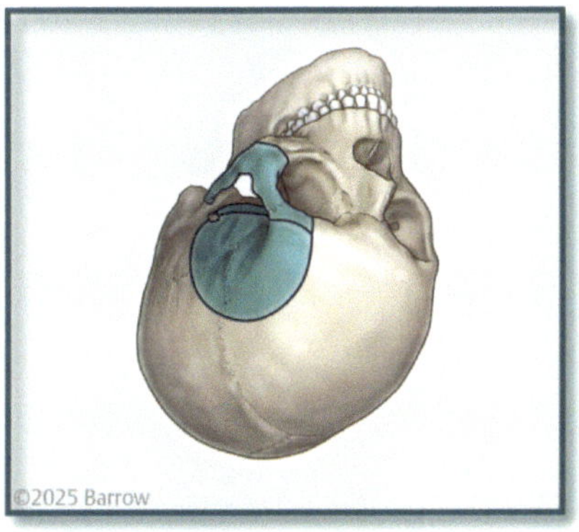

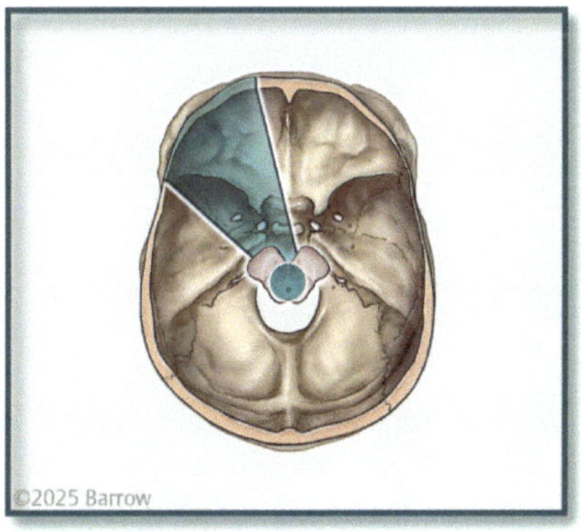

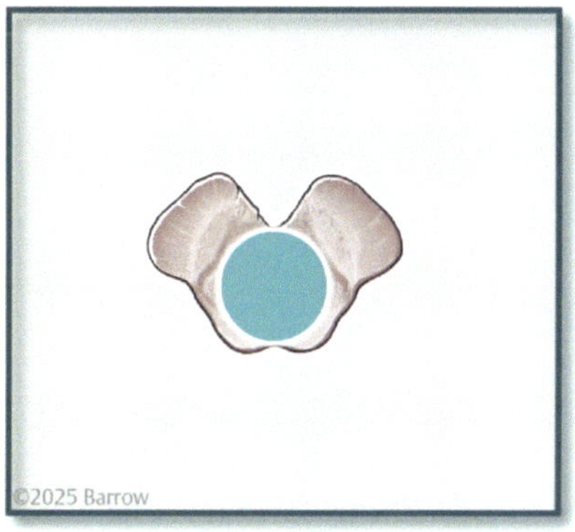

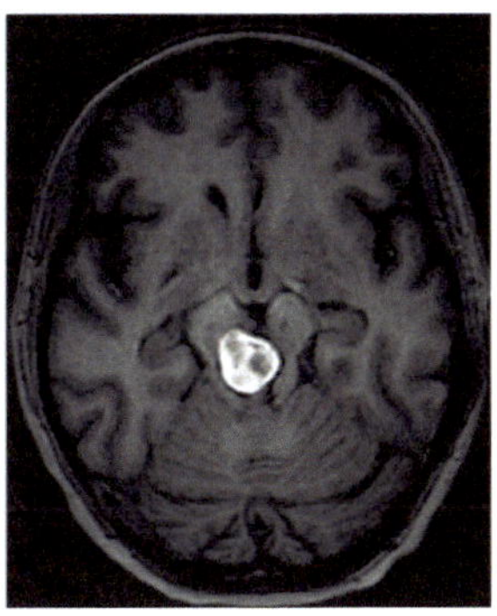

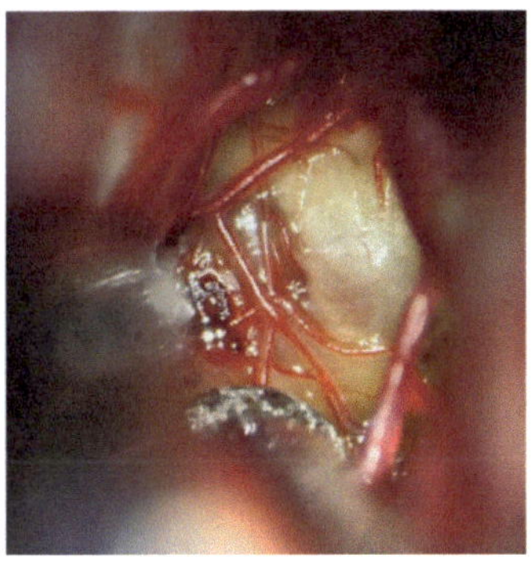

Video 14.2
Transsylvian-Interpeduncular Approach for Interpeduncular Midbrain Cavernous Malformation Resection (Reproduced with permission from Barrow Neurological Institute, Phoenix, AZ.)

14

Surgical Case 14.3

MIDBRAIN

Cavernoma Subtype: Interpeduncular

Position: Supine
Craniotomy: Left orbitozygomatic-pterional
Approach: Contralateral transsylvian-interpeduncular (cTSyl-IntPed)
Triangle: Carotid-oculomotor
SEZ: Interpeduncular
Artery: P1 PCA

Video: Resection of a right interpeduncular midbrain cavernoma

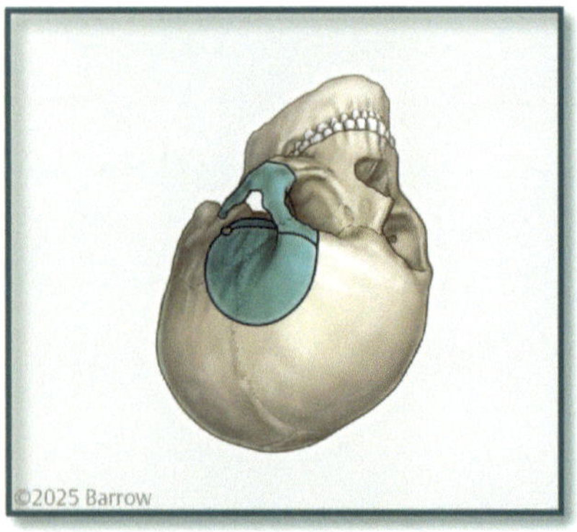

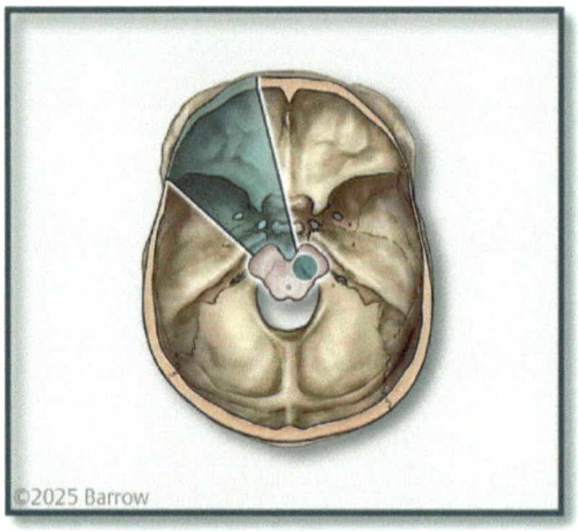

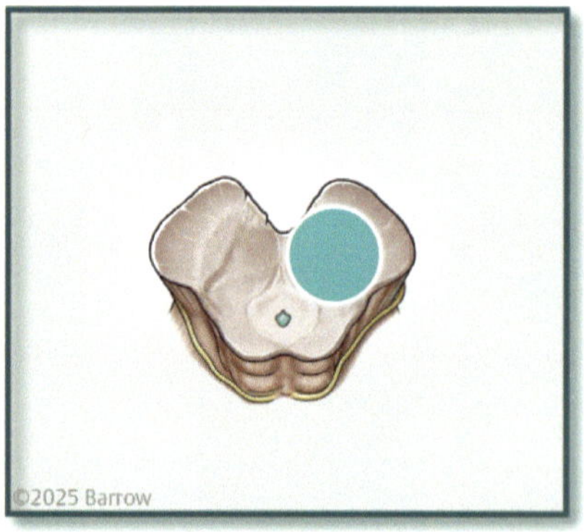

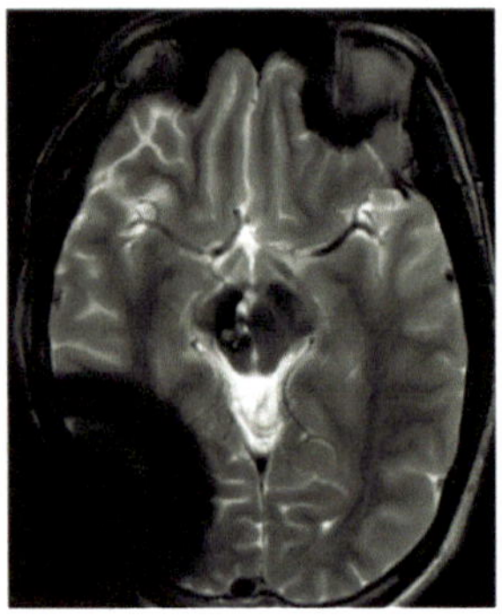

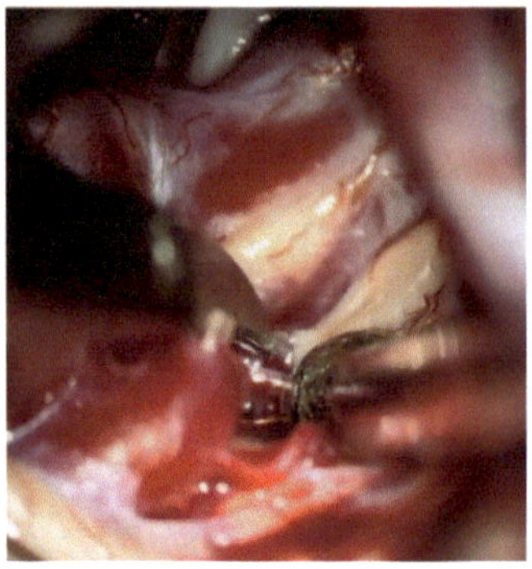

Video 14.3
Contralateral Transsylvian-Interpeduncular Approach for Recurrent Interpeduncular Midbrain Cavernous Malformation Resection (Reproduced with permission from Barrow Neurological Institute, Phoenix, AZ.)

Surgical Case 14.4

MIDBRAIN

Cavernoma Subtype: Interpeduncular

Position: Supine
Craniotomy: Right orbitozygomatic-pterional
Approach: Contralateral transsylvian-interpeduncular (cTSyl-IntPed)
Triangle: Carotid-oculomotor
SEZ: Interpeduncular
Artery: P1 PCA

Video: Resection of a left interpeduncular midbrain cavernoma

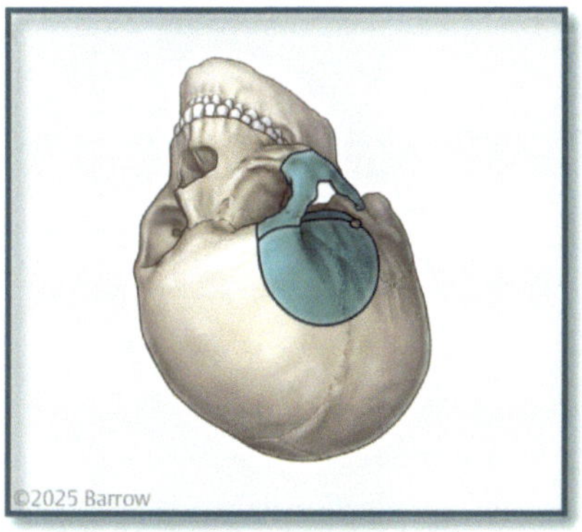

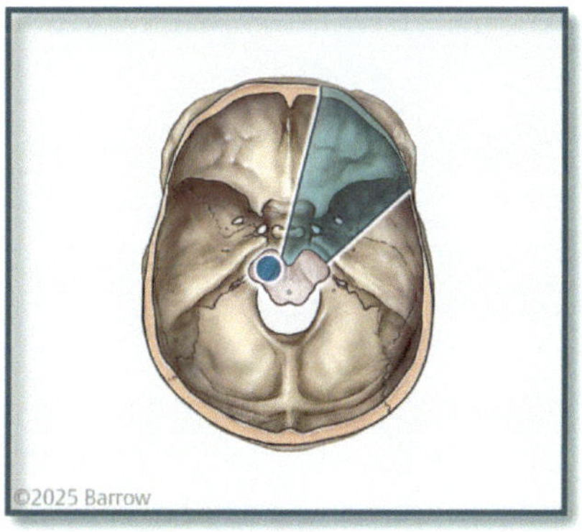

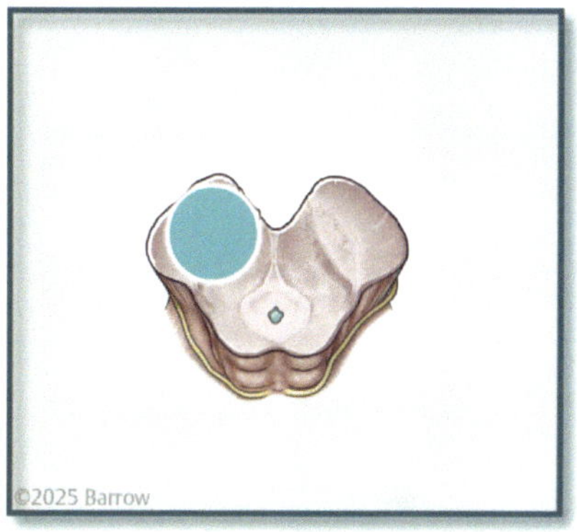

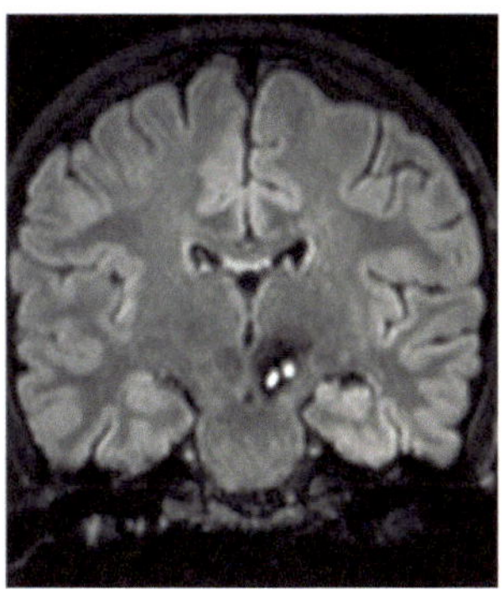

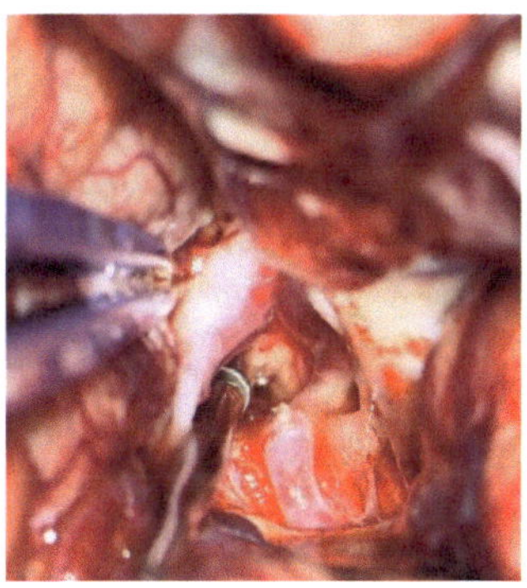

Video 14.4
Contralateral Transsylvian-Interpeduncular Approach for Interpeduncular Midbrain Cavernous Malformation Resection (Reproduced with permission from Barrow Neurological Institute, Phoenix, AZ.)

14

Peduncular Midbrain Cavernoma

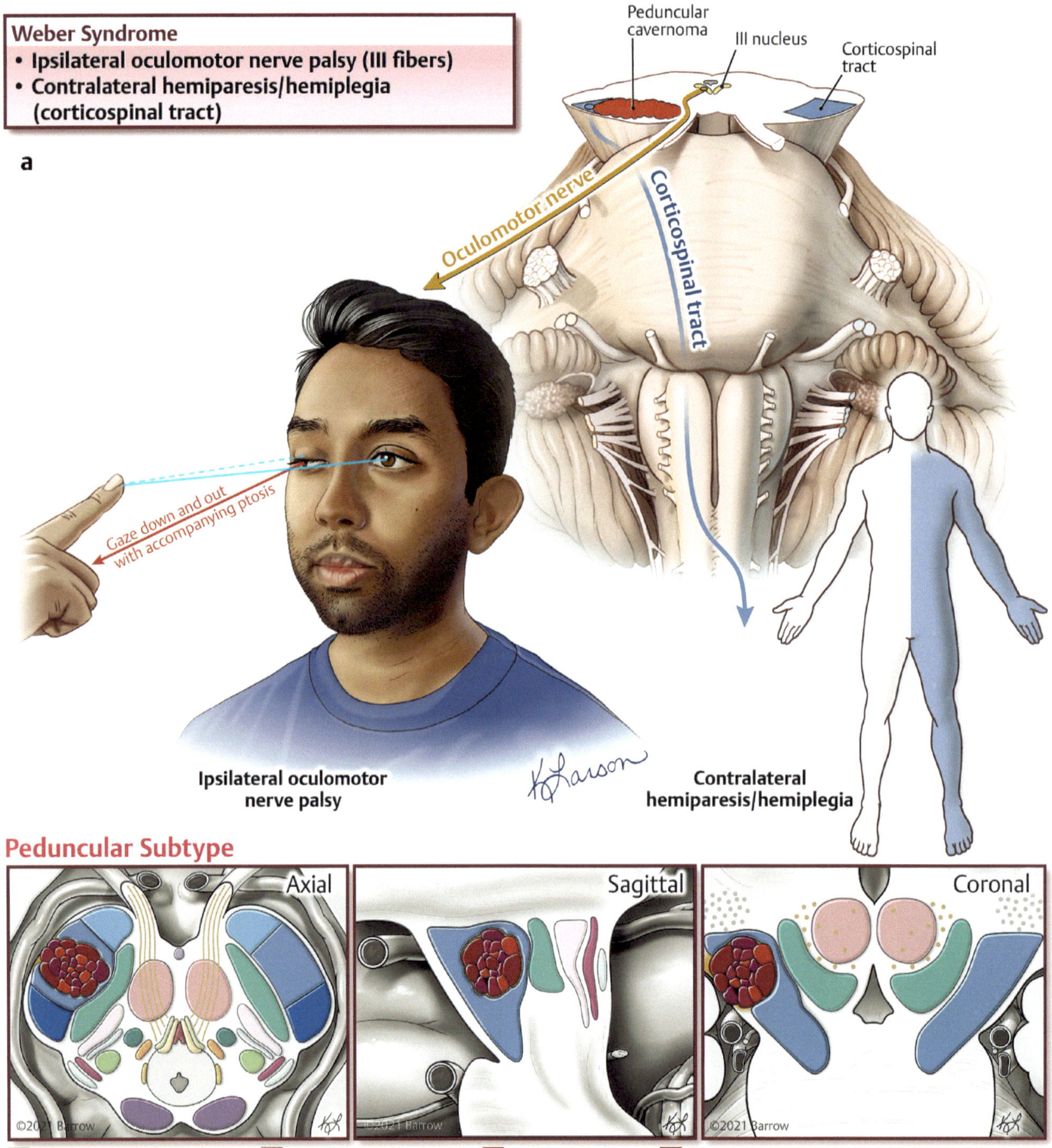

Fig. 14.4 Peduncular midbrain CMs. **(a)** Patients with peduncular midbrain CMs present with Weber syndrome (contralateral hemiparesis or hemiplegia and ipsilateral oculomotor nerve palsy). The relationships between this right-sided CM and the corticospinal tract, oculomotor nerve, substantia nigra, and red nucleus are shown in axial, sagittal, and coronal views (*lower insets*).

(Continued)

Surgical Approach

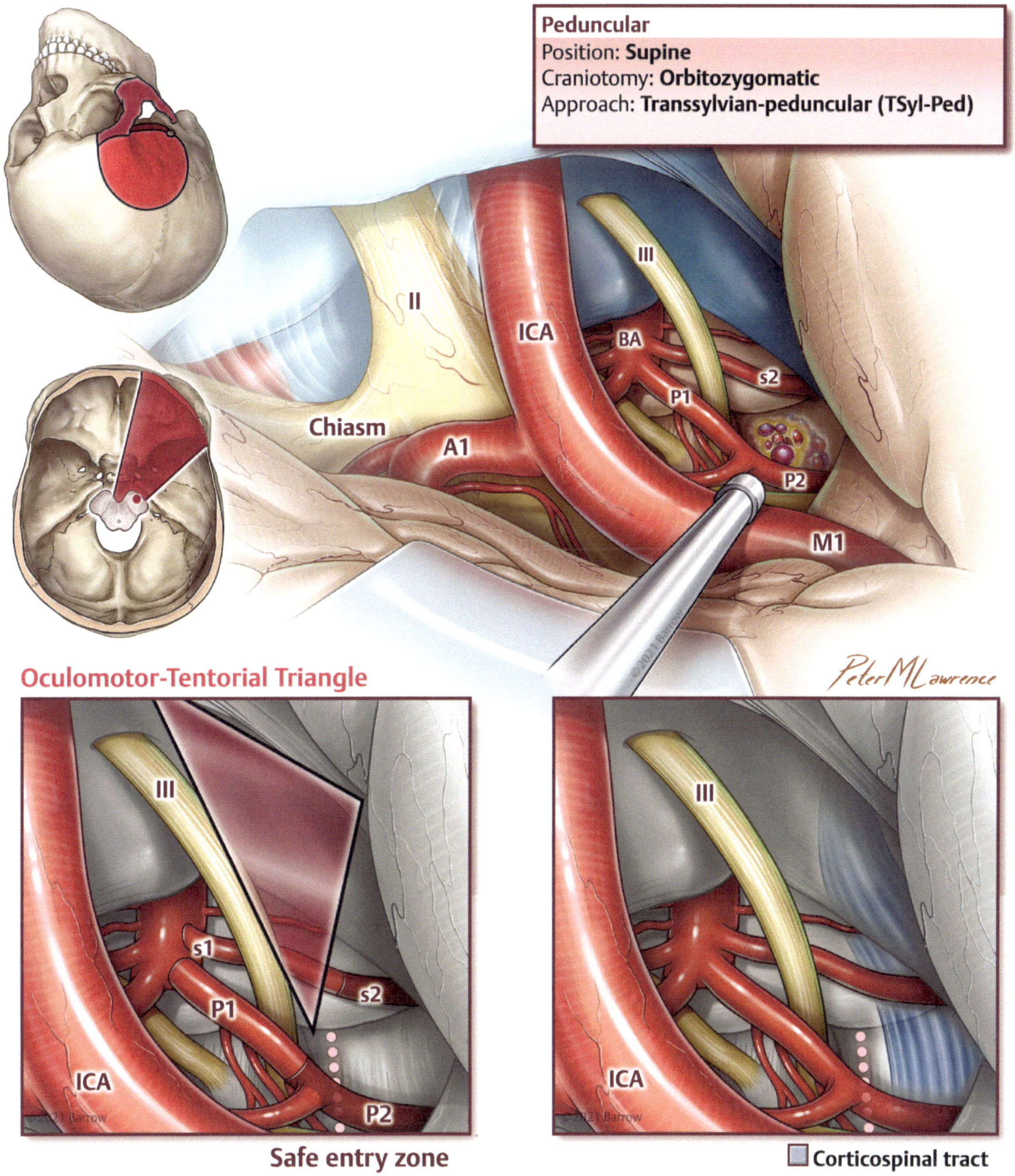

Fig. 14.4 (*Continued*) **(b)** The orbitozygomatic craniotomy (*upper left inset*) and TSyl-Ped approach with CM (*middle left inset*; *red circle*) are preferred for peduncular CMs. The approach is lateral to the oculomotor nerve and requires mobilization of the temporal pole to open the oculomotor-tentorial triangle (*lower left inset*; *red triangle*). Peduncular lesions present to the surface of the upper peduncle above the P2A segment of the PCA or in the lower peduncle between the P2A segment of the PCA and s2 segment of the SCA. The anterior mesencephalic SEZ (*lower left and right insets*; *pink dotted line*) entails a vertical incision in the medial one-third of the peduncle, lateral to the oculomotor nerve and medial to the corticospinal tract (*lower right inset*; *ghosted structure*) (surgical cases; ▶ Video 14.5, ▶ Video 14.6, ▶ Video 14.7, QR codes). Roman numerals denote CNs. (Reproduced with permission from Barrow Neurological Institute, Phoenix, AZ).

Surgical Case 14.5

MIDBRAIN

Cavernoma Subtype: Peduncular

Position: Supine
Craniotomy: Left orbitozygomatic-pterional
Approach: Transsylvian-transpeduncular (TSyl-Ped)
Triangle: Oculomotor-tentorial
SEZ: Anterior mesencephalic
Artery: P2A PCA and s1 SCA

Video: Resection of a left peduncular midbrain cavernoma

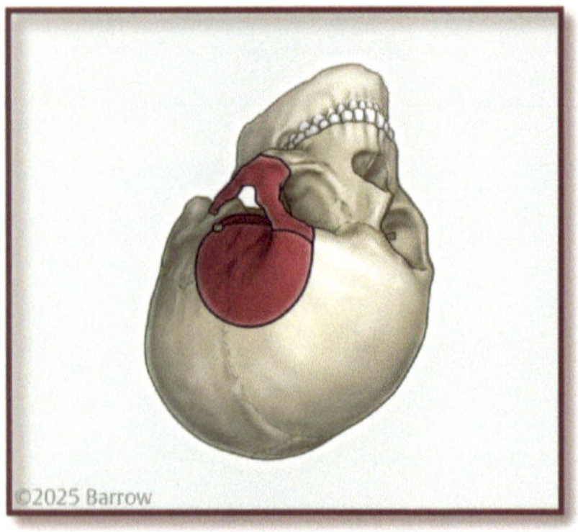

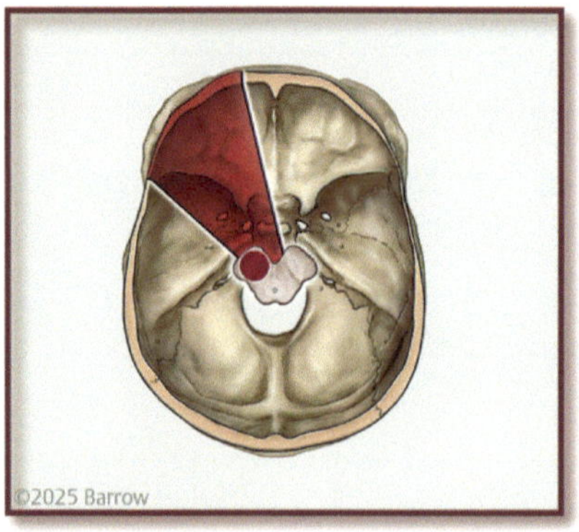

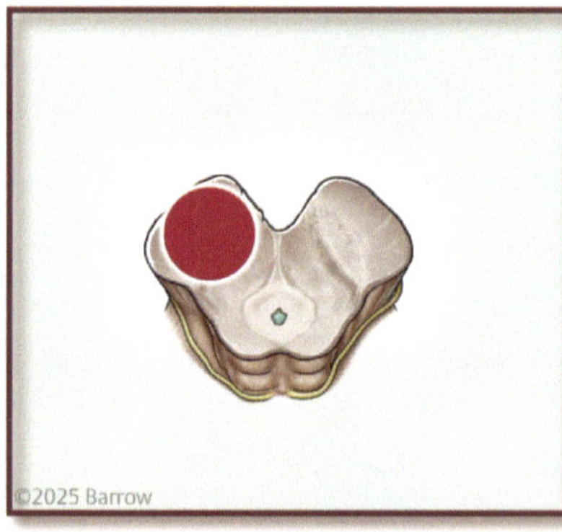

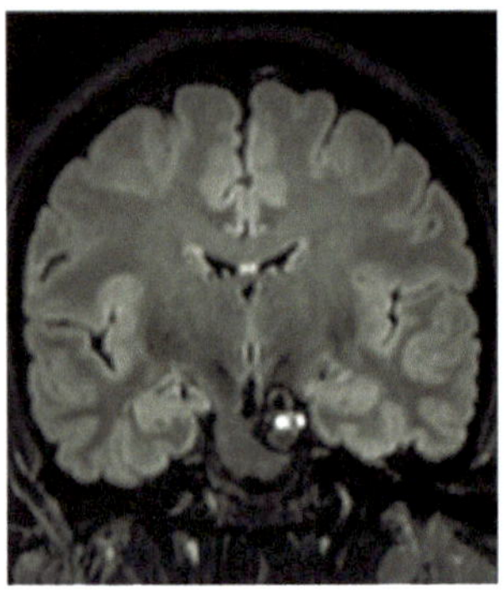

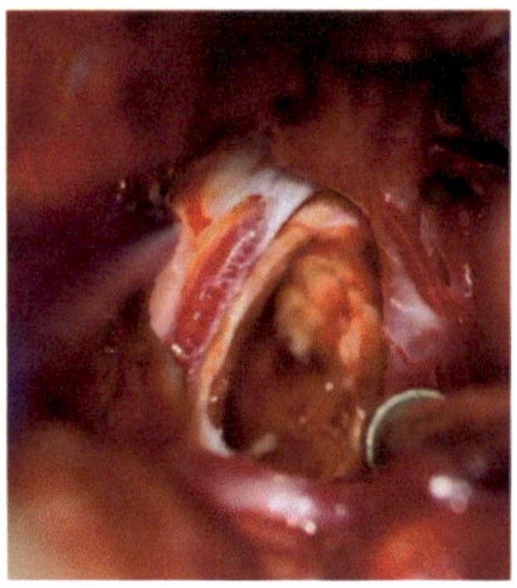

Video 14.5
Transsylvian-Transpeduncular Approach for Peduncular Midbrain and Peritrigeminal Pontine Cavernous Malformation Resection (Reproduced with permission from Barrow Neurological Institute, Phoenix, AZ.)

14

Surgical Case 14.6

MIDBRAIN

Cavernoma Subtype: Peduncular

Position: Supine
Craniotomy: Right orbitozygomatic-pterional
Approach: Transsylvian-transpeduncular (TSyl-Ped)
Triangle: Oculomotor-tentorial
SEZ: Anterior mesencephalic
Artery: P2A PCA

Video: Resection of a right peduncular midbrain cavernoma

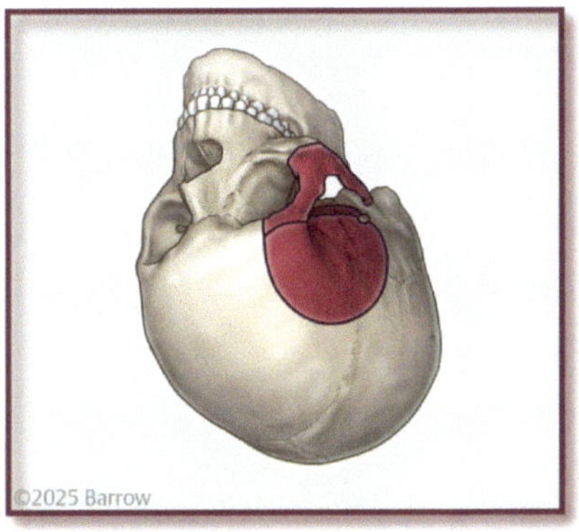

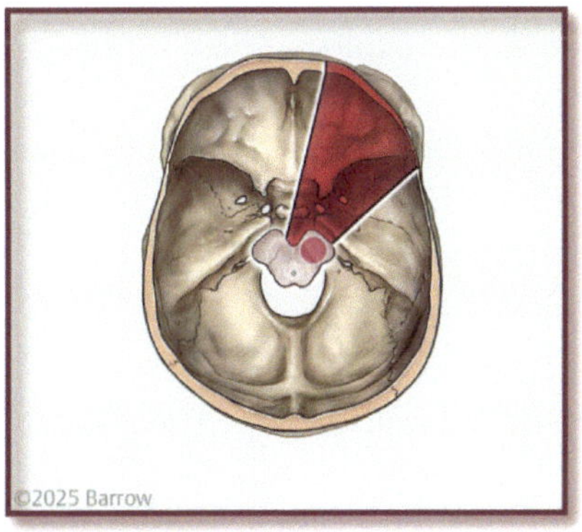

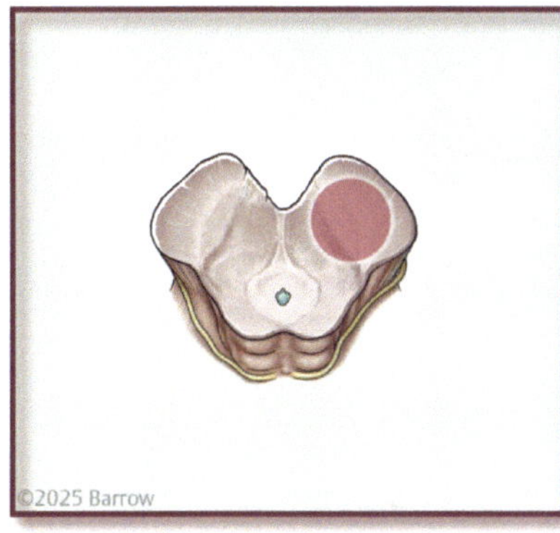

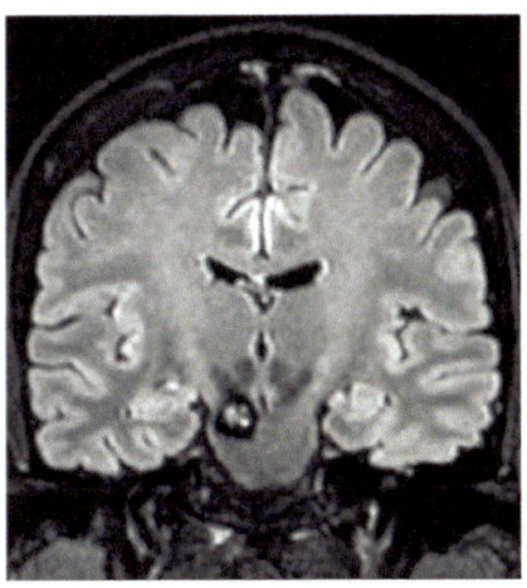

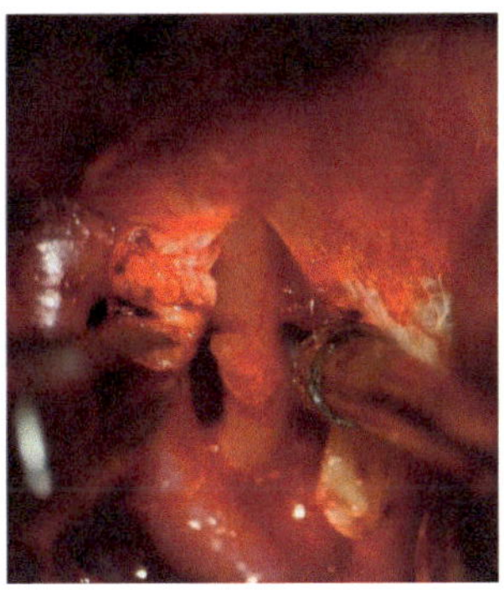

Video 14.6
Transsylvian-Transpeduncular Approach for Peduncular Midbrain Cavernous Malformation Resection (Reproduced with permission from Barrow Neurological Institute, Phoenix, AZ.)

Surgical Case 14.7

MIDBRAIN

Cavernoma Subtype: Peduncular

Position: Supine
Craniotomy: Left orbitozygomatic-pterional
Approach: Transsylvian-transpeduncular (TSyl-Ped)
Triangle: Oculomotor-tentorial
SEZ: Anterior mesencephalic
Artery: P2A PCA and s2 SCA

Video: Resection of a left peduncular midbrain cavernoma

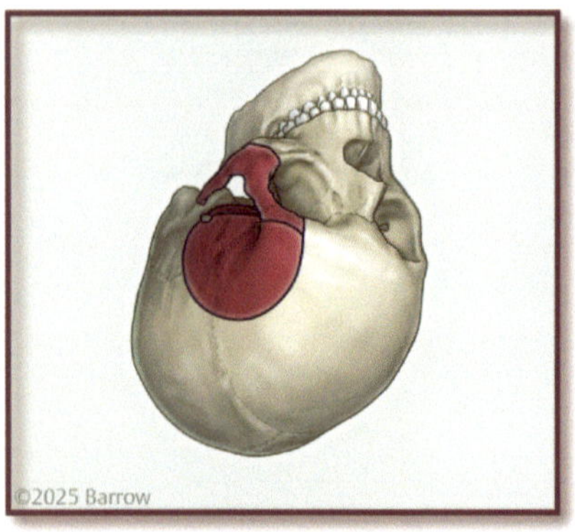

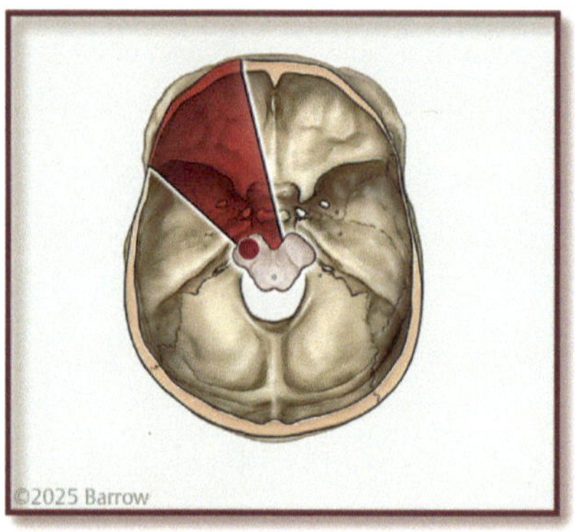

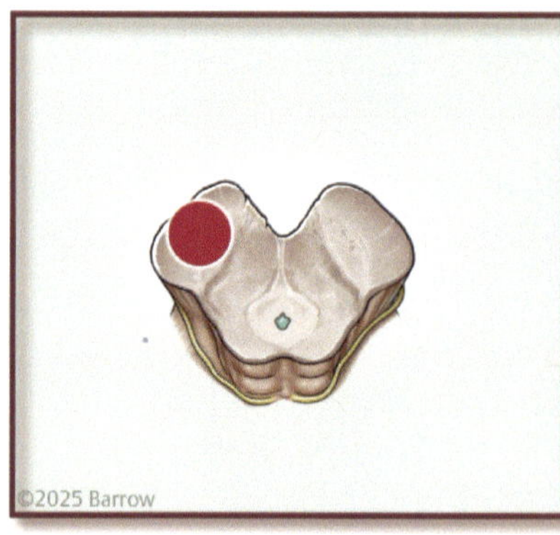

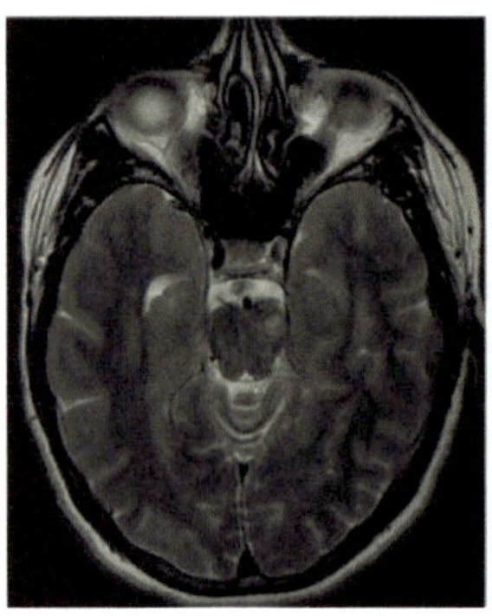

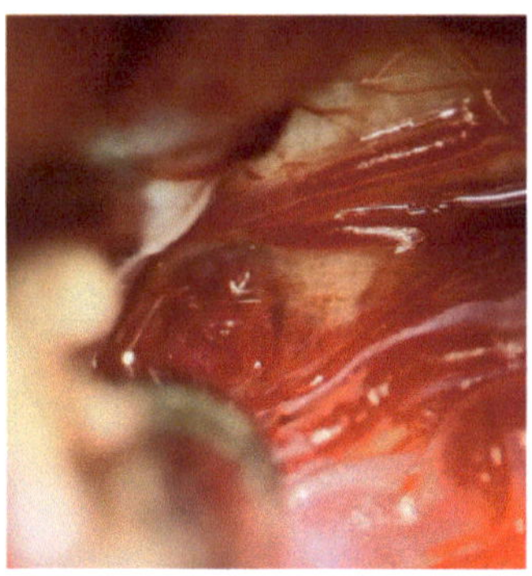

Video 14.7
Transsylvian-Transpeduncular Approach for Peduncular Midbrain Cavernous Malformation Resection (Reproduced with permission from Barrow Neurological Institute, Phoenix, AZ.)

frontopontine fibers spares the corticospinal tract. The substantia nigra and red nucleus are the posterior limits of this incision.

14.4.3 Tegmental

The midbrain tegmentum extends from the substantia nigra anteriorly to the cerebral aqueduct and tectum posteriorly. Tegmental midbrain CMs occur only in the lateral tegmentum beneath the posterolateral midbrain surface, which forms the medial boundary of the ambient cistern. This subtype is located lateral to the red nucleus and periaqueductal gray matter. Tegmental CMs were the most common subtype encountered, accounting for nearly half of all midbrain lesions (73 of 151, 48%). Patients with these lesions do not have an eponymous clinical syndrome but have what I consider to be a "lemniscal syndrome" due to the involvement of the three lemniscal tracts (medial, trigeminal, and lateral lemnisci), as well as the spinothalamic tract. They present with contralateral sensory disturbances of proprioception, vibration, fine touch, and two-point discrimination, as well as pain, temperature, and crude touch disturbances because the medial lemniscus and spinothalamic tract are centrally located in this region (▶ Fig. 14.5a). Medial to these tracts, the trigeminal lemniscus relays contralateral facial pain, temperature, and touch signals to the thalamus, making contralateral facial numbness part of the tegmental syndrome. These tegmental CMs can cause hearing impairment and contralateral tinnitus because the lateral lemniscus carries auditory information from the cochlear nuclei to the contralateral inferior colliculus and brachium.

Tegmental CMs are exposed preferentially through a retrosigmoid craniotomy and SCIT-Lat approach (▶ Fig. 14.5b; ▶ Video 14.8, ▶ Video 14.9, ▶ Video 14.10). The approach can be performed with the patient in a supine or lateral position. The sitting position exploits gravity to allow sagging of the cerebellum, widening of the supracerebellar corridor, and opening of the ambient cistern. The free edge of the tentorium and trochlear nerve are key orienting landmarks in the ambient cistern. The s3 segment of the SCA courses inferior and parallel to the trochlear nerve, often bifurcating into rostral and caudal trunks before diving into the cerebellomesencephalic fissure to find the superior cerebellar peduncle. Dissection downward in this fissure along the arteries extends the exposure inferiorly. Although the lemniscal trigone (Reil's trigone) is not a triangular space for routing dissection, it is a surface landmark formed by the inferior colliculus and its brachium superiorly, lateral mesencephalic sulcus anteriorly, and superior cerebellar peduncle (brachium conjunctivum) inferiorly, with the trochlear nerve coursing through it. The lemniscal trigone forms the medial wall of the cerebellomesencephalic fissure, but the inferior colliculus brachium lies above the trochlear nerve, hidden from view by the tentorium. The lateral mesencephalic sulcus subtly marks the posterior border of the cerebral peduncle, and the lateral mesencephalic vein is a prominent landmark that typically overlies the lateral mesencephalic sulcus as it courses supratentorially upward to join the basal vein of Rosenthal (BVR). The tegmentum can be safely entered with a vertical incision through the lateral mesencephalic sulcus, with a vertical deepening in an anteromedial direction that parallels the substantia nigra and medial lemniscus. This SEZ extends from the medial geniculate body superiorly to the trochlear nerve inferiorly. Entry through this sulcus more inferiorly risks injury to the superior cerebellar peduncle, which can cause disabling cerebellar ataxia and tremor. The narrow window of the supracerebellar corridor can be enlarged superiorly by cutting the tentorium and inferiorly by resecting the quadrangular lobule of the cerebellum.

14.4.4 Quadrigeminal

The superior and inferior colliculi orient the head and eyes toward visual and auditory inputs. The superior colliculus receives visual signals from the optic tract and lateral geniculate body and projects to the pulvinar. The inferior colliculus receives auditory signals from the cochlear nuclei and lateral lemniscus and projects to the medial geniculate body and auditory cortex. Patients with quadrigeminal midbrain CMs present with Parinaud syndrome or any combination of impaired upward or downward gaze, setting sun sign (downward gaze at

Tegmental Midbrain Cavernoma

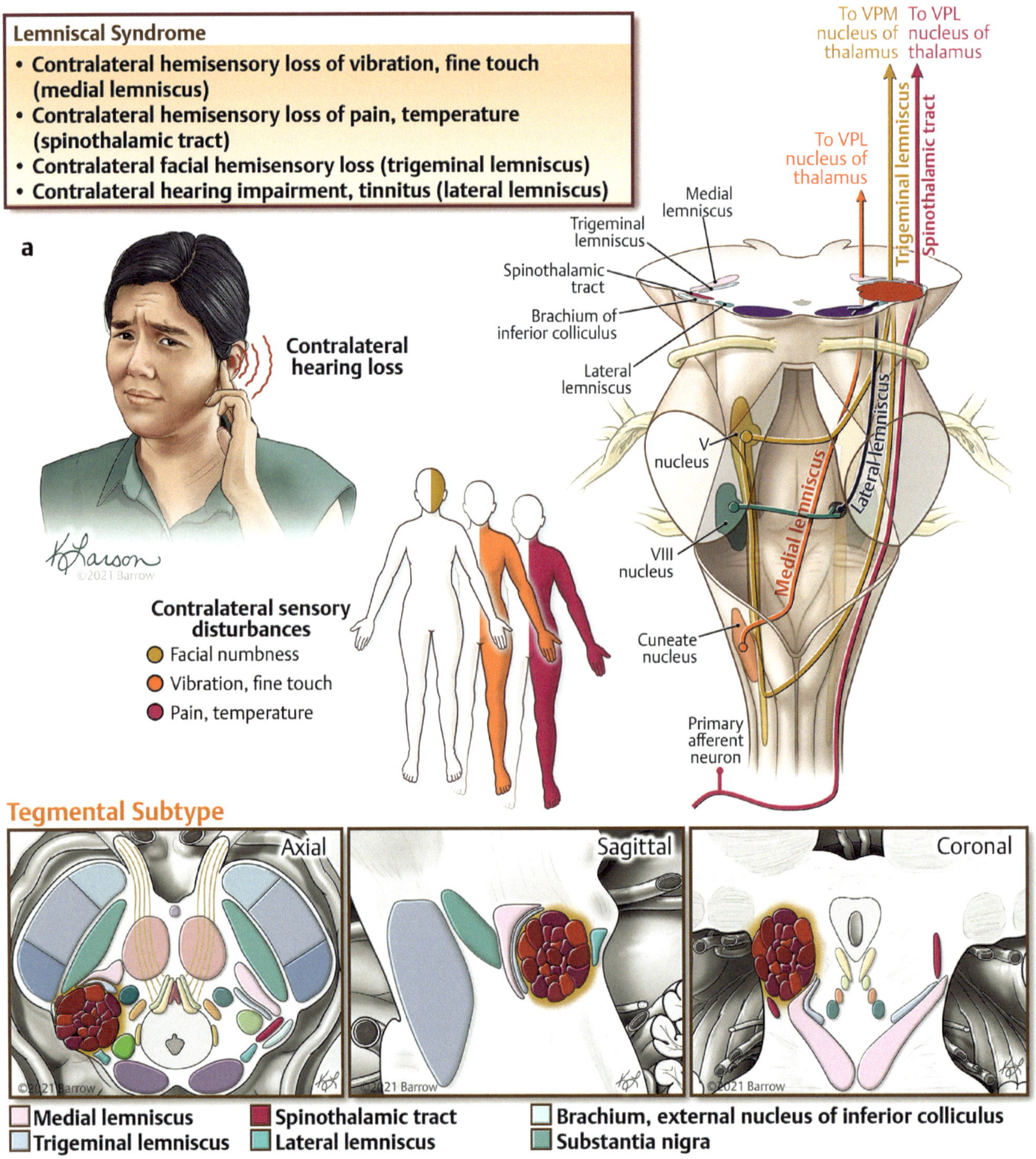

Fig. 14.5 Tegmental midbrain CMs. **(a)** Patients with tegmental midbrain CMs present with contralateral sensory disturbances of proprioception, vibration, fine touch, and two-point discrimination, as well as pain, temperature, and crude touch because the medial lemniscus and spinothalamic tract are centrally located in this region. Patients may also present with contralateral facial numbness to pain, temperature, and touch from the involvement of the trigeminal lemniscus as well as hearing impairment and contralateral tinnitus from the involvement of the lateral lemniscus. The involvement of these four sensory fiber bundles suggests that this clinical syndrome could be called the lemniscal syndrome. The relationships between this right-sided tegmental CM and the three lemnisci and spinothalamic tract are shown in axial, sagittal, and coronal views (*lower insets*).

(Continued)

Surgical Approach

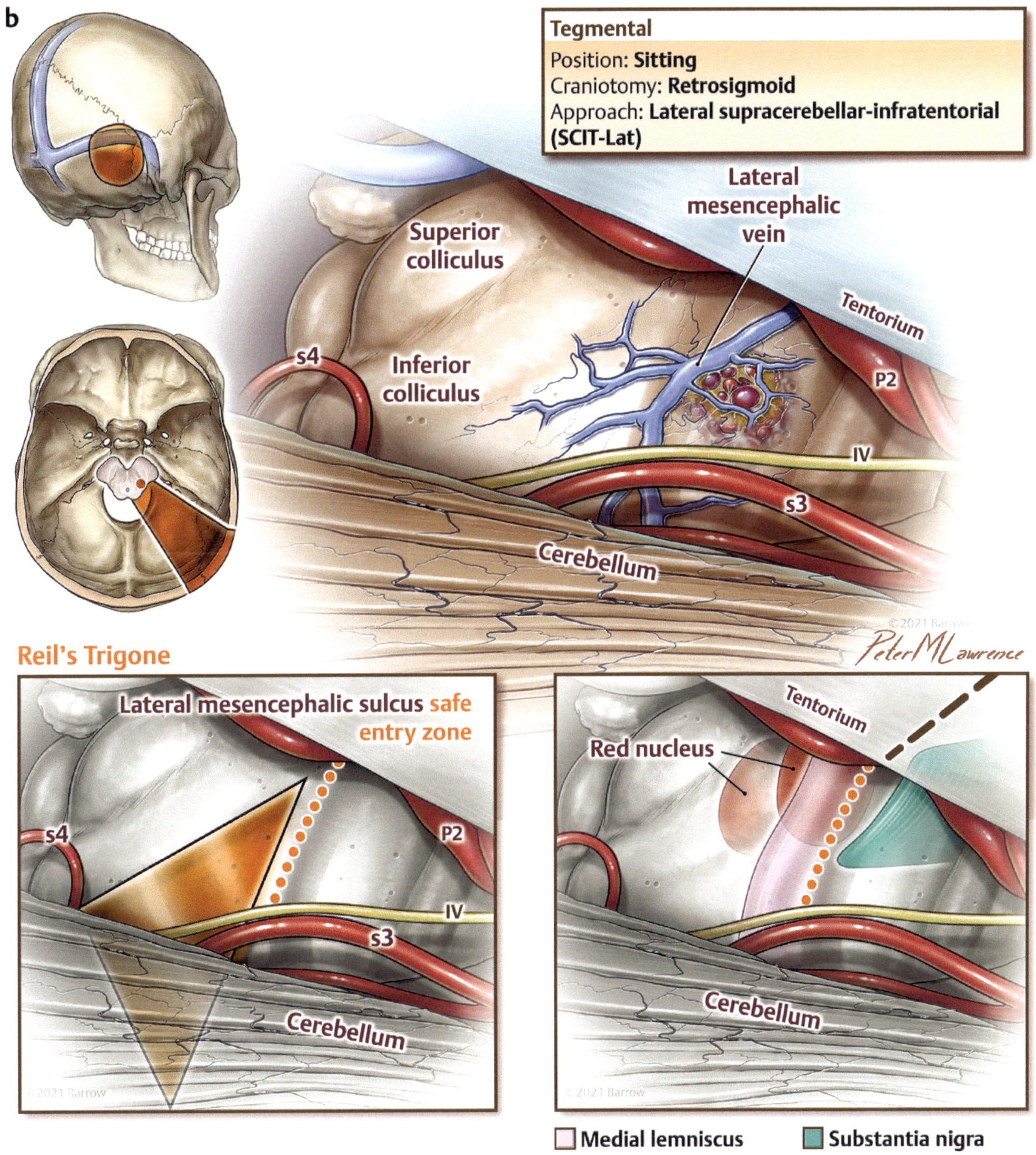

Fig. 14.5 *(Continued)* **(b)** Tegmental CMs are exposed through a retrosigmoid craniotomy (*upper left inset*). The SCIT-Lat approach exposes the CM (*middle left inset*; *orange circle*). The patient is positioned in the sitting posture for gravity retraction of the cerebellum. The free edge of the tentorium, trochlear nerve, and s3 SCA are orienting landmarks in the ambient cistern and cerebellomesencephalic fissure. The lemniscal trigone (Reil's trigone) is a surface landmark formed by the inferior colliculus and its brachium superiorly, lateral mesencephalic sulcus anteriorly, and superior cerebellar peduncle (brachium conjunctivum) inferiorly, with the trochlear nerve coursing through it (*lower left inset*; *orange triangle*). The tegmentum can be entered safely through the lateral mesencephalic sulcus, which is often marked by the lateral mesencephalic vein coursing vertically upward to join the BVR supratentorially. A vertically oriented incision (*lower left and right insets*; *orange dotted line*) extends from the medial geniculate body superiorly to the trochlear nerve inferiorly. It is deepened in an anteromedial direction that parallels the substantia nigra and medial lemniscus (*lower right inset*; *ghosted structures*). The narrow window of the supracerebellar corridor can be enlarged superiorly by cutting the tentorium (*black dashed line*) and inferiorly by resecting the quadrangular lobule (surgical cases; ▶ Video 14.8, ▶ Video 14.9, ▶ Video 14.10, QR codes). Roman numerals denote CNs. (Reproduced with permission from Barrow Neurological Institute, Phoenix, AZ).

Surgical Case 14.8

MIDBRAIN

Cavernoma Subtype: Tegmental

Position: Sitting
Craniotomy: Retrosigmoid
Approach: Lateral supracerebellar-infratentorial (SCIT-Lat)
Triangle: Supratrochlear
SEZ: Lateral Mesencephalic sulcus
Artery: s3 SCA

Video: Resection of a left tegmental midbrain cavernoma

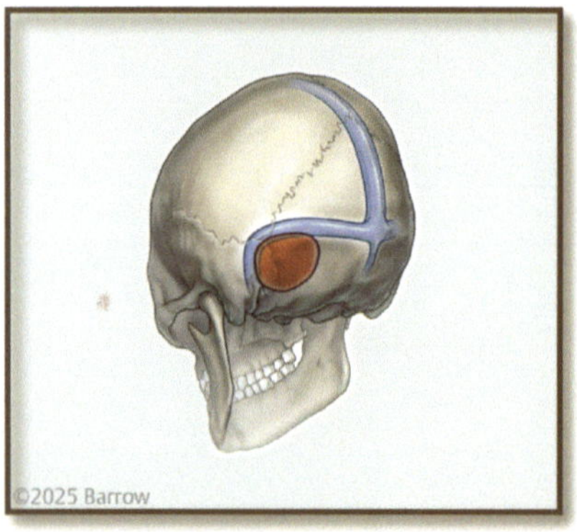

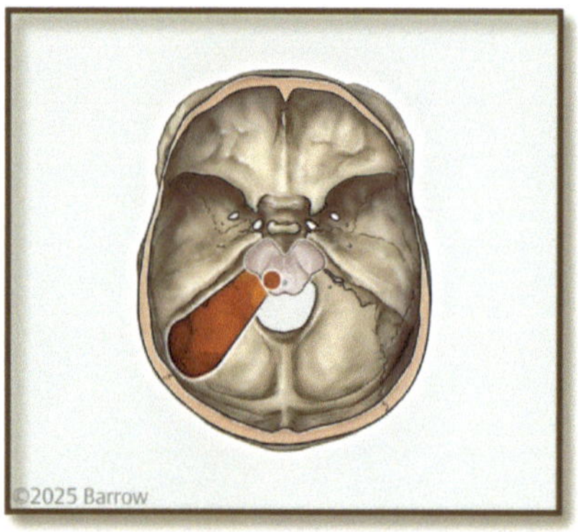

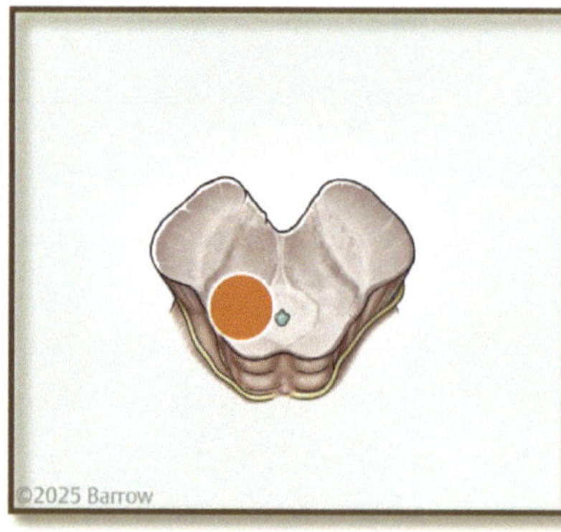

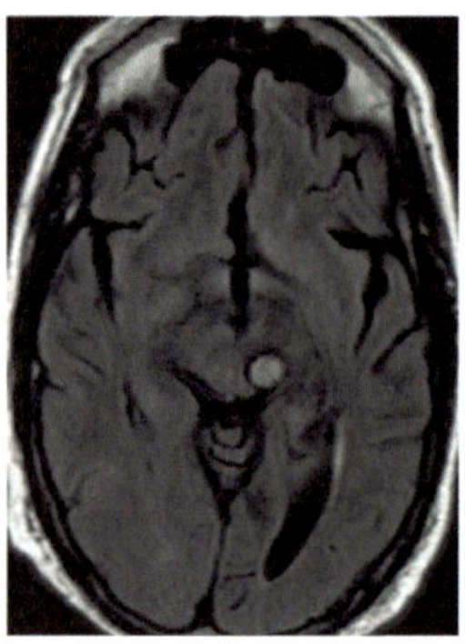

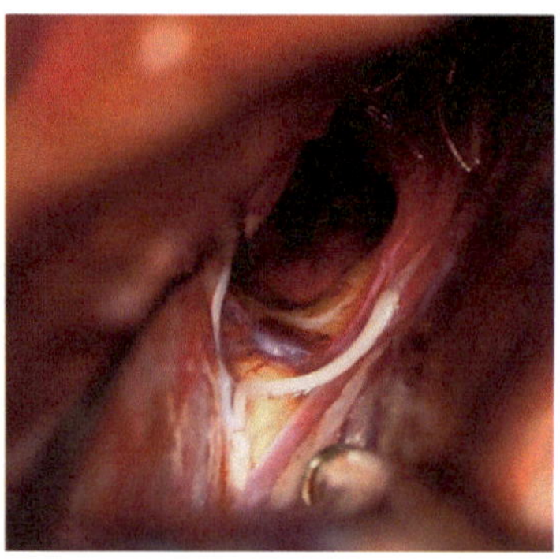

Video 14.8
Lateral Supracerebellar-Infratentorial Approach for Tegmental Midbrain Cavernous Malformation Resection (Reproduced with permission from Barrow Neurological Institute, Phoenix, AZ.)

Surgical Case 14.9

MIDBRAIN

Cavernoma Subtype: Tegmental

Position: Sitting
Craniotomy: Retrosigmoid
Approach: Lateral supracerebellar-transtentorial (SCTT-Lat)
Triangle: Supratrochlear
SEZ: Lateral mesencephalic sulcus
Artery: s3 SCA

Video: Resection of a left tegmental midbrain cavernoma

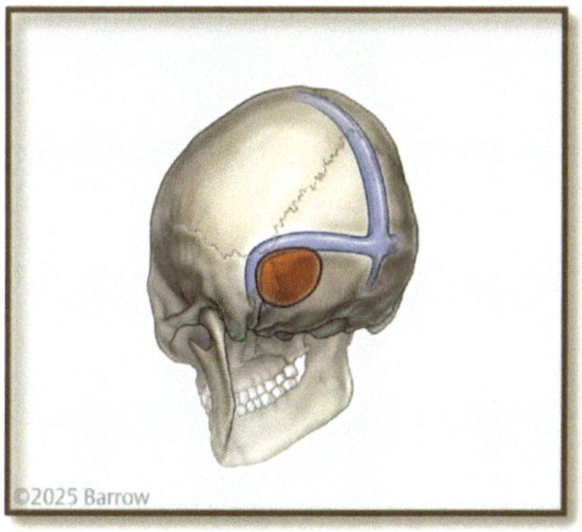

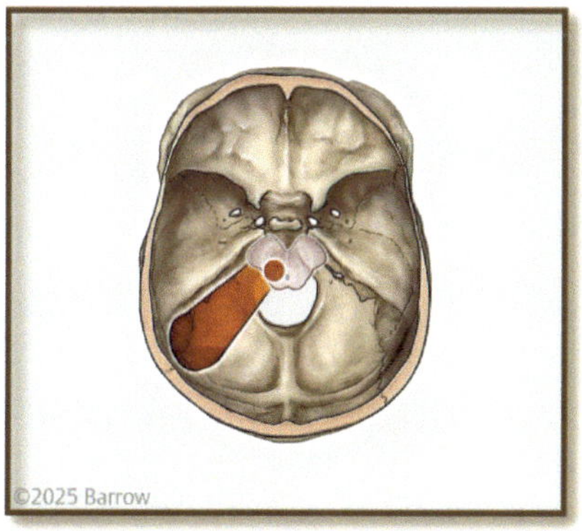

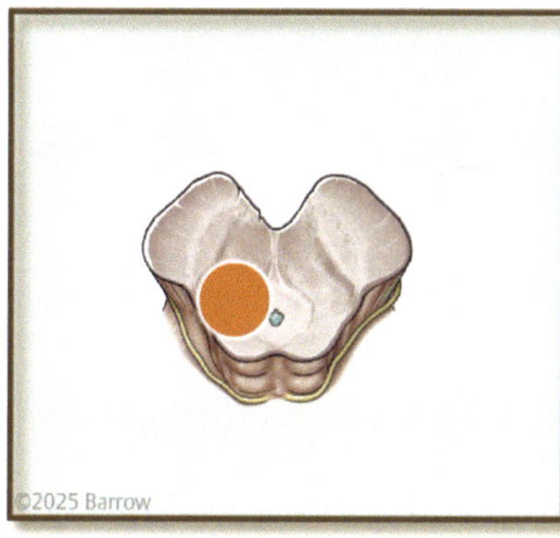

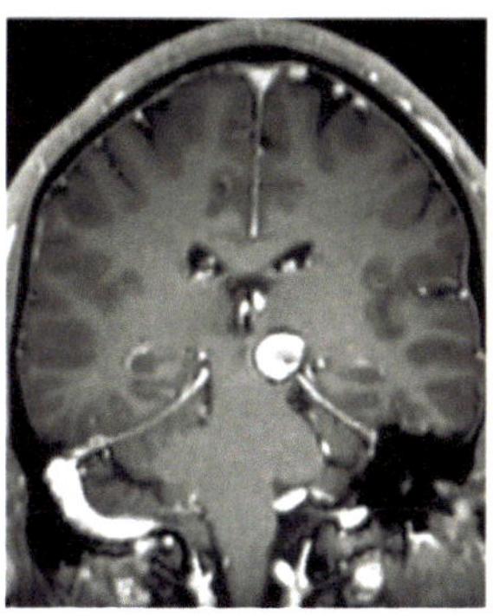

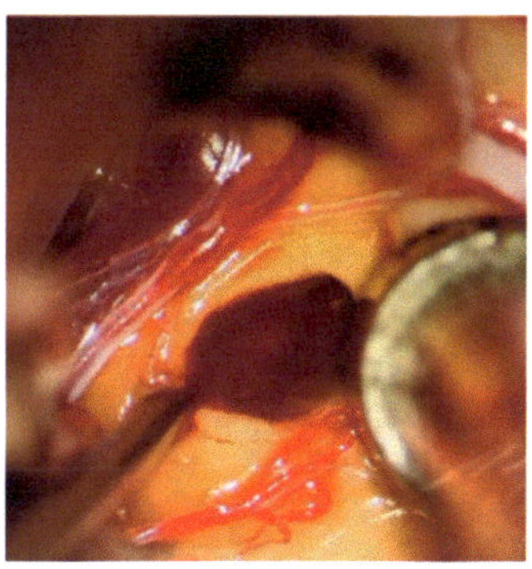

Video 14.9
Lateral Supracerebellar-Transtentorial Approach for Tegmental Midbrain Cavernous Malformation Resection (Reproduced with permission from Barrow Neurological Institute, Phoenix, AZ.)

Surgical Case 14.10

MIDBRAIN

Cavernoma Subtype: Tegmental

Position: Sitting
Craniotomy: Retrosigmoid
Approach: Lateral supracerebellar-infratentorial (SCIT-Lat)
Triangle: Infratrochlear
SEZ: Lateral mesencephalic sulcus
Artery: s3 SCA

Video: Resection of a right tegmental midbrain cavernoma

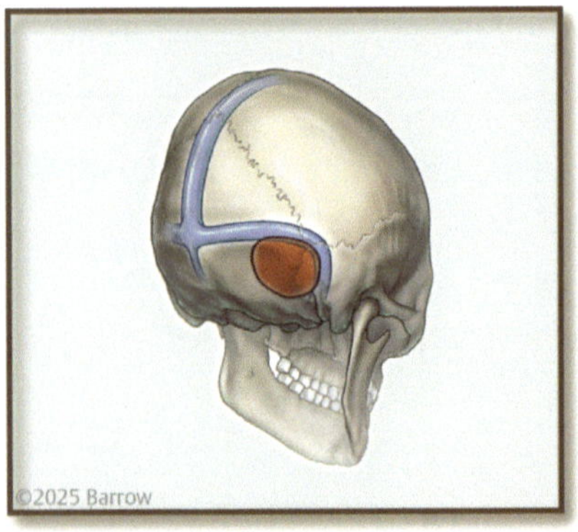

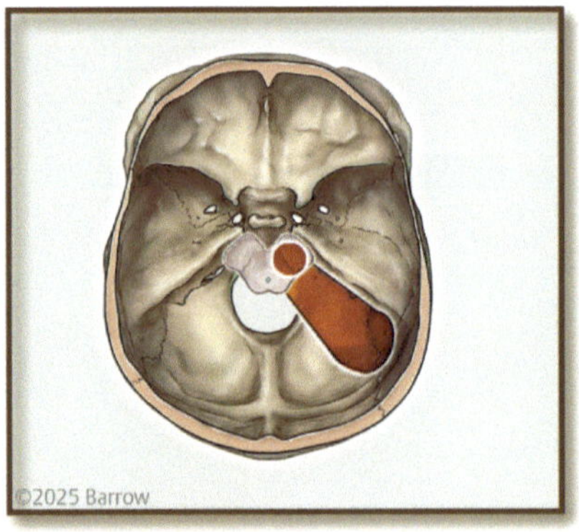

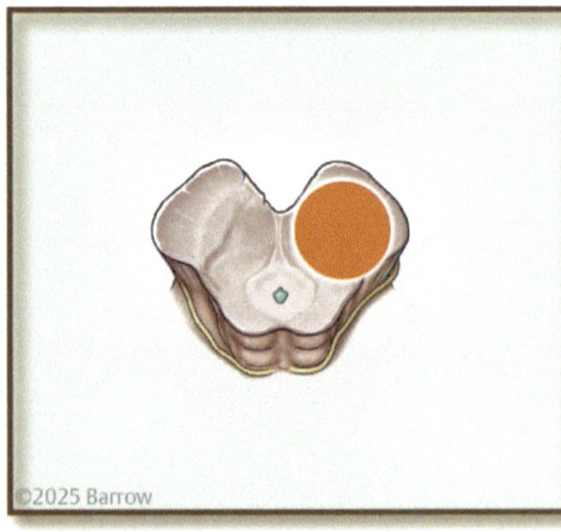

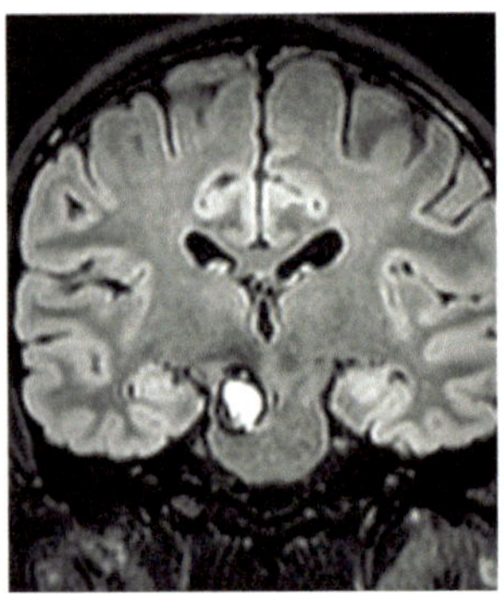

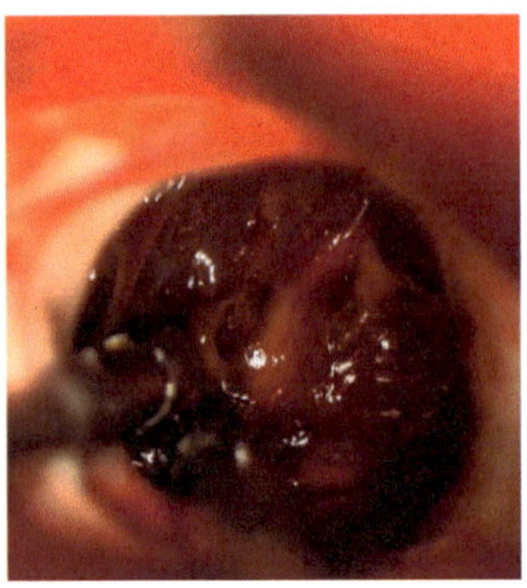

Video 14.10
Lateral Supracerebellar-Infratentorial Approach for Pontomesencephalic Cavernous Malformation Resection (Reproduced with permission from Barrow Neurological Institute, Phoenix, AZ.)

14

rest), pupillary abnormality, or accommodation reflex loss (▸ Fig. 14.6a). A loss of upward gaze with fixed, dilated pupils suggests a lesion in the superior colliculus. In contrast, a loss of downward gaze, pupillary reactivity, and convergence suggest a lesion in the inferior colliculus. Patients with large lesions obstructing the aqueduct present with hydrocephalus.

The SCIT-Mid approach with the patient in the sitting position is preferred for quadrigeminal midbrain CMs. A torcular craniotomy, gravity retraction of the cerebellum, and cerebrospinal fluid release from the cisterna magna and quadrigeminal cisterns maximize the supracerebellar exposure (▸ Fig. 14.6b; ▸ Video 14.11, ▸ Video 14.12). The keys to accessing these CMs include (1) the release of arachnoid granulations between the cerebellum and transverse sinuses, (2) upward traction on the dural flap to elevate the torcular, (3) division of superior hemispheric veins when necessary, and (4) dissection of the five tributaries of the galenic venous complex overlying the tectum (precentral cerebellar vein, two BVRs, two internal cerebral veins, and the vein of Galen). The confluence of the precentral cerebellar vein, BVR, and vein of Galen forms a working triangle underneath the venous complex in line with the approach trajectory, which we call the infragalenic triangle. Arrival at the collicular plate requires mobilization of long circumflex perforators from the P1 and P2 (postcommunicating) segments of the PCAs, the medial posterior choroidal artery, and any loops of the P3 (quadrigeminal) segments of the PCA away from the lesion. Surface landmarks include the superior colliculi, inferior colliculi, pineal gland, and trochlear nerves. Three SEZs are described.

First, the intercollicular SEZ lies in the vertical midline between the colliculi. It extends anteriorly to the aqueduct and inferiorly to just above the trochlear nerves, avoiding their decussation behind the periaqueductal gray matter. Second, the supracollicular entry zone courses horizontally above the superior colliculus, below the posterior and habenular commissures, laterally to the habenula, and anteriorly to the periaqueductal gray matter. Third, the infracollicular entry zone courses horizontally at the level of the frenulum veli, below the inferior colliculus, above and between the origin of the trochlear nerves, and anteriorly to the periaqueductal gray matter. SEZ selection depends on whether the lesion is located in the midline or upper or lower tectum.

14.4.5 Periaqueductal

The periaqueductal gray matter forms a midline hollow cylinder in the posterior tegmentum that interfaces between the forebrain and lower brainstem to respond to internal (e.g., pain) and external stressors (e.g., threat). Patients with periaqueductal CMs present with Nothnagel syndrome comprising ipsilateral oculomotor nerve palsy and ipsilateral cerebellar ataxia resulting from the involvement of the fascicular midbrain portion of the oculomotor nerve and the superior cerebellar peduncle (▸ Fig. 14.7a). Patients with lesions located above the decussation of the superior cerebellar peduncles can present with contralateral ataxia and Claude syndrome. A periaqueductal lesion can block the aqueduct to cause obstructive hydrocephalus, as found in two of seven patients in our study.

The central midbrain location and its important surrounding structures make periaqueductal lesions difficult to access. Nonetheless, access is made less challenging due to the proximity of the third ventricular floor reached from above through the ventricular system. Periaqueductal CMs are exposed with a TCal-TChor approach, best performed through a bifrontal craniotomy with the patient's head turned laterally to the right and the right hemisphere in the dependent position with the midline oriented horizontally (▸ Fig. 14.7b; ▸ Video 14.13). This position avoids the dominant hemisphere, allows gravity to retract the right hemisphere, and widens the interhemispheric fissure. The corpus callosum is divided over the foramen of Monro, and the thalamostriate vein is followed around the venous angle to the internal cerebral vein in the velum interpositum. The choroidal fissure is opened along the tenia fornicea, and the foramen of Monro is enlarged. The third ventricle is traversed to arrive at the funnel-shaped inlet of the aqueduct. Third ventricle landmarks include the optic chiasm, infundibular recess, tuber cinereum, and mammillary bodies anteriorly and the habenular commissure, pineal recess, and posterior commissure posteriorly. This region does not have an anatomical triangle or SEZ. However, these lesions present with an exophytic component at the inlet to the aqueduct, at the ependymal surface, or are accessible more distally through the aqueduct.

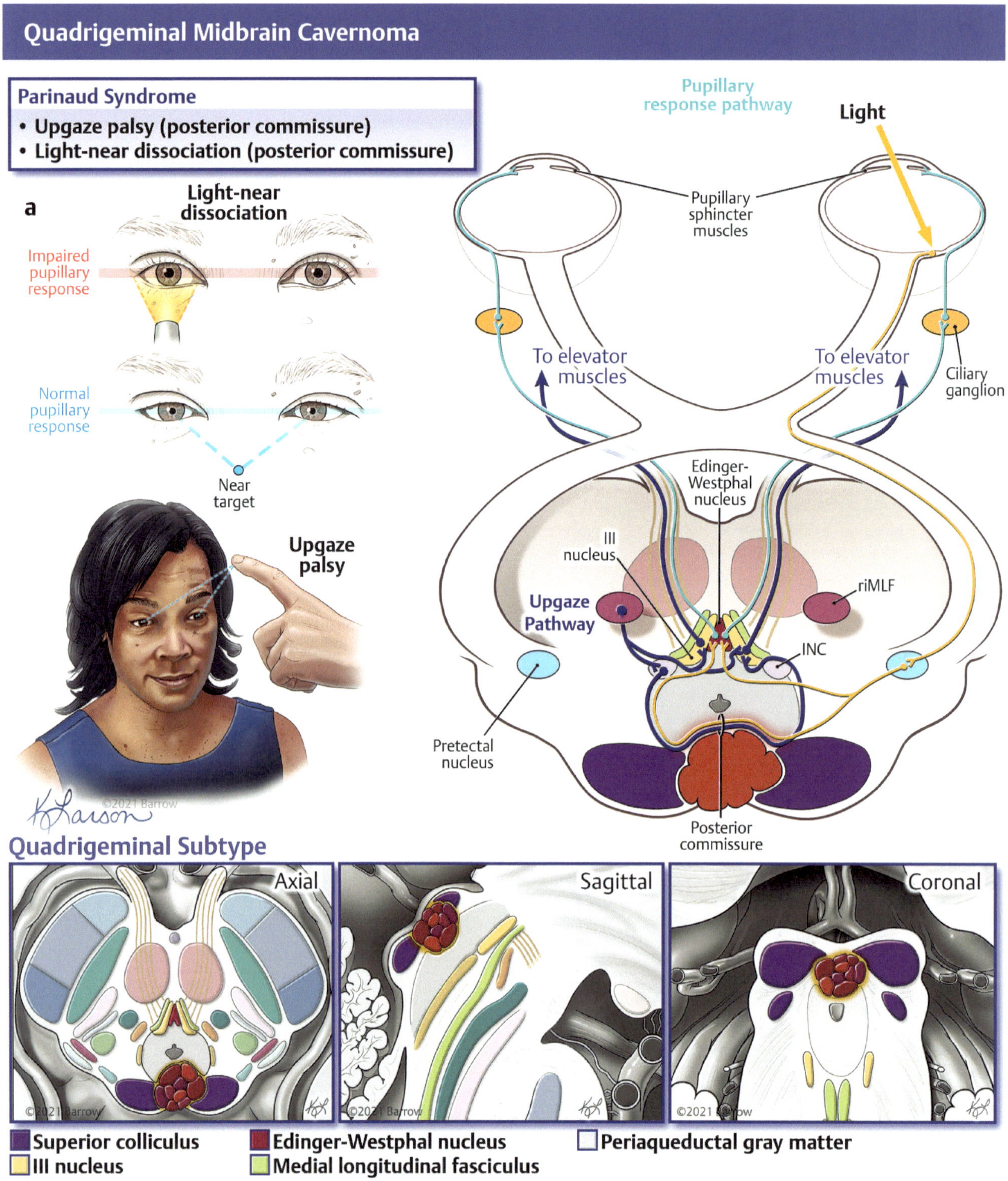

Fig. 14.6 Quadrigeminal midbrain CMs. **(a)** Patients with quadrigeminal midbrain CMs present with Parinaud syndrome or any combination of impaired upward gaze, impaired downward gaze, setting sun sign, pupillary abnormality, or loss of accommodation reflex. These symptoms and signs reflect the involvement of the superior colliculi and posterior commissure. The relationships between this midline CM and the oculomotor nerve nuclei, superior colliculi, and posterior commissure are shown in axial, sagittal, and coronal views (*lower insets*).

(Continued)

14

Surgical Approach

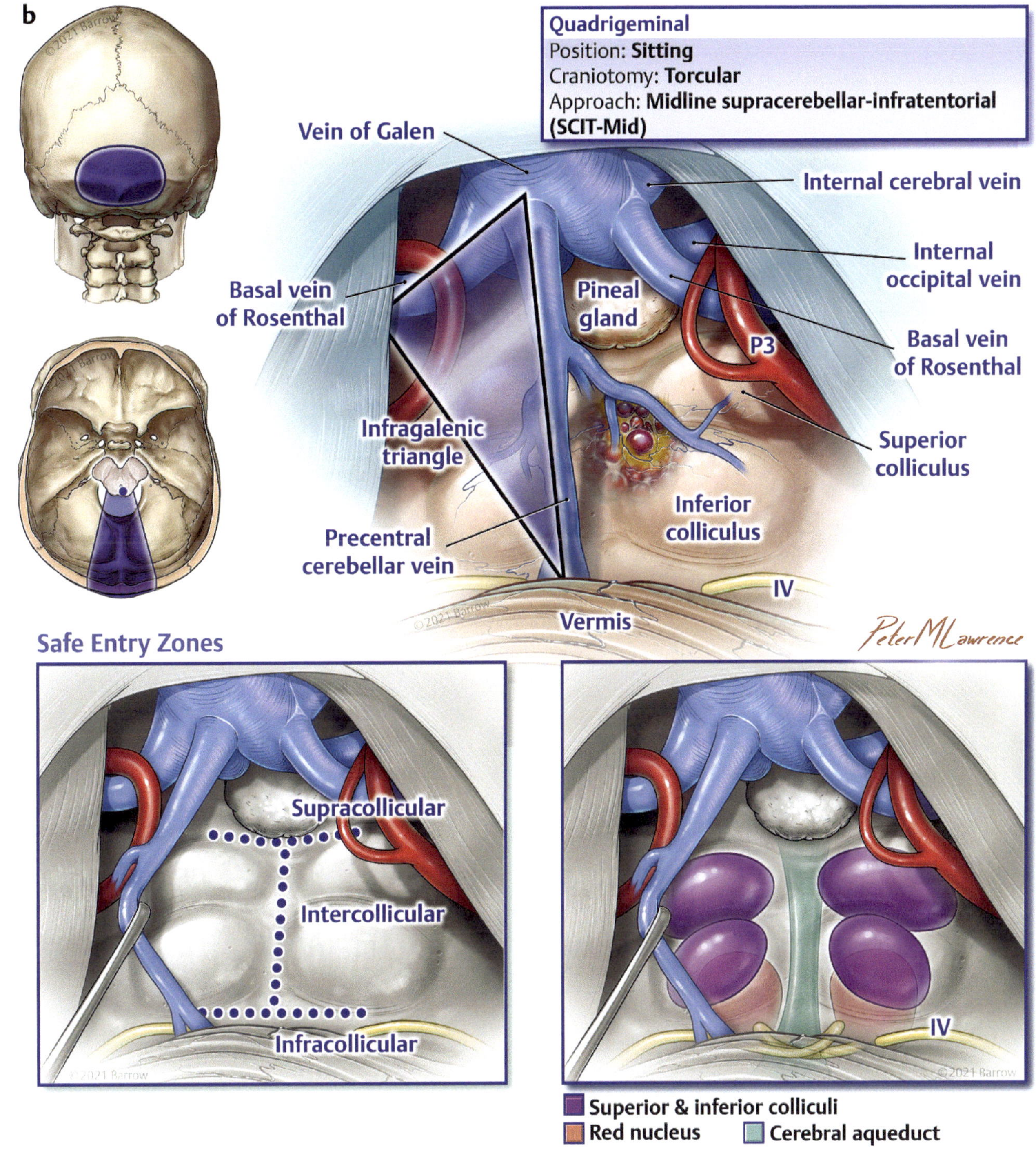

Fig. 14.6 (*Continued*) **(b)** A torcular craniotomy (*upper left inset*) and the SCIT-Mid approach is preferred for quadrigeminal CMs (*middle left inset*; *purple circle*). The patient is positioned in the sitting posture for gravity retraction of the cerebellum. The confluence of the precentral cerebellar vein, the BVR, and the vein of Galen form a working triangle underneath the venous complex (infragalenic triangle). Arterial landmarks include long circumflex perforators from the P1 and P2 segments of the PCAs, the medial posterior choroidal artery, and loops of the P3 PCA, and surface landmarks include the superior colliculi, inferior colliculi, pineal gland, and trochlear nerves. Three SEZs are described for this region: intercollicular, supracollicular, and infracollicular (*lower left inset*; *purple dotted lines*). Entry in the midline or upper or lower tectum must avoid the colliculi and decussation of the trochlear nerves (*lower right inset*; *ghosted structures*) (surgical cases; ▶ Video 14.11, ▶ Video 14.12, QR codes). Roman numerals denote CNs. (Reproduced with permission from Barrow Neurological Institute, Phoenix, AZ).

Surgical Case 14.11

MIDBRAIN

Cavernoma Subtype: Quadrigeminal

Position: Sitting
Craniotomy: Torcular
Approach: Midline supracerebellar-infratentorial (SCIT-Mid)
Triangle: Infragalenic
SEZ: Supracollicular
Artery: mPChA

Video: Resection of a right quadrigeminal midbrain cavernoma

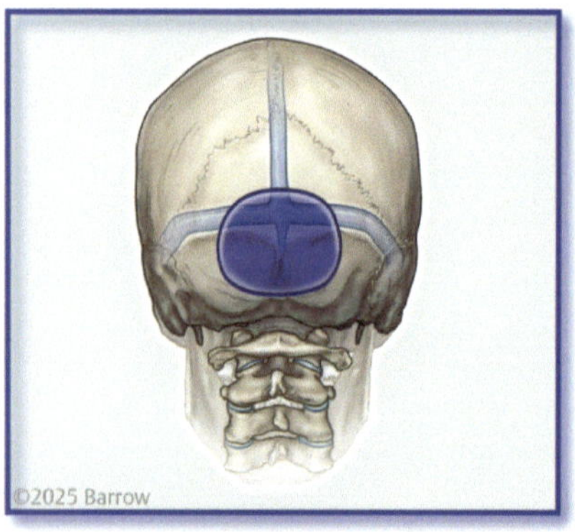

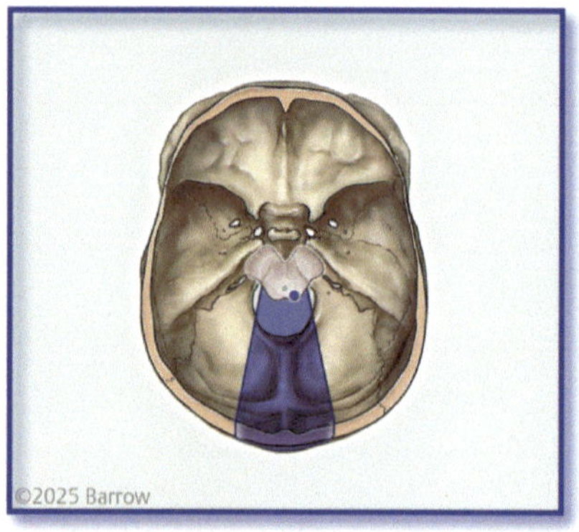

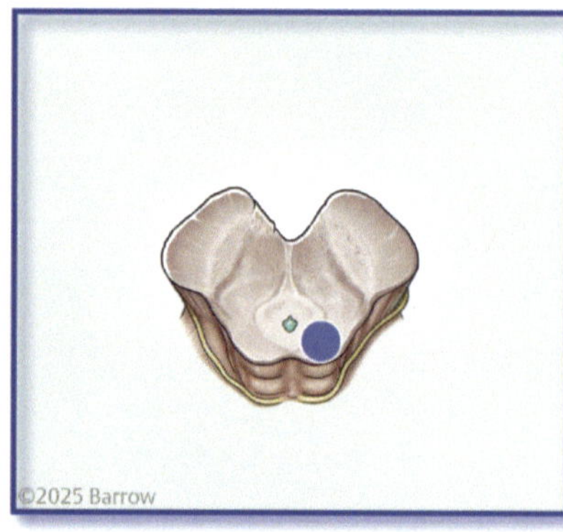

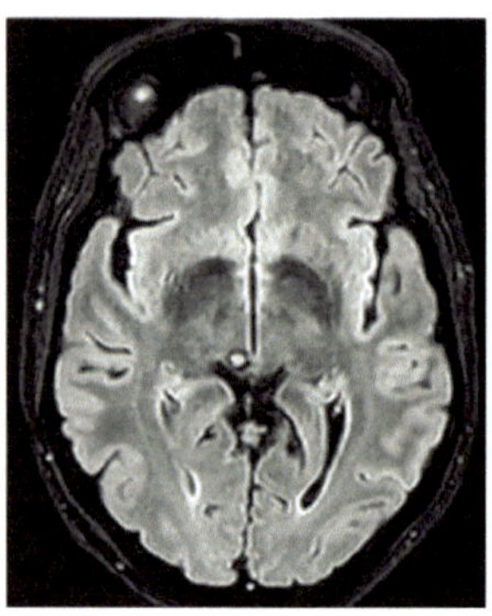

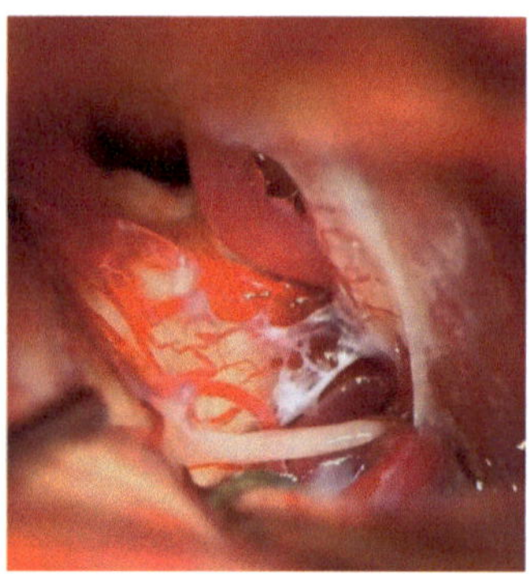

Video 14.11
Midline Supracerebellar-Infratentorial Approach for Quadrigeminal Midbrain Cavernous Malformation Resection (Reproduced with permission from Barrow Neurological Institute, Phoenix, AZ.)

Surgical Case 14.12

MIDBRAIN

Cavernoma Subtype: Quadrigeminal

Position: Sitting
Craniotomy: Torcular
Approach: Midline supracerebellar-infratentorial (SCIT-Mid)
Triangle: Infragalenic
SEZ: Intercollicular
Artery: mPChA, s4 SCA

Video: Resection of a left quadrigeminal midbrain cavernoma

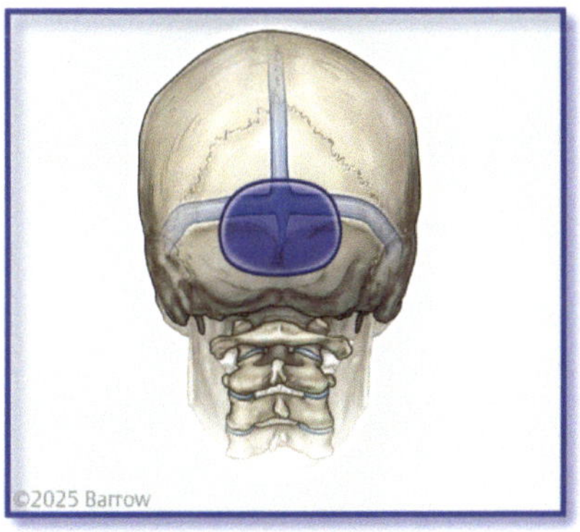

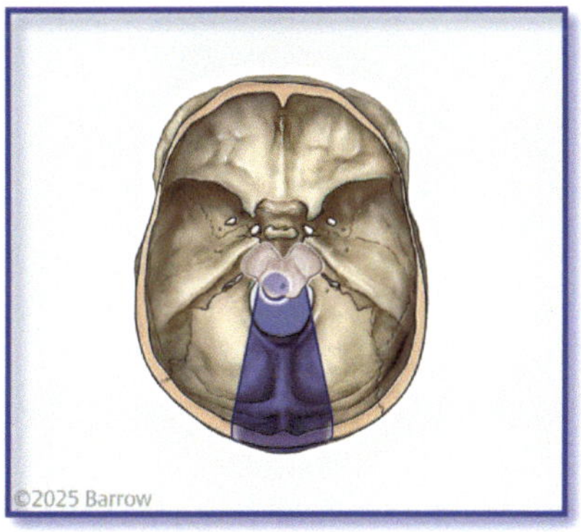

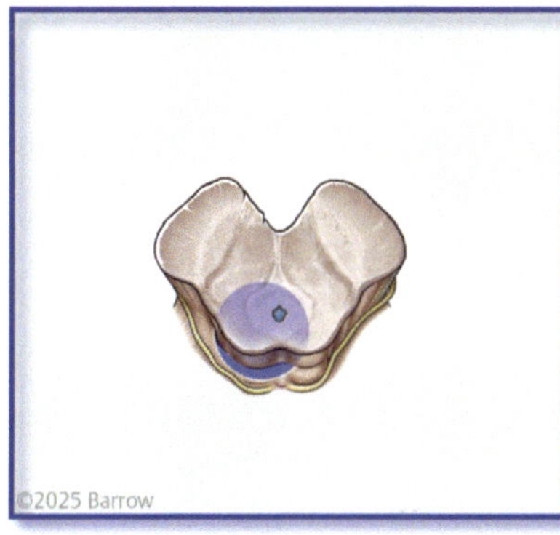

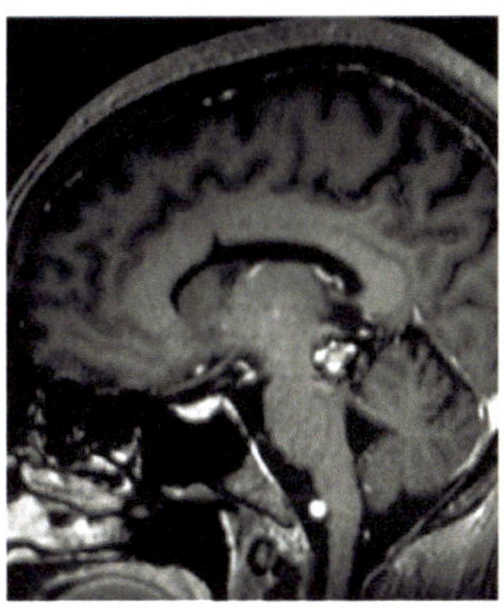

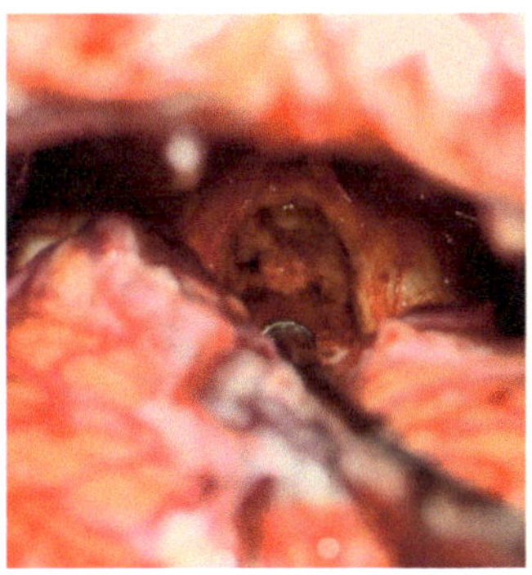

Video 14.12
Midline Supracerebellar-Infratentorial Approach for Quadrigeminal Midbrain Cavernous Malformation Resection (Reproduced with permission from Barrow Neurological Institute, Phoenix, AZ.)

14

Periaqueductal Midbrain Cavernoma

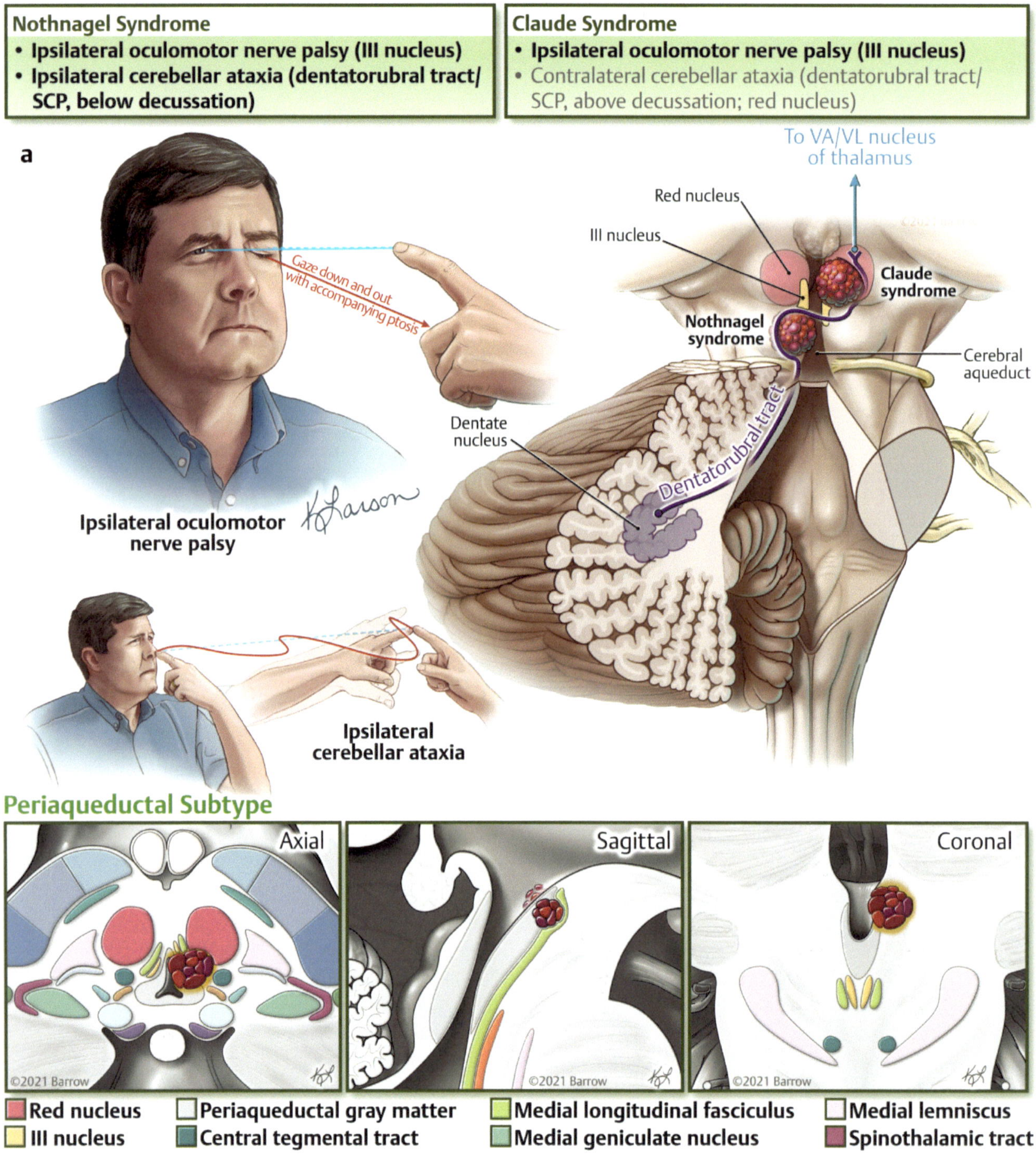

Fig. 14.7 Periaqueductal midbrain CMs. **(a)** Patients with the periaqueductal CM subtype present with Nothnagel syndrome comprising ipsilateral oculomotor nerve palsy and ipsilateral cerebellar ataxia from the involvement of the fascicular midbrain portion of the oculomotor nerve and superior cerebellar peduncle (SCP). Patients with lesions located more superiorly, above the decussation of the SCPs, may present with Claude syndrome (contralateral ataxia). The relationships between this left-sided CM and the oculomotor nerve nuclei and fascicle, red nucleus, and medial longitudinal fasciculus are shown in axial, sagittal, and coronal views (*lower insets*).

(Continued)

Surgical Approach

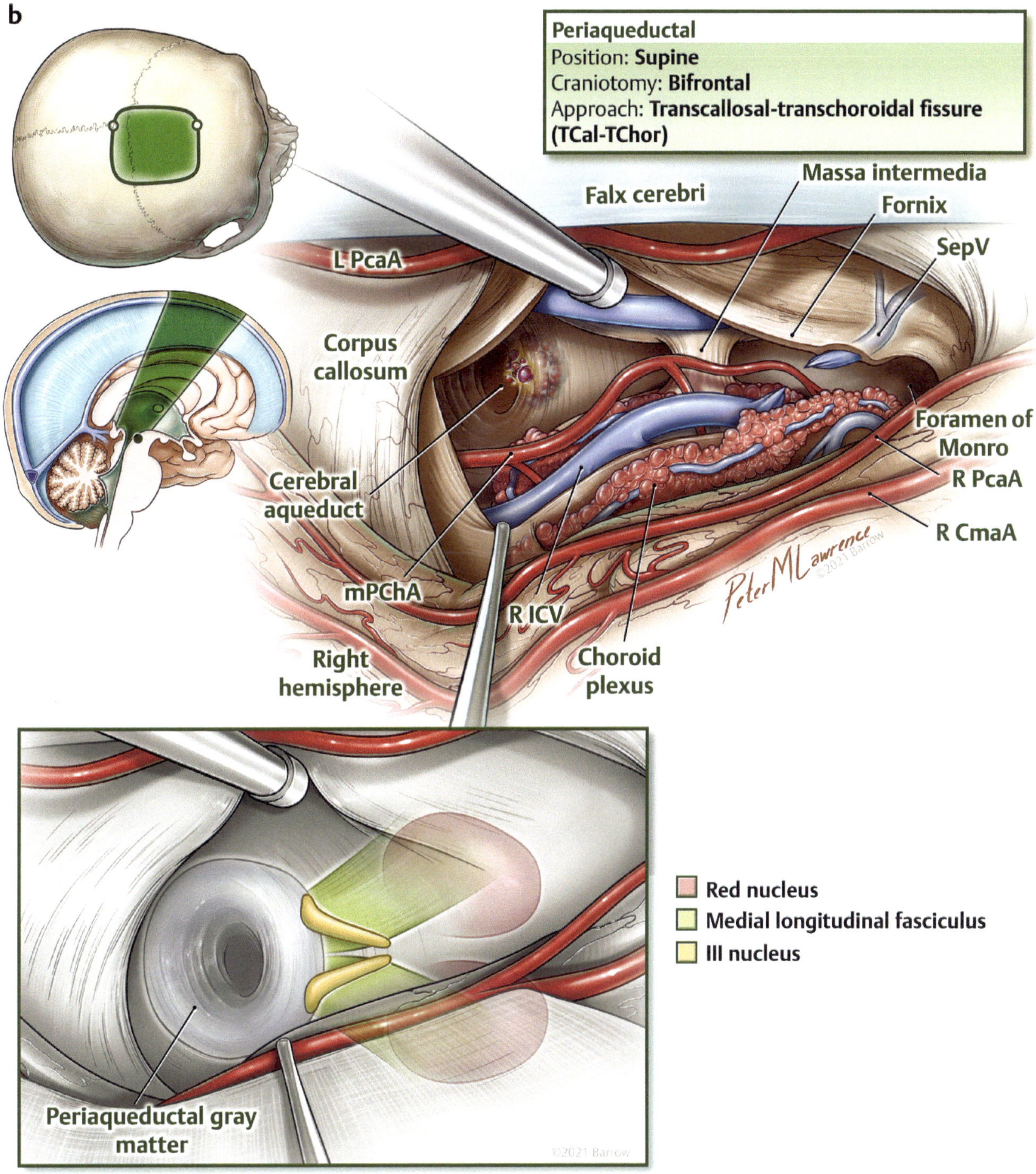

Fig. 14.7 *(Continued)* **(b)** Periaqueductal CMs are exposed through a bifrontal craniotomy (*upper left inset*) with the patient's head turned laterally to the right to avoid the dominant hemisphere and allow gravity to widen the interhemispheric fissure. A TCal-TChor approach showing CM (*middle left inset; green circle*) enlarges the foramen of Monro and traverses the third ventricle to arrive at the inlet of the aqueduct. This region does not have an anatomical triangle or SEZ. However, exophytic lesions are accessible at the inlet to the aqueduct or distally through the aqueduct (*lower left inset; ghosted structures*) (surgical case; ▶ Video 14.13, QR code). Roman numerals denote CNs. (Reproduced with permission from Barrow Neurological Institute, Phoenix, AZ).

Surgical Case 14.13

MIDBRAIN

Cavernoma Subtype: Periaqueductal

Position: Supine, with head lateral and midline horizontal
Craniotomy: Bifrontal
Approach: Contralateral transcallosal-transchoroidal (cTCal-TChor)
Triangle: None
SEZ: None
Artery: None

Video: Resection of a midline periaqueductal midbrain cavernoma

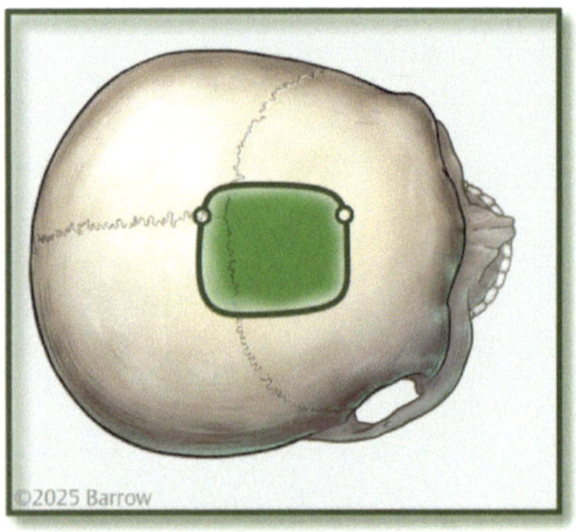

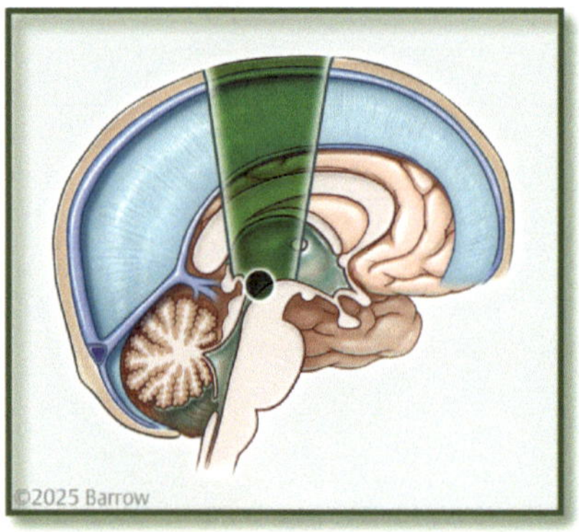

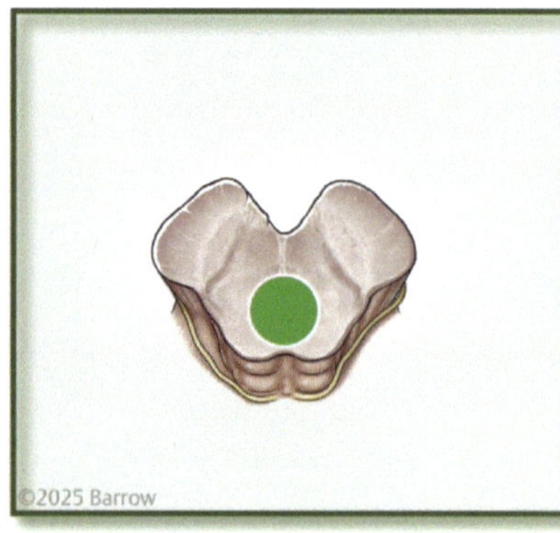

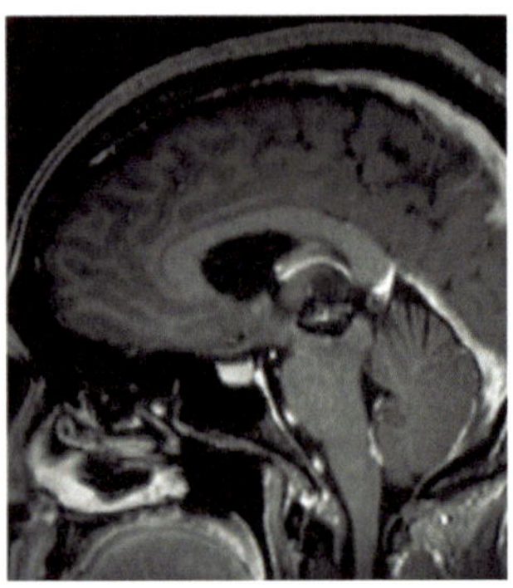

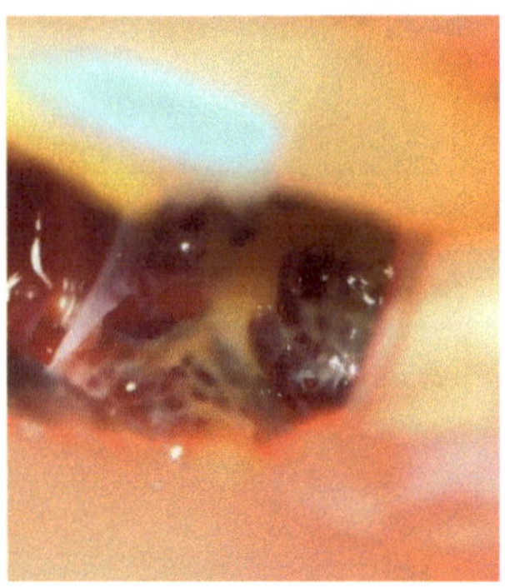

Video 14.13
Contralateral Transcallosal-Transchoroidal Approach for Periaqueductal Midbrain Cavernous Malformation Resection (Reproduced with permission from Barrow Neurological Institute, Phoenix, AZ.)

14

14.5 Conclusion

The anatomical taxonomy for brainstem CMs based on type or location (midbrain, pons, or medulla) and subtype or surface presentation (anterior, posterior, lateral, anterolateral, posterolateral) meaningfully guided the selection of the surgical approach and resection strategies. Five midbrain subtypes were defined by surface presentation, including interpeduncular, peduncular, tegmental, quadrigeminal, and periaqueductal. A single surgical approach for each midbrain CM subtype was preferred in more than 90% of patients. The constellation of neurologic symptoms and signs associated with a hemorrhagic midbrain CM subtype also helped define clinically recognizable neurologic syndromes at the bedside, even before seeing the pathoanatomy on MRI. The taxonomy increased diagnostic acumen and helped identify preferred surgical approaches for these rare midbrain CMs that can cause devastating neurologic deficits upon hemorrhaging. Taxonomy-guided surgery for patients with these lesions offers an interventional alternative to this difficult and destructive natural history.

15 PONS

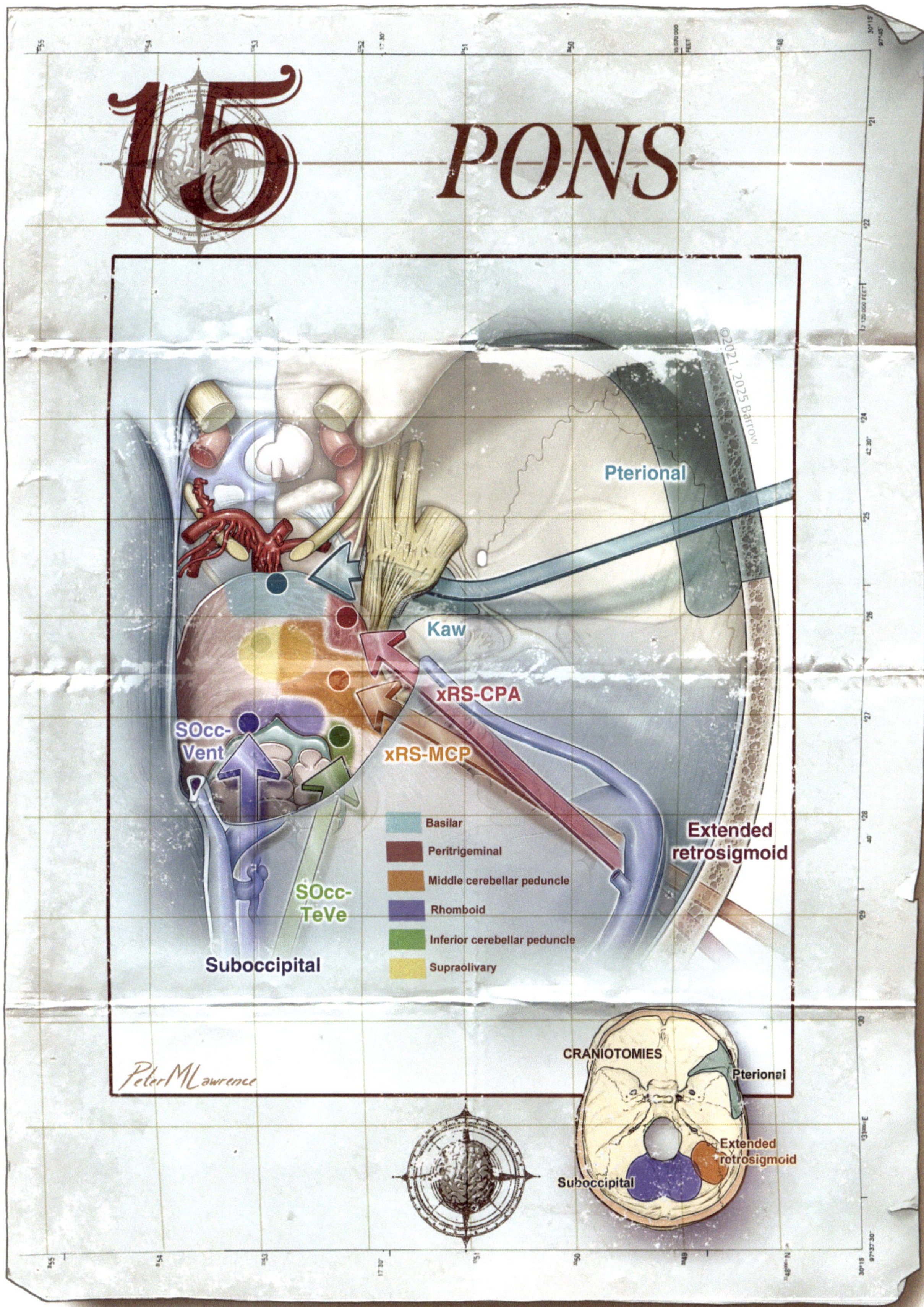

Reproduced with permission from Barrow Neurological Institute, Phoenix, AZ.

15 Pontine Cavernous Malformations

Summary

The pons is the most common site of brainstem cavernous malformations (CMs), accounting for nearly 60% of lesions. Six pontine CM subtypes are defined: basilar, peritrigeminal, middle cerebellar peduncular, inferior cerebellar peduncular, rhomboid, and supraolivary. Approaches to pontine CMs are selected on the basis of where the lesion presents to a pial or ependymal surface. The choice of the approach has a critical influence on successful lesion exposure, complete resection, and patient outcome. The brainstem CM taxonomy helps guide the choice of approach. This taxonomy was applied to a 2-surgeon microsurgical experience of 323 pontine CMs over a 30-year period. Of the 323 patients, 6 (2%) had basilar CMs, 53 (16%) had peritrigeminal CMs, and 100 (31%) had middle cerebellar peduncle (MCP) CMs. Another 47 (15%) patients had inferior cerebellar peduncle (ICP) CMs, 80 (25%) had rhomboid CMs, and 37 (12%) had supraolivary CMs. A single surgical approach and resection strategy were preferred for each subtype. For basilar CMs, a pterional craniotomy and an anterior transpetrous approach were preferred. For peritrigeminal CMs, an extended retrosigmoid craniotomy and trans-cerebellopontine angle approach were preferred. For MCP CMs, an extended retrosigmoid craniotomy and trans-MCP approach were preferred. For ICP CMs, a suboccipital craniotomy and telovelar approach were preferred. For rhomboid CMs, a suboccipital craniotomy and transventricular approach were preferred, and for supraolivary CMs, a far lateral craniotomy and trans-pontomedullary sulcus approach were preferred. Favorable outcomes were observed in 255 of 293 (87%) patients with follow-up. Most patients had improved or unchanged postoperative modified Rankin Scale scores (252/293, 86%). The pontine taxonomy meaningfully guided the selection of surgical approaches and resection strategies. It increased diagnostic acumen at the bedside because the constellation of neurological symptoms and signs associated with hemorrhagic pontine CMs helped define the subtype clinically with recognizable neurological signs before magnetic resonance imaging could be reviewed.

Keywords: basilar, brainstem, cavernoma, inferior cerebellar peduncle, medulla, midbrain, middle cerebellar peduncle, peritrigeminal, rhomboid, supraolivary

15.1 Introduction

The pons lies between the midbrain and the medulla and is the largest of these three brainstem structures. The pons contains descending pathways to the medulla and spinal cord, tracts that relay sensory signals upward to the thalamus, the termination or origination of four cranial nerves (CNs), and extra layers of transverse nerve fibers that connect the cerebral cortex and medulla with the cerebellum through the cerebellar peduncles. The pons is the most common site of brainstem cavernous malformations (CMs), accounting for nearly 60% of such lesions in the experience reported here. Approaches to pontine CMs are based on where the lesion presents to a pial or ependymal surface. Many nuanced surgical options exist, including lateral (transpetrous), posterior (transventricular), anterolateral (transcavernous), and even anterior (transclival) approaches. Simple concepts like the two-point method were previously used to determine the optimal surgical approach. The choice of the approach has a critical influence on successful lesion exposure, complete resection, and patient outcome. The taxonomy based on brainstem CM anatomy can now help guide the choice of the approach. With the dense packing of tracts and CN nuclei in the pons, the constellation of neurological symptoms and signs associated with a hemorrhagic brainstem CM subtype provides a unique clinical definition, just as the location of a brainstem CM on magnetic resonance imaging (MRI) provides an anatomical definition. Therefore, pontine CMs are associated with recognizable neurological syndromes and characteristic radiographic anatomy.

15.2 Neuroanatomy of the Six Pontine Cavernous Malformation Subtypes

Six pontine CM subtypes are defined on the basis of their locations on MRI: (1) basilar, (2) peritrigeminal, (3) middle cerebellar peduncular, (4) inferior cerebellar peduncular, (5) rhomboid, and (6) supraolivary (▶ Fig. 15.1).

15.2.1 Basilar

Basilar pontine CMs occur anteriorly in the pons, midline or off the midline directly opposite the clivus. They lie behind the basilar artery, its pontine perforators, and the s1 (anterior pontomesencephalic) segments of the superior cerebellar artery (SCA) and the a1 (precommunicating) segments of the anterior inferior cerebellar artery (AICA). This anterior surface extends between vertical lines drawn through the long axis of the inferior olive extended upward on the pons, which is the same landmark Rhoton defined as the dividing line between the a1 anterior pontine and the a2 lateral pontine segments of the AICA. The abducens nerve (CN VI) lies at the inferior border of this surface and ascends to the Dorello canal as a recognizable surgical landmark approximating this transolivary line. This anterior pontine surface extends from the pontomesencephalic sulcus superiorly to the pontomedullary sulcus inferiorly, with the basilar sulcus in the midline. The corticospinal tracts and transverse pontine fibers are below this surface and course to the middle cerebellar peduncles (MCPs).

15.2.2 Peritrigeminal

Peritrigeminal pontine CMs are located anterolaterally above, below, and medial to the trigeminal nerve root. These lesions lie between two vertical lines: the transolivary line medially and the transtrigeminal line laterally. They also lie between two horizontal sulci: the pontomesencephalic sulcus superiorly and the pontomedullary sulcus inferiorly. The s2 (lateral pontomesencephalic) segments of the SCA and a2 (lateral pontine) segments of the AICA approximate the superior and inferior

15

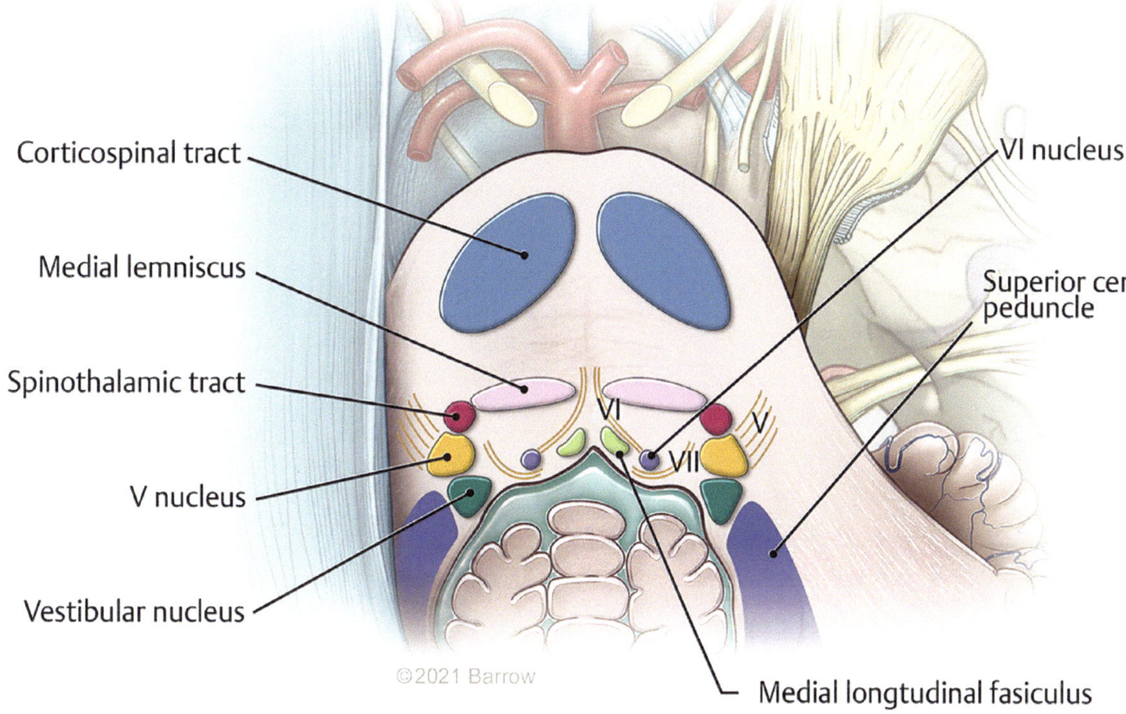

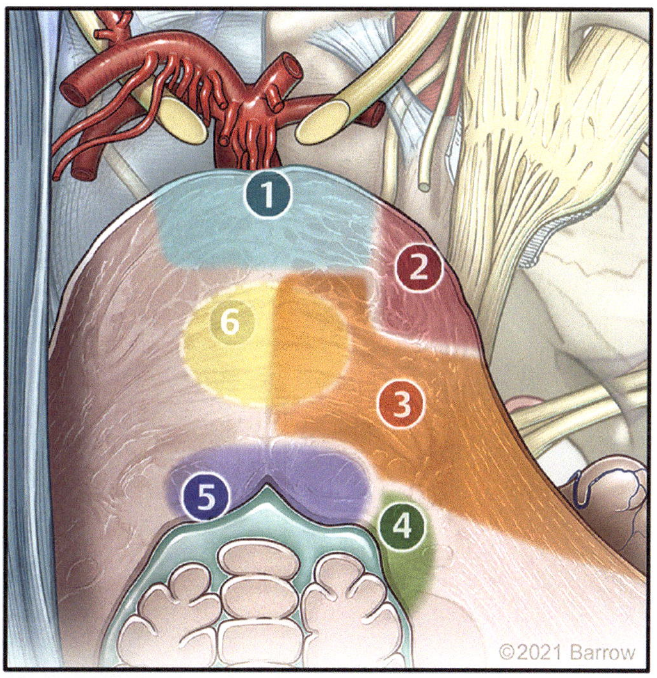

Fig. 15.1 Overview of pontine anatomy and CM subtypes. The anatomy of pontine nuclei and tracts is shown in axial cross-section. The subtype locations (*inset*; *colored circles*) within the pons are (1) basilar (*teal*), (2) peritrigeminal (*red*), (3) middle peduncular (*orange*), (4) inferior peduncular (*green*), (5) rhomboid (*purple*), and (6) the inferiorly located supraolivary subtype (*yellow*), ghosted through the pons. Roman numerals denote CNs. (Reproduced with permission from Barrow Neurological Institute, Phoenix, AZ.)

15

borders of this region, respectively. The vestibulocochlear nerve complex (CN VIII) lies at the inferolateral corner of this surface. Peritrigeminal CMs lie lateral to the corticospinal tracts and within the transverse pontine fibers.

15.2.3 Middle Peduncular

MCP pontine CMs are located in the lateral pons. This lateral border of the pons lacks a pial or subarachnoid surface because the MCP (brachium pontis) envelops it. These lesions lie posterior to the trigeminal root entry zone and medial to the MCP, flocculus, and superior and inferior limbs of the cerebellopontine fissures. The lateral pons contains the spinothalamic tract, lateral lemniscus, motor nucleus of the facial nerve, spinal nucleus and tract of the trigeminal nerve, ventral spinocerebellar tract, rubrospinal tract, and superior olivary nucleus.

15.2.4 Inferior Peduncular

Inferior cerebellar peduncle (ICP) pontine CMs are located in the posterolateral pons, just anterior to the lateral recess of the fourth ventricle. The stria medullaris delineates the pons above and the medulla below, forming the lower limit of ICP lesions. These lesions reside anterior to the stria and above the foramen of Luschka, distinct from rhomboid CMs on the floor of the fourth ventricle. ICP CMs lie lateral to the internal genu of the facial nerve (CN VII) and its intrapontine course. These CMs can involve the medial and lateral vestibular nuclei, cochlear nucleus, spinal nucleus and tract of the trigeminal nerve, superior salivatory nucleus, nucleus solitarius, and restiform and juxtarestiform bodies.

15.2.5 Rhomboid

Rhomboid pontine CMs are located in the posterior pons and present on the surface of the floor of the fourth ventricle. The ventricular floor, also known as the rhomboid fossa, has three parts: a pontine part extending from the aqueduct triangularly down to an imaginary line connecting the lower margin of the cerebellar peduncles, a junctional or intermediate part forming a thin strip between the lateral recesses, and a medullary part extending triangularly down to the obex. Surface landmarks in the rhomboid fossa's pontine part include the following: (1) the median sulcus, which divides the floor longitudinally in the midline; (2) the median eminence, a raised strip paralleling the median sulcus; (3) the facial colliculus, which is centered in the median eminence; (4) the sulcus limitans, another longitudinal sulcus on the lateral border of median eminence; (5) the locus ceruleus, a bluish-gray area at the rostral end of the sulcus limitans in the lateral margin of the floor; and (6) the superior foveae, which are dimples in the sulcus limitans just lateral to the facial colliculus. The facial colliculus overlies the abducens nucleus and the ascending root of CN VII. The striae medullaris, which are white strands traversing the junctional part of the floor from the lateral recess to the sulcus limitans, overlie the vestibular nuclei. Rhomboid CMs lie above the stria medullaris, whereas lesions at the level of the stria or below are considered medullary trigonal lesions. Critical structures below the floor include the medial longitudinal fasciculus (MLF), the dorsal longitudinal fasciculus, the reticular formation, the tectospinal tract, the central tegmental tract, the ventral trigeminothalamic tract, the medial lemniscus, the lateral lemniscus, and the trapezoid body.

15.2.6 Supraolivary

Supraolivary pontine CMs are located in the inferior pons and project downward to a pial surface at the pontomedullary junction. The intersection of the pons and the medulla creates a pontine underbelly or basis pontis overhang that enables CMs in the central pons to be entered from below. This anatomical protuberance allows the surgeon access to a region otherwise surrounded by eloquent tracts and nuclei. The location lies above the inferior olivary nucleus, lateral to the exit of the abducens nerve, medial to the exit of the facial nerve, and above the distal a1 and proximal a2 segments of the AICA. These CMs lie lateral to the corticospinal tract and transpontine course of the abducens nerve within the lower transverse pontine fibers. The supraolivary trajectory leads to the center of the pons near the medial lemniscus, lateral lemniscus, spinothalamic tract, superior olivary nucleus, rubrospinal tract, and trapezoid body.

15.3 Clinical Evidence

The brainstem CM taxonomy was applied to a 2-surgeon experience of 323 pontine CMs that Robert F. Spetzler and I treated microsurgically over a 30-year period (1990–2019) (▸ Table 15.1). These pontine CMs were classified into 6 distinct subtypes: (1) basilar (6/323, 2%), (2) peritrigeminal (53/323, 16%), (3) middle cerebellar peduncular (100/323, 31%), (4) inferior cerebellar peduncular (47/323, 15%), (5) rhomboid (80/323, 25%), and (6) supraolivary (37/323, 12%) (▸ Fig. 15.1).

Basilar lesions are located in the anteromedial pons and are associated with contralateral hemiparesis. Peritrigeminal lesions are located in the anterolateral pons and are associated with hemiparesis and sensory changes. Patients with MCP lesions presented with mild AICA syndrome with contralateral hemisensory loss, ipsilateral ataxia, ipsilateral facial numbness, and hemiparesis without cranial neuropathies. ICP lesions are located in the inferolateral pons and are associated with acute vestibular syndrome. Rhomboid lesions on the fourth ventricle floor are associated with dysconjugate eye movements. Larger lesions may cause ipsilateral facial weakness. Supraolivary lesions present to the surface at the ventral pontine underbelly, and ipsilateral abducens palsy was a strong localizing sign for this subtype. The heat map summarizes patients' symptoms by subtype (▸ Fig. 15.2).

The Lawton brainstem CM grades were determined for 178 patients: 66 (37%) had low-grade brainstem CMs (grades 0–II), 100 (56%) had intermediate-grade brainstem CMs (grades III–V), and 12 (7%) had high-grade brainstem CMs (grades VI and VII). A single surgical approach and resection strategy were preferred for each subtype. For basilar CMs, a pterional craniotomy and an anterior transpetrous approach were preferred. For peritrigeminal CMs, an extended retrosigmoid craniotomy and a trans-cerebellopontine angle approach were preferred. For CMs in the MCP, an extended retrosigmoid craniotomy and a trans-MCP approach were preferred. For CMs in the ICP, a

Table 15.1 Preoperative and postoperative outcome measures for patients who underwent resection of pontine CMs by subtype

Variable	All (*N* = 323)	Basilar (*n* = 6)	Peritrigeminal (*n* = 53)	Middle peduncular (*n* = 100)	Inferior peduncular (*n* = 47)	Rhomboid (*n* = 80)	Supraolivary (*n* = 37)	*p*-value
Brainstem CM grade								
Patients with data available, *n*	178	3	40	51	25	35	24	
Low (0-II)	66/178 (37)	1/66 (2)	13/66 (20)	19/66 (29)	7/66 (11)	10/66 (29)	16/66 (67)	0.20
Intermediate (III–V)	100/178 (56)	1/100 (1)	25/100 (25)	30/100 (30)	16/100 (16)	21/100 (21)	7/100 (1)	
High (VI, VII)	12/178 (7)	1/12 (8)	2/12 (17)	2/12 (17)	2/12 (17)	4/12 (33)	1/12 (8)	
Follow-up								
Mean (SD), mo	29 (39)	17 (9)	26 (38)	31 (39)	28 (36)	32 (49)	19 (22)	0.58
> 30 d	279/323 (86)	6/279 (2)	46/279 (16)	84/279 (30)	42/279 (15)	68/279 (24)	33/279 (12)	0.91
Pre-op mRS score								
Median (IQR)	2 (1–2)	2 (2–3)	1 (1–2)	1 (1–2)	1 (1–2)	2 (1–2)	2 (1–2)	0.73
> 2	54/323 (17)	2/54 (4)	6/54 (11)	20/54 (37)	7/54 (13)	15/54 (28)	4/54 (7)	0.73
Post-op mRS score								
Median (IQR)	2 (1–2)	2 (2–2)	1 (1–2)	2 (1–3)	2 (1–3)	2 (2–3)	2 (1–2)	0.31
> 2	75/323 (23)	1/75 (1)	6/75 (8)	25/75 (33)	13/75 (17)	22/75 (29)	8/75 (11)	0.31
Final mRS score								
Patients with data available, *n*	293	6	49	88	41	74	35	
Median (IQR)	1 (1–2)	1 (1–1)	1 (1–2)	1 (1–2)	1 (1–2)	1 (1–2)	1 (1–2)	0.30
> 2	38/293 (13)	0/38 (0)	5/38 (13)	15/38 (39)	6/38 (16)	11/38 (29)	1/38 (3)	0.35
≤ 2	255/293 (87)	6/255 (2)	44/255 (17)	73/255 (29)	35/255 (14)	63/255 (25)	34/255 (13)	0.35
Worsened vs. pre-op mRS score	41/293 (14)	0/41 (0)	8/41 (20)	11/41 (27)	7/41 (17)	10/41 (24)	5/41 (12)	0.98

Note: Data are presented as n (%) unless otherwise indicated. Percentages might not total 100% due to rounding.

	Subtype					
Symptom	Basilar (n=6)	Peritrigeminal (n=53)	MCP (n=100)	ICP (n=47)	Rhomboid (n=80)	Supraolivary (n=37)
Hemisensory deficit	1 (17%)	18 (34%)	42 (42%)	21 (45%)	41 (51%)	18 (49%)
Hemiparesis	4 (67%)	22 (42%)	28 (28%)	9 (19%)	15 (19%)	17 (46%)
Ataxia	1 (17%)	15 (28%)	34 (34%)	22 (47%)	24 (30%)	7 (19%)
N/V, vertigo	0 (0%)	6 (11%)	20 (20%)	14 (30%)	16 (20%)	2 (5%)
Abducens nerve palsy	1 (17%)	10 (19%)	15 (15%)	11 (23%)	37 (46%)	26 (70%)
Facial weakness	2 (33%)	2 (4%)	17 (17%)	11 (23%)	29 (36%)	11 (30%)

Fig. 15.2 Heat map showing symptoms of patients with pontine CMs by subtype. Percentages were calculated as the frequency of a particular symptom or sign within a given midbrain subtype population. The sensitivity and specificity of neurological findings are known to vary significantly. Hemiparesis is more likely to be accurately documented in medical records than trochlear nerve palsy. Thus, for each symptom or sign, rates were sorted according to their relative frequency across the six subtypes. Conditional formatting was applied on a scale of least common (*red*) to most common (*green*). Well-defined syndromes associated with each subtype aligned most closely with cells with *green* formatting. (Reproduced with permission from Catapano JS, Rumalla K, Srinivasan VM, Lawrence PM, Larson Keil K, Lawton MT. A taxonomy for brainstem cavernous malformations: subtypes of pontine lesions. Part 1: basilar, peritrigeminal, and middle peduncular. J Neurosurg 2022;137(5):1462–1476).

suboccipital craniotomy and a telovelar approach were preferred. For rhomboid CMs, a suboccipital craniotomy and a transventricular approach were preferred, and for supraolivary CMs, a far lateral craniotomy and a trans-pontomedullary sulcus approach were preferred. Favorable outcomes were observed in 255 of 293 (87%) patients with follow-up. Most patients had improved or unchanged postoperative modified Rankin Scale (mRS) scores (252/293, 86%). There were no significant differences in outcomes between the subtypes.

15.4 Resection Strategies for Pontine Cavernous Malformations

The taxonomy for pontine CM subtypes guides the selection of surgical approaches and resection strategies (▶ Fig. 15.3). In addition, the constellation of neurological symptoms and signs associated with a hemorrhagic pontine CM subtype helped define that subtype clinically with recognizable neurological signs, even before pathological anatomy findings on MRI were available.

15.4.1 Basilar Subtype

The basis pontis is the ventral two-thirds of the pons and contains descending corticospinal tracts and transverse pontine fibers. These tracts and fibers run anterior to the pontine tegmentum, the dorsal one-third of the pons that contains other nuclei and tracts. Basilar pontine CMs occupy the midline or paramedian strip of the ventral pontine surface (▶ Fig. 15.4a). Some patients with unilateral CMs present with medial pontine syndrome or contralateral hemiparesis, whereas those with larger bilateral lesions present with locked-in syndrome comprising quadriplegia and paralysis of the lower CNs with preserved consciousness.

We treated only a few patients with basilar pontine CMs in our surgical experience, which reflects the difficulty of access to the region surrounded by the clival portion of the occipital bone anteriorly and the petrous parts of the temporal bones laterally. These lesions displace the descending corticospinal tract laterally, placing it in harm's way for posterolateral approaches like the extended retrosigmoid craniotomy and trans-cerebellopontine angle or trans-MCP approaches. The Kawase approach through the medial petrous bone provides a safer anterolateral exposure (▶ Fig. 15.4b; ▶ Video 15.1, ▶ Video 15.2). The dura propria of the temporal lobe is peeled from the lateral wall of the cavernous sinus, exposing the branches of the trigeminal nerve. The petrous bone is drilled in the Kawase triangle between the lateral border of V3 (mandibular branch of the trigeminal nerve), the greater superficial petrosal nerve, and the internal auditory canal between the superior and inferior petrosal sinuses. Opening the petrous dura transitions this extradural approach to an intradural one. The basilar artery, pontine perforators, and a1 segments of the AICA are typically medial to the pontine surface exposed through the Kawase approach. The surface anatomy comprises a prominent basilar groove or sulcus and superficial transverse pontine fibers. No safe entry zone (SEZ) guides the dissection. The ideal lesion presentation is to the anterior pia. The Kawase approach provides oblique anterolateral access to the basilar surface. This approach is adequate when lesions are eccentric or exophytic and finessed into the surgical field. However, misaligning this long, narrow, bony surgical corridor with the lesion's axis may lead to blind corners and incomplete resections. The Kawase approach, first introduced for AICA aneurysms on the proximal basilar trunk, is ideal for lesions below the trigeminal nerve in the lower half of the basilar pontine region. Lesions above the trigeminal nerve in the upper half of the basilar pontine region require a transsylvian-transcavernous approach, providing an anterolateral trajectory to the lesion. The basilar pontine CM may be amenable to midline transclival approaches with further advances in endoscopic-endonasal visualization and refinements in instrumentation. However, our experience with these endoscopic-endonasal approaches is limited because we did not perform them.

15.4.2 Peritrigeminal Subtype

The peritrigeminal territory encompasses the anterolateral pontine surface as it bends from the ventral pons to the MCP or between the transolivary and transtrigeminal lines. Peritrigeminal pontine CMs are the second most common pontine subtype. Despite the name, they rarely cause trigeminal symptoms or signs because they sit anteromedial to the transpontine nerve fascicles, principal sensory nucleus, mesencephalic nucleus, and spinal nucleus and tract (▶ Fig. 15.5a). Instead, this subtype is most associated with contralateral hemiparesis due to its proximity to the corticospinal tract. These lesions cause ipsilateral ataxia and contralateral hemisensory loss, affecting touch and pain or temperature sensations in approximately one-third of patients due to the involvement of the MCP, medial lemniscus, and spinothalamic tract. Nonetheless, these signs are not specific to peritrigeminal lesions.

The extended retrosigmoid approach was the most used approach to enter the cerebellopontine cistern (▶ Fig. 15.5b; ▶ Video 15.3, ▶ Video 15.4, ▶ Video 15.5, ▶ Video 15.6). This approach relies on the complete skeletonization of the sigmoid sinus from the transverse–sigmoid sinus junction superiorly to the jugular bulb inferiorly. It widens the craniocaudal exposure and retracts the sigmoid sinus anteriorly for improved access to the anterolateral pons. Dissection through the cerebellopontine angle exposes the three CN complexes of the posterior fossa: CN V (trigeminal) in the upper complex, CNs VII/VIII in the middle complex, and CNs IX/X/XI (glossopharyngeal, vagus, and accessory) in the lower complex. These nerve complexes define three triangular dissection routes: (1) the supratrigeminal triangle, superior to the trigeminal nerve and inferior to the tentorium and trochlear nerve; (2) the infratrigeminal triangle, inferior to the trigeminal nerve and superior to the vestibular nerve; and (3) the glossopharyngeal-cochlear triangle, inferior to the cochlear nerve and superior to the glossopharyngeal nerve.

The supratrigeminal triangle provides a good trajectory to superiorly located lesions despite its small size and limited room between CN V and the tentorium. The infratrigeminal triangle provides the largest corridor and best exposure of the anterolateral pontine surface, with the low origin of the vestibulocochlear nerves and the high position of the trigeminal nerve. The glossopharyngeal-cochlear triangle provides access to the inferomedial peritrigeminal region containing the abducens nerve

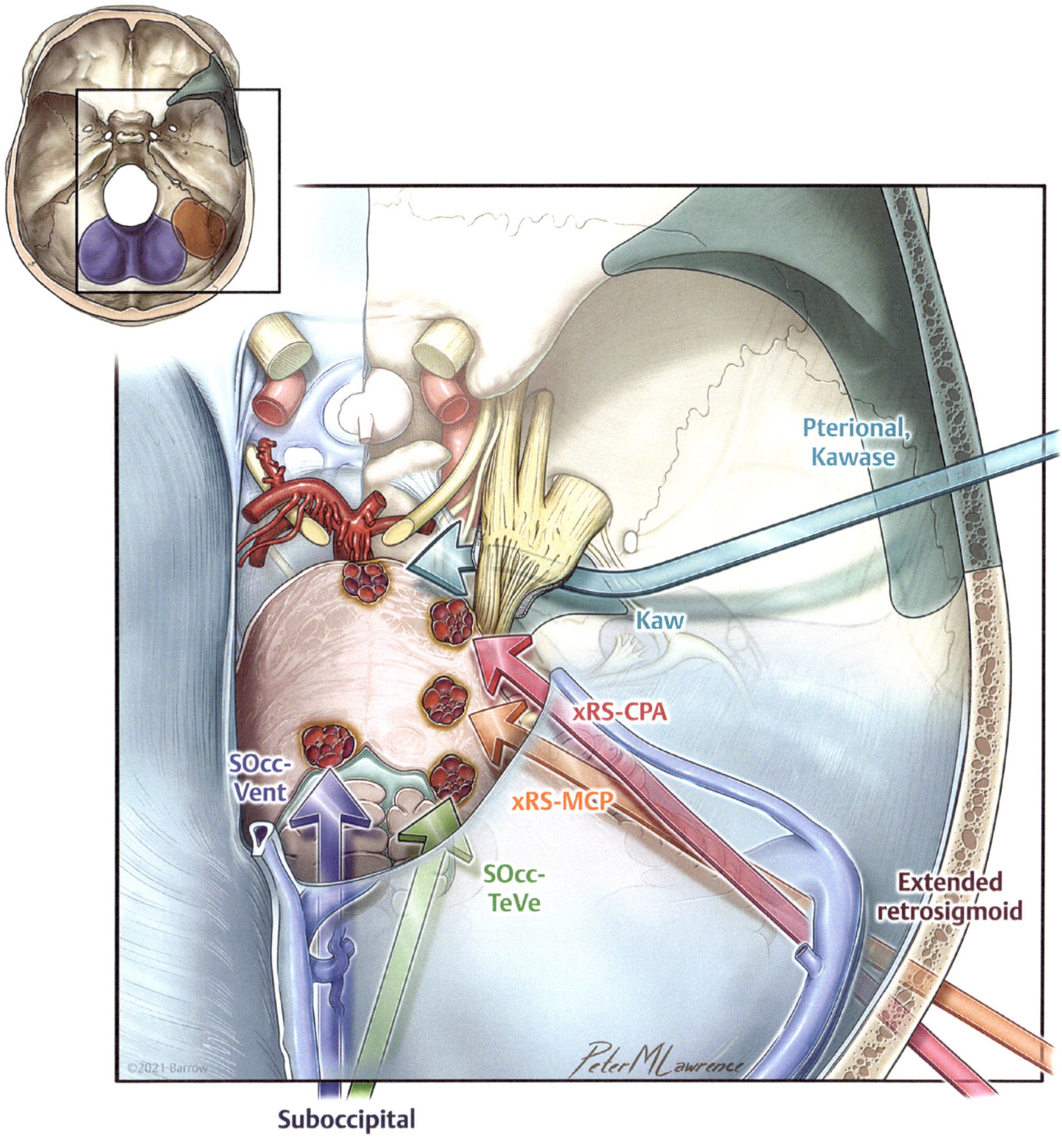

Fig. 15.3 Overview of surgical approaches to pontine CMs shown in axial cross-section viewed from above. Craniotomies associated with these approaches are shown in relation to the skull base (*inset*). The pterional craniotomy and anterior transpetrous (Kawase) approach is used for basilar CMs (Kaw; *teal arrow*). The extended retrosigmoid craniotomy and xRS-CPA approach (*red arrow*) is used for peritrigeminal CMs, and the extended retrosigmoid and xRS-MCP approach (*orange arrow*) is used for middle peduncular CMs. The SOcc-Vent approach (*purple arrow*) is used for rhomboid lesions, and the SOcc-TeVe approach (*green arrow*) is used for inferior peduncular lesions. The far lateral craniotomy trans-pontomedullary sulcus approach (not shown) is used for supraolivary lesions located more inferiorly in the pons. (Reproduced with permission from Barrow Neurological Institute, Phoenix, AZ.)

Basilar Pontine Cavernoma

Medial Pontine Syndrome

- **Contralateral hemiparesis (unilateral corticospinal tract)**

Locked-in Syndrome

- Quadriplegia and paralysis of lower CNs (bilateral corticospinal tract)

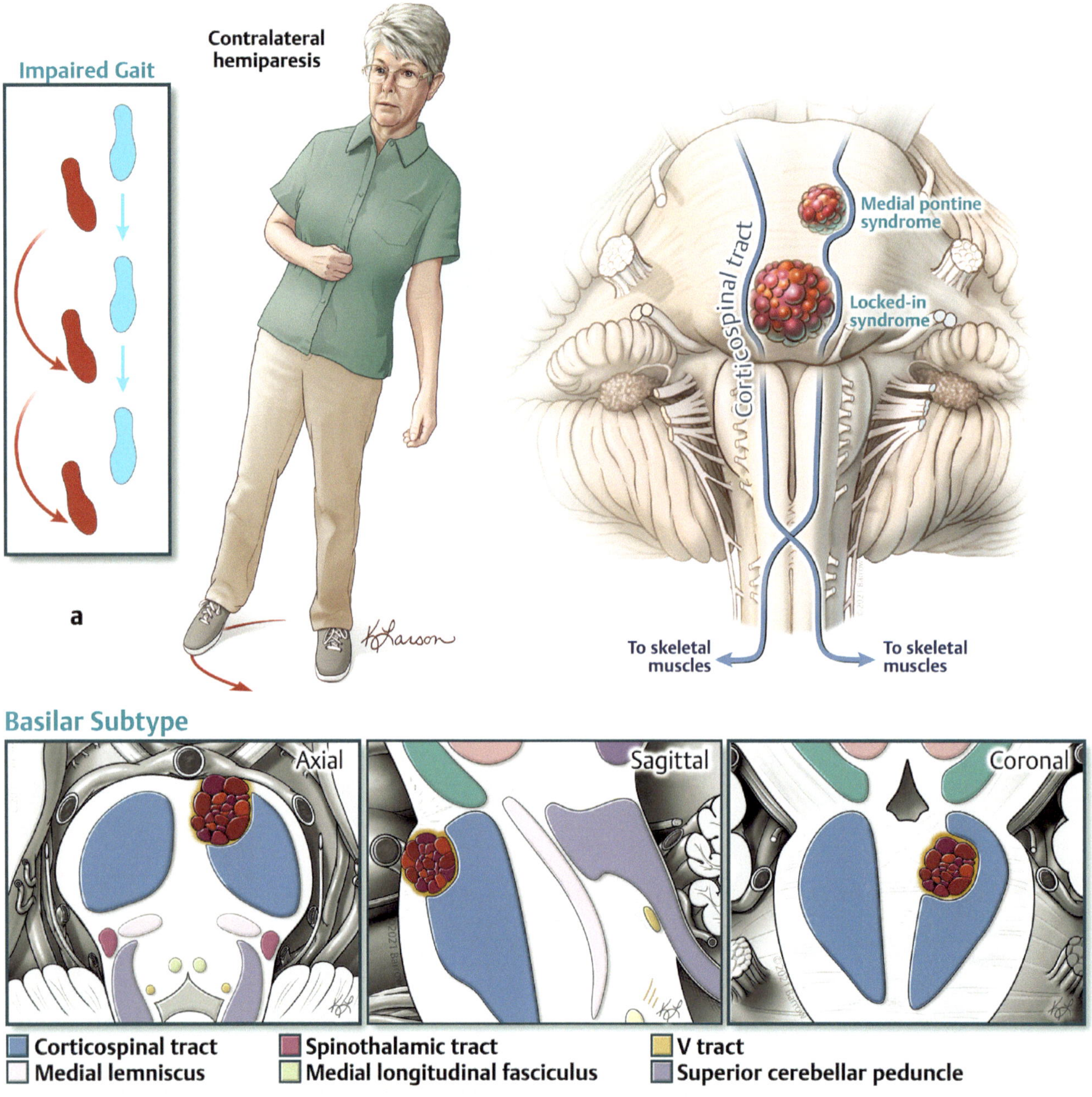

Fig. 15.4 Clinical syndromes and surgical approaches for basilar pontine CMs. **(a)** Patients with small unilateral basilar pontine CMs present with contralateral hemiparesis and impaired gait (medial pontine syndrome), whereas patients with large bilateral basilar pontine CMs present with quadriplegia and paralysis of lower CN targets (locked-in syndrome; not shown). This left-sided basilar CM resides anteriorly in the pons behind the basilar trunk and involves the corticospinal tract, as shown in axial, sagittal, and coronal views (*lower insets*).

(Continued)

Surgical Approach

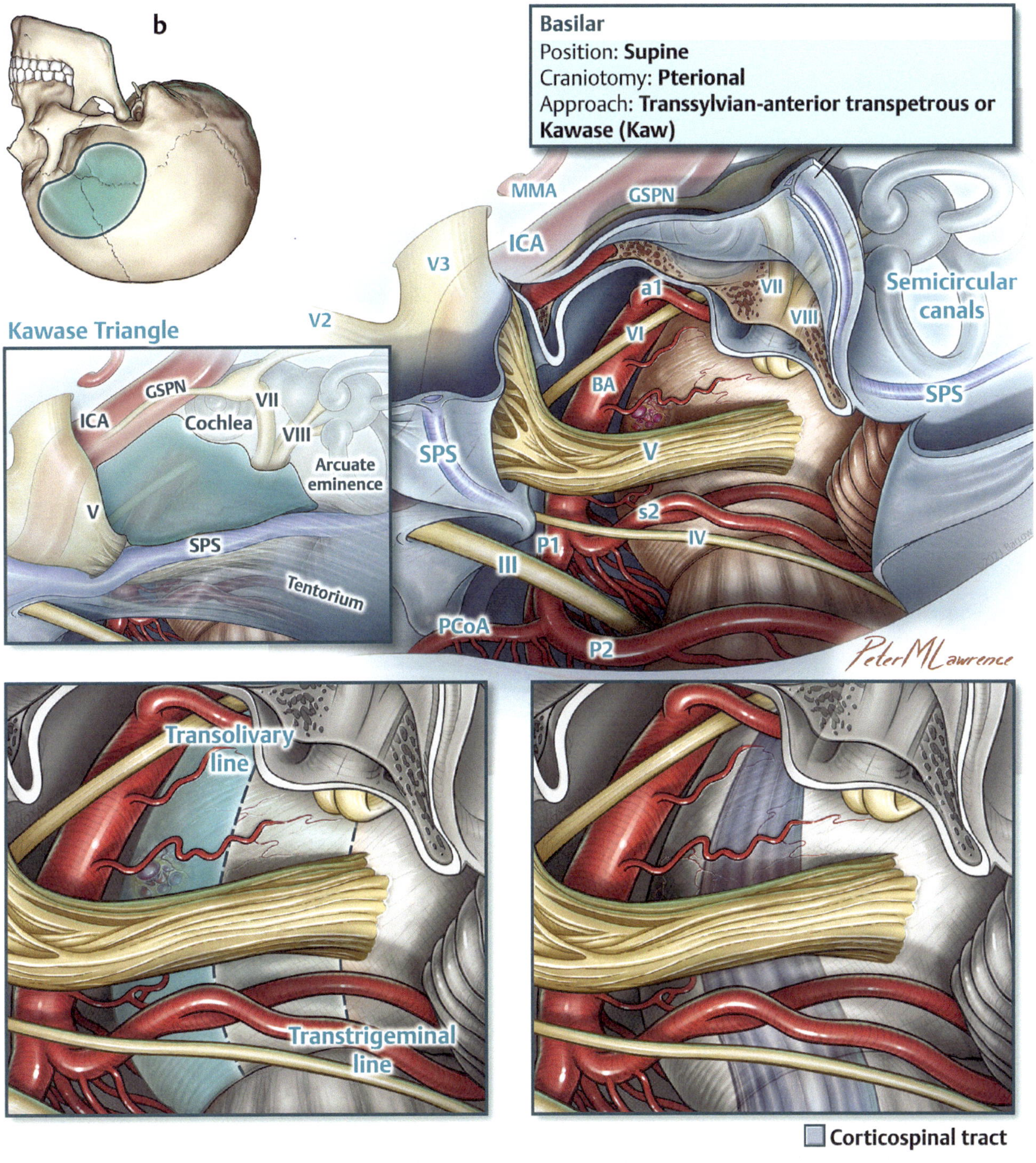

Fig. 15.4 *(Continued)* **(b)** Basilar pontine CMs are exposed surgically through a pterional craniotomy (*upper left inset*) and anterior transpetrous approach. The anterior petrous bone is exposed extradurally by peeling the dura propria of the temporal lobe from the lateral wall of the cavernous sinus and exposing the branches of the trigeminal nerve (*middle left inset*). The petrous bone is drilled in the Kawase triangle (*teal quadrangle*) between the lateral border of V3, the GSPN, the internal auditory canal, and the superior and inferior petrosal sinuses. Opening the petrous dura and resecting a portion of the tentorium exposes the anterior pons. The dissection route travels through the Kawase triangle, under the trigeminal nerve, above the facial nerve, medial to CN VI or the transolivary line, and lateral to the basilar trunk to reach the targeted basilar CM (*lower left inset*; *ghosted below the anterior pontine surface*; *teal*). The transolivary line (*dashed line*) is approximately midway between the basilar artery and the transtrigeminal line (*dashed line*). The corticospinal tract (*lower right inset*; *ghosted in blue*) lies beneath the pontine surface (surgical cases; ▶ Video 15.1, ▶ Video 15.2; QR codes). Roman numerals denote CNs. (Reproduced with permission from Barrow Neurological Institute, Phoenix, AZ.)

Surgical Case 15.1

PONTINE

Cavernoma Subtype: Basilar

Position: Supine
Craniotomy: Orbitozygomatic-pterional
Approach: Transsylvian-transpontine (TSyl-Pon)
Triangle: Oculomotor-tentorial
SEZ: None
Artery: s1 SCA

Video: Resection of a right basilar pontine cavernoma

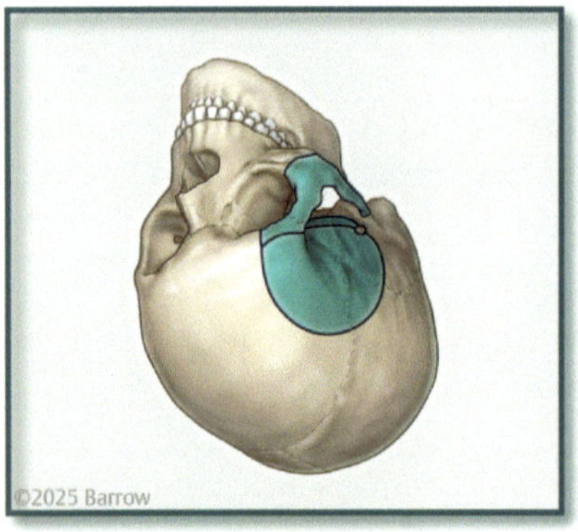

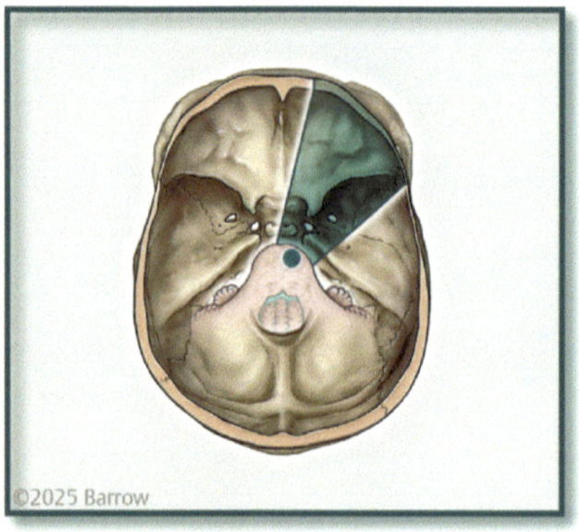

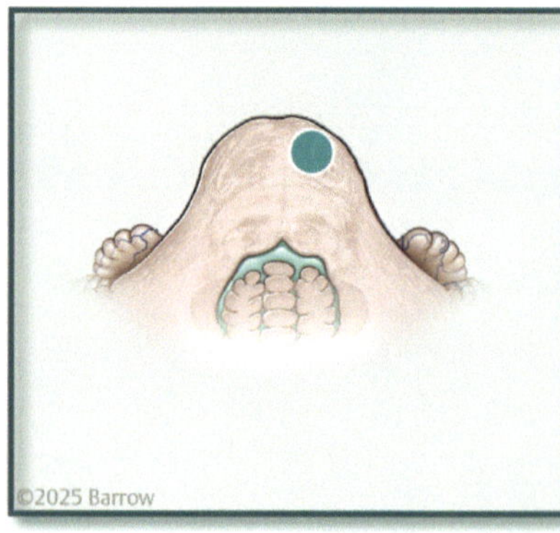

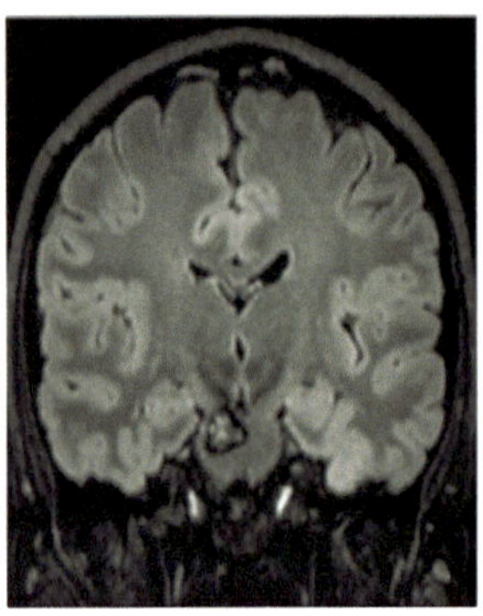

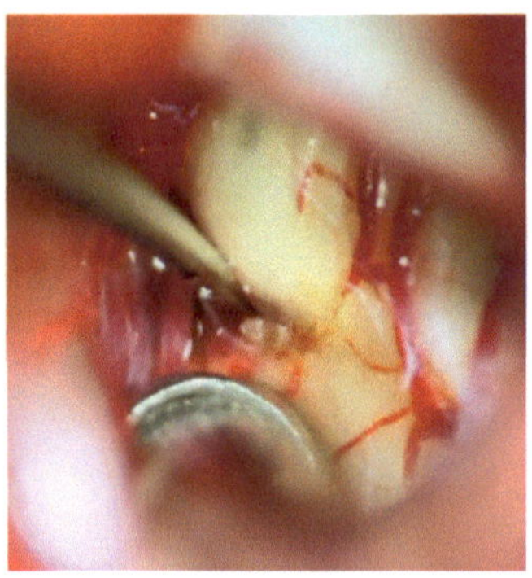

Video 15.1
Transsylvian-Transpontine Approach for Superior Basilar Pontine Cavernous Malformation Resection (Reproduced with permission from Barrow Neurological Institute, Phoenix, AZ.)

Surgical Case 15.2

PONTINE

Cavernoma Subtype: Basilar

Position: Supine
Craniotomy: Orbitozygomatic-pterional
Approach: Transsylvian-transpontine (TSyl-Pon)
Triangle: Carotid-oculomotor and oculomotor-tentorial
SEZ: None
Artery: s1 SCA

Video: Resection of a left basilar pontine cavernoma

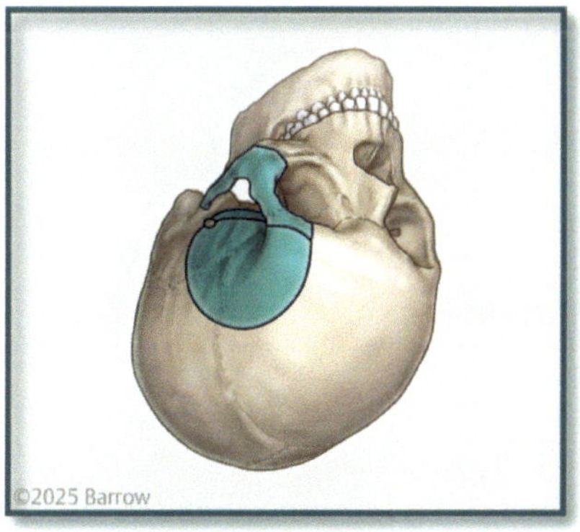

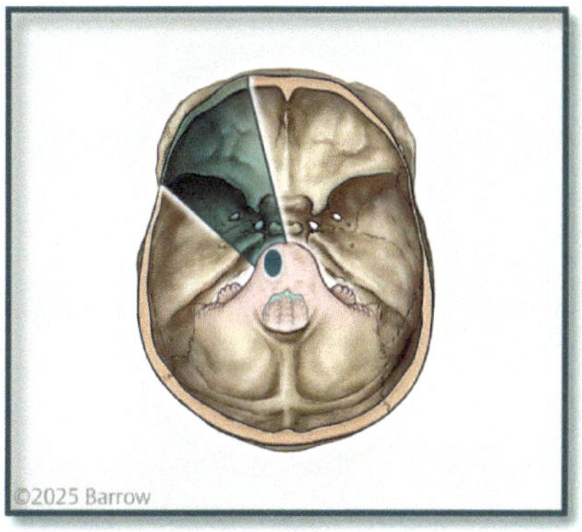

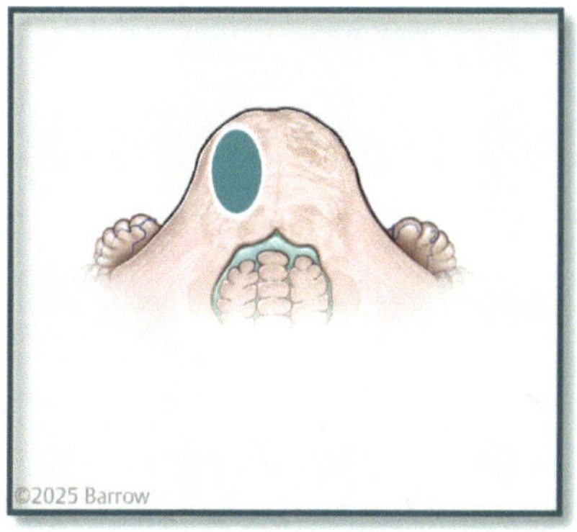

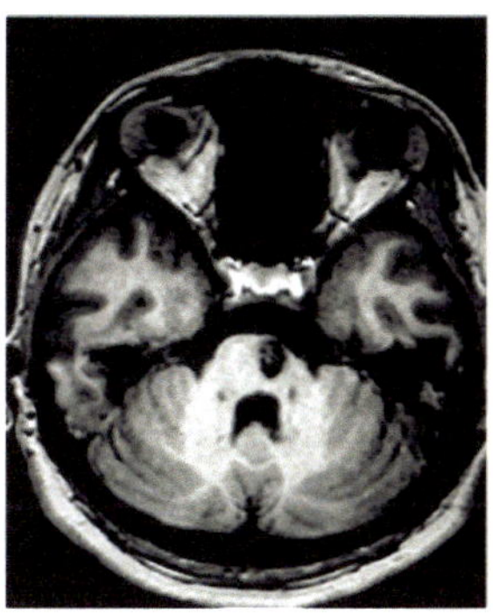

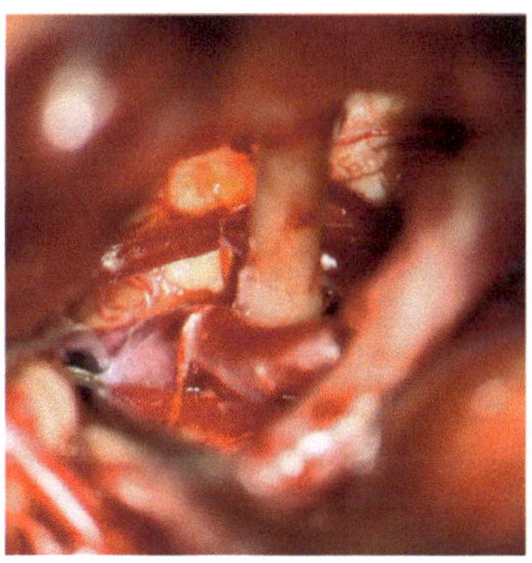

Video 15.2
Transsylvian-Transpontine Approach for Superior Basilar Pontine Cavernous Malformation Resection (Reproduced with permission from Barrow Neurological Institute, Phoenix, AZ.)

Peritrigeminal Pontine Cavernoma

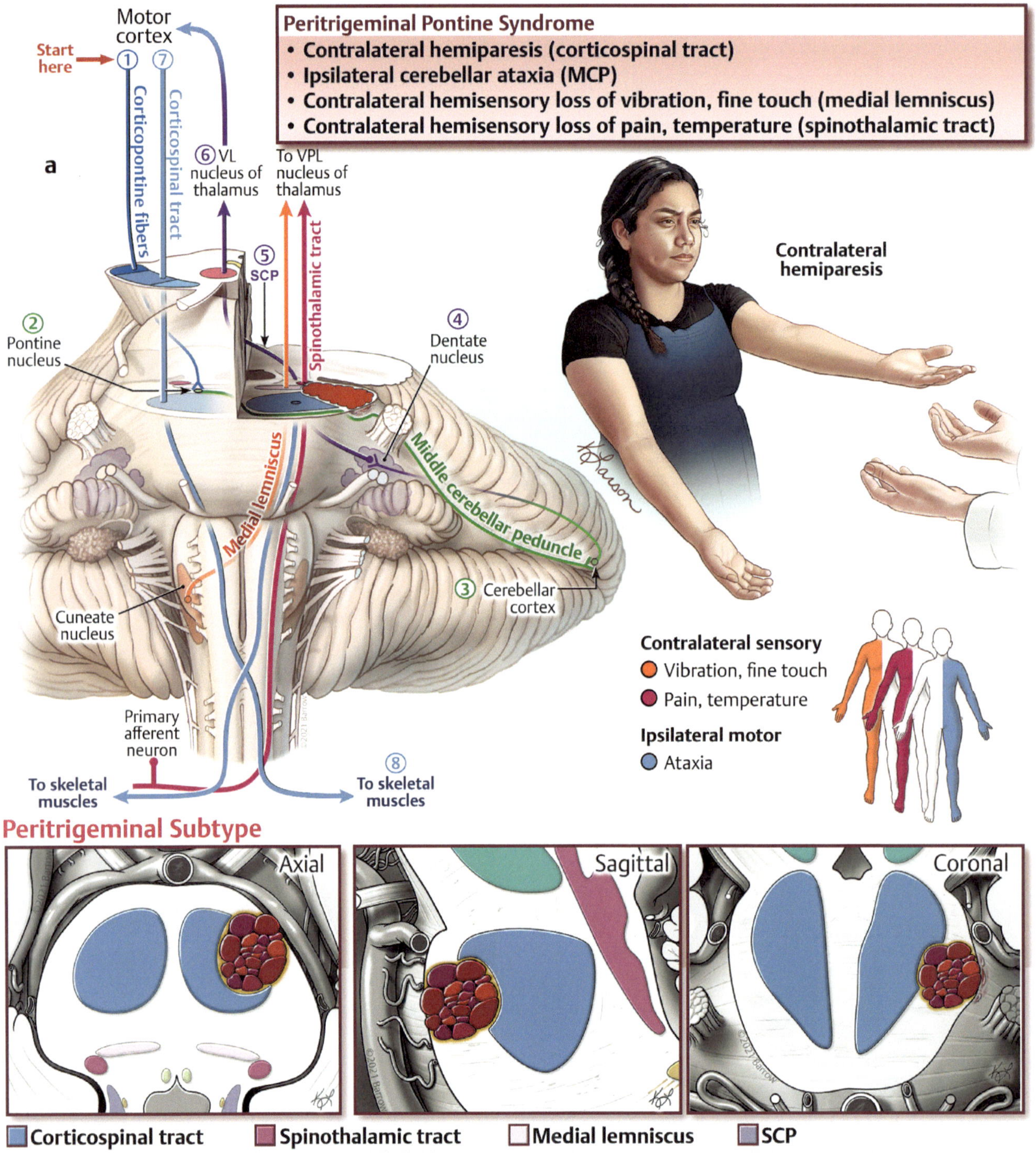

Fig. 15.5 Clinical syndromes and surgical approaches for peritrigeminal pontine CMs. **(a)** Patients with peritrigeminal pontine CMs present with contralateral hemiparesis, ipsilateral cerebellar ataxia, and contralateral loss of fine touch, proprioception, vibration, pain, and temperature sensation. This constellation of crossed and uncrossed symptoms and signs results from involvement of the corticospinal tract, MCP, medial lemniscus, and spinothalamic tract. Peritrigeminal CMs are based anterolaterally and involve the corticospinal tract and MCP, as shown for the left-sided CM in the axial, sagittal, and coronal views (*lower insets*). They are large and extend posteriorly and sometimes involve the medial lemniscus and spinothalamic tract.

(Continued)

Surgical Approach

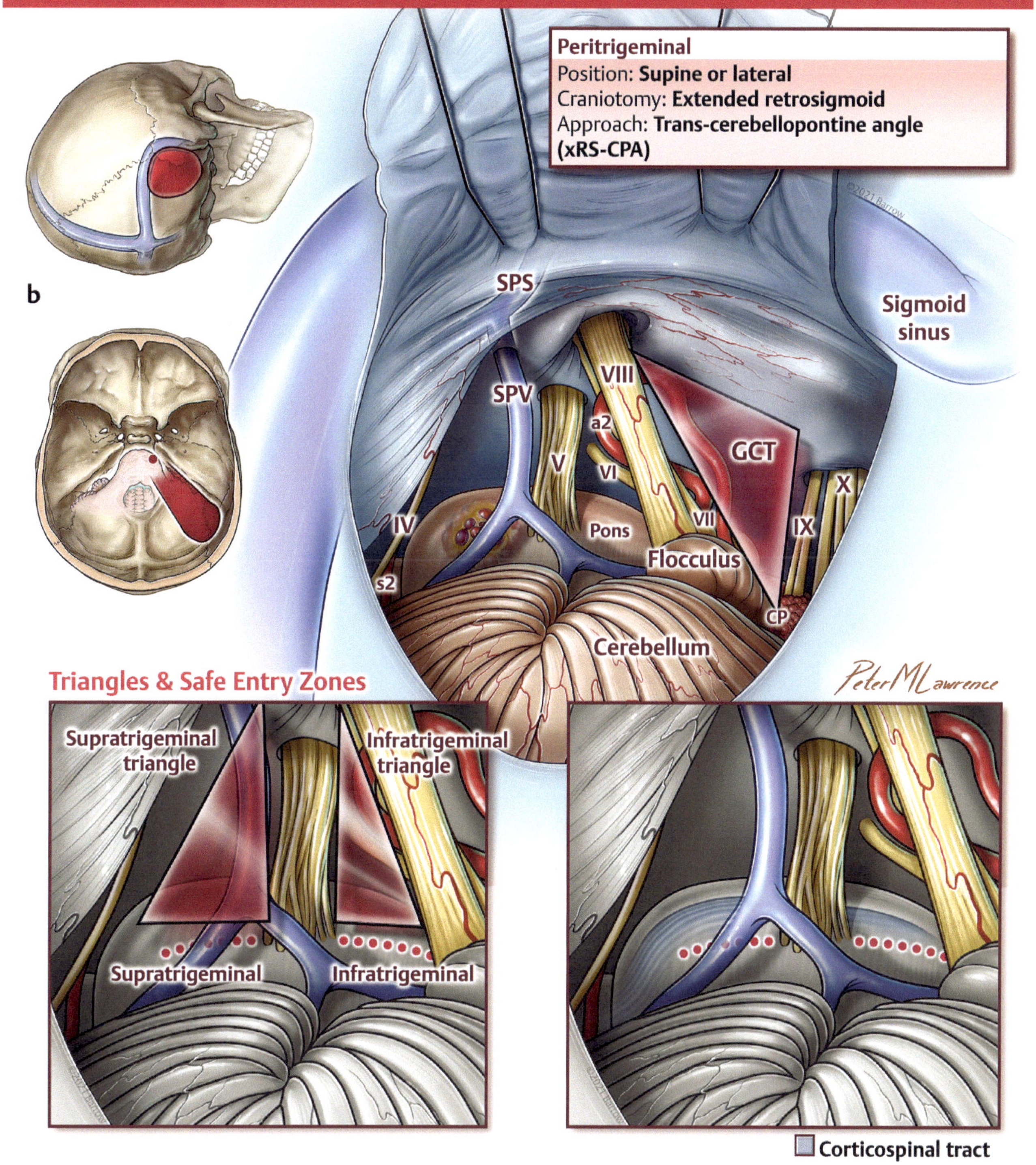

Fig. 15.5 *(Continued)* **(b)** Peritrigeminal pontine CMs are exposed surgically through an xRS-CPA (*upper left inset*) that opens a corridor into the cerebellopontine cistern parallel to the posterior petrous bone (*middle left inset; red circle*). Dissection through this cistern exposes the upper (CN V), middle (CNs VII and VIII), and lower (CNs IX, X, and XI) CN complexes that define the supratrigeminal, infratrigeminal, and glossopharyngeal-cochlear triangles (*lower left inset*). The vertical transtrigeminal line defines the SEZs: the supratrigeminal SEZ runs from the shoulder of the trigeminal nerve to the pontomesencephalic sulcus, and the infratrigeminal SEZ runs from the axilla of the trigeminal root to the shoulder of the vestibulocochlear nerve (*lower left and right insets; dotted red lines*). Lateral entry at these sites provides access to lesions in the territory of peritrigeminal CMs while avoiding the corticospinal tract located more anteriorly and medially (*lower right inset; ghosted in blue*) (surgical cases; ▶ Video 15.3, ▶ Video 15.4, ▶ Video 15.5, ▶ Video 15.6; QR codes). Roman numerals denote CNs. (Reproduced with permission from Barrow Neurological Institute, Phoenix, AZ.)

15

Surgical Case 15.3

PONTINE

Cavernoma Subtype: Peritrigeminal

Position: Supine
Craniotomy: Extended retrosigmoid
Approach: Trans-cerebellopontine angle (xRS-CPA)
Triangle: Infratrigeminal
SEZ: Infratrigeminal
Artery: s2 SCA

Video: Resection of a right peritrigeminal pontine cavernoma

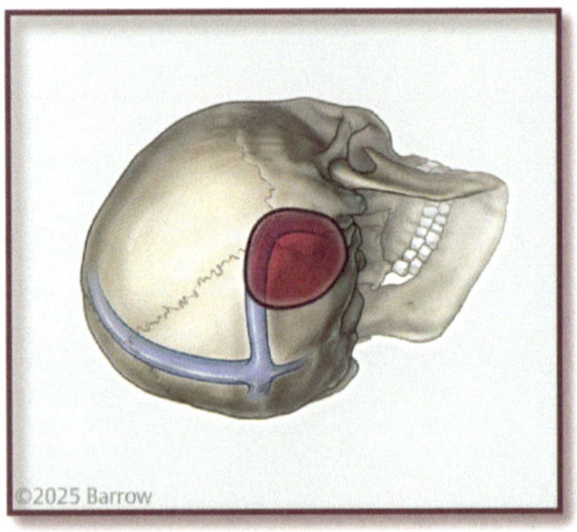

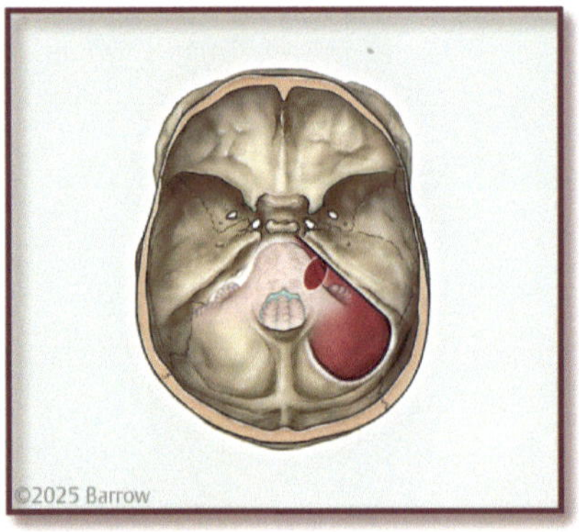

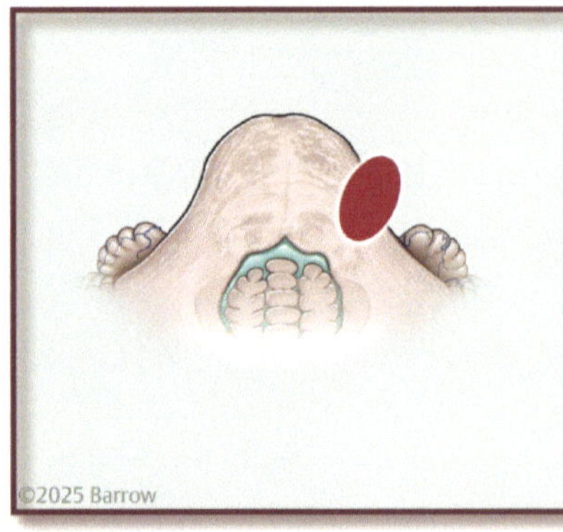

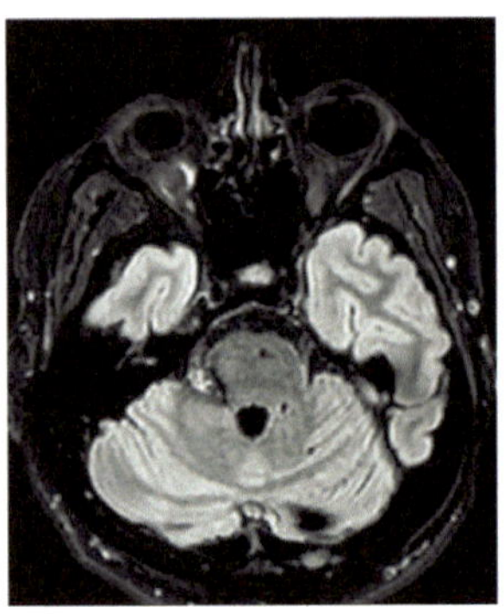

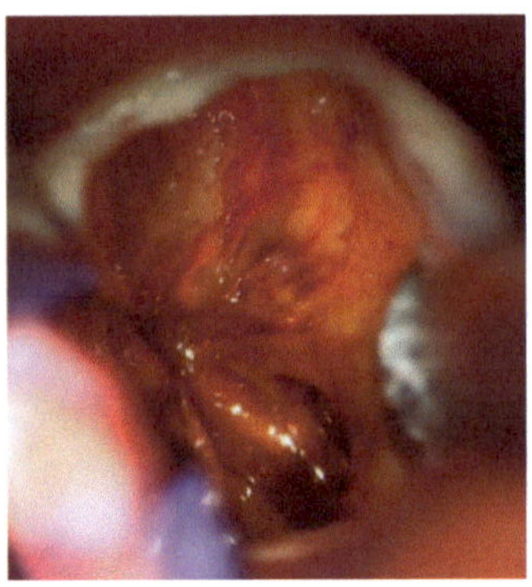

Video 15.3
Extended Retrosigmoid Craniotomy with Trans-Cerebellopontine Angle Approach for Peritrigeminal and Trigeminal Pontine Cavernous Malformation Resection (Reproduced with permission from Barrow Neurological Institute, Phoenix, AZ.)

15

Surgical Case 15.4

PONTINE

Cavernoma Subtype: Peritrigeminal

Position: Supine
Craniotomy: Extended retrosigmoid
Approach: Trans-cerebellopontine angle (xRS-CPA)
Triangle: Supratrigeminal and infratrigeminal
SEZ: Supratrigeminal and infratrigeminal
Artery: s2 SCA

Video: Resection of a left peritrigeminal pontine cavernoma

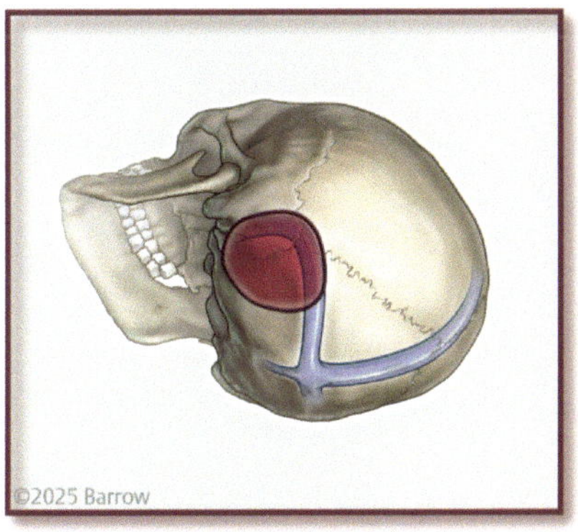

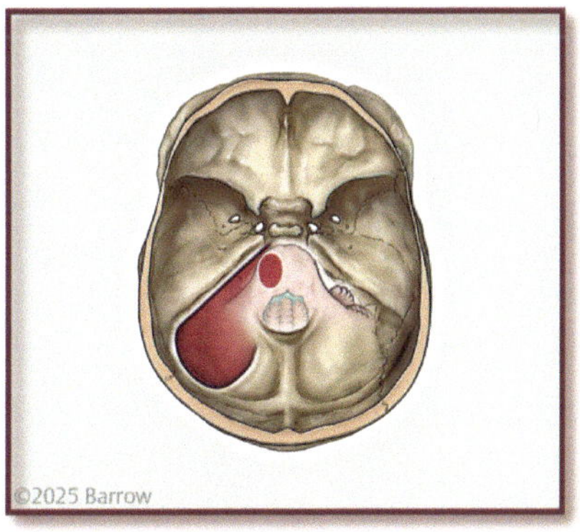

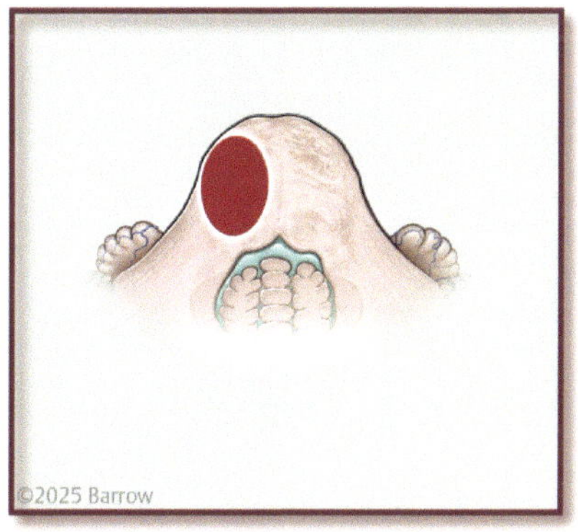

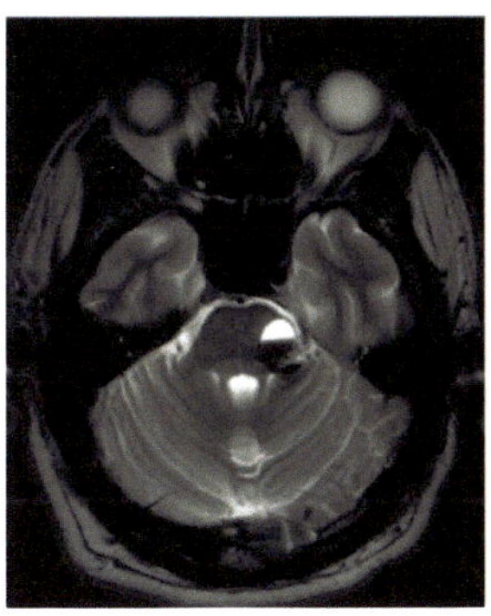

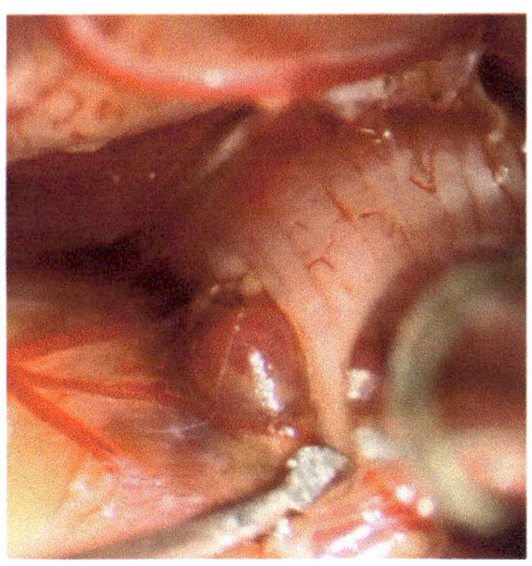

Video 15.4
Extended Retrosigmoid Craniotomy with Trans-Cerebellopontine Angle Approach for Peritrigeminal Pontine Cavernous Malformation Resection (Reproduced with permission from Barrow Neurological Institute, Phoenix, AZ.)

Surgical Case 15.5

PONTINE

Cavernoma Subtype: Peritrigeminal

Position: Supine
Craniotomy: Extended retrosigmoid
Approach: Trans-cerebellopontine angle (xRS-CPA)
Triangle: Glossopharyngeal-cochlear
SEZ: Infratrigeminal
Artery: a2 AICA

Video: Resection of a left peritrigeminal pontine cavernoma

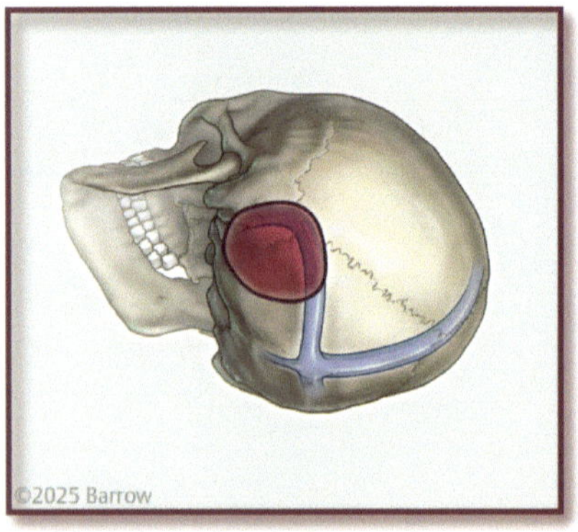

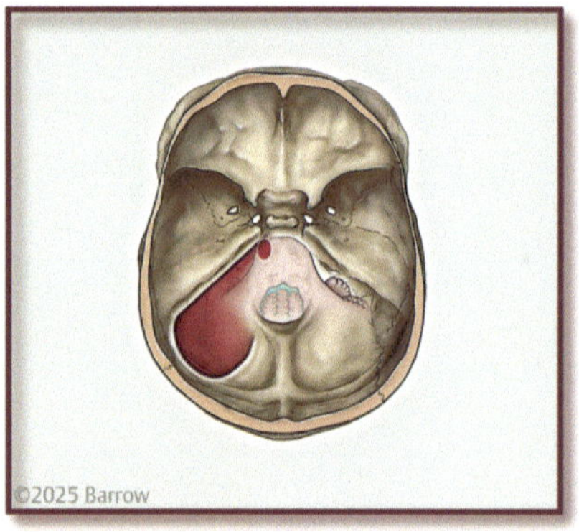

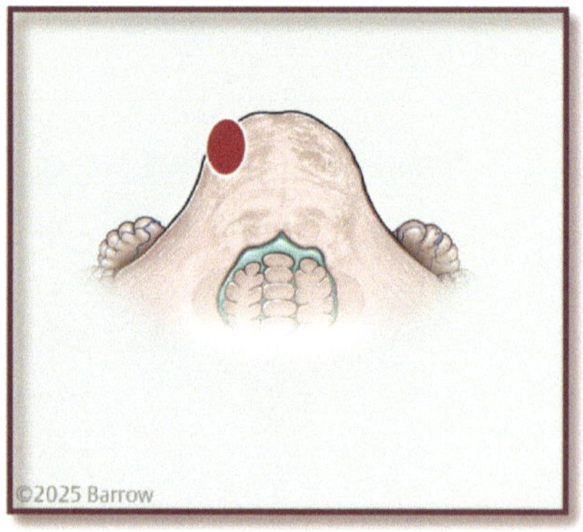

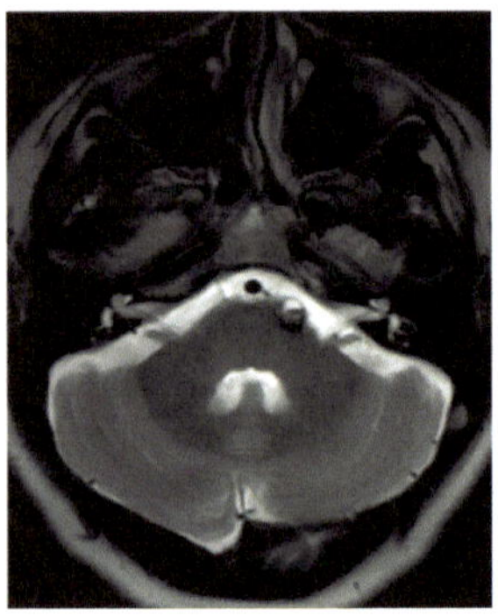

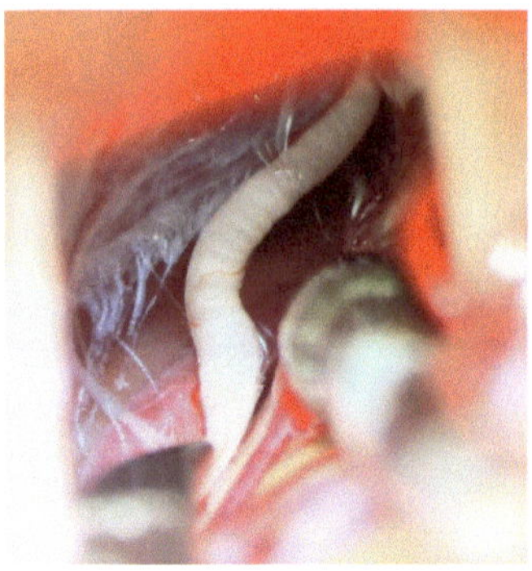

Video 15.5
Extended Retrosigmoid Craniotomy with Trans-Cerebellopontine Angle Approach for Peritrigeminal Cavernous Malformation Resection (Reproduced with permission from Barrow Neurological Institute, Phoenix, AZ.)

15

Surgical Case 15.6

PONTINE

Cavernoma Subtype: Basilar and Peritrigeminal

Position: Supine
Craniotomy: Extended retrosigmoid
Approach: Trans-cerebellopontine angle (xRS-CPA)
Triangle: Glossopharyngeal-cochlear
SEZ: Infratrigeminal
Artery: a2 AICA

Video: Resection of a right basilar and peritrigeminal pontine cavernoma

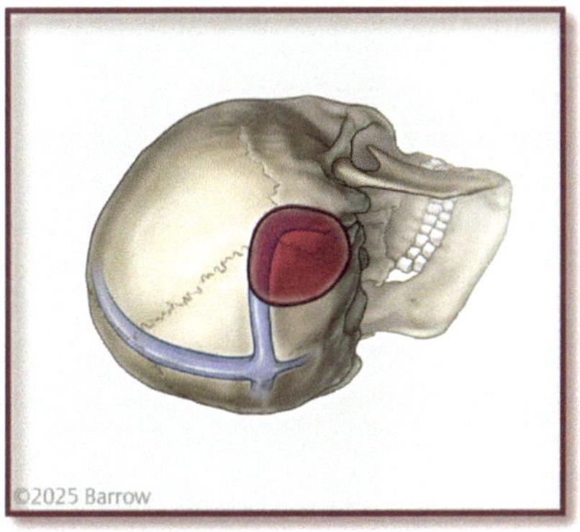

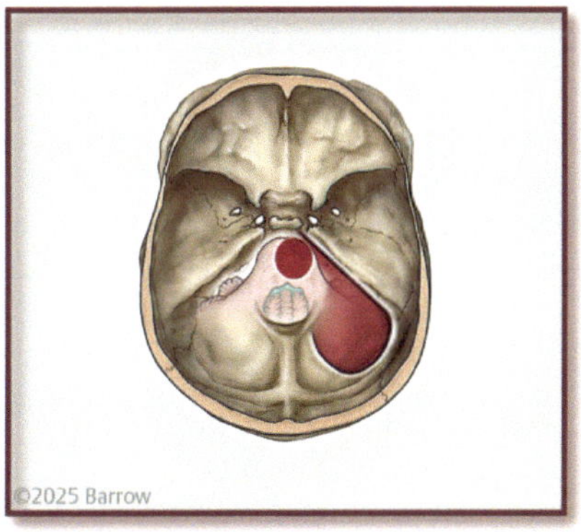

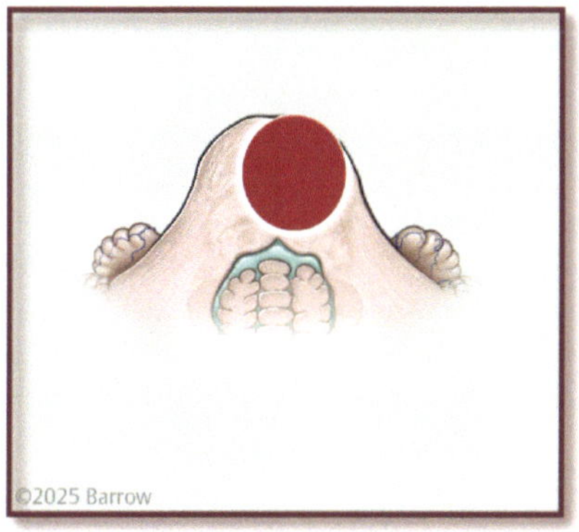

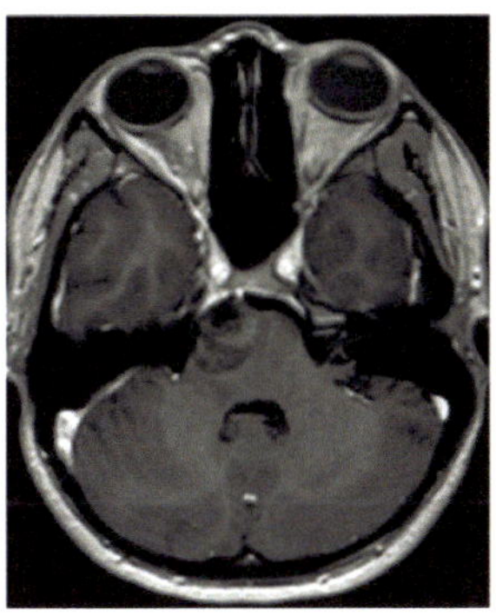

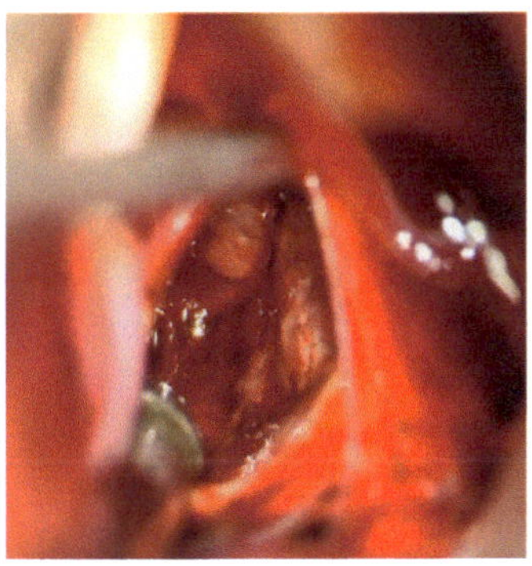

Video 15.6
Extended Retrosigmoid Craniotomy with Trans-Cerebellopontine Angle Approach for Basilar and Peritrigeminal Pontine Cavernous Malformation Resection (Reproduced with permission from Barrow Neurological Institute, Phoenix, AZ.)

and basilar artery deep to the nerve. The ascending courses of CNs VII and VIII relative to the lower CNs form this small access triangle.

The approach through the cerebellopontine cistern provides oblique or tangential lesion exposure not aligned with the lesion's axis. However, opening SEZs helps compensate. The peri- or infratrigeminal SEZ runs in the vertical transtrigeminal line from the axilla of the trigeminal root to the shoulder of the vestibulocochlear nerve. Entry at this lateral border of the peritrigeminal region exposes medially located lesions because of the anterior protuberance of the pons. The entry should parallel the fascicles of the trigeminal nerve as the incision deepens and moves obliquely posteriorly, which positions it almost perpendicular to the approach's trajectory and away from the anterolateral pons. A supratrigeminal SEZ has also been described from the shoulder of the trigeminal nerve to the pontomesencephalic sulcus for more superior peritrigeminal pontine lesions. We used this approach through peritrigeminal SEZs as a corridor for more medial access to mixed basilar-peritrigeminal lesions.

15.4.3 Middle Peduncular Subtype

The MCPs connect the cerebellum to the pons and transmit afferent fibers from the pontine nuclei to the opposite cerebellar hemisphere. Patients with pontine MCP CMs present with a mild version of Marie–Foix syndrome with contralateral hemisensory loss (medial lemniscus and spinothalamic tract), ipsilateral ataxia (MCP), ipsilateral facial numbness (CN V), and contralateral hemiparesis (corticospinal tract), without cranial neuropathies (▶ Fig. 15.6a). The classic Marie–Foix syndrome is a lateral pontine stroke resulting from AICA occlusion that involves more territory posteriorly, including the facial, solitary, vestibular, and cochlear nuclei. In contrast to peritrigeminal CMs, MCP lesions are associated with a lower incidence of hemiparesis and a higher incidence of hemifacial numbness. They reside posterolateral to the corticospinal tract and adjacent to the principal sensory and spinal nuclei of the trigeminal nerve.

Although the MCPs encase the lateral pons and deprive it of a subarachnoid surface, this peduncle contains the safest of the SEZs. It provides generous access to the lateral and central pons. The extended retrosigmoid craniotomy and trans-MCP approach combine to provide robust exposure to pontine CMs (▶ Fig. 15.6b; ▶ Video 15.7, ▶ Video 15.8, ▶ Video 15.9). This approach is the most common for surgical treatment of these lesions in our experience. The extended retrosigmoid craniotomy is the same for both peritrigeminal and MCP cavernomas, but the approaches differ significantly. MCP lesions require parenchymal dissection through the MCP, with entry as lateral as possible to arrive at the lateral pons behind the corticospinal tracts. In contrast, peritrigeminal lesions are deep to the CNs and require subarachnoid dissection through the supratrigeminal, infratrigeminal, or glossopharyngeal-cochlear triangles. This lateral entry through the MCP is made possible by splitting the petrosal (horizontal) fissure where the semilunar lobules wrap around the MCP from above (superior limb) and below (inferior limb).

The AICA and its branches travel in the petrosal fissure. They are followed inward to separate the superior and inferior semilunar lobules, earning the petrosal fissure the nickname of the *cerebellar sylvian fissure*. Splitting the petrosal fissure opens the interlobular triangle and exposes the SEZ of the MCP. The flocculus sits in the cerebellopontine angle between the superior and inferior limbs of the cerebellopontine fissures and medial to the apex of the petrosal fissure. The flocculus is mobilized inferiorly away from the vestibulocochlear nerve to expose the full course of the MCP. By entering the MCP laterally at the apex of the interlobular triangle (apical SEZ), the dissection parallels the course of the MCP fibers. It continues toward the lateral pons, well lateral, posterior, and inferior to the root entry zone of the trigeminal nerve. Access through the MCP changes the retrosigmoid approach from a trajectory paralleling the petrous bone and arriving at the anterolateral pons through the cerebellopontine cistern to a transparenchymal trajectory tunneling to the lateral pons with minimal cisternal travel. Once the MCP is entered, there are no landmarks or triangles. Navigation and hemosiderin staining guide the dissection to the lesion.

15.4.4 Inferior Peduncular Subtype

The ICP carries afferent posterior spinocerebellar, vestibulocerebellar, olivocerebellar, and reticulocerebellar tracts; its efferent fibers integrate proprioceptive sensory input with motor vestibular functions such as balance and posture. Unlike the MCP, which contains only afferent fibers, the ICP contains both afferent and efferent fibers. The ICP occupies the inferolateral corner of the pons, ventral to the lateral recess of the fourth ventricle, as it courses upward before turning posteriorly under the MCP and superior cerebellar peduncle (▶ Fig. 15.7a). Patients with CMs in this location present with an acute vestibular syndrome of nausea and vomiting, with vertigo, ataxia, imbalance, and nystagmus related to the involvement of the adjacent vestibular nuclei. No other pontine syndrome is associated with nausea, vomiting, and vestibular symptoms, making these symptoms a localizing sign. Larger lesions that extend beyond the vestibular nuclei and ICP cause diplopia and ipsilateral facial hemisensory loss related to the paramedian pontine reticular formation and spinal trigeminal nucleus and tract.

The suboccipital craniotomy and the telovelar approach were the only methods selected to treat ICP lesions on the basis of the brainstem CM taxonomy (▶ Fig. 15.7b; ▶ Video 15.10, ▶ Video 15.11). A generous midline suboccipital craniotomy is used with C1 laminectomy to increase the exposure of the cisterna magna and fourth ventricle. The cerebellar tonsils are liberated to open the vallecula and mobilize the ipsilateral tonsil laterally. The p3 tonsillomedullary segment of the posterior inferior cerebellar artery and its caudal loop are mobilized off the posterior medulla and repositioned laterally to access the inferior medullary velum. The incision of the velum from the foramen of Magendie superolaterally to the foramen of Luschka along the tela choroidea unroofs the fourth ventricle and leads to the lateral recess. A fixed retractor holds the tonsil laterally, thus forming a natural working triangle between the incised attachment of the velum inferiorly, the retracted tonsil superiorly, and the midline (subtonsillar triangle). The stria medullaris provides an obvious surface landmark on the fourth ventricular floor, spotlighting the foramen of Luschka and revealing the inferior limit of the pons. The area acustica, defined as the floor of the lateral recess overlying the cochlear

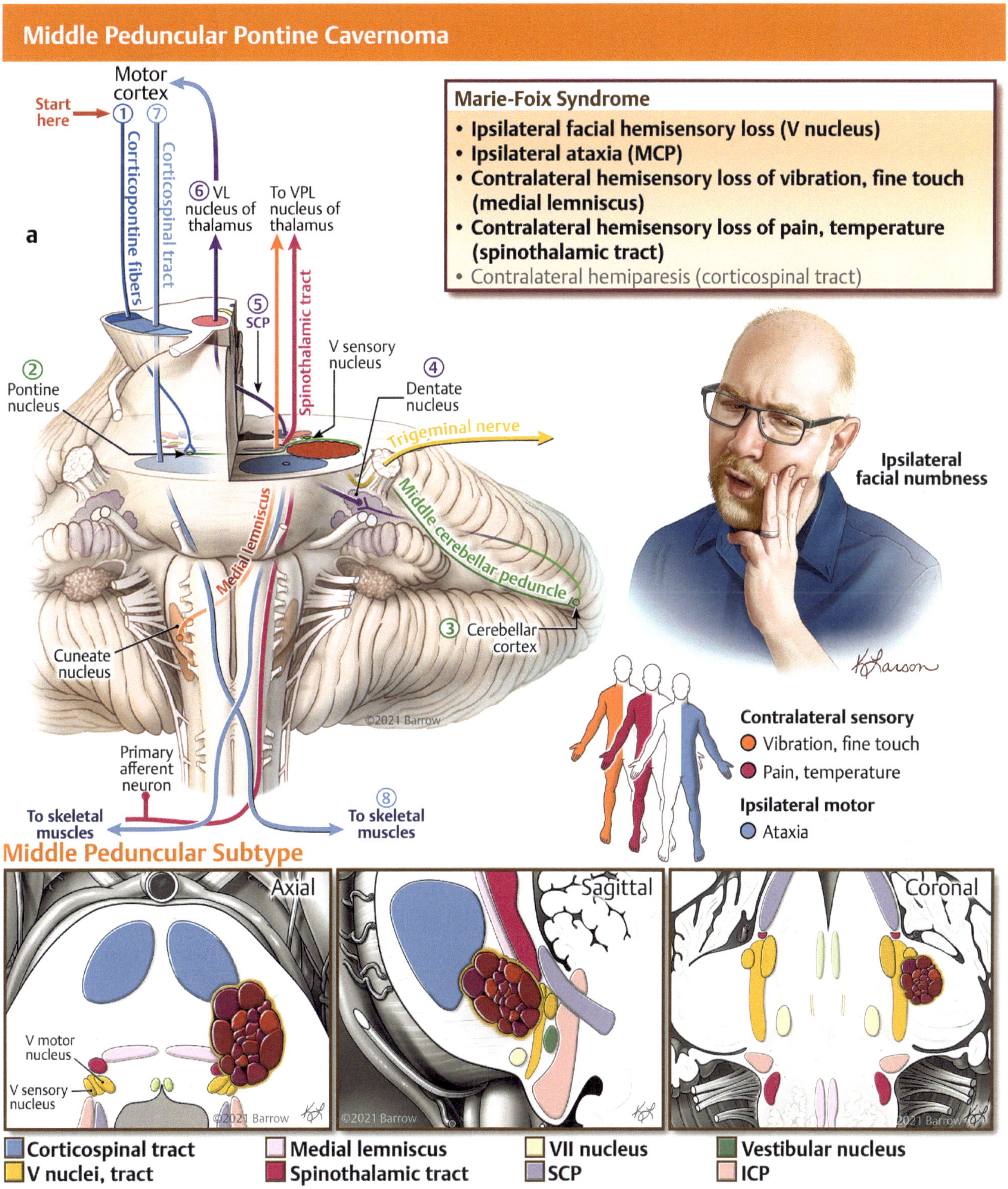

Fig. 15.6 Clinical syndromes and surgical approaches for middle peduncular pontine CMs. **(a)** Patients with middle peduncular pontine CMs present with ipsilateral facial numbness, ipsilateral cerebellar ataxia, and contralateral loss of fine touch, proprioception, vibration, pain, and temperature sensation. This constellation of symptoms is similar to Marie–Foix syndrome but lacks involvement of the facial, solitary, vestibular, and cochlear nuclei. Middle peduncular CMs are located more lateral and posterior than peritrigeminal CMs, which positions them behind the corticospinal tract and closer to trigeminal nuclei, medial lemniscus, and spinothalamic tract, as seen with this left-sided CM in axial, sagittal, and coronal views (*lower insets*).

(Continued)

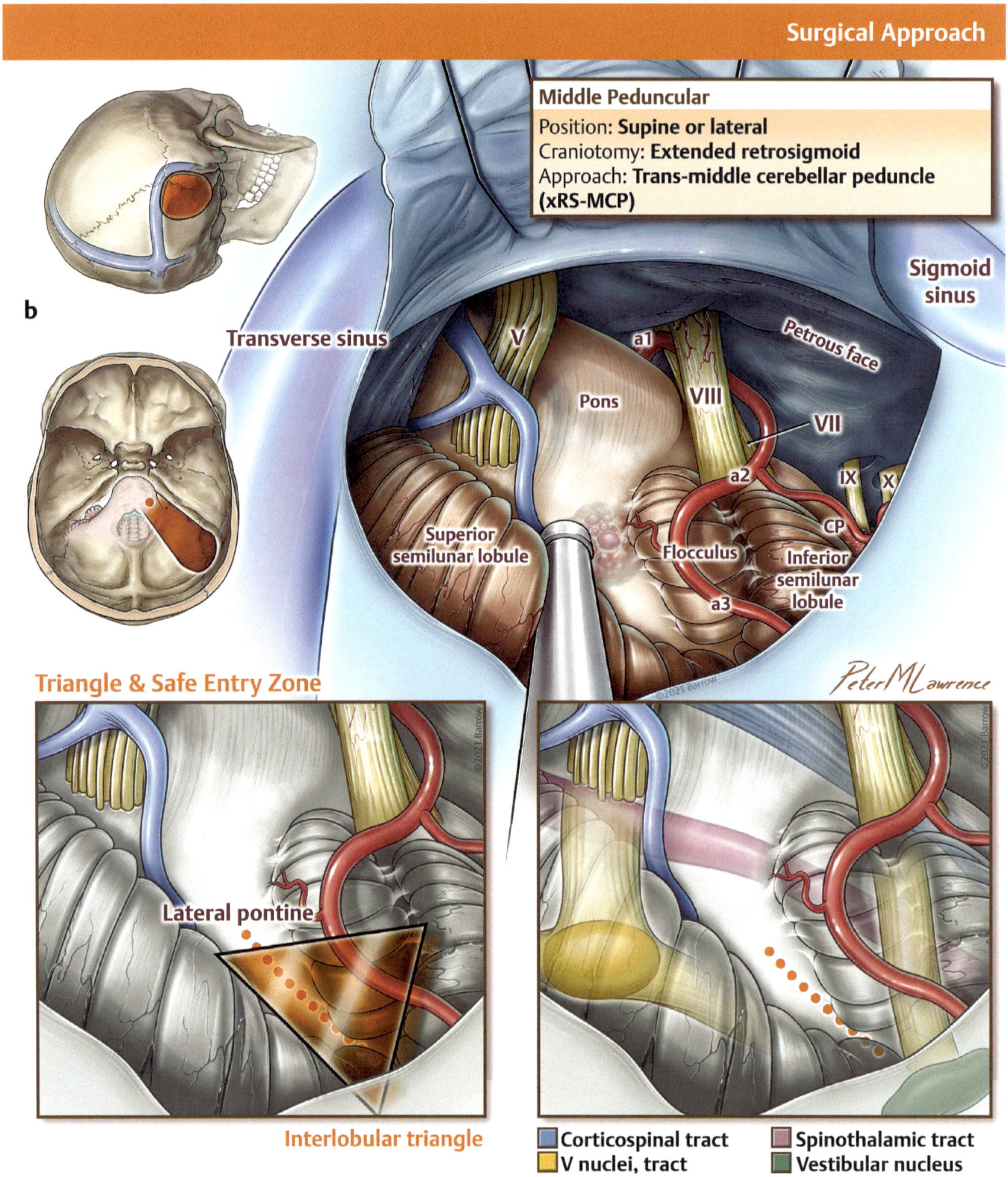

Fig. 15.6 *(Continued)* **(b)** Middle peduncular pontine CMs are exposed surgically through an extended retrosigmoid craniotomy (*upper left inset*) that opens a corridor into the cerebellopontine cistern paralleling the posterior petrous bone (*middle left inset*; *orange circle*). However, middle peduncular lesions require parenchymal dissection through the MCP, with entry into its most lateral point. The petrosal fissure is opened by dissecting the a3 (flocculopeduncular) segment of the AICA in a distal-to-proximal direction, separating the superior and inferior semilunar lobules, and mobilizing the flocculus inferiorly away from the vestibulocochlear nerve. By opening the interlobular triangle, the full course of the MCP is exposed and the MCP or lateral pontine SEZ is visualized (*lower left and right insets*; *dotted orange line*). Transparenchymal dissection into the lateral pons courses behind the corticospinal tract (*lower right inset*; *ghosted in blue*) and anterior to the trigeminal nuclei and tract (*ghosted in yellow*) and spinothalamic tract (*ghosted in red*) (surgical cases; ▶ Video 15.7, ▶ Video 15.8, ▶ Video 15.9; QR codes). Roman numerals denote CNs. (Reproduced with permission from Barrow Neurological Institute, Phoenix, AZ.)

Surgical Case 15.7

PONTINE

Cavernoma Subtype: Middle Peduncular

Position: Supine
Craniotomy: Extended retrosigmoid
Approach: Trans-middle cerebellar peduncle (xRS-MCP)
Triangle: Interlobular
SEZ: MCP (lateral pontine)
Artery: a3 AICA

Video: Resection of a left middle peduncular pontine cavernoma

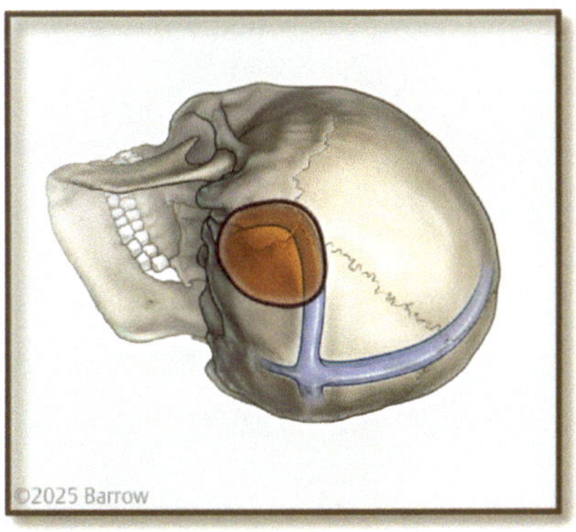

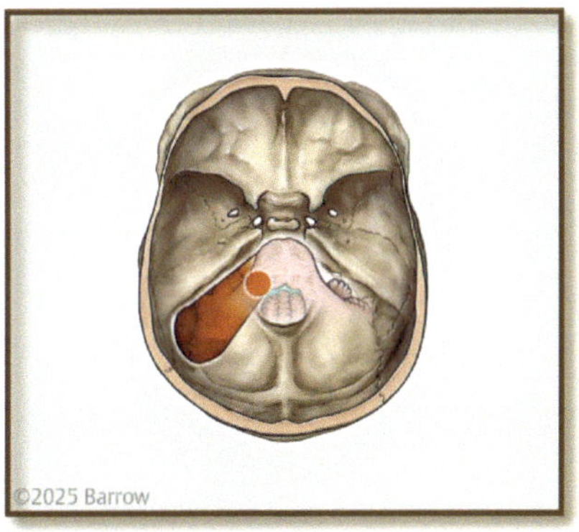

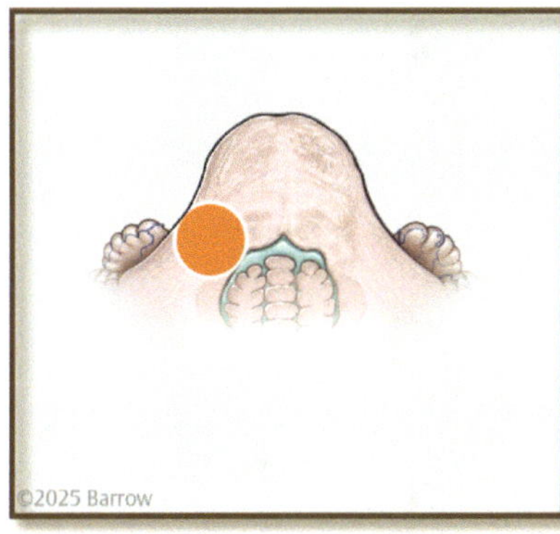

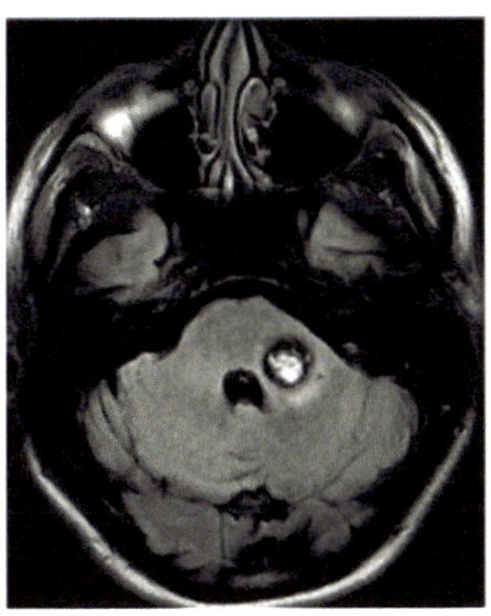

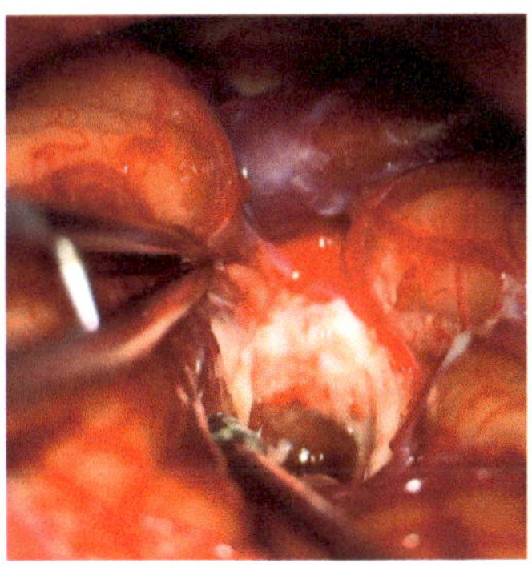

Video 15.7
Trans–Middle Cerebellar Peduncle Approach for Middle Peduncular Pontine Cavernous Malformation Resection (Reproduced with permission from Barrow Neurological Institute, Phoenix, AZ.)

Surgical Case 15.8

PONTINE

Cavernoma Subtype: Middle Peduncular

Position: Supine
Craniotomy: Extended retrosigmoid
Approach: Trans-middle cerebellar peduncle (xRS-MCP)
Triangle: Interlobular
SEZ: MCP (lateral pontine)
Artery: a3 AICA

Video: Resection of a midline middle peduncular pontine cavernoma

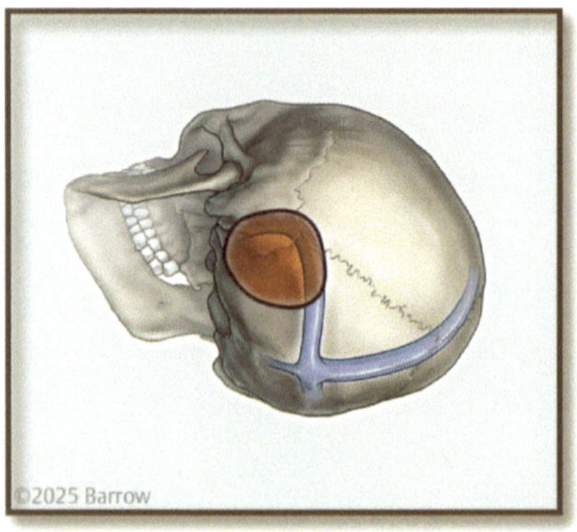

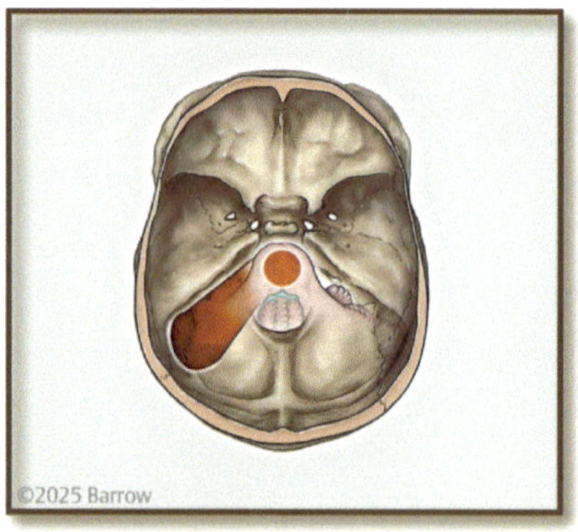

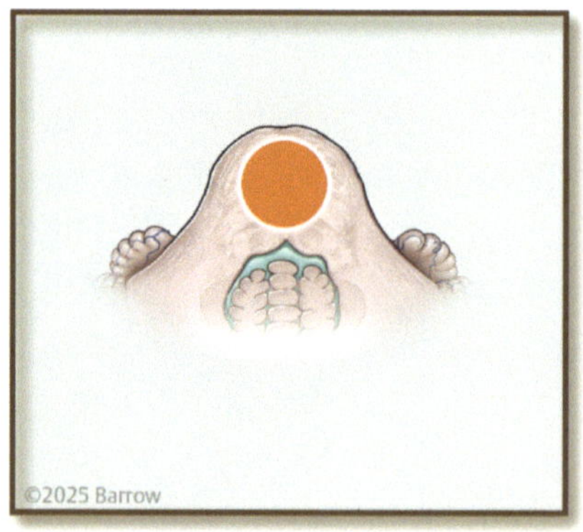

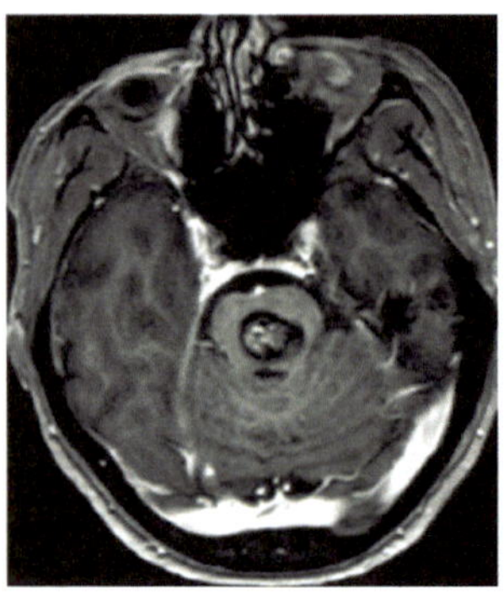

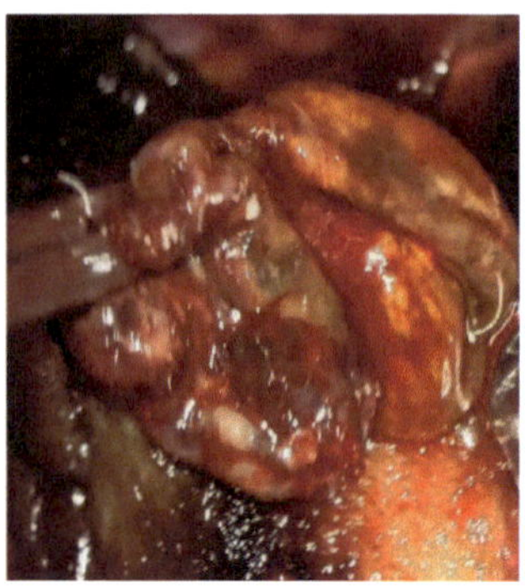

Video 15.8
Trans–Middle Cerebellar Peduncle Approach for Middle Peduncular Pontine Cavernous Malformation Resection (Reproduced with permission from Barrow Neurological Institute, Phoenix, AZ.)

15

Surgical Case 15.9

PONTINE & MIDBRAIN

Cavernoma Subtype: Middle Peduncular and Tegmental

Position: Supine
Craniotomy: Extended retrosigmoid
Approach: Trans-middle cerebellar peduncle (xRS-MCP) and lateral supracerebellar-infratentorial (SCIT-Lat)
Triangle: Interlobular
SEZ: MCP (lateral pontine)
Artery: a3 AICA

Video: Resection of a giant right middle peduncular pontine and tegmental midbrain cavernoma

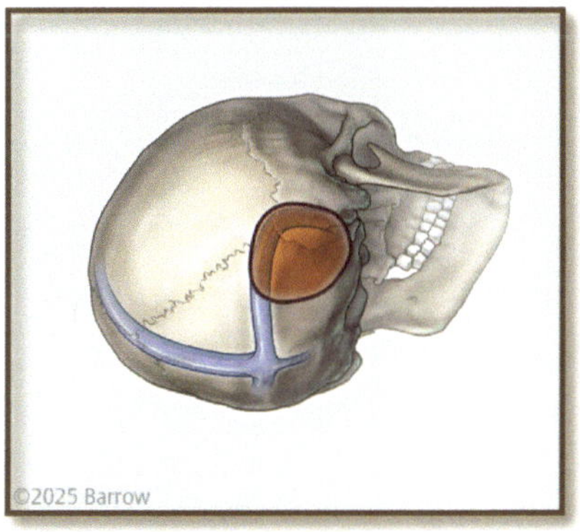

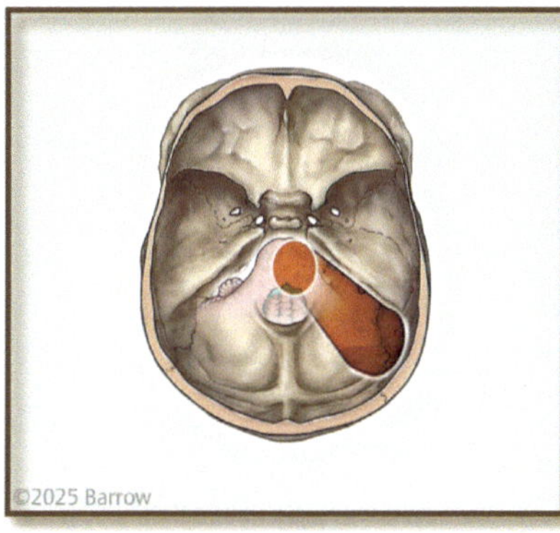

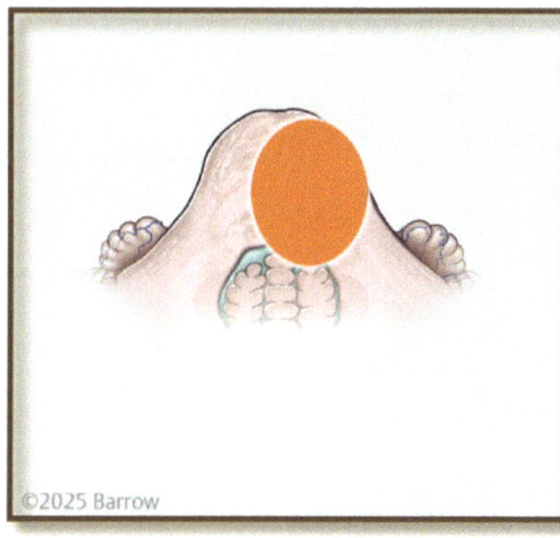

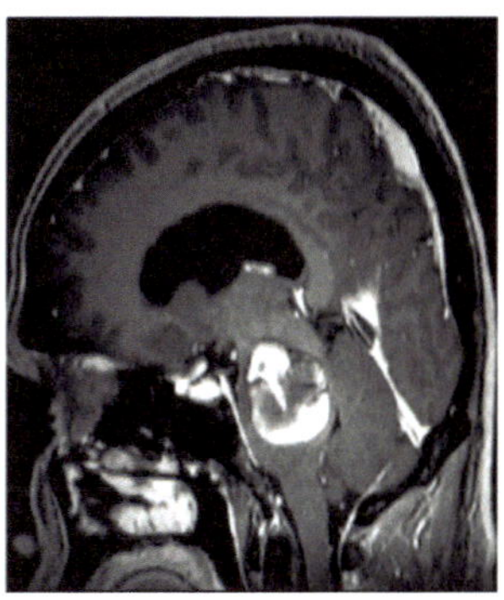

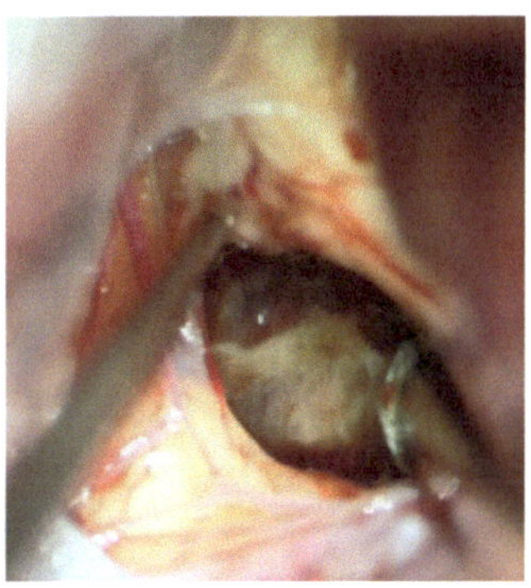

Video 15.9
Combined Trans–Middle Cerebellar Peduncle and Lateral Supracerebellar-Infratentorial Approach for Giant Middle Peduncular Pontine and Tegmental Midbrain Cavernous Malformation Resection (Reproduced with permission from Barrow Neurological Institute, Phoenix, AZ.)

Inferior Peduncular Pontine Cavernoma

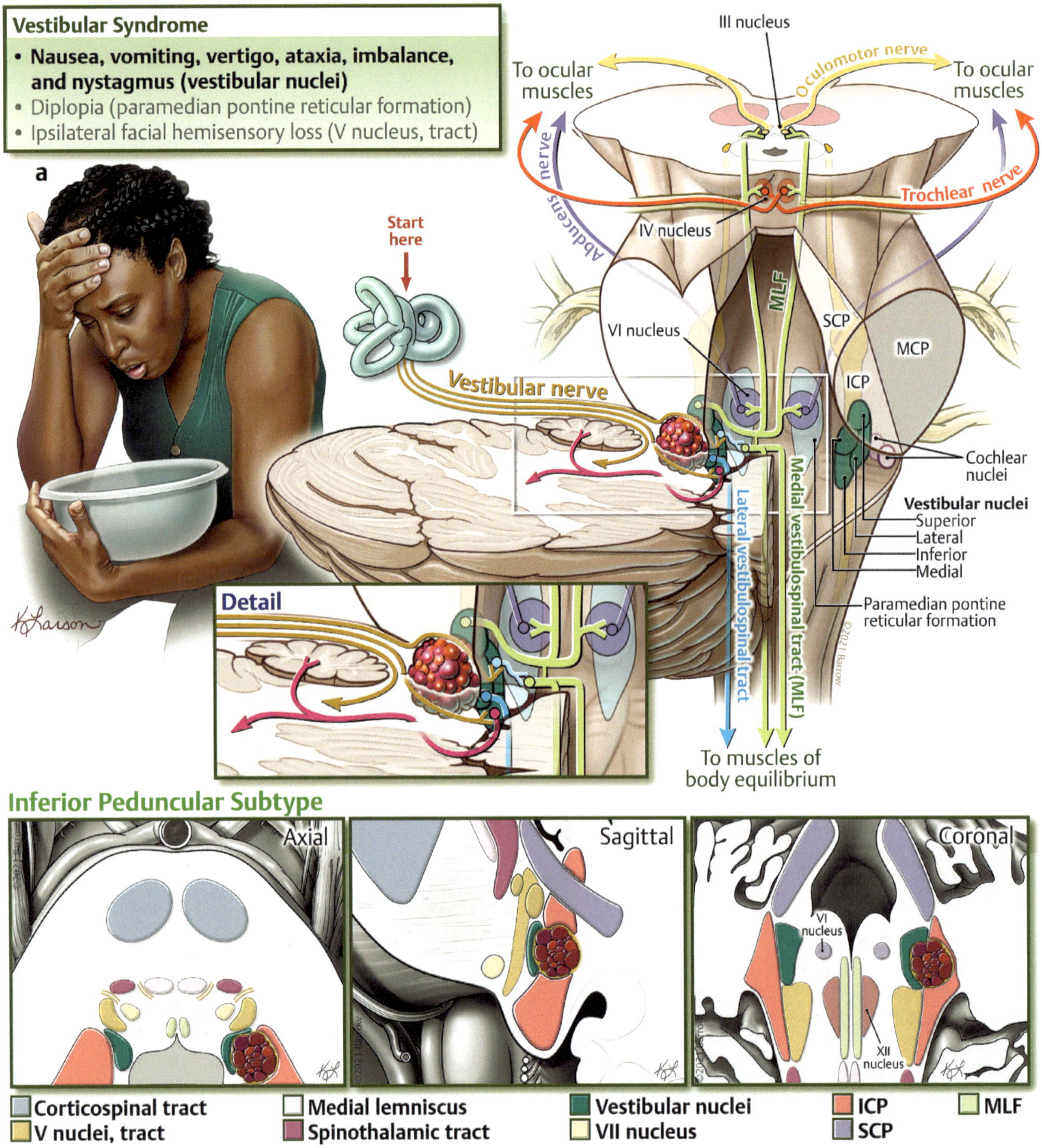

Fig. 15.7 Clinical syndromes and surgical approaches for inferior peduncular pontine CMs. **(a)** Patients with inferior peduncular pontine CMs present with an acute vestibular syndrome of nausea, vomiting, vertigo, ataxia, imbalance, and nystagmus related to the involvement of adjacent vestibular nuclei. Larger lesions cause diplopia and ipsilateral facial numbness (not shown) related to the paramedian pontine reticular formation and spinal trigeminal nucleus and tract (*detail inset*). This left-sided inferior peduncular CM resides posterolaterally in the pons, above the lateral recess of the fourth ventricle, and involves the inferior cerebellar peduncle and vestibular nuclei, as shown in the axial, sagittal, and coronal views (*lower insets*).

(*Continued*)

Surgical Approach

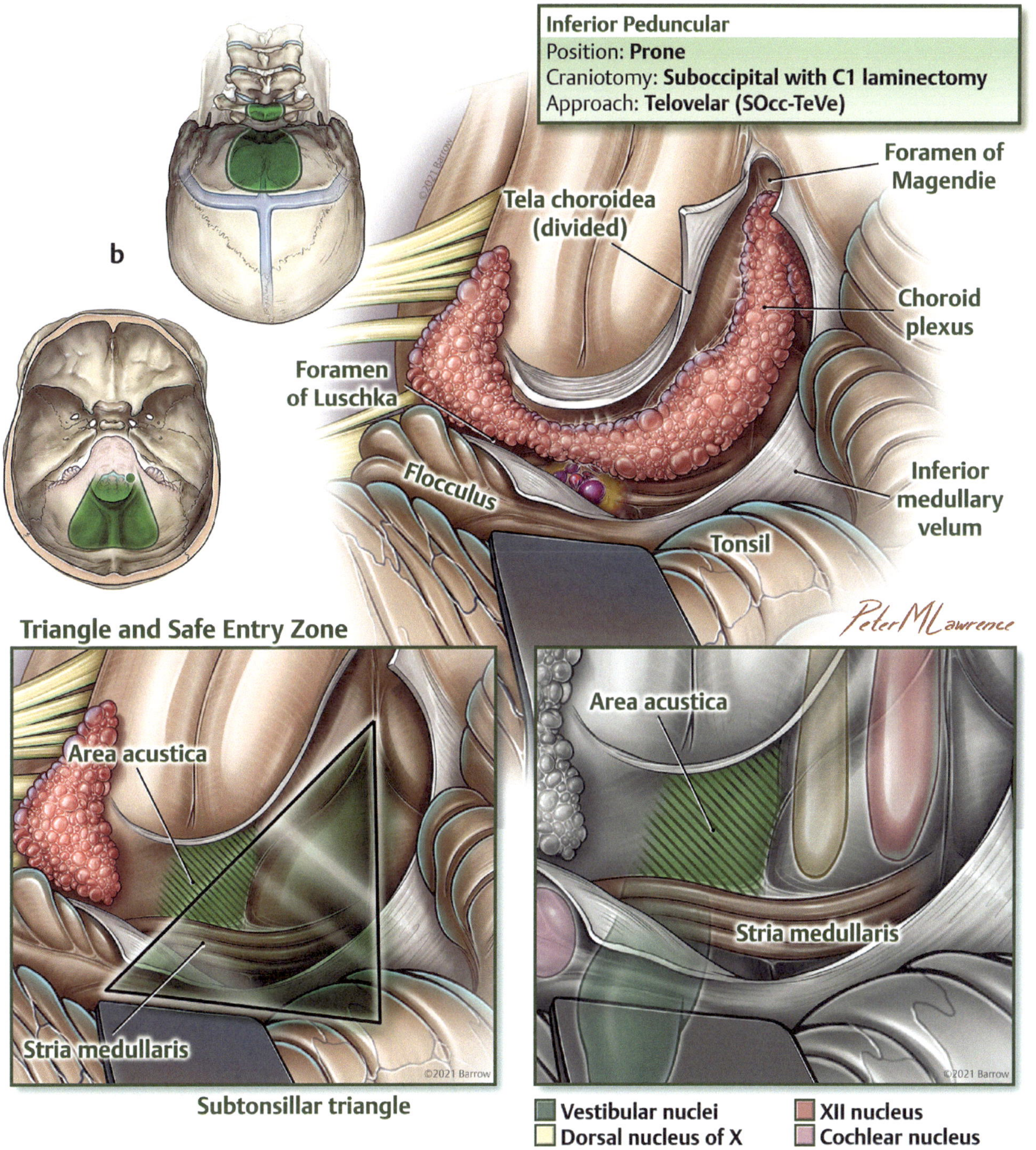

Fig. 15.7 *(Continued)* **(b)** Inferior peduncular pontine CMs are exposed surgically through a suboccipital craniotomy, C1 laminectomy (*upper left inset*), and telovelar approach (*middle left inset*; *green circle*). Retraction of the cerebellar tonsil superiorly and incision of the inferior medullary velum along the tela choroidea opens the subtonsillar triangle, through which the fourth ventricle is entered. Removal of the choroid plexus gives an overview of the ventricular floor, stria medullaris, lateral recess, foramen of Luschka, area acustica, and inferior peduncular CM (*lower left inset*). The area acustica overlying the cochlear and vestibular nuclei creates an SEZ for accessing inferior peduncular lesions located deep to the ependyma. Careful dissection protects the cochlear nuclei laterally and the vestibular nuclei, paramedian pontine reticular formation, and spinal trigeminal nucleus and tract medially (*lower right inset*) (surgical cases; ▶ Video 15.10, ▶ Video 15.11; QR codes). Roman numerals denote CNs. (Reproduced with permission from Barrow Neurological Institute, Phoenix, AZ.)

Surgical Case 15.10

PONTINE

Cavernoma Subtype: Inferior Peduncular

Position: Prone
Craniotomy: Suboccipital
Approach: Telovelar (SOcc-TeVe)
Triangle: Subtonsillar
SEZ: Area acustica
Artery: p4 PICA

Video: Resection of a left inferior peduncular pontine cavernoma

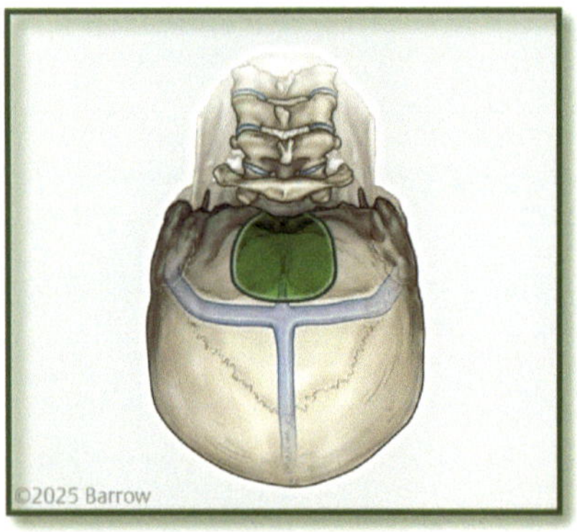

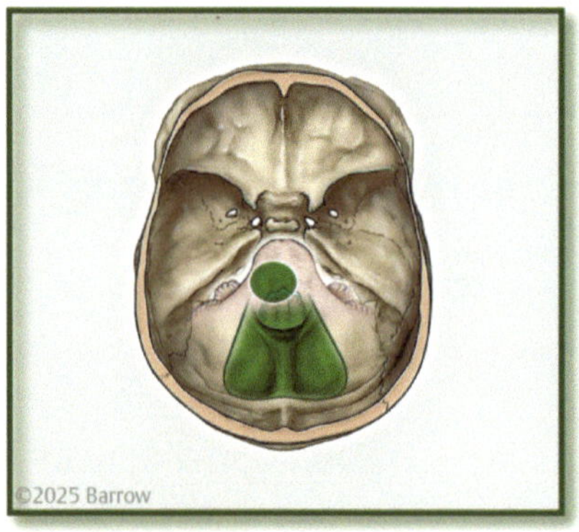

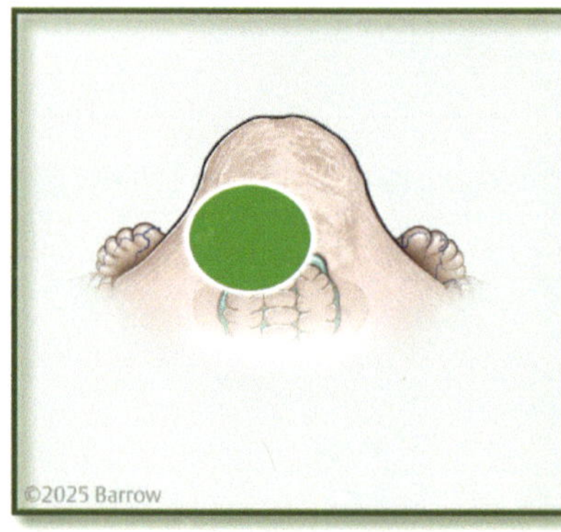

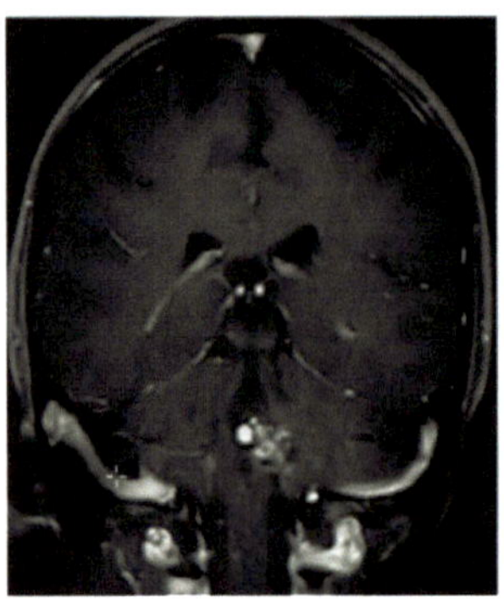

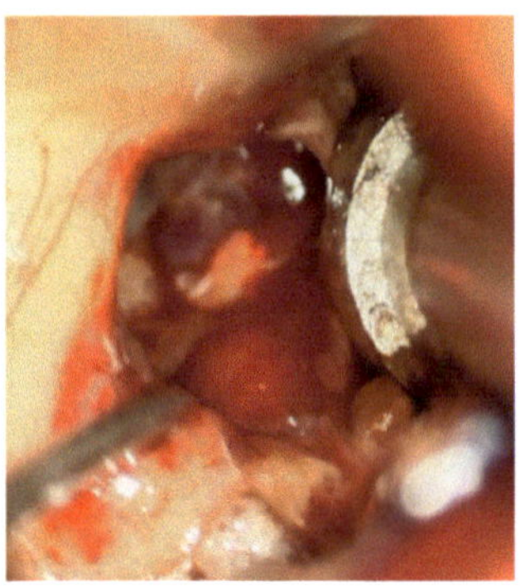

Video 15.10
Suboccipital Craniotomy with Telovelar Approach for Inferior Peduncular Pontine Cavernous Malformation Resection (Reproduced with permission from Barrow Neurological Institute, Phoenix, AZ.)

15

Surgical Case 15.11

PONTINE

Cavernoma Subtype: Inferior Peduncular

Position: Prone
Craniotomy: Suboccipital with C1 laminectomy
Approach: Telovelar (SOcc-TeVe)
Triangle: Subtonsillar
SEZ: Area acustica
Artery: p4 PICA

Video: Resection of a left inferior peduncular pontine cavernoma

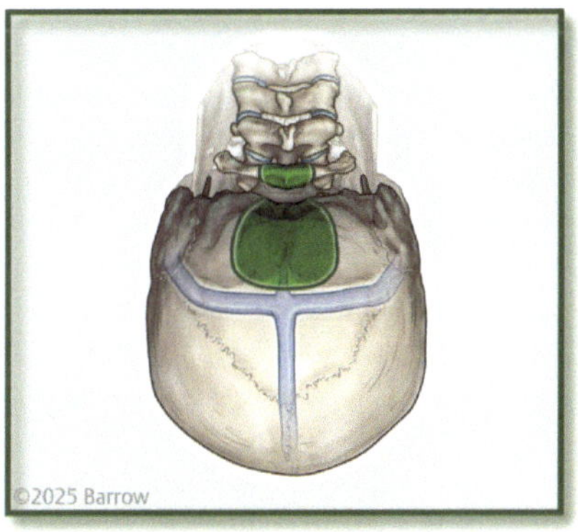

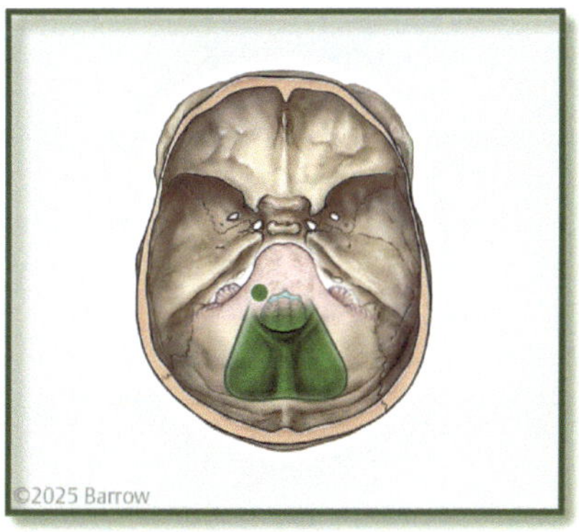

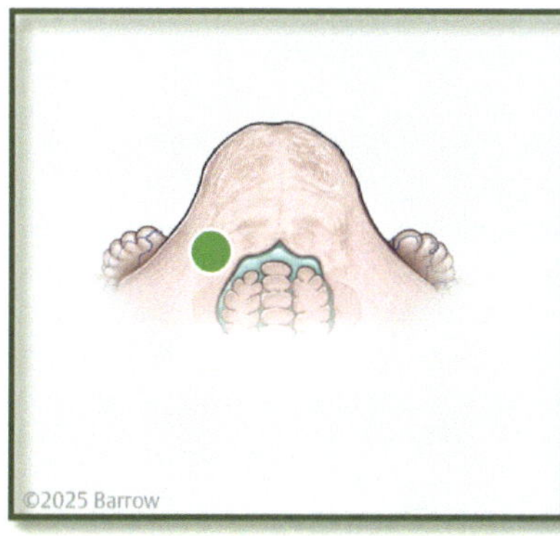

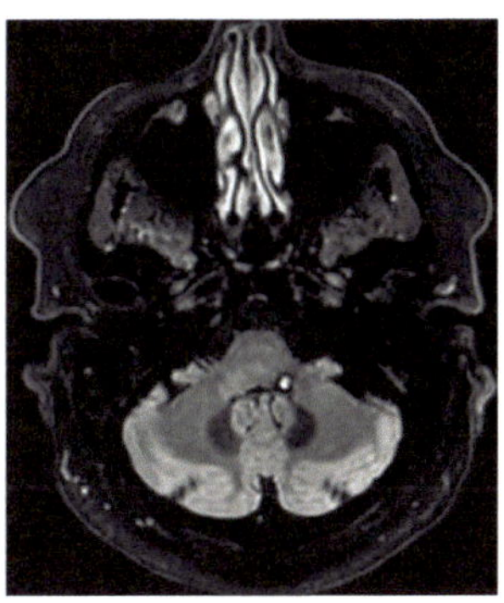

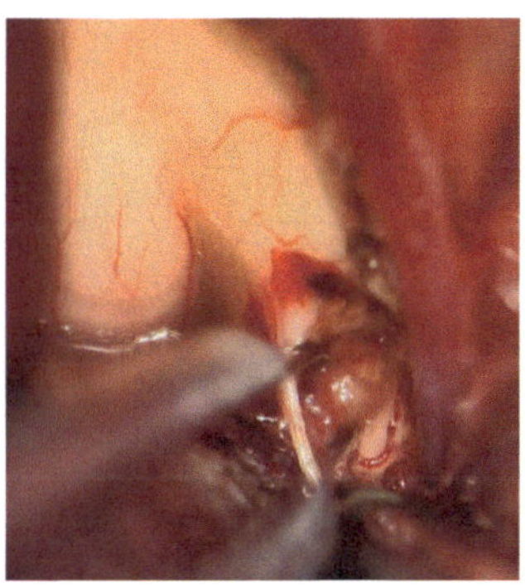

Video 15.11
Suboccipital Craniotomy with Telovelar Approach for Inferior Peduncular Pontine Cavernous Malformation Resection (Reproduced with permission from Barrow Neurological Institute, Phoenix, AZ.)

and vestibular nuclei and inferior to stria medullaris, is one of the pontine SEZs available for accessing subependymal lesions.

15.4.5 Rhomboid Subtype

Surgical access through the floor of the fourth ventricle requires caution and care because of the dense concentration of CNs and nuclei nearby. It is called the rhomboid fossa because of its shape, with its upper triangular part from the outlet of the sylvian aqueduct to the striae medullaris forming the posterior surface of the pons. Rhomboid CMs presenting to the fourth ventricular floor constitute rhomboid lesions when they reside in the posterior pons. Patients with rhomboid lesions present with dysconjugate eye movement caused by injuries to the abducens nerve nucleus, MLF, and paramedian pontine reticular formation (▶ Fig. 15.8a). Syndromes vary depending on lesion size and midline or eccentric location. Syndromes associated with midline lesions include classic internuclear ophthalmoplegia (INO) with MLF damage and failure of the medial recti to move synchronously with the lateral recti on attempted lateral gaze. Reverse INO with intact MLF also occurs with bilateral damage affecting the relay to the abducens nuclei and failure of the lateral recti to move synchronously with the medial recti on attempted lateral gaze. Two syndromes are associated with eccentric lesions. The first is unilateral INO with impaired adduction on attempted gaze away from the lesion and normal abduction in the contralateral eye due to a unilateral MLF lesion. The second is the one-and-a-half syndrome with no movement of one eye ipsilateral to the lesion and only outward movement of the other eye (conjugate gaze palsy toward the lesion and INO away from the lesion) due to unilateral paramedian pontine reticular formation and MLF damage. Larger eccentric lesions cause facial colliculus syndrome, described as ipsilateral horizontal gaze palsy and ipsilateral facial weakness (lower motor neuron pattern) caused by damage affecting the abducens nerve nuclei and the internal genu of the facial nerve.

A suboccipital craniotomy with C1 laminectomy and transventricular approach exposes the rhomboid fossa (▶ Fig. 15.8b; ▶ Video 15.12, ▶ Video 15.13, ▶ Video 15.14). The natural trajectory of this approach is typically too low for most pontine lesions. However, head flexion in the prone position with a tucked chin steepens the trajectory upward to reach the upper rhomboid fossa. Dissection along the p3 segments of the posterior inferior cerebellar artery opens the tonsillomedullary fissures, liberates the tonsils from the medulla, and widens the vallecula (vallecular triangle). The inferior vermis (uvula and nodule deep to it) can still obscure visualization. Thus, limited resection of the vermis could be required for high-riding lesions in the upper pons. Eccentric lesions lying off midline may require the release of the inferior medullary velum, as in a telovelar approach. The median sulcus, facial colliculus, superior foveae, and striae medullaris are landmarks on the upper floor.

The facial colliculi and MLF are forbidden zones. The SEZs include the median sulcus and supra- and infrafacial collicular SEZs. The median sulcus runs in the midline. Careful entry for small lesions preserves the MLF, which is immediately lateral. The supra- and infrafacial collicular SEZs are off the midline within the median eminence. The superior foveal SEZ is a fourth site lateral to the facial colliculus in the sulcus limitans. The superior fovea is just a dimple in the sulcus limitans, giving the superior foveal triangle its name. The working triangle is defined superolaterally by the superior cerebellar peduncle, inferolaterally by the vestibular area, and medially by the sulcus limitans. The apex of the triangle maps at the transverse level to the upper edge of the facial colliculus. The motor and main sensory nuclei of the trigeminal nerve lie beneath the superolateral border. Therefore, this triangle provides landmarks for the motor nuclei of the trigeminal, abducens, and facial nerves. A vertical incision in the superior foveal triangle provides safe access to more laterally placed lesions. Hemosiderin staining or lesion presentation on the ependymal floor guides the ultimate entry site to open the corridor to the lesion. Stimulation mapping is helpful when the entry is not obvious or the lesion distorts the anatomy.

15.4.6 Supraolivary Subtype

The ventral pontine underbelly creates a supraolivary access portal for inferolateral pontine CMs that lie lateral to the pyramidal tract and abducens nerve, medial to the lower CNs, and project upward in the central pons (▶ Fig. 15.9a). Ipsilateral abducens nerve palsy was a strong localizing sign for this subtype, with more than two-thirds of patients presenting with this finding. Patients with supraolivary lesions present with mild Millard–Gubler syndrome, one of the classic pontine crossed syndromes. It consists of the ipsilateral abducens and facial nerve palsies as well as contralateral hemiparesis and hemiplegia. Supraolivary CMs displace the pyramidal tract and, thus, are associated with milder motor deficits. The medial lemniscus and spinothalamic tracts were spared in half of these patients. Nonetheless, they were present in those with larger lesions that extended dorsally, involving the pontine tegmentum and producing the contralateral hemisensory deficits of Foville's syndrome.

A far lateral craniotomy and a trans-pontomedullary sulcus approach are ideal for reaching the pontine underbelly (▶ Fig. 15.9b; ▶ Video 15.15, ▶ Video 15.16). The park bench position used for this approach orients the clivus and vertebral artery vertically for viewing along the axis of the brainstem anterolaterally. An extensive condylectomy opens the cerebellomedullary cistern and exposes the vagoaccessory triangle, revealing the olivary nucleus. The vagus nerve is separated from the medullary rootlets of the accessory nerve to widen the triangle. The V4 (intradural) segment of the vertebral artery resides at the depths of this triangle, and the hypoglossal nerve rootlets drape the segment. With the steep upward trajectory to the pontine underbelly, the trans-pontomedullary sulcus approach moves superiorly through the vagoaccessory triangle into its suprahypoglossal portion. Deepening the dissection through these triangles moves the surgeon medially toward the lower CN complex (CNs IX–XI). The p2 (lateral medullary) segment of the posterior inferior cerebellar artery often travels in this working window. The contours of the superior olive and inferior pons intersect at the pontomedullary sulcus, which is the SEZ for these lesions. CN VI also exits from this sulcus, and its cisternal segment can be traced in the retrograde direction to identify the sulcus. Entry lateral to CN VI protects the corticospinal tract. The superior pole of the olive, rather than the pontomedullary sulcus, can be entered if a more posterior trajectory is needed.

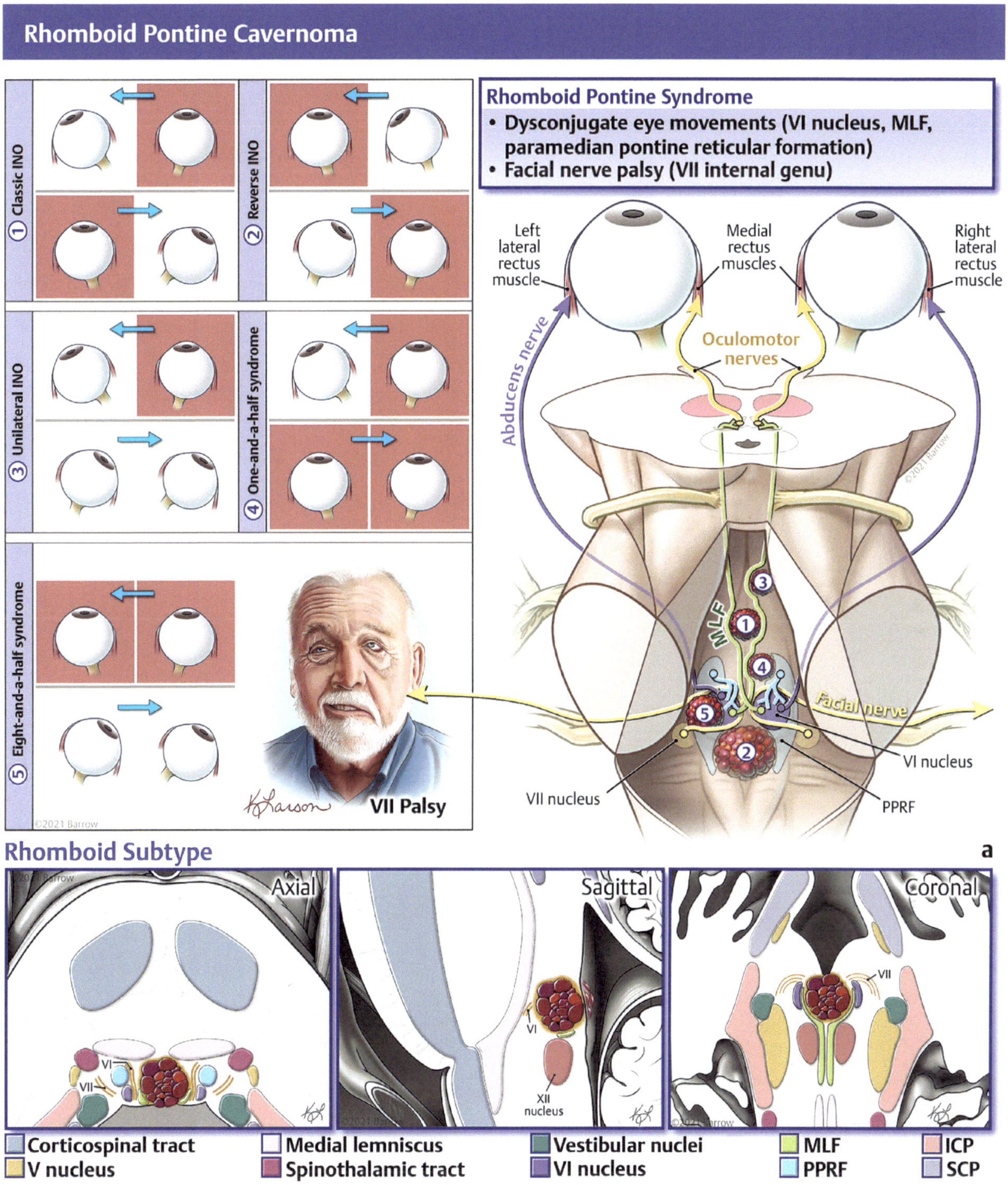

Fig. 15.8 Clinical syndromes and surgical approaches for rhomboid pontine CMs. **(a)** Patients with rhomboid pontine CMs present with dysconjugate eye movements and INOs caused by injuries to the MLF, abducens nerve nucleus, and paramedian pontine reticular formation. Syndromes associated with midline lesions include (1) classic INO, defined as MLF damage and failure of the medial rectus muscle to move synchronously with the lateral rectus muscle during attempted lateral gaze, and (2) reverse INO, defined as bilateral abducens nuclei injury with intact MLF and failure of the lateral rectus muscle to move synchronously with the medial rectus muscle during attempted lateral gaze. Eccentric rhomboid CMs can cause (3) unilateral INO, defined as a unilateral MLF lesion with impaired adduction during attempted gaze away from the lesion and normal abduction in the contralateral eye, and (4) one-and-a-half syndrome, defined as unilateral paramedian pontine reticular formation and an MLF lesion, with no movement of the eye ipsilateral to the lesion and only outward movement of the other eye (conjugate gaze palsy toward the lesion and INO away from the lesion). Larger eccentric lesions affecting the abducens nerve nucleus and internal genu of the facial nerve cause facial colliculus syndrome or (5) eight-and-a-half syndrome, defined as ipsilateral horizontal gaze palsy and ipsilateral facial weakness. *Blue arrows* in the *left insets* indicate the direction of the patient's attempted lateral gaze. The *red background* indicates abnormal eye findings, and the *white background* indicates normal eye movements. This midline rhomboid CM resides in the posterior pons and floor of the fourth ventricle adjacent to the MLF, CN VI nuclei, and paramedian pontine reticular formation (PPRF), as shown in the axial, sagittal, and coronal views (*lower insets*).

(Continued)

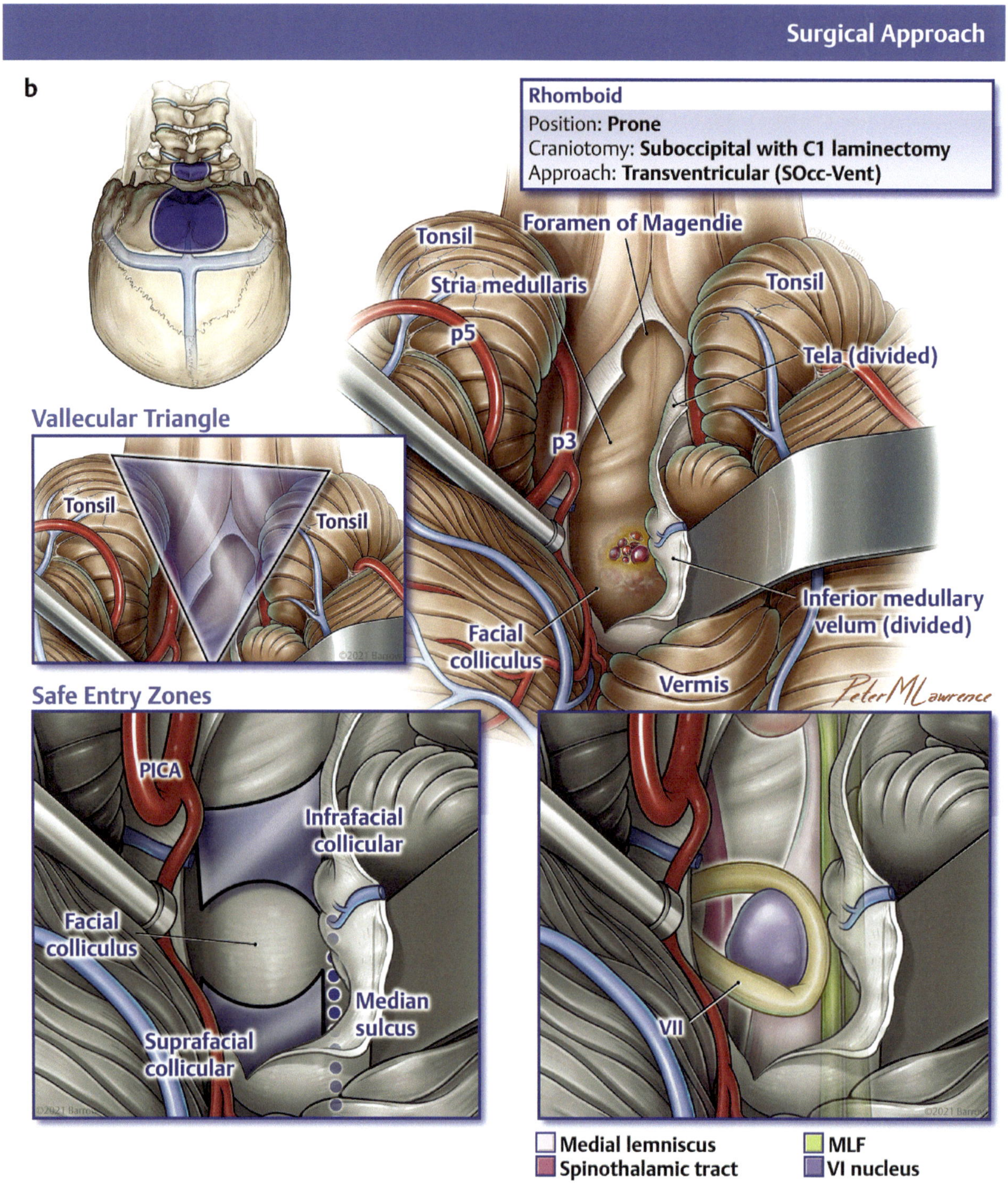

Fig. 15.8 *(Continued)* **(b)** Rhomboid pontine CMs are exposed with a suboccipital craniotomy, C1 laminectomy (*upper left inset*), and transventricular approach. Dissection into the tonsillomedullary fissures bilaterally and liberation of the tonsils opens the vallecular triangle (*middle left inset*). Incision and release of the inferior medullary velum, as with a telovelar approach, extends exposure superiorly and allows the surgeon to reach the pontine portion of the rhomboid fossa where the stria medullaris, median sulcus, median eminence, sulcus limitans, facial colliculus, and superior foveae are visualized. The fourth ventricular floor can be entered safely at four locations (*lower left inset*): the median sulcus (*purple dotted line*), the suprafacial and infrafacial collicular SEZs (*purple shapes*), and the superior foveal SEZ (not shown). Safe entry avoids the MLF (*lower right inset*; *green*), abducens nerve nuclei (*purple*), and internal genu of the facial nerve (*yellow*) (surgical cases; ▶ Video 15.12, ▶ Video 15.13, ▶ Video 15.14; QR codes). Roman numerals denote CNs. (Reproduced with permission from Barrow Neurological Institute, Phoenix, AZ.)

Surgical Case 15.12

PONTINE

Cavernoma Subtype: Rhomboid

Position: Prone
Craniotomy: Suboccipital with C1 laminectomy
Approach: Transventricular (SOcc-Vent)
Triangle: Vallecular
SEZ: None (exophytic)
Artery: p3 PICA

Video: Resection of left rhomboid pontine cavernomas

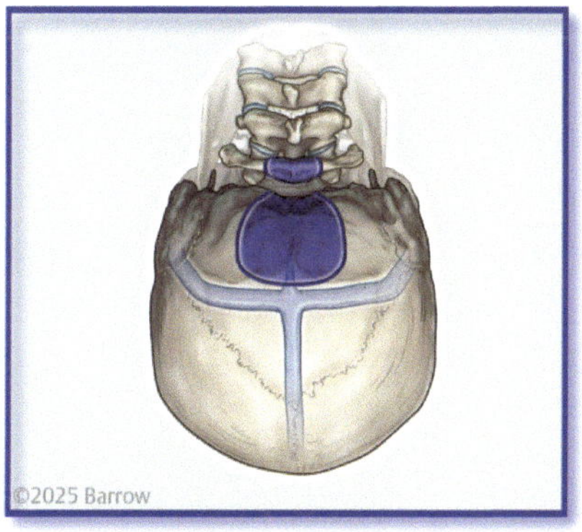

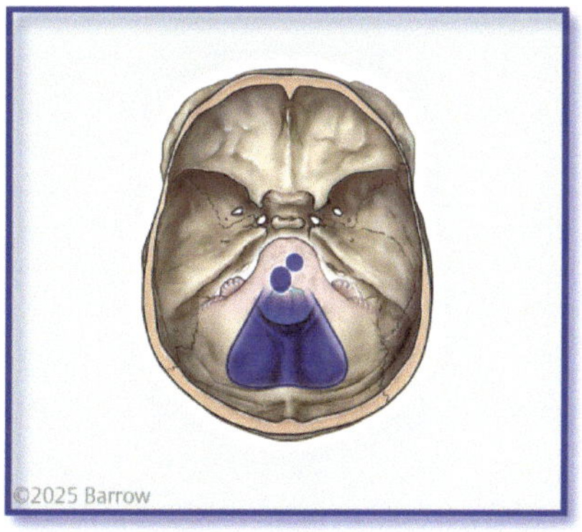

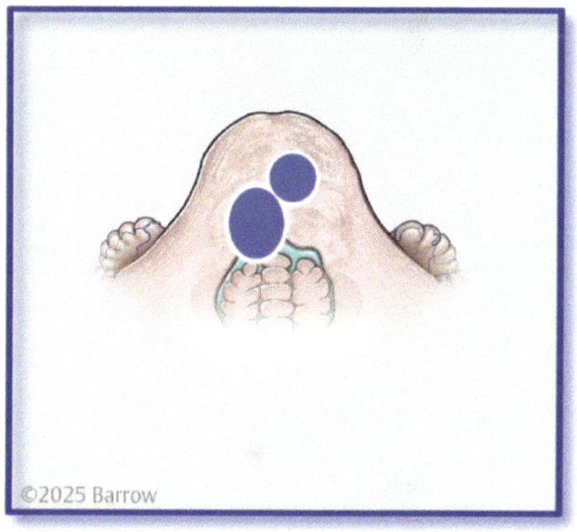

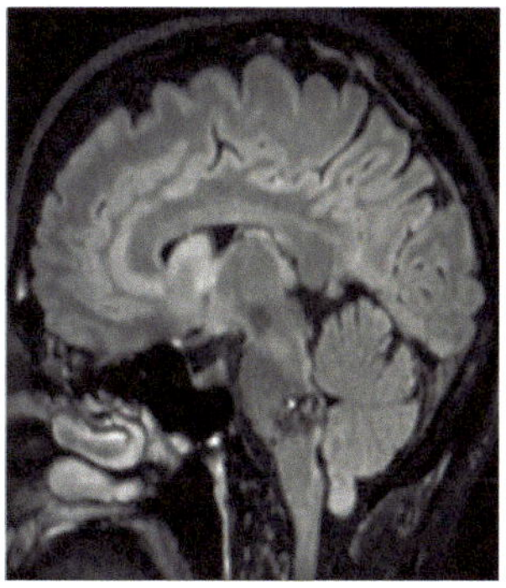

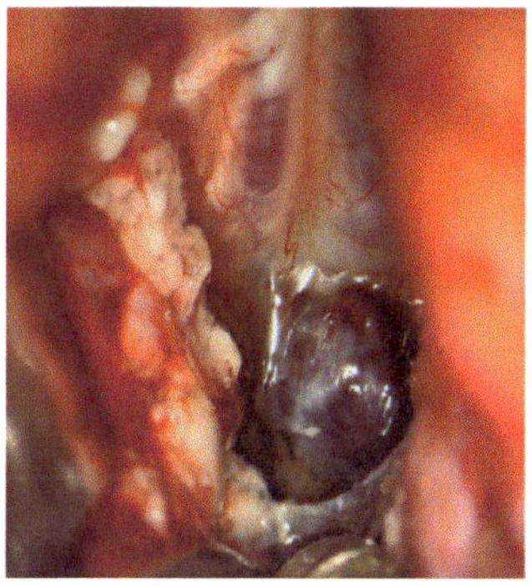

Video 15.12
Suboccipital Craniotomy with Transventricular Approach for Rhomboid Pontine Cavernous Malformation Resection (Reproduced with permission from Barrow Neurological Institute, Phoenix, AZ.)

Surgical Case 15.13

PONTINE

Cavernoma Subtype: Rhomboid

Position: Prone
Craniotomy: Suboccipital with C1 laminectomy
Approach: Transventricular (SOcc-Vent)
Triangle: Vallecular
SEZ: Suprafacial collicular
Artery: p3 PICA

Video: Resection of left rhomboid pontine cavernoma

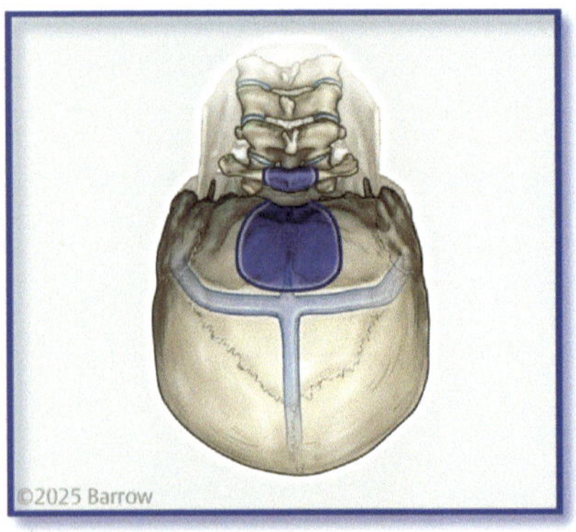

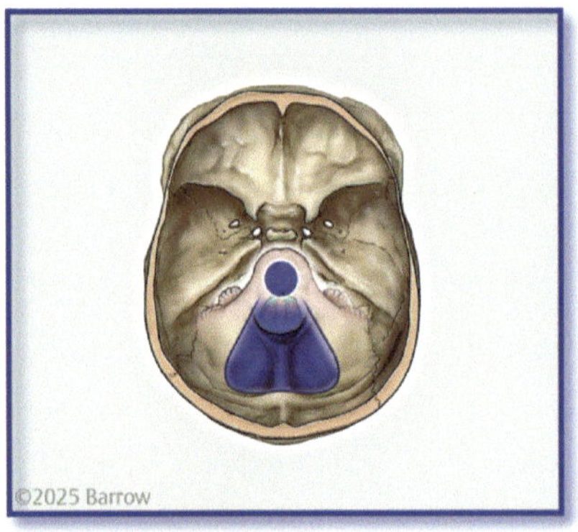

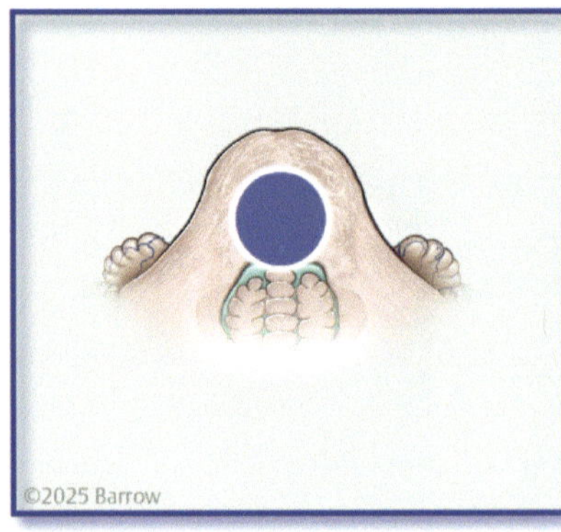

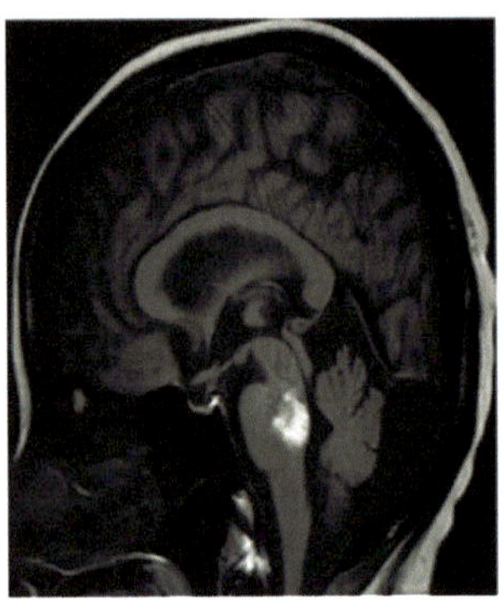

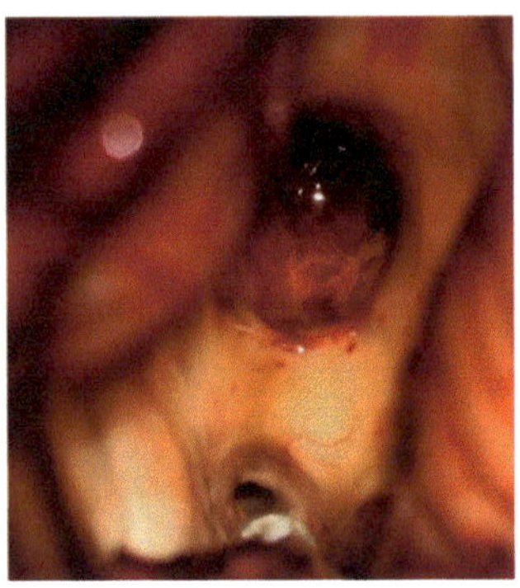

Video 15.13
Suboccipital Craniotomy with Transventricular Approach for Rhomboid Pontine Cavernous Malformation Resection (Reproduced with permission from Barrow Neurological Institute, Phoenix, AZ.)

Surgical Case 15.14

PONTINE

Cavernoma Subtype: Rhomboid

Position: Prone
Craniotomy: Suboccipital with C1 laminectomy
Approach: Transventricular (SOcc-Vent)
Triangle: Vallecular
SEZ: Median sulcus
Artery: p3 PICA

Video: Resection of a midline rhomboid pontine cavernoma

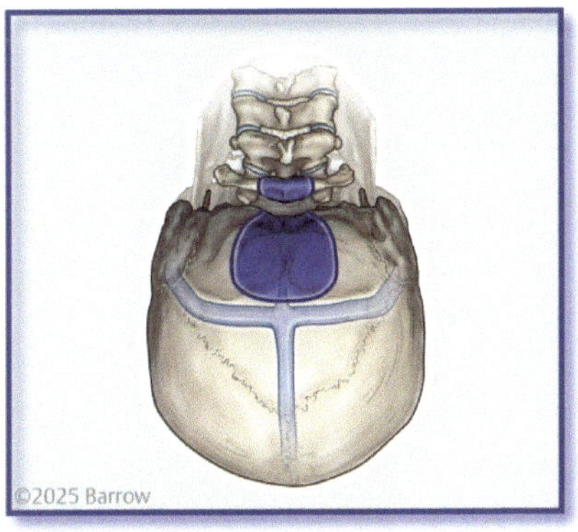

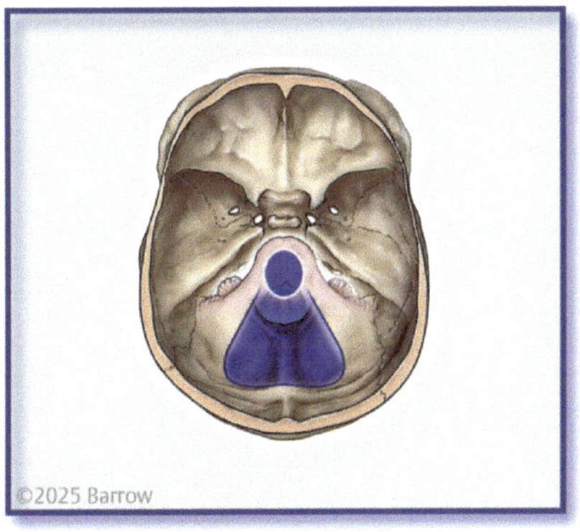

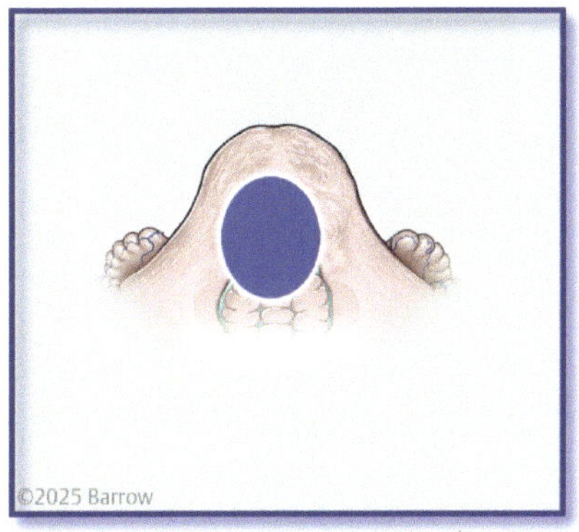

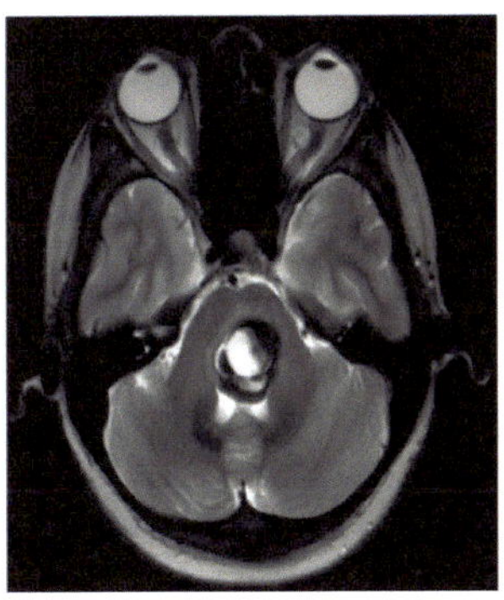

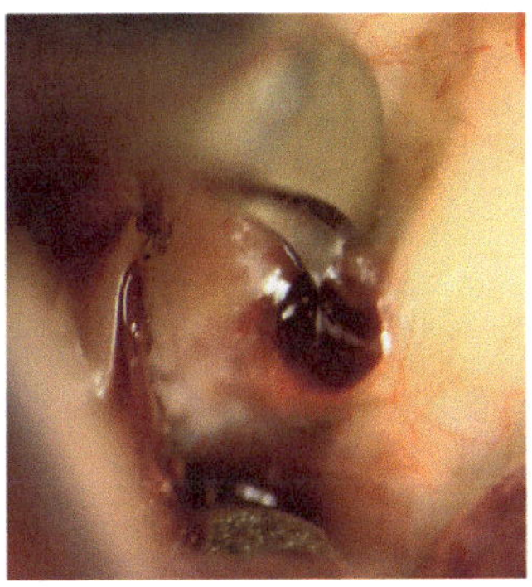

Video 15.14
Suboccipital Craniotomy with Transventricular Approach for Rhomboid Pontine Cavernous Malformation Resection (Reproduced with permission from Barrow Neurological Institute, Phoenix, AZ.)

15

Supraolivary Pontine Cavernoma

Millard-Gubler Syndrome

- **Ipsilateral abducens nerve palsy (VI tract)**
- **Ipsilateral facial nerve palsy (VII tract)**
- **Contralateral hemiparesis/hemiplegia (pyramidal tract)**

Foville Syndrome

- **Millard-Gubler Syndrome symptoms**
- Contralateral hemisensory loss (medial lemniscus, spinothalamic tract)

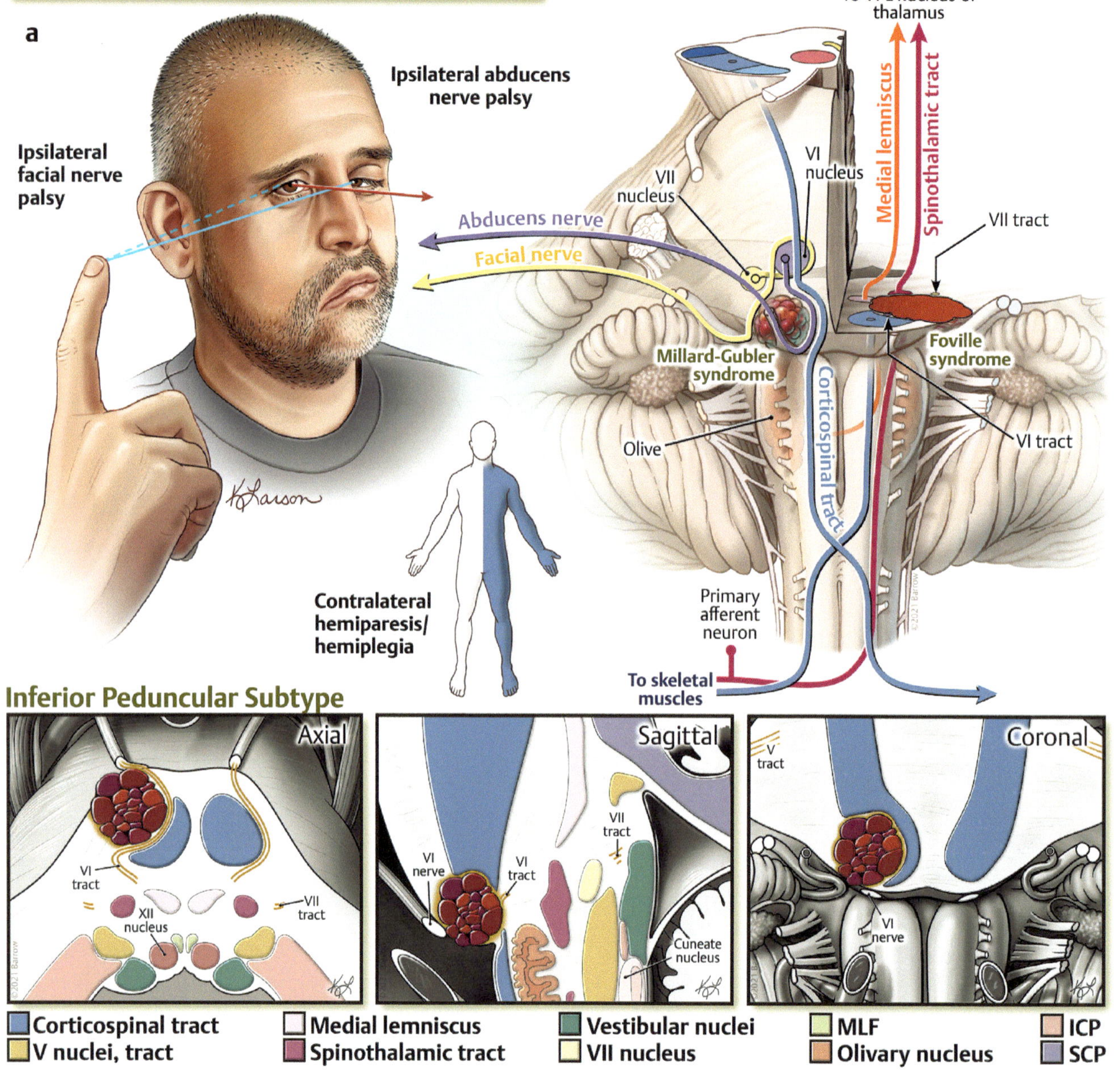

Fig. 15.9 Clinical syndromes and surgical approaches for supraolivary pontine CMs. **(a)** Patients with supraolivary pontine CMs present with ipsilateral abducens nerve palsy. These patients may also have ipsilateral facial palsy and contralateral hemiparesis or hemiplegia due to involvement of the transpontine facial nerve fibers and pyramidal tract (mild Millard–Gubler syndrome). Larger lesions may also cause contralateral hemisensory deficits due to involvement of the medial lemniscus and spinothalamic tracts (Foville syndrome). This left-sided supraolivary CM resides in the underbelly of the pons adjacent to CN VI, CN VII, corticospinal tract, medial lemniscus, and spinothalamic tract, as shown in axial, sagittal, and coronal views (*lower insets*).

(Continued)

Surgical Approach

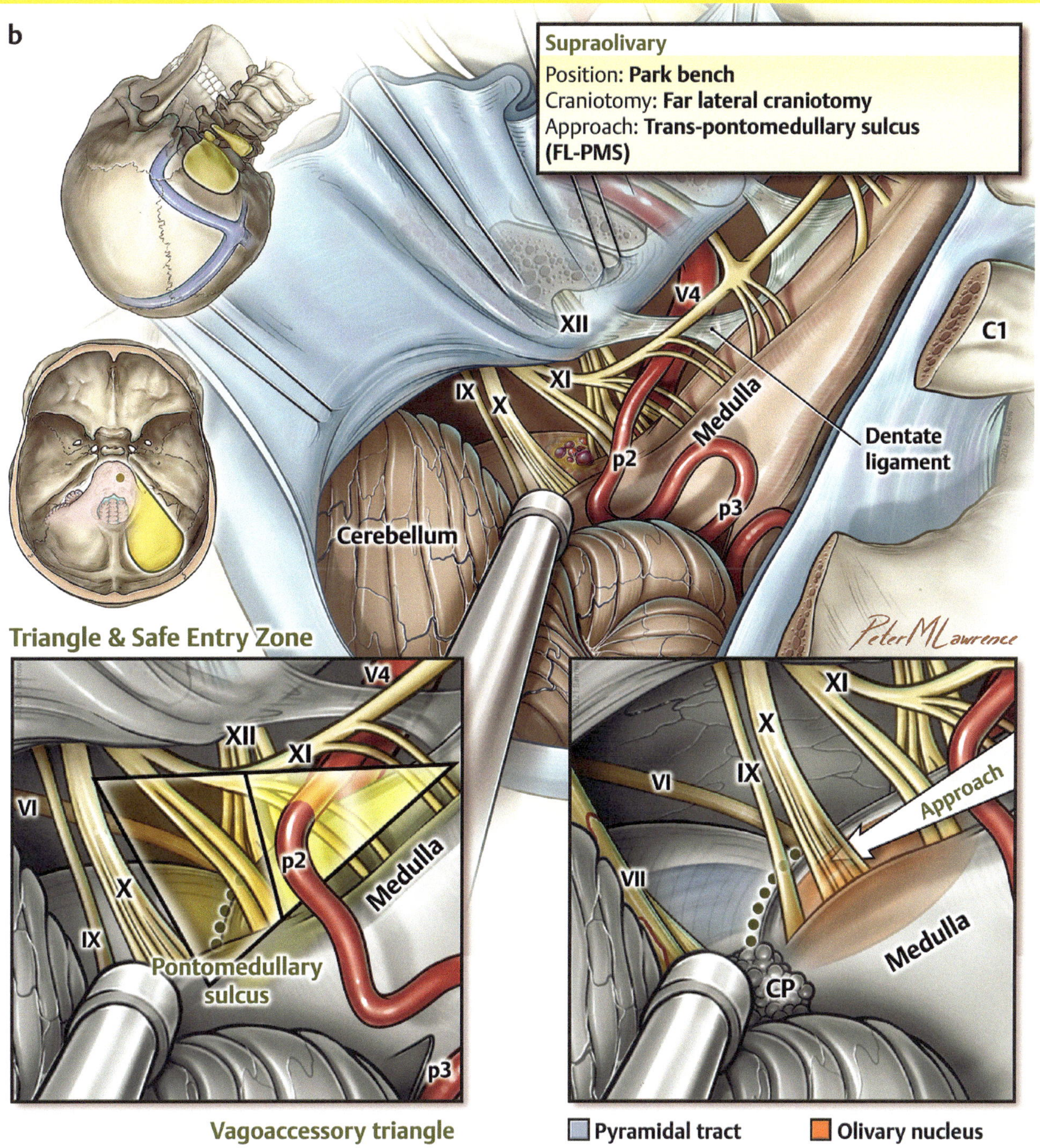

Fig. 15.9 *(Continued)* **(b)** Supraolivary pontine CMs are exposed with a far lateral craniotomy (*upper left inset*). The trans-pontomedullary sulcus approach exposes the CM (*middle left inset; yellow circle*). The patient is placed in the park bench position to orient the clivus and vertebral artery vertically for viewing along the axis of the anterolateral brainstem. Condylectomy opens the cerebellomedullary cistern and exposes the tonsil, lower CNs, V4 (intradural) segment of the vertebral artery, p1 (anterior medullary segment) and p2 (lateral medullary segment) of the PICA, and lateral brainstem. Dissection into the suprahypoglossal portion (superior to CN XII) of the vagoaccessory triangle (*lower left inset; yellow triangle*) leads to the olivary nucleus, pontine underbelly, and pontomedullary sulcus (*gray dotted line*) at their intersection. Supraolivary lesions surface at the pontomedullary sulcus, lateral to the exit of the abducens nerve. Sulcal entry lateral to the abducens nerve protects the pyramidal tract of the corticospinal tract (*lower right inset; ghosted in blue*). The superior pole of the olive (*olivary nucleus ghosted in orange*) meets the inferior pons and forms the pontomedullary sulcus (*gray dotted line*), which is an SEZ for a more posterior trajectory to reach central pontine lesions (surgical cases; ▸ Video 15.15, ▸ Video 15.16; QR codes). Roman numerals denote CNs. (Reproduced with permission from Barrow Neurological Institute, Phoenix, AZ.)

Surgical Case 15.15

PONTINE

Cavernoma Subtype: Supraolivary

Position: Park bench (3/4 prone)
Craniotomy: Far lateral
Approach: Trans-pontomedullary sulcus (FL-PMS)
Triangle: Vagoaccessory
SEZ: Pontomedullary sulcus
Artery: a2 AICA

Video: Resection of a right supraolivary pontine cavernoma

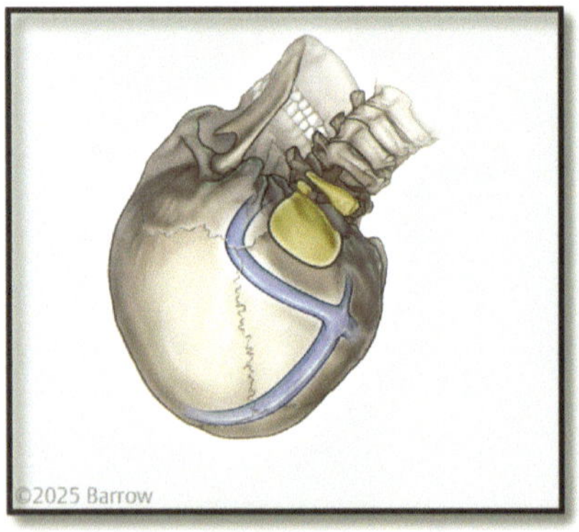

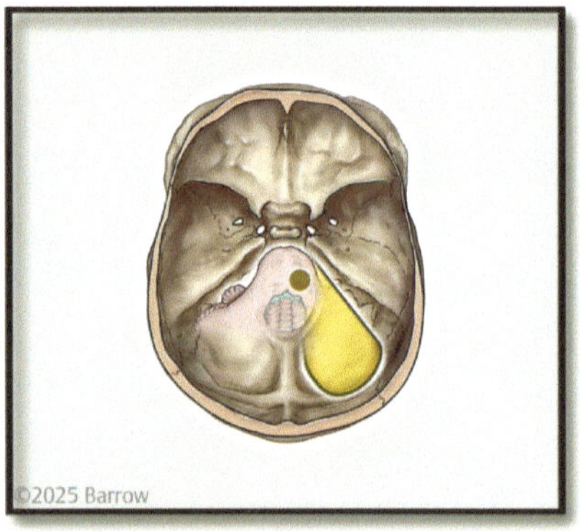

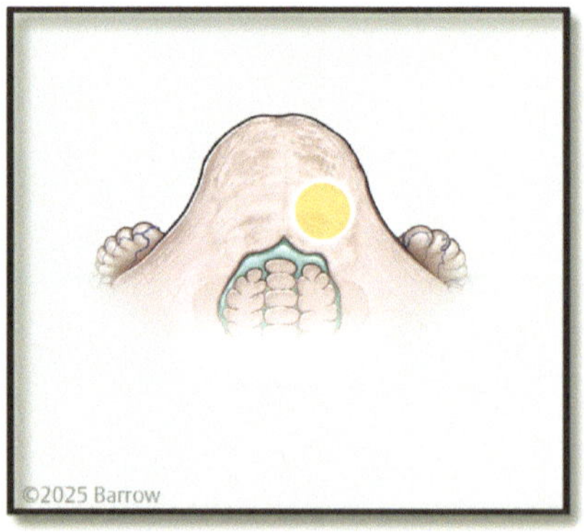

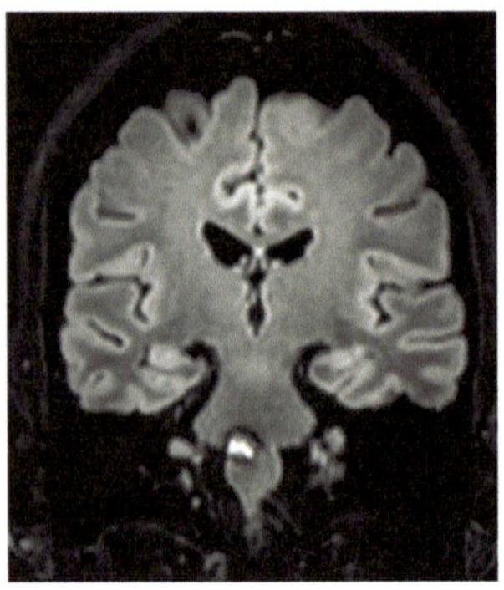

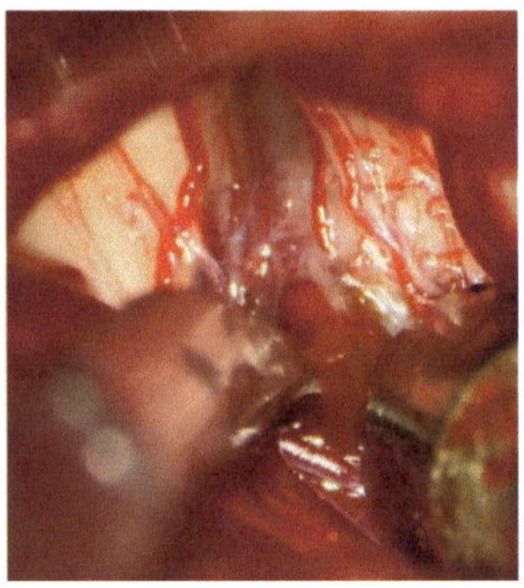

Video 15.15
Far Lateral Craniotomy with Trans-Pontomedullary Sulcus Approach for Supraolivary Pontine Cavernous Malformation Resection (Reproduced with permission from Barrow Neurological Institute, Phoenix, AZ.)

Surgical Case 15.16

PONTINE

Cavernoma Subtype: Supraolivary

Position: Park bench (3/4 prone)
Craniotomy: Far lateral
Approach: Trans-pontomedullary sulcus (FL-PMS)
Triangle: Vagoaccessory
SEZ: Pontomedullary sulcus
Artery: a2 AICA

Video: Resection of a right supraolivary pontine cavernoma

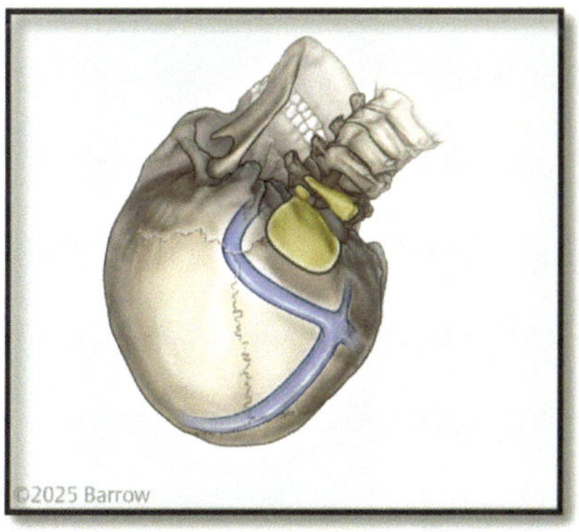

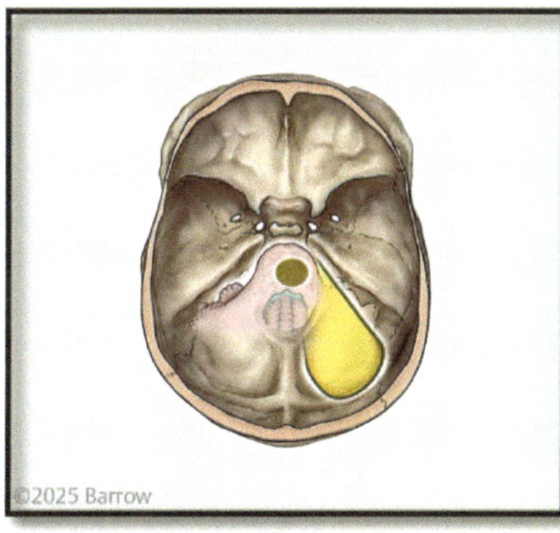

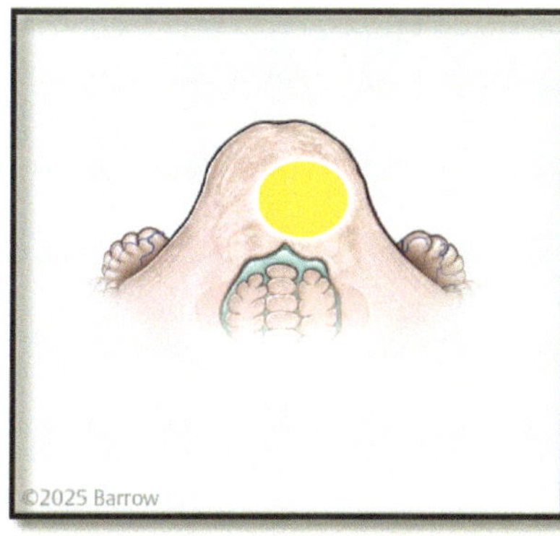

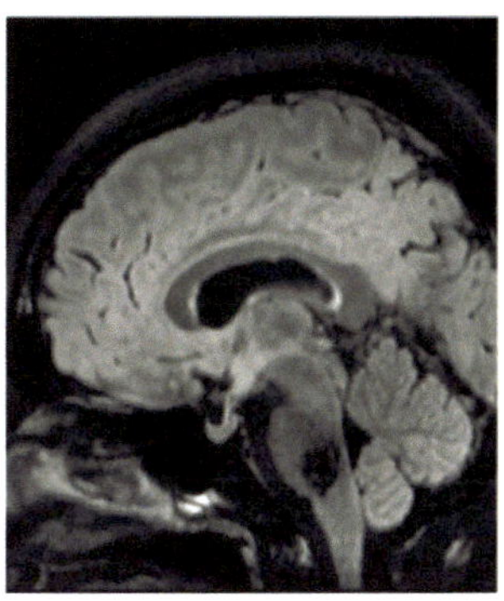

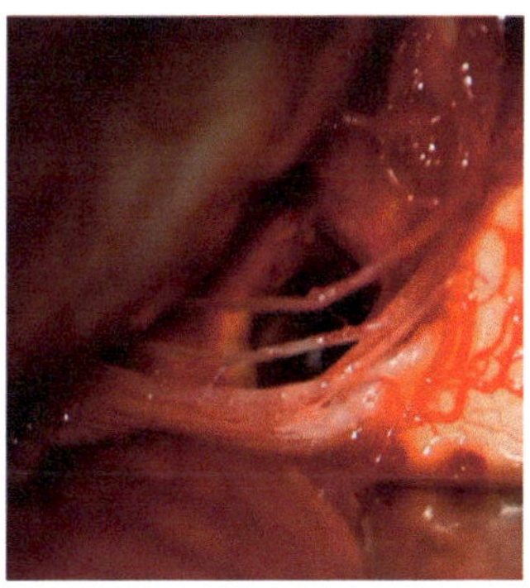

Video 15.16
Far Lateral Craniotomy with Trans-Pontomedullary Sulcus Approach for Supraolivary Pontine Cavernous Malformation Resection (Reproduced with permission from Barrow Neurological Institute, Phoenix, AZ.)

15.5 Signs and Syndromes

The taxonomy for pontine CMs guided the selection of surgical approaches and resection strategies. In addition, the constellation of neurological symptoms and signs associated with a hemorrhagic pontine CM subtype helped define that subtype clinically with recognizable neurological signs, even before pathological anatomy findings on MRI. Pontine CMs have key localizing signs and syndromes, but eponymous pontine vascular syndromes may not be appropriate for describing all presentations of pontine CMs. Perforator infarctions can extend across the entire anteroposterior wedge of the pons and involve CN nuclei in the pontine tegmentum, producing larger constellations of symptoms and signs. In contrast, CMs with spherical capsules limit the extent of neurological injury. For example, Foville syndrome is the result of an inferomedial pontine infarction. It causes contralateral hemiparesis and hemisensory loss, similar to peritrigeminal syndrome, with abducens, facial, and vestibulocochlear nerve palsies and a trigeminal sensory nuclear palsy not seen with peritrigeminal cavernomas. Therefore, specific constellations of signs may be more useful than classic stroke syndromes in localizing pontine CMs. For example, ipsilateral abducens palsy is associated with supraolivary lesions, facial weakness and INO with rhomboid lesions, contralateral hemiparesis with peritrigeminal or basilar lesions, and nausea and vomiting with ICP lesions. Thus, the proposed taxonomy increases bedside diagnostic acumen.

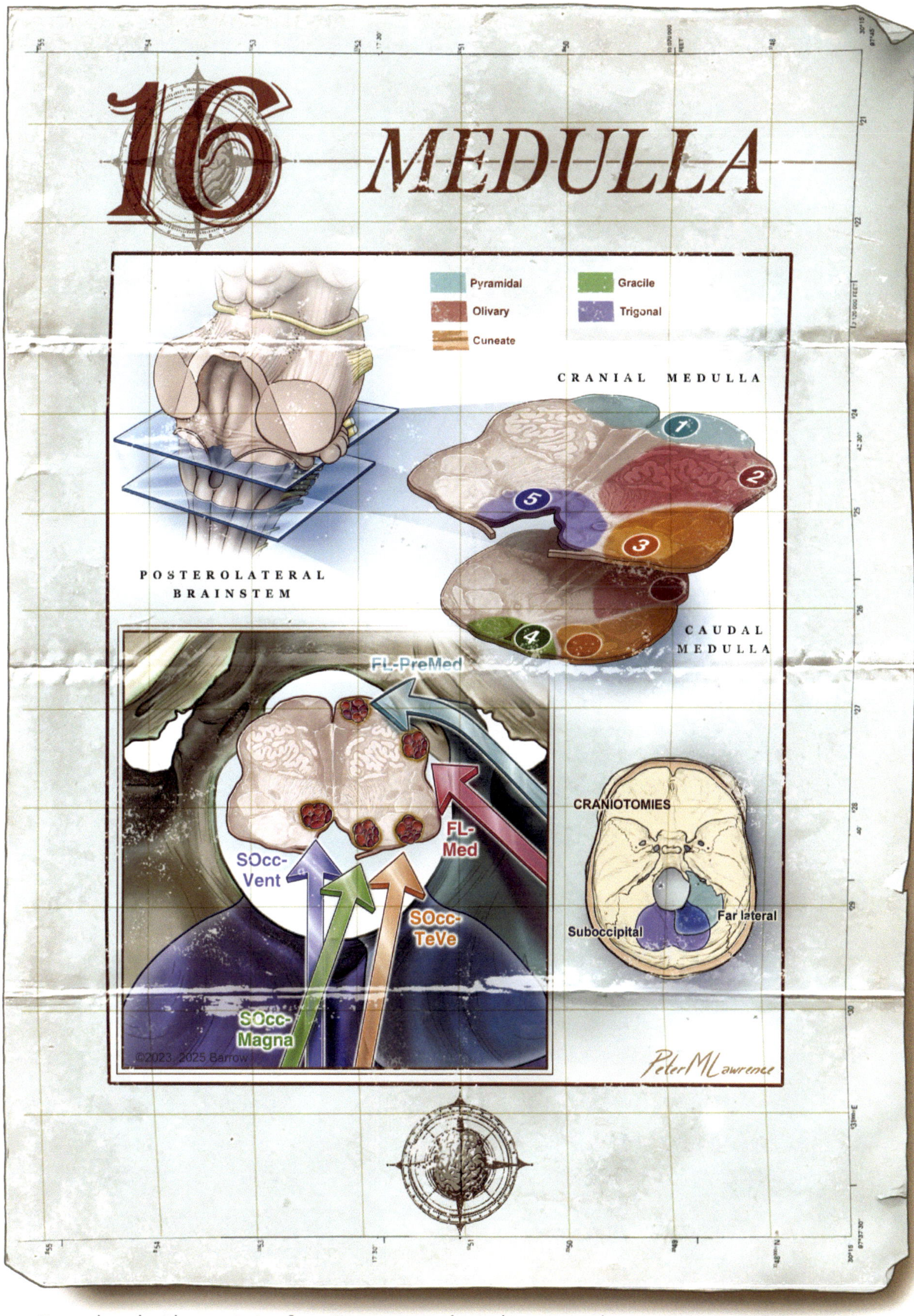

Reproduced with permission from Barrow Neurological Institute, Phoenix, AZ.

16 Medullary Cavernous Malformations

Summary
Medullary cavernous malformations (CMs) are the least commonly occurring subtype of brainstem CMs, accounting for only 14% of lesions in our surgical experience. The brainstem CM taxonomy describes five medullary subtypes: pyramidal, olivary, cuneate, gracile, and trigonal CMs. The CM subtypes are defined on the basis of their medullary surface presentations: anterior, anterolateral, posterolateral, posteroinferior, or posterosuperior. The brainstem CM taxonomy was applied to a surgical series of 77 patients with medullary CMs treated over a 30-year period. Three patients (4%) had pyramidal CMs. Thirty-five (46%) had olivary CMs, and 24 (31%) had cuneate CMs. Another 5 (7%) had gracile CMs, and 10 (13%) had trigonal CMs. A single surgical approach was preferred for each medullary subtype in more than 90% of patients. The far lateral approach was preferred for pyramidal and olivary CMs. The suboccipital-telovelar approach was preferred for cuneate CMs. The suboccipital–trans-cisterna magna approach was preferred for gracile CMs, and the suboccipital-transventricular approach was preferred for trigonal CMs. Of the 73 patients for whom follow-up data were available, 63 (86%) had favorable outcomes, and 67 (92%) had unchanged or improved functional status. Favorable outcomes did not differ significantly among the medullary subtypes. The constellation of neurological signs and symptoms associated with a hemorrhagic subtype defines it clinically as a neurological syndrome recognizable at the bedside. The taxonomy offers a useful scheme for classifying medullary CMs into subtypes, deciphering their clinical presentations at the bedside, and guiding surgical decision-making.

Keywords: cavernoma, cuneate, gracile, hemorrhagic, hemosiderin, olivary, pyramidal, taxonomy, trigonal

16.1 Introduction

The medulla oblongata, the oblong enlargement of the top of the spinal cord, comprises the lower third of the brainstem and is responsible for autonomic functions ranging from breathing and heartbeat to vomiting and sneezing. Medullary cavernous malformations (CMs) are the least commonly occurring subtype of brainstem CMs, accounting for only 14% of lesions in our surgical experience. Unlike CMs in the midbrain and pons that can be accessed from many trajectories through various approaches, medullary CMs are accessed posteriorly through a suboccipital-transventricular approach or laterally through a far lateral approach. Although these two approaches have important variations, the limited options make the selection of surgical approaches simpler for medullary CMs than for other brainstem CMs. Anatomical taxonomy for these lesions, like other brainstem CMs, would also improve clinical decision-making and resection strategy for improved patient outcomes. Like other brainstem regions, the dense packing of tracts and cranial nerve (CN) nuclei in the medulla yields unique constellations of neurological signs and symptoms associated with hemorrhagic lesions. Therefore, a brainstem CM in an individual patient would have a recognizable neurological syndrome upon examination at the patient's bedside and characteristic radiographic anatomy on magnetic resonance imaging, as observed in our experience.

16.2 Neuroanatomy of the Five Medullary Cavernous Malformation Subtypes

The brainstem CM taxonomy describes five medullary subtypes: (1) pyramidal, (2) olivary, (3) cuneate, (4) gracile, and (5) trigonal (▶ Fig. 16.1). The CM subtypes are defined on the basis of their medullary surface presentations: anterior, anterolateral, posterolateral, posteroinferior, or posterosuperior.

16.2.1 Pyramidal

Pyramidal CMs are located in the anterior medulla, within or alongside the pyramidal tracts. They lie on the anterior surface in the midline, centered on the anteromedian fissure, or eccentric to the fissure. The anterolateral sulcus defines the lateral extent of these CMs. The lesions localize medial to the CN XII (hypoglossal) rootlets that exit the anterolateral sulcus and lie between the pontomedullary sulcus superiorly and the decussation of the pyramids inferiorly. This surface sits behind the distal V4 (intradural) segments of the vertebral arteries, vertebrobasilar junction, proximal basilar trunk, and anterior spinal arteries. Pyramidal CMs affect the corticospinal tracts, pyramidal decussation, medial lemnisci, arcuate nuclei, and medial accessory olivary nuclei.

16.2.2 Olivary

Olivary CMs can occur in the anterolateral medulla in or just posterior to the olivary nucleus. They lie between the anterolateral or preolivary sulcus, from which the CN XII (hypoglossal) rootlets arise, and the posterolateral or retro-olivary sulcus, from which the rootlets of CNs IX (glossopharyngeal), X (vagus), and XI (spinal accessory) arise. This surface is intimately associated with the p2 (lateral medullary) segment of the posterior inferior cerebellar artery (PICA), localized by the same landmarks. The olivary nucleus is an easily identifiable surface landmark made more identifiable by the nerve rootlets on either side. These lesions lie between the pontomedullary sulcus and CN VI (abducens) superiorly and the foramen magnum inferiorly. Deep to this surface lies the olivary nucleus, vestibulospinal fibers, reticulospinal fibers, ventral spinocerebellar tract, spinothalamic tract, rubrospinal tract, and lateral reticular nucleus.

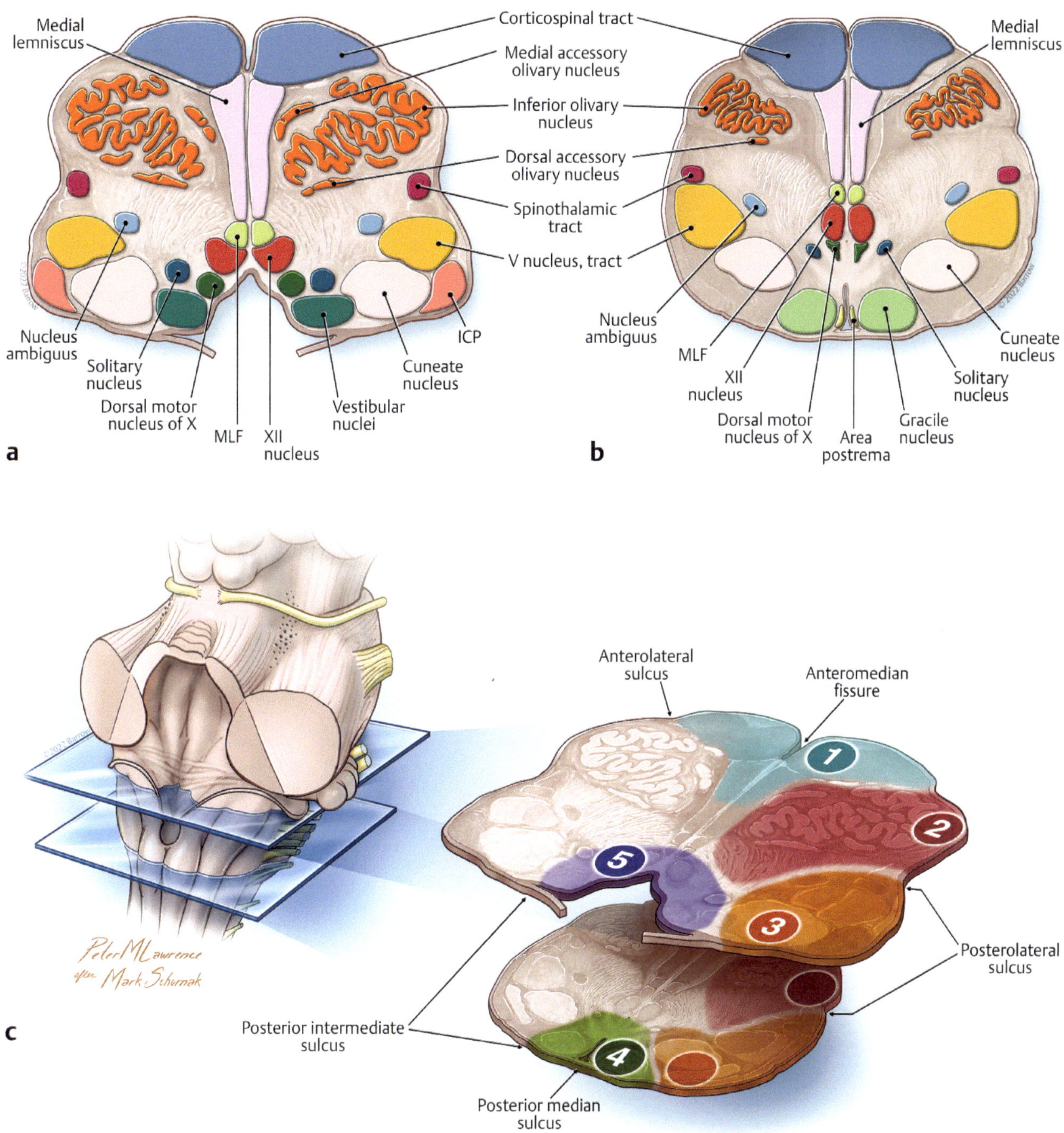

Fig. 16.1 Overview of medullary anatomy and CM subtypes. The anatomy of medullary nuclei and tracts is shown in axial cross-section **(a)** through the upper medulla and fourth ventricle and **(b)** through the lower medulla below the ventricle. **(c)** The locations of the five subtypes are shown in upper and lower axial cross-sections: (1) pyramidal (*teal*), (2) olivary (*red*), (3) cuneate (*orange*), (4) gracile (*green*), and (5) trigonal (*purple*).

(Continued)

16.2.3 Cuneate

Cuneate CMs are located in the posterolateral medulla outside the fourth ventricle. They are lateral to the gracile nucleus between the posterior intermediate sulcus and the posterolateral or retro-olivary sulcus. This region lies below the lateral recess and is almost the mirror image of the inferior peduncular pontine subtype that lies above the lateral recess. Cuneate lesions are found posterior to the medullary rootlets of CN XI. The posterolateral sulcus, one of only a few surface landmarks, runs through this region lateral to the cuneate tubercle and in front of the trigeminal tubercle. The proximal p3

d

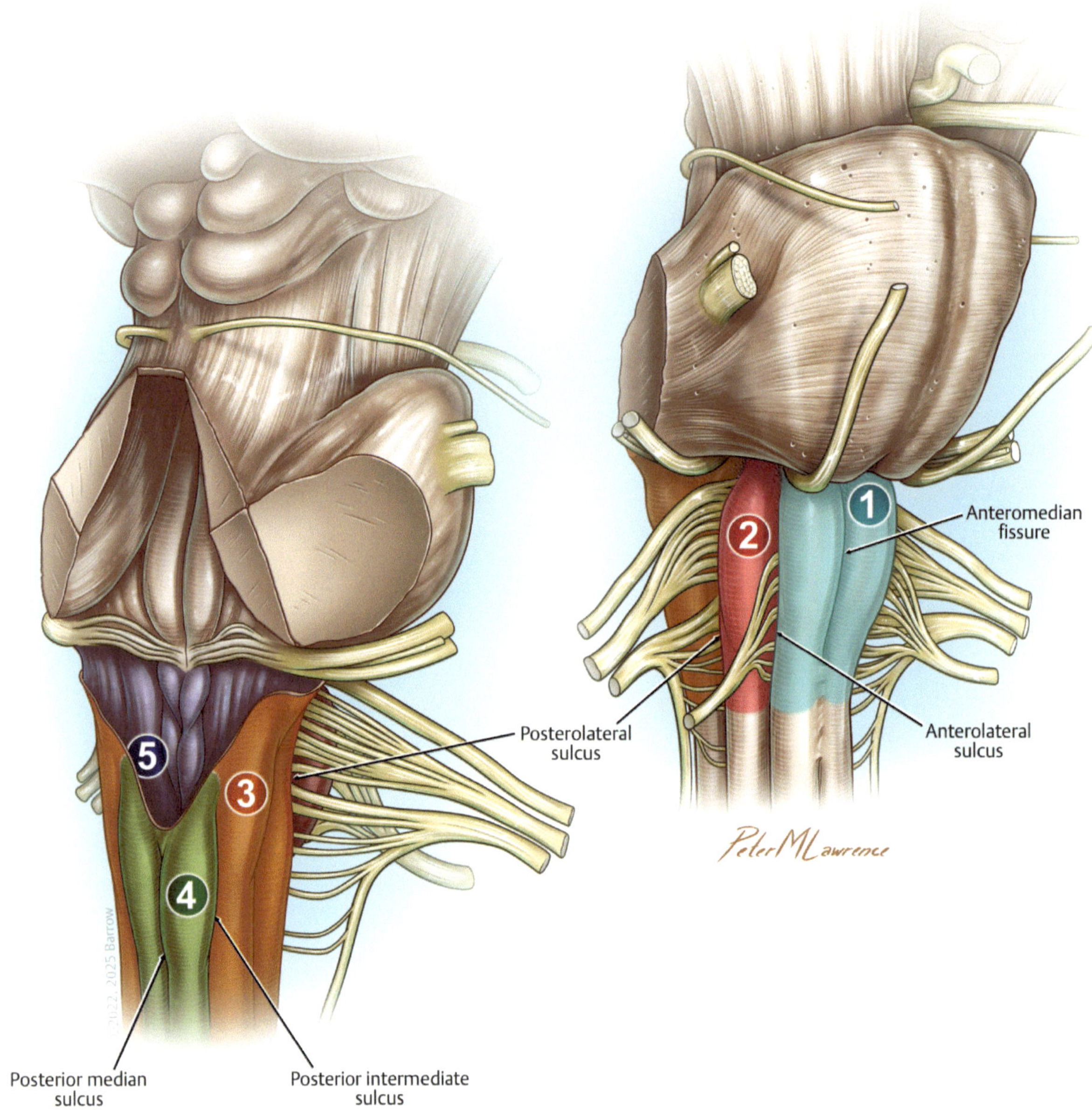

Fig. 16.1 (*Continued*) **(d)** The locations of the five subtypes are shown in posterolateral and anterolateral views. Roman numerals denote CNs. (Reproduced with permission from Barrow Neurological Institute, Phoenix, AZ).

(tonsillomedullary) segment of the PICA overlies this area. Deep structures in this region include the spinal nucleus and tract of the trigeminal nerve; dorsal spinocerebellar, rubrospinal, spinothalamic, and ventral spinocerebellar tracts; the nucleus ambiguus and lateral reticular nucleus; the reticular formation; and the vestibulospinal and reticulospinal fibers.

16.2.4 Gracile

Gracile medullary CMs are located in the posteroinferior aspect of the medulla, outside the fourth ventricle, and below the medullary part of the rhomboid fossa. They are named for their relationship to the gracile tubercles and fasciculi, which parallel the midline on both sides of the posterior median sulcus below the obex and tela choroidea of the fourth ventricle. The posterior intermediate sulcus separates the gracile and cuneate tubercles and forms the lateral limit of a gracile medullary CM. These CMs lie underneath the caudal p3 loop of the PICA. Beneath the gracile tubercles lie the area postrema, the dorsal motor nucleus of CN X, the solitary nucleus and tract, and the dorsal longitudinal fasciculi.

16.2.5 Trigonal

Trigonal CMs are located in the posterosuperior medulla at the surface of the fourth ventricular floor. The medullary part of the rhomboid fossa is smaller than the pontine part, and it extends inferiorly from the stria medullaris to the obex and laterally between the teniae choroidea of the fourth ventricle. These CMs are named after the three triangular areas of the caudal median eminence: the hypoglossal trigone, vagal trigone, and area postrema, which collectively form the calamus scriptorius. The hypoglossal trigone overlies the hypoglossal nucleus. Just below it, the vagal trigone overlies the dorsal nucleus of CN X and the solitary nucleus. The area postrema is at the lower limit of the median eminence and is immediately rostral to the obex.

16.3 Clinical Evidence

The brainstem CM taxonomy system was applied to a two-surgeon surgical series of 77 patients with medullary CMs that Robert F. Spetzler and I treated over a 30-year period (1990–2019; ▸ Table 16.1). Five distinct medullary CM subtypes were defined: pyramidal (3, 3.9%), olivary (35, 46%), cuneate (24, 31%), gracile (5, 6.5%), and trigonal (10, 13%). Pyramidal CMs were located in the anterior medulla and were associated with hemiparesis and hypoglossal nerve palsy (▸ Fig. 16.2). Olivary CMs were found in the anterolateral medulla and were associated with ataxia. Cuneate CMs were located in the posterolateral medulla and were associated with ipsilateral upper extremity sensory deficits. Gracile CMs were found outside the fourth ventricle in the posteroinferior medulla and were associated with ipsilateral lower extremity sensory deficits. Trigonal CMs in the ventricular floor were associated with nausea, vomiting, and diplopia.

Table 16.1 Preoperative and postoperative outcome measures for patients who underwent resection of medullary CMs by subtype

Variable	All subtypes (*N* = 73)	Pyramidal (*n* = 3)	Olivary (*n* = 34)	Trigonal (*n* = 10)	Gracile (*n* = 5)	Cuneate (*n* = 21)	*p*-value
Brainstem CM grade							
Patients with data available	42	3	13	6	4	16	0.32
Low	28/42 (67)	3/28 (11)	9/28 (32)	2/28 (7)	3/28 (11)	11/28 (39)	
Intermediate	13/42 (31)	0/13 (0)	4/13 (31)	3/13 (23)	1/13 (8)	5/13 (38)	
High	1/42 (2)	0/1 (0)	0/1 (0)	1/1 (100)	0/1 (0)	0/1 (0)	
Follow-up							
Mean (SD), mo	37 (47)	27 (21)	41 (49)	42 (67)	17 (11)	35 (44)	0.93
> 30 d	73/73 (100)	3/73(4)	34/73 (46)	10/73 (14)	5/73 (7)	21/73 (29)	0.36
Pre-op mRS score							
Median (IQR)	2 (1–2)	2 (2–2)	1 (1–2)	2 (1–4)	1 (1–1)	1 (1–2)	**0.02**
> 2	11/73 (15)	0/11 (0)	6/11 (54)	3/11 (27)	0/11 (0)	2/11 (18)	0.39
Post-op mRS score							
Median (IQR)	2 (1–2)	2 (2–4)	1 (1–3)	2 (2–4)	1 (1–1.5)	1 (1–2)	0.07
> 2	15/73 (20)	1/15 (7)	10/15 (67)	3/15 (20)	0/15 (0)	1/15 (7)	0.11
Final mRS score							
Median (IQR)	1 (1–2)	2 (2–2)	1 (1–2)	1.5 (1–2.4)	1 (1–1)	1 (1–1.5)	0.14
> 2	10/73 (14)	0/10 (0)	7/10 (70)	2/10 (20)	0/10 (0)	1/10 (10)	0.36
≤ 2	63/73 (86)	2/63 (3)	27/63 (43)	8/63 (13)	5/63 (8)	20/63 (32)	0.36
Worsened vs. pre-op mRS score	6/73 (8)	0/6 (0)	3/6 (50)	1/6 (17)	0/6 (0)	2/6 (33)	0.93

Note: Data are presented as n (%) unless otherwise indicated. Percentages might not total 100% due to rounding. Bold p-values indicate statistical significance ($p < 0.05$).

16

Symptom	Subtype				
	Pyramidal (n=3)	Olivary (n=35)	Cuneate (n=24)	Gracile (n=5)	Trigonal (n=10)
Hemisensory deficit	2 (67%)	18 (51%)	15 (63%)	3 (60%)	4 (40%)
Ataxia, dysmetria	0 (0%)	15 (43%)	7 (29%)	2 (20%)	3 (30%)
Hemiparesis	3 (100%)	11 (31%)	2 (8%)	0 (0%)	4 (40%)
N/V, vertigo	0 (0%)	9 (26%)	7 (29%)	0 (0%)	3 (30%)
Diplopia	0 (0%)	12 (34%)	2 (8%)	0 (0%)	4 (40%)
Dysphagia	0 (0%)	4 (11%)	5 (21%)	1 (20%)	3 (30%)
Tongue weakness	2 (67%)	2 (6%)	1 (4%)	0 (0%)	2 (20%)

Fig. 16.2 Heat map illustrating the symptoms of patients with medullary CMs by subtype. Percentages were calculated as the frequency of patients with a particular symptom or sign of a given medullary subtype. Conditional formatting was applied on a scale of least common (*red*) to most common (*green*). Well-defined syndromes associated with each subtype aligned most closely with cells with *green* formatting. (Reproduced with permission from Catapano JS, Rumalla K, Srinivasan VM, Lawrence PM, Larson Keil K, Lawton MT. A taxonomy for brainstem cavernous malformations: subtypes of medullary lesions. J Neurosurg 2022;138(1):128–146).

Lawton brainstem CM grades were determined in 42 patients: 28 patients (67%) had low-grade CMs (grades 0–II), 13 (31%) had intermediate-grade CMs (grades III–V), and 1 (2%) had a high-grade CM (grade VI or VII). A single surgical approach was preferred for each medullary subtype in more than 90% of patients. The far lateral approach was preferred for pyramidal and olivary CMs. The suboccipital-telovelar approach was preferred for cuneate CMs. The suboccipital–trans-cisterna magna approach was preferred for gracile CMs, and the suboccipital-transventricular approach was preferred for trigonal CMs. Of the 73 patients for whom follow-up data were available, 63 (86%) had favorable outcomes, and 67 (92%) had unchanged or improved functional status. Favorable outcomes did not differ significantly among the medullary subtypes ($p = 0.36$).

16.4 Resection Strategies for Medullary Cavernous Malformations

The brainstem CM taxonomy was used as a guide for the selection of surgical approaches to medullary CM subtypes. Medullary CMs are accessed posteriorly through a suboccipital-transventricular approach or laterally through a far lateral approach. These two approaches have essential variations, but these options make the selection of surgical approaches simpler for medullary CMs than for other brainstem CMs (▶ Fig. 16.3). A single surgical approach was preferred for each medullary subtype in more than 90% of patients.

16.4.1 Pyramidal Subtype

The pyramids are paired white matter structures on the ventral medulla that appear triangular in cross-section and decussate at the base of the pyramids to mark the border between the medulla and the spinal cord. They contain the motor fibers of the outgoing corticospinal tracts. Patients with a unilateral pyramidal CM presented with Dejerine's syndrome, a medial medullary syndrome defined by contralateral hemiparesis due to corticospinal tract involvement, hemisensory loss due to medial lemniscus involvement, and ipsilateral tongue weakness due to CN XII involvement (▶ Fig. 16.4a). Larger midline CMs can be associated with bilateral medial medullary syndrome; however, we did not observe this presentation among our patients.

Pyramidal lesions were approached via a far lateral craniotomy and dissection through the premedullary cistern (▶ Fig. 16.4b; ▶ Video 16.1). Aggressive condylectomy opened the lateral corridor, and incising the dentate ligaments helped mobilize the ventral surface into view. Dissection ventral to CN XI in front of the vagoaccessory triangle gave a view down the long axis of V4 to the vertebrobasilar junction and the origin of the anterior spinal artery. The ipsilateral and contralateral V4 and CN XI define the vertebrobasilar junctional triangle, with the vertebrobasilar junction at the triangle's superior apex. The transverse medullary vein can be traced medially to the median anterior medullary vein, marking the midline. The anterior median fissure and anterolateral sulcus are surface landmarks, but the lateral view makes only the anterolateral sulcus visible. The CN XII rootlets are easily identified in the cerebellomedullary cistern and lead back to the anterolateral sulcus. This surgical trajectory brings the clivus and arterial anatomy into view but is tangential to the anterior medullary surface and not aligned with pyramidal CMs. The lesion must be moved gently from the parenchyma into the surgical corridor. The anterolateral sulcus provides a safe entry zone (SEZ) to access more medially located CMs below the anterior surface of the medulla. The malalignment of the far lateral trajectory and pyramidal lesion axis is another example where a transclival approach may provide better exposure for resection, particularly with further advancement in endoscopic endonasal

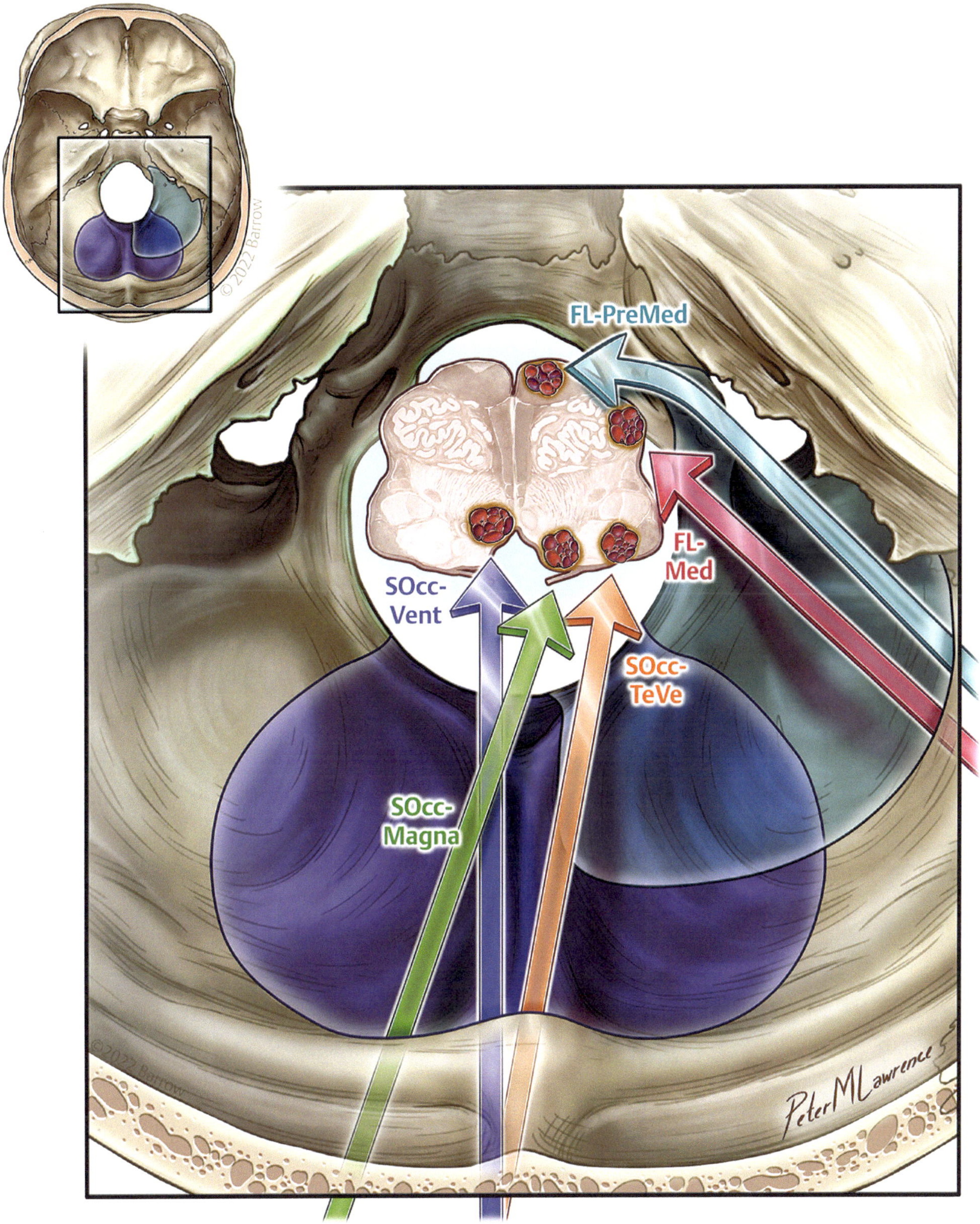

Fig. 16.3 Overview of surgical approaches to medullary CMs shown in axial cross-section viewed from above. The FL-PreMed approach (*teal arrow*) is used for pyramidal CMs, the FL-Med approach (*red arrow*) is used for olivary CMs, and the SOcc-TeVe approach (*orange arrow*) is used for cuneate CMs. The SOcc-Magna approach (*green arrow*) is used for gracile CMs, and the SOcc-Vent approach (*purple arrow*) is used for trigonal CMs. The far lateral craniotomy is used for FL-PreMed and FL-Med approaches (*inset, teal*), and the suboccipital craniotomy is used for SOcc-Vent, SOcc-TeVe, and SOcc-Magna approaches (*inset, purple*). (Reproduced with permission from Barrow Neurological Institute, Phoenix, AZ).

Pyramidal Medullary Cavernoma

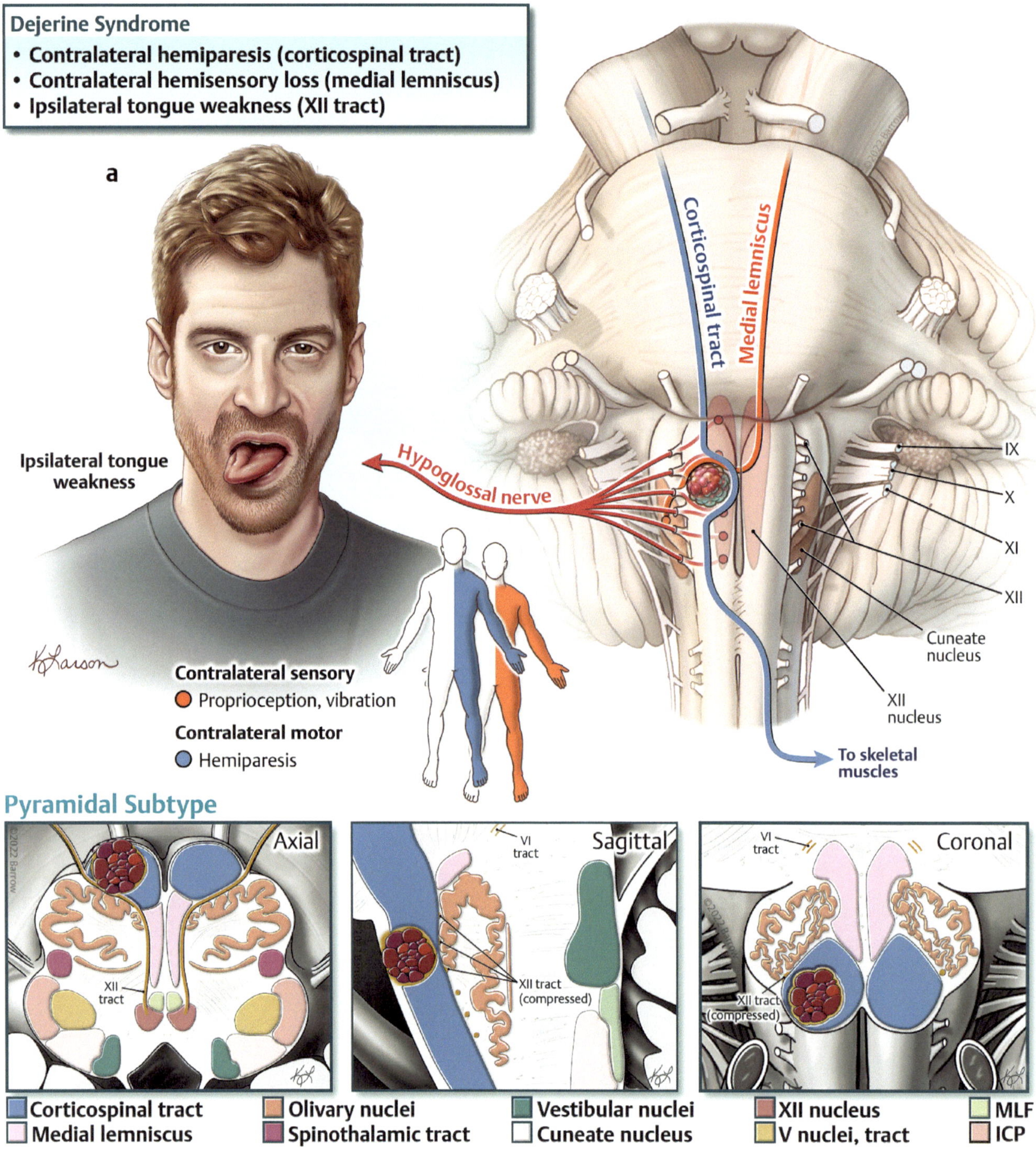

Fig. 16.4 Pyramidal medullary clinical syndromes and surgical approaches. **(a)** Patients with pyramidal CMs present with Dejerine's syndrome (contralateral hemiparesis, contralateral hemisensory loss, and ipsilateral tongue weakness). The relationships between this right-sided medullary CM and the corticospinal tract, medial lemniscus, and intramedullary tract of CN XII are shown in axial, sagittal, and coronal views (*lower insets*).

(Continued)

Surgical Approach

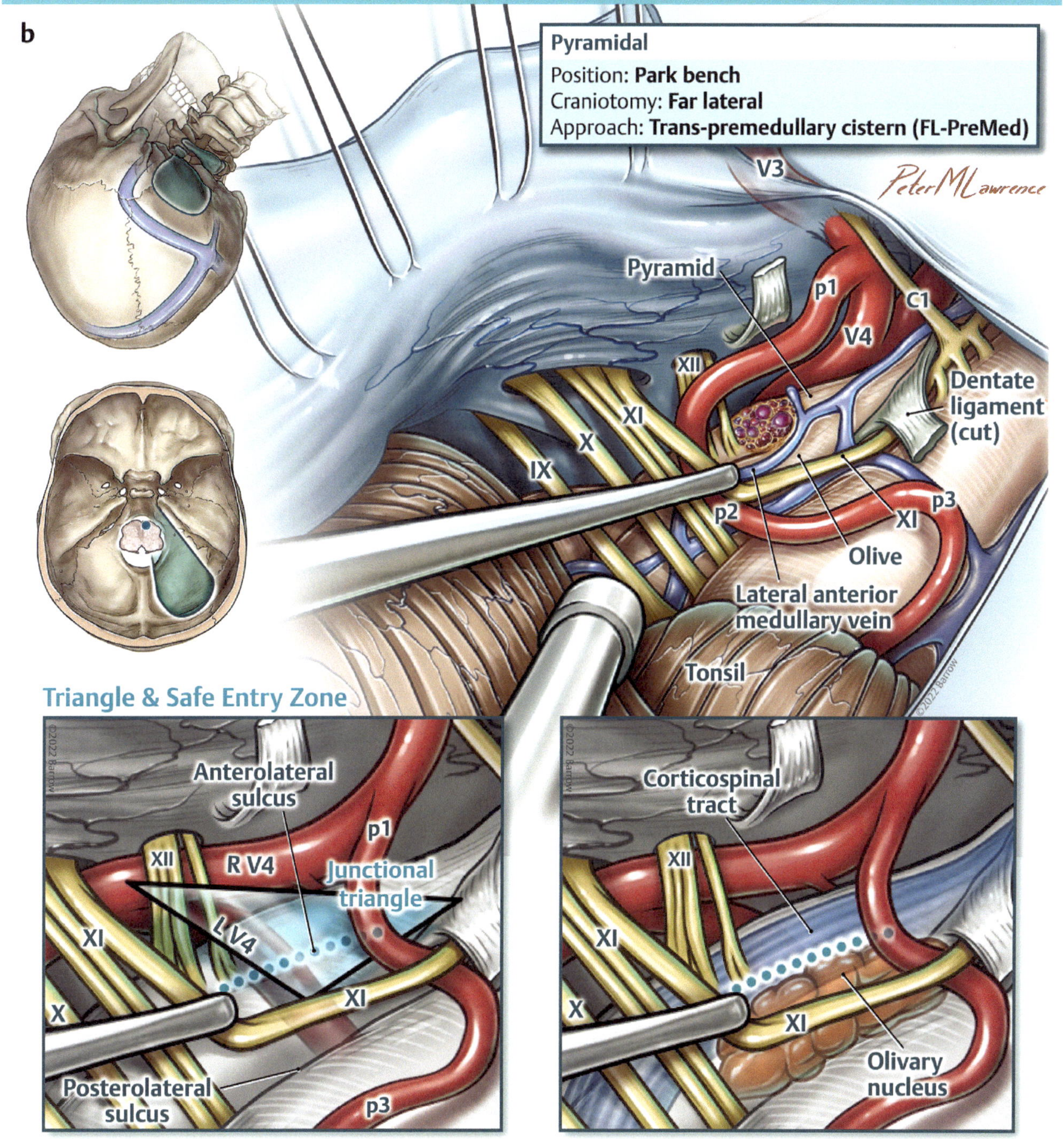

Fig. 16.4 *(Continued)* **(b)** Pyramidal CMs are approached through a far lateral craniotomy (*upper left inset*) and trans-premedullary cistern approach (*middle left inset, teal circle*). The patient is placed in the park bench or three-quarter prone position. Incising the dentate ligaments and dissecting ventral to CN XI (spinal accessory) opens a view into the vertebrobasilar junction triangle formed by ipsilateral and contralateral V4 segments of the vertebral artery and the spinal accessory nerve, with the vertebrobasilar junction at the superior apex of the triangle (*lower left inset*). The transverse medullary vein can be traced medially to the median anterior medullary vein, marking the midline. The CN XII (hypoglossal) rootlets are easily identified in the cerebellomedullary cistern and lead back to the anterolateral sulcus. The anterolateral sulcus SEZ (*teal dotted line*) provides access to more medially located CMs below the anterior surface (*lower left and right insets*; *ghosted structures*) (surgical case; ▸ Video 16.1; QR code). Roman numerals denote CNs. (Reproduced with permission from Barrow Neurological Institute, Phoenix, AZ.)

Surgical Case 16.1

MEDULLARY

Cavernoma Subtype: Pyramidal

Position: Park bench (3/4 prone)
Craniotomy: Far lateral
Approach: Trans-premedullary cistern (FL-PreMed)
Triangle: Junctional
SEZ: Anterolateral sulcus
Artery: VBJ

Video: Resection of a left pyramidal medullary cavernoma

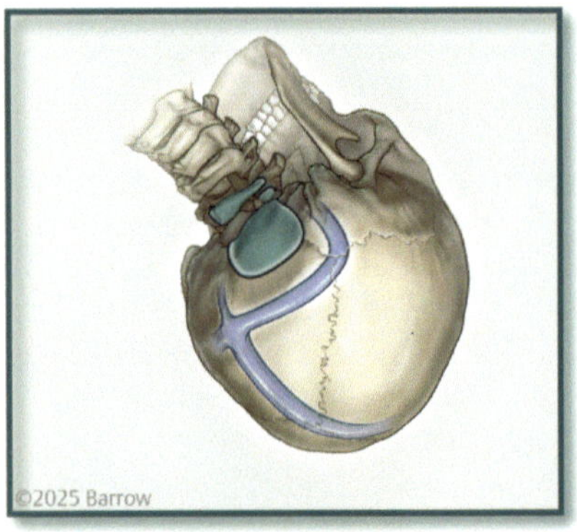

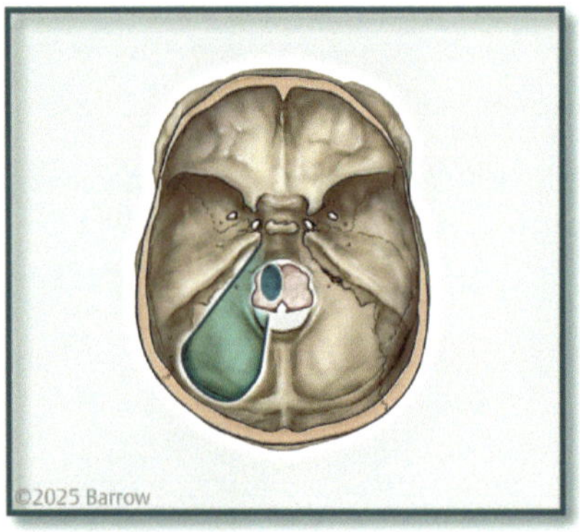

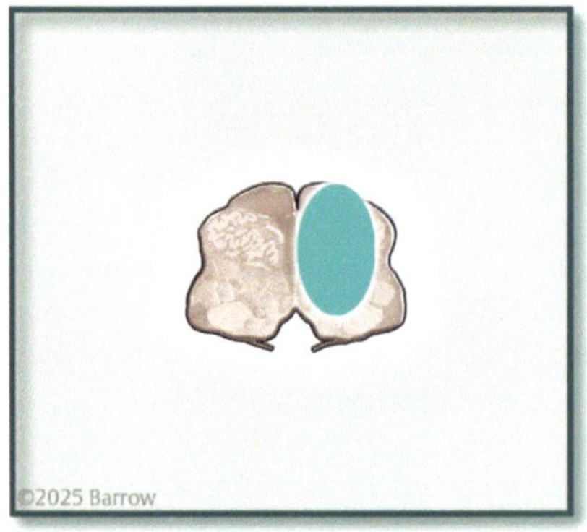

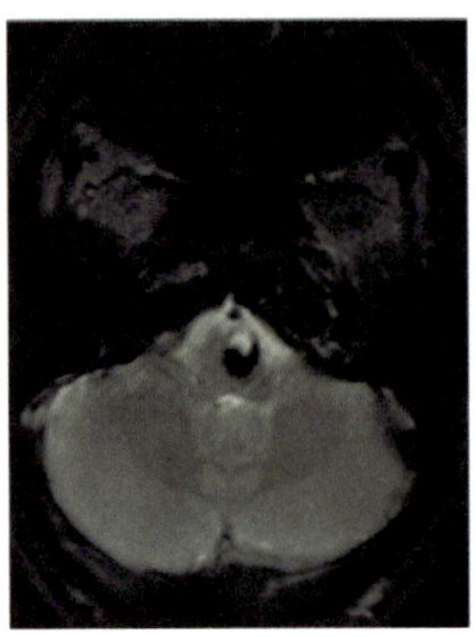

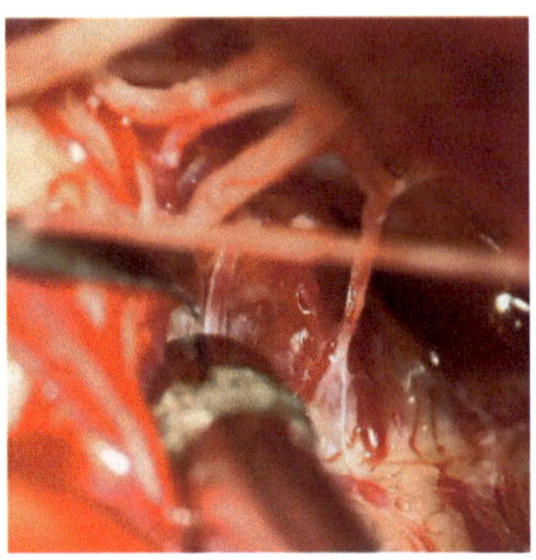

Video 16.1
Far Lateral Craniotomy with Transpremedullary Approach for Pyramidal Medullary Cavernous Malformation Resection (Reproduced with permission from Barrow Neurological Institute, Phoenix, AZ.)

visualization and refinements in instrumentation. Although transclival approaches to this CM subtype were not performed in our patient series, this lesion may be amenable to an endoscopic endonasal approach, and taxonomic subtyping would guide the selection of this approach.

16.4.2 Olivary Subtype

The olivary body is a prominent oval structure on the lateral medulla that measures approximately 1.25 cm in length and contains the superior and inferior olivary nuclei. The superior olivary nucleus resides in the pons and is associated with the auditory system. In contrast, the inferior olivary complex resides in the medulla and contains the primary olivary nucleus, medial accessory olivary nucleus, and dorsal accessory olivary nucleus. The inferior olive sends climbing fibers to Purkinje's cells in the cerebellar cortex and is involved in motor coordination, timing, and learning. Patients with olivary CMs present with ataxia due to inferior olive and anterior spinocerebellar tract involvement, contralateral hemisensory pain and temperature loss due to spinothalamic tract involvement, and ipsilateral hemisensory loss due to involvement of the internal arcuate fibers to the medial lemniscus. To a lesser degree, patients present with contralateral hemiparesis due to pyramid or decussation involvement and dysphagia and dysphonia due to nucleus ambiguus, CN IX, and CN X involvement (▶ Fig. 16.5a). In the classic Wallenberg syndromes or lateral medullary syndromes, PICA infarctions involve the entire lateral medulla, including the inferior cerebellar peduncle (ICP), spinal trigeminal nucleus and tract, vestibular nuclei, dorsal motor nucleus of CN X, solitary nucleus, and nucleus ambiguus, which are all located more posteriorly in the distal PICA territory. Because olivary CMs occur in the anterior portion of the lateral medulla, their constellation of signs and symptoms includes only some of the symptoms of Wallenberg's syndrome. Together, olivary and cuneate CMs produce the classic Wallenberg syndrome; however, individually, each produces either the anterior or posterior signs and symptoms of Wallenberg's syndrome, respectively.

Like pyramidal CMs, olivary lesions were reached microsurgically through a far lateral craniotomy with an aggressive condylectomy, and the olive was visualized through the vagoaccessory triangle (▶ Fig. 16.5b; ▶ Video 16.2, ▶ Video 16.3, ▶ Video 16.4, ▶ Video 16.5). Dissection in the cerebellomedullary fissure liberated the tonsil for upward retraction and a clear view into the suprahypoglossal triangle in the upper half of the vagoaccessory triangle. The V4 and the p1 (anterior medullary) segment of the PICA are found anterior and deep to the olive. However, the p2 segment coursed over the olive and often needed to be mobilized. These CMs typically accentuate the olive's prominence and discolor it yellow (hemosiderin staining), and entry is typically at this surface. Deeper lesions without superficial presentation are accessed through the posterolateral (retro-olivary) sulcus SEZ, identified by the exiting rootlets of CNs X and XI.

16.4.3 Cuneate Subtype

The cuneate nucleus and gracile nucleus form the paired dorsal column nuclei. The cuneate nucleus receives ipsilateral touch and proprioceptive information from the upper body (above T6, except for the face). Consequently, patients with cuneate CMs present with ipsilateral sensory loss in the arm. However, the cuneate nucleus occupies only half of this posterolateral medullary surface, and cuneate lesions may involve more than this cuneate tubercle. Cuneate CMs can extend medially to the posterior intermediate sulcus and gracile tubercle; laterally to the posterolateral sulcus and rootlets of CNs IX, X, and XI; and superiorly to the lateral recess and tenia choroidea of the fourth ventricle. CMs in this territory affect the spinal trigeminal nucleus and tract to cause ipsilateral facial numbness. Hemorrhage here can also cause diplopia (CN VI nucleus involvement); nausea, vertigo, or dizziness (inferior vestibular nuclei involvement); and dysphagia or dysphonia (nucleus ambiguus and CN IX and X involvement), as well as cerebellar ataxia (ICP involvement) and Horner's syndrome (sympathetic tract involvement) (▶ Fig. 16.6a). These findings are also associated with Wallenberg's syndrome when paired with olivary CMs. Cuneate lesions are responsible for a posterior Wallenberg syndrome (the classic Wallenberg syndrome minus the ataxia and contralateral hemisensory pain and temperature loss associated with more anteriorly located olivary CMs).

The surgical exposure of cuneate CMs is through a midline suboccipital craniotomy with C1 laminectomy and telovelar approach (▶ Fig. 16.6b; ▶ Video 16.6, ▶ Video 16.7, ▶ Video 16.8). Although this approach is usually used to access ventricular lesions in the lateral recess and inferior peduncular CMs in the pons, it is also suited to cuneate CMs located inferiorly outside the ventricle. These lesions are found in the cerebellomedullary cistern anterior to the tonsil, and thorough dissection of the p3 segment brings them into full view. The inferior medullary velum was incised superolaterally to enter the lateral recess, as with most telovelar approaches, and liberate the tonsil and visualize the cuneate nucleus. Dissection of the velum and retraction of the tonsil open the subtonsillar triangle, an anatomical triangle formed by the insertion of the tela choroidea of the fourth ventricle inferolaterally, the medial border of the tonsil superolaterally, and the medullary midline. Cuneate lesions reside lateral to the subtonsillar triangle and cannot be accessed without thoroughly opening this triangle. Although cuneate lesions are extraventricular, the choroid plexus protruding through the foramen of Luschka on top of CN IX is a landmark for the superolateral extent of this region. The CN XI rootlets mark the inferolateral border. This subtonsillar space lies posterior to the vagoaccessory triangle. Exophytic and superficial cuneate CMs enlarge the posterolateral medulla. They are accessed through the lateral medullary SEZ. The posterior intermediate sulcus SEZ is entered between the gracile and cuneate nuclei to access deeper lesions. The posterolateral sulcus SEZ was not used in treating our patients with cuneate lesions because entry from the telovelar trajectory would take the dissection into the olivary region.

16.4.4 Gracile Subtype

The gracile nucleus is the other of the paired dorsal column nuclei at the junction between the medulla and the spinal cord, with the two gracile nuclei forming twin tubercles on either side of the midline at the foramen of Magendie. These nuclei receive input from dorsal root ganglia sensory neurons subserving the legs and lower trunk (below T6). Patients with gracile

Olivary Medullary Cavernoma

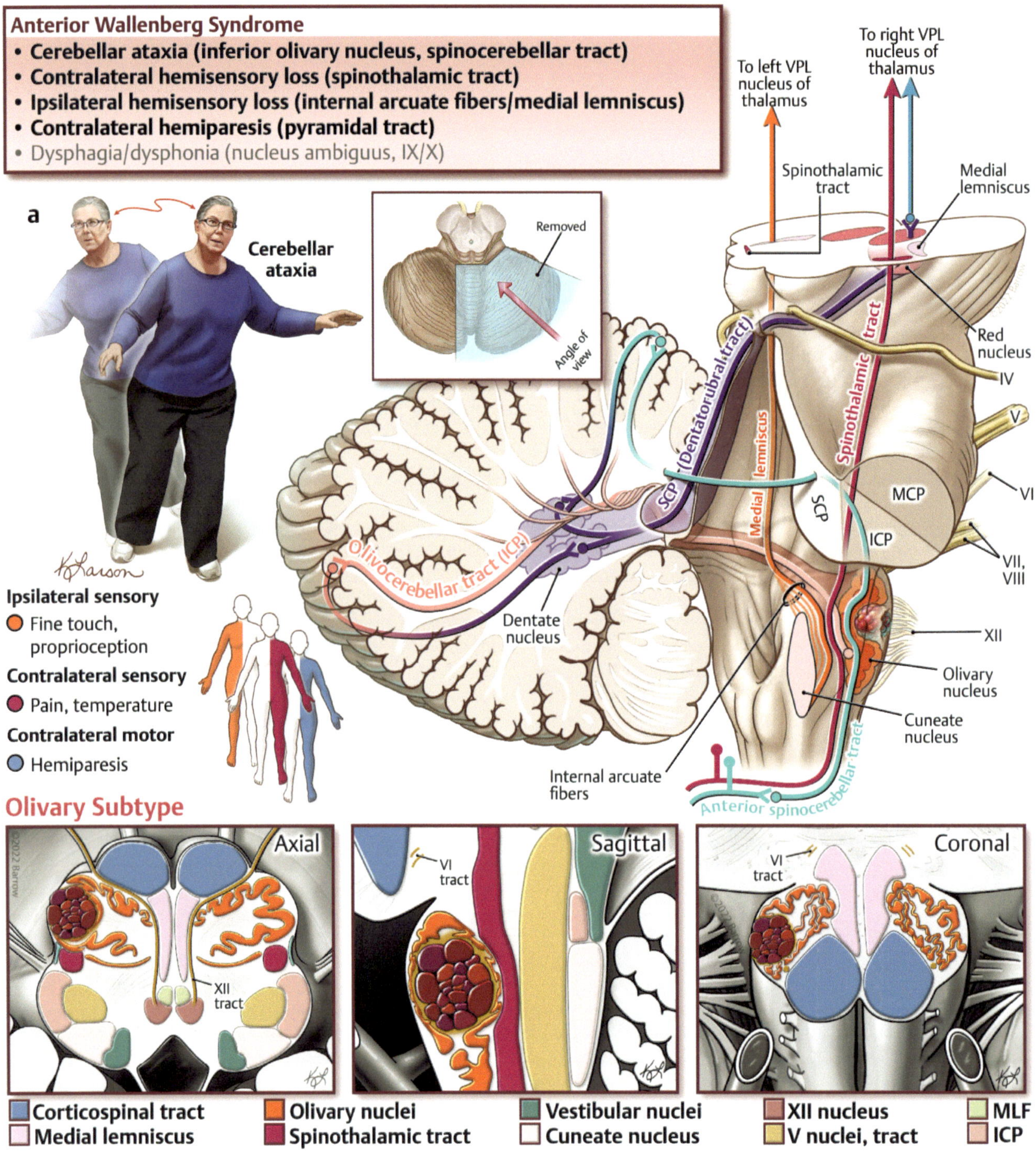

Fig. 16.5 Olivary medullary clinical syndromes and surgical approaches. **(a)** Patients with olivary CMs present with an anterior Wallenberg syndrome (contralateral cerebellar ataxia, contralateral loss of pain and temperature sensation, ipsilateral loss of fine touch and proprioception, contralateral hemiparesis, dysphagia, and dysphonia). The relationships between this right-sided medullary CM and the inferior olivary nucleus, spinocerebellar tract, spinothalamic tract, internal arcuate fibers, medial lemniscus, corticospinal tract, nucleus ambiguus, and the intramedullary tracts of the vagus and accessory nerves are shown in axial, sagittal, and coronal views (*lower insets*).

(Continued)

Surgical Approach

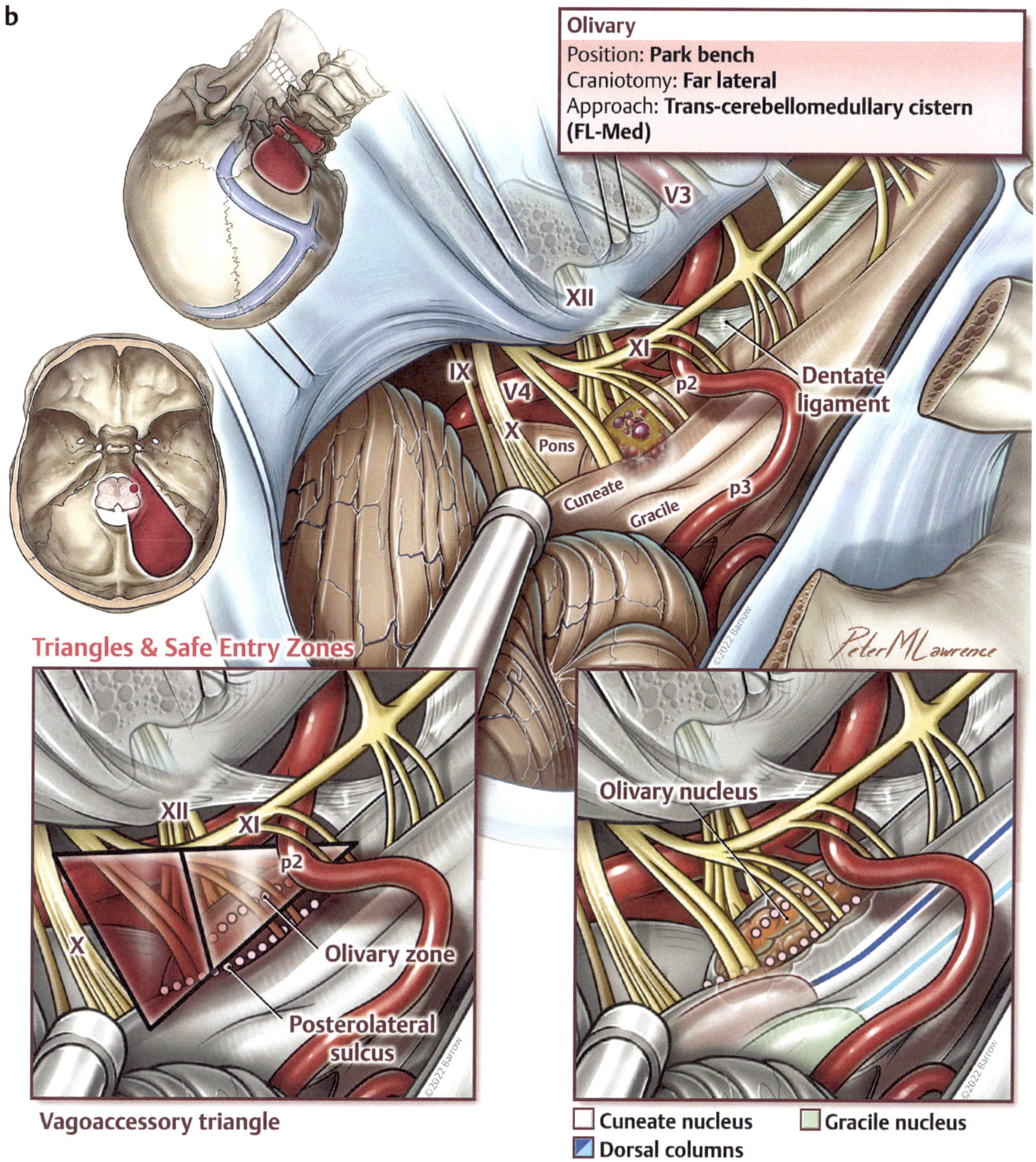

Fig. 16.5 *(Continued)* **(b)** Olivary medullary CMs are exposed through a far lateral craniotomy (*upper left inset*) and trans-cerebellomedullary cistern approach (*middle left inset*; *red circle*). The patient is placed in the park bench or three-quarter prone position. Dissection in the cerebellomedullary fissure liberates the tonsil for upward retraction, and the olive is visualized through the vagoaccessory triangle (*lower left inset*). The V4 segment of the vertebral artery and the p1 segment of the posterior inferior cerebellar artery are anterior and deep to the olive and CN XII rootlets, but the p2 segment courses over the olive. The olive can be entered safely through its discolored prominence between the anterolateral and posterolateral sulci (*lower left and right insets*; *olivary SEZ*; *pink dotted line*) or accessed more deeply through the posterolateral sulcus SEZ (*lower left and right insets*; *pink dotted line*), which is identified by the exiting rootlets of the vagus and accessory nerves. The olivary SEZ transgresses the inferior olivary nucleus, and the posterolateral SEZ courses lateral to the cuneate nucleus and dorsal columns (*lower right inset*; *ghosted structures*) (surgical cases; ▶ Video 16.2, ▶ Video 16.3, ▶ Video 16.4, ▶ Video 16.5; QR codes). Roman numerals denote CNs. (Reproduced with permission from Barrow Neurological Institute, Phoenix, AZ.)

Surgical Case 16.2

MEDULLARY

Cavernoma Subtype: Olivary

Position: Park bench (3/4 prone)
Craniotomy: Far lateral
Approach: Trans-cerebellomedullary cistern (FL-Med)
Triangle: Vagoaccessory (infrahypoglossal)
SEZ: Olivary zone
Artery: p2 PICA

Video: Resection of a right olivary medullary cavernoma

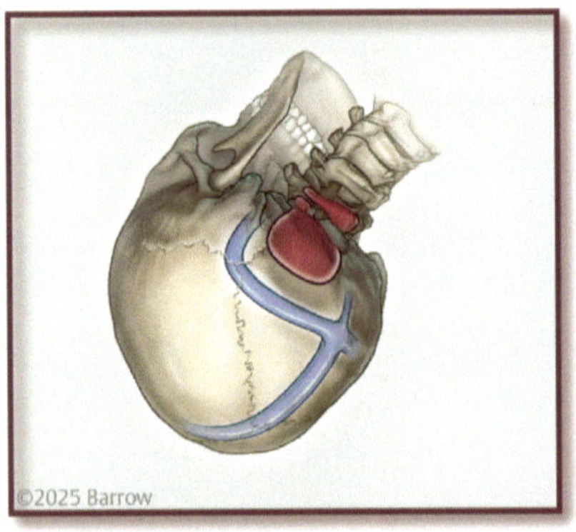

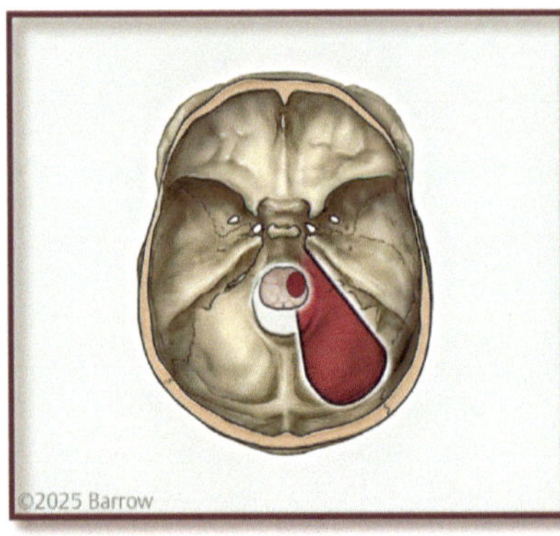

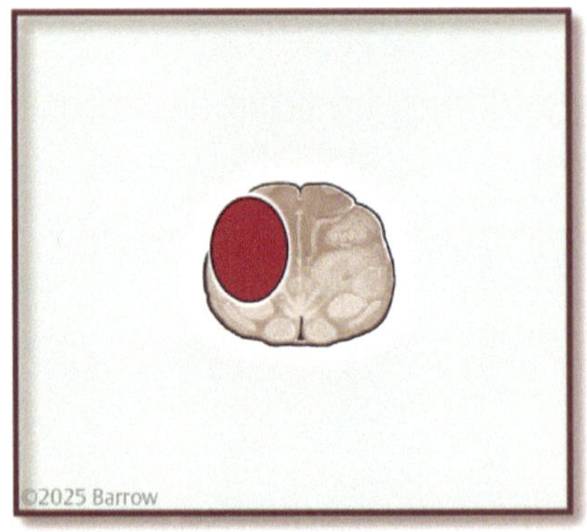

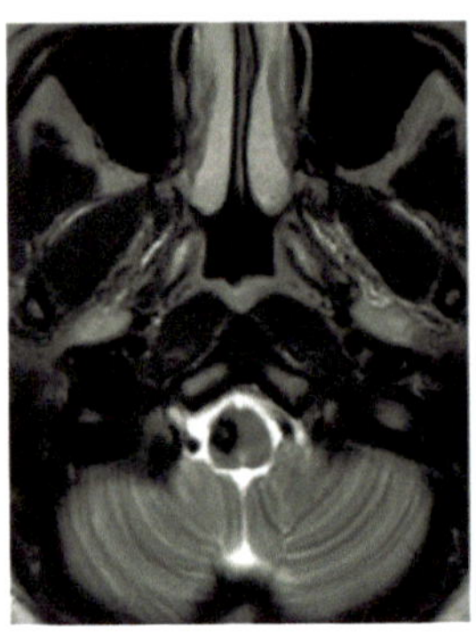
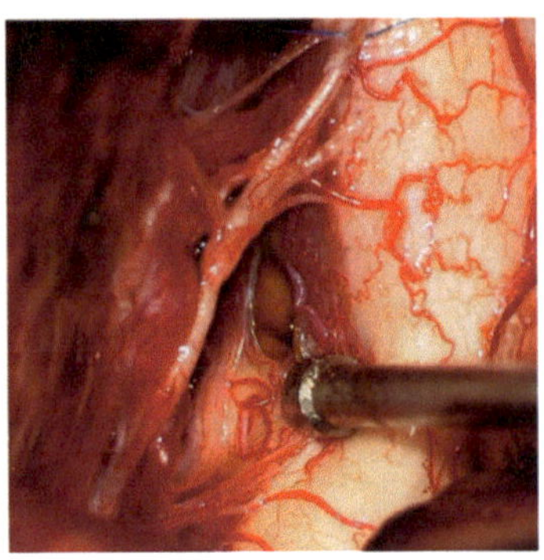

Video 16.2
Far Lateral Craniotomy with Transcerebellomedullary Approach for Olivary Medullary Cavernous Malformation Resection (Reproduced with permission from Barrow Neurological Institute, Phoenix, AZ.)

16

Surgical Case 16.3

MEDULLARY

Cavernoma Subtype: Olivary

Position: Park bench (3/4 prone)
Craniotomy: Far lateral
Approach: Trans-cerebellomedullary cistern (FL-Med)
Triangle: Vagoaccessory (suprahypoglossal)
SEZ: Olivary zone
Artery: p2 PICA

Video: Resection of a left olivary medullary cavernoma

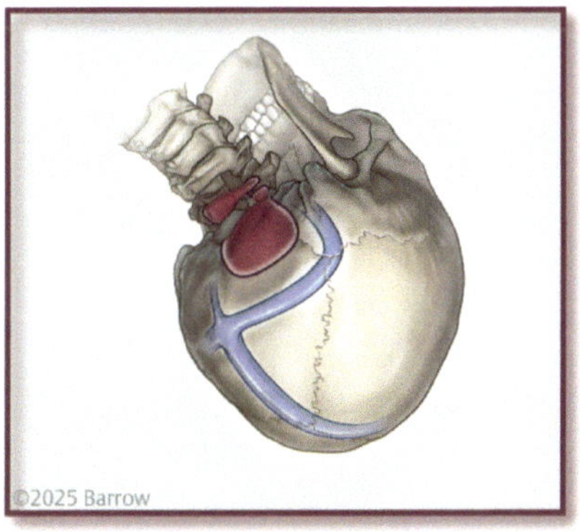

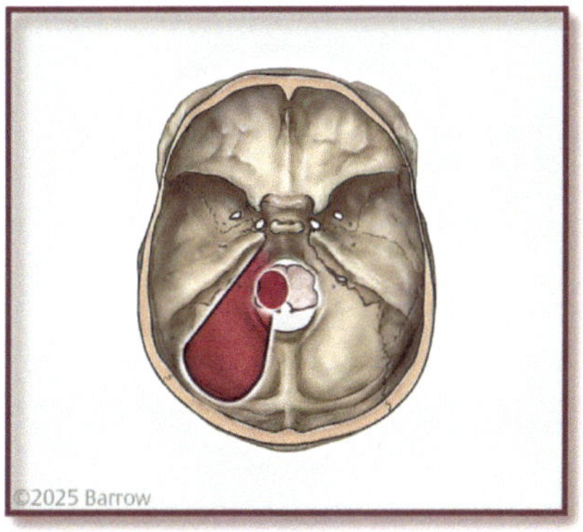

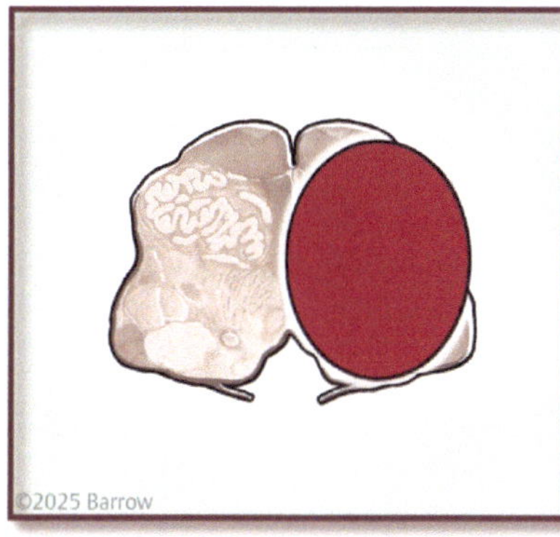

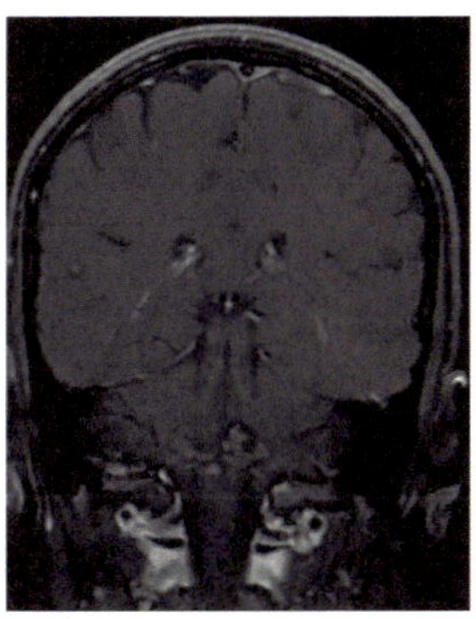

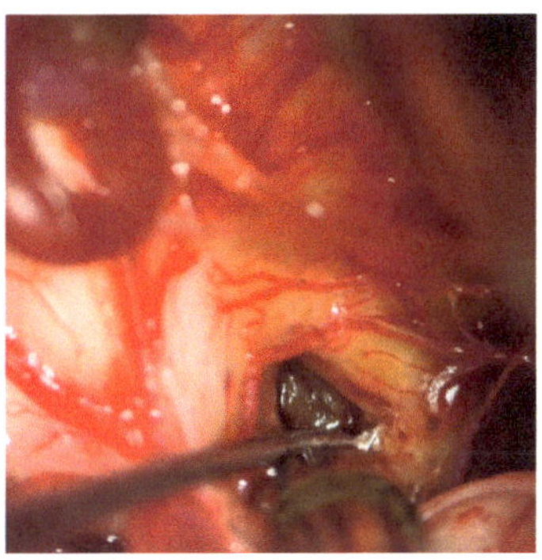

Video 16.3
Far Lateral Craniotomy with Transcerebellomedullary Approach for Olivary Medullary Cavernous Malformation Resection (Reproduced with permission from Barrow Neurological Institute, Phoenix, AZ.)

Surgical Case 16.4

MEDULLARY

Cavernoma Subtype: Olivary

Position: Park bench (3/4 prone)
Craniotomy: Far lateral
Approach: Trans-cerebellomedullary cistern (FL-Med)
Triangle: Vagoaccessory (infrahypoglossal)
SEZ: Olivary zone
Artery: p2 PICA

Video: Resection of a left olivary medullary cavernoma

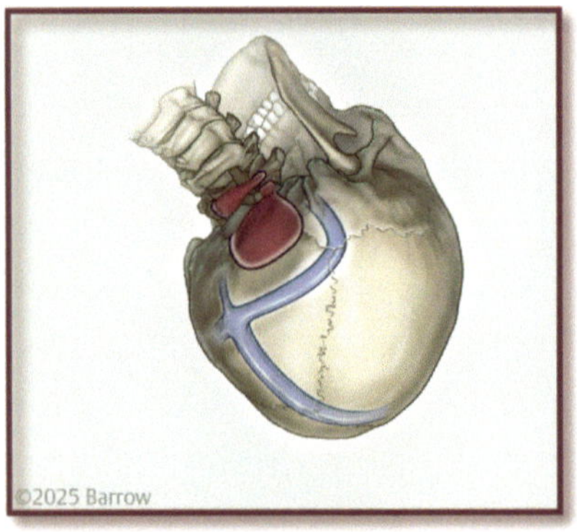

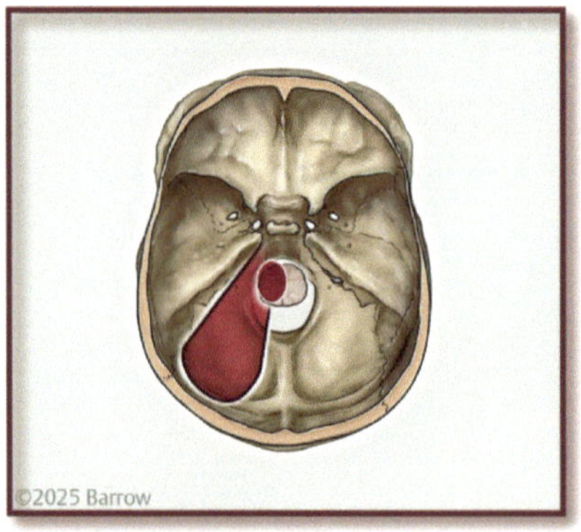

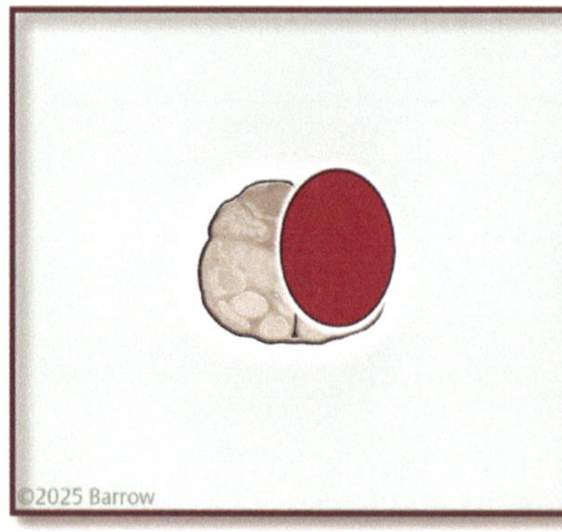

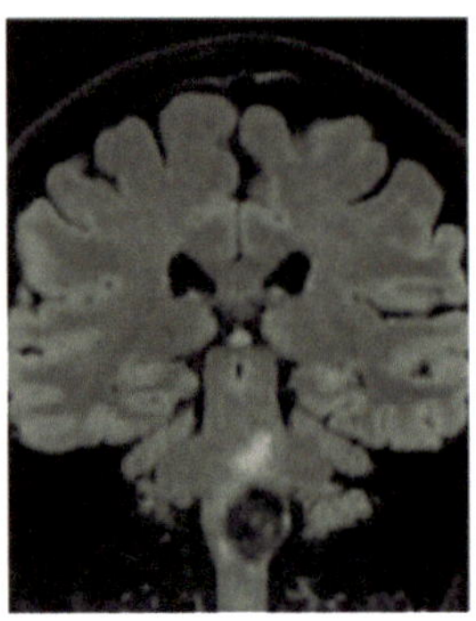

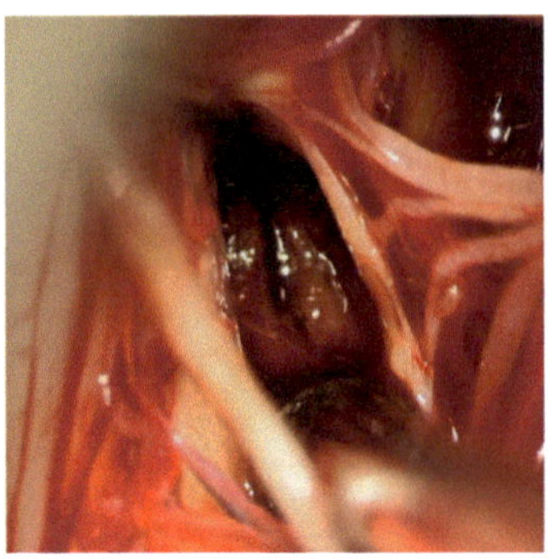

Video 16.4
Far Lateral Craniotomy with Transcerebellomedullary Approach for Olivary Medullary Cavernous Malformation Resection (Reproduced with permission from Barrow Neurological Institute, Phoenix, AZ.)

Surgical Case 16.5

MEDULLARY

Cavernoma Subtype: Olivary

Position: Park bench (3/4 prone)
Craniotomy: Far lateral
Approach: Trans-cerebellomedullary cistern (FL-Med)
Triangle: Vagoaccessory (hypoglossal-hypoglossal)
SEZ: Olivary zone
Artery: p2 PICA

Video: Resection of a left olivary medullary cavernoma

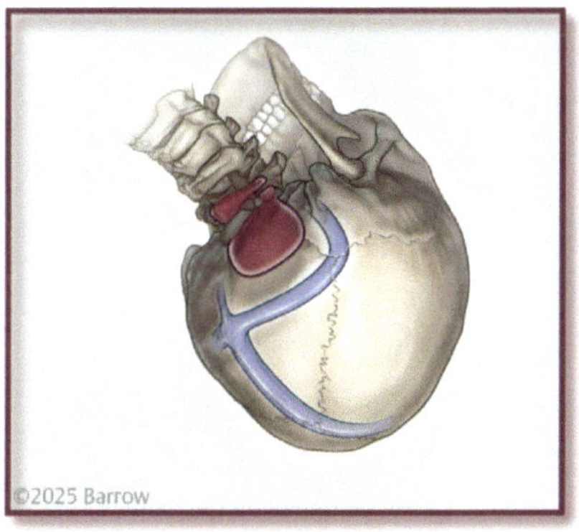

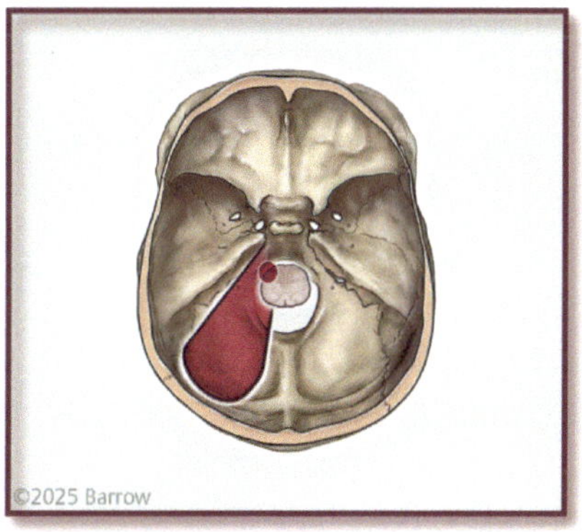

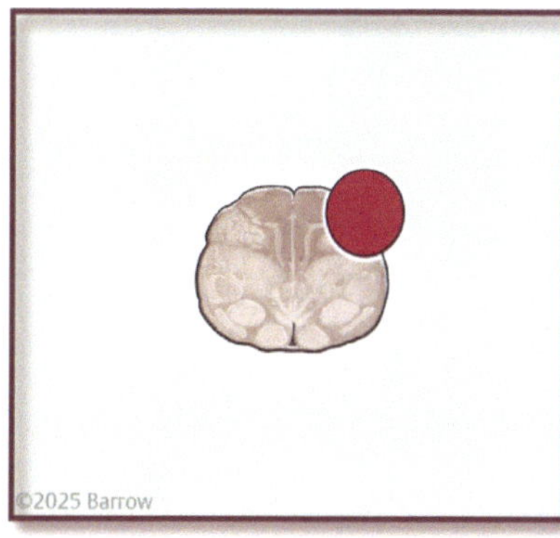

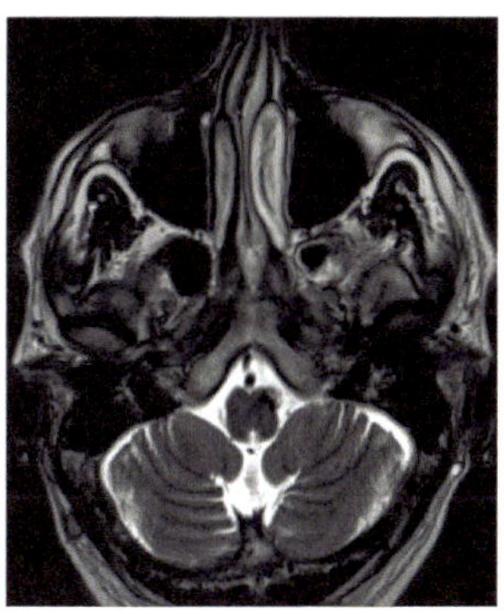

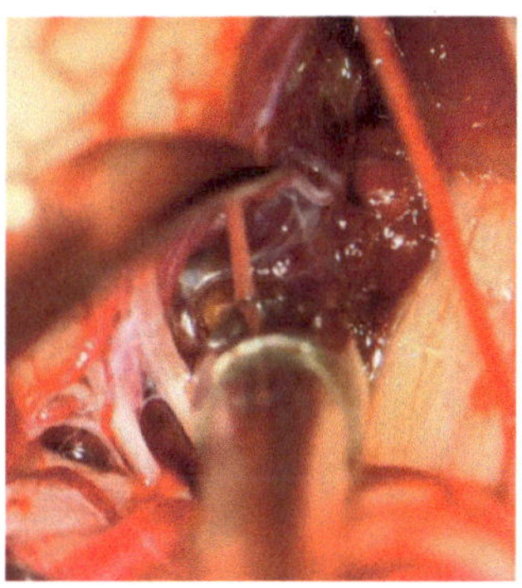

Video 16.5
Far Lateral Craniotomy with Transcerebellomedullary Approach for Olivary Medullary Cavernous Malformation Resection (Reproduced with permission from Barrow Neurological Institute, Phoenix, AZ.)

16

Cuneate Medullary Cavernoma

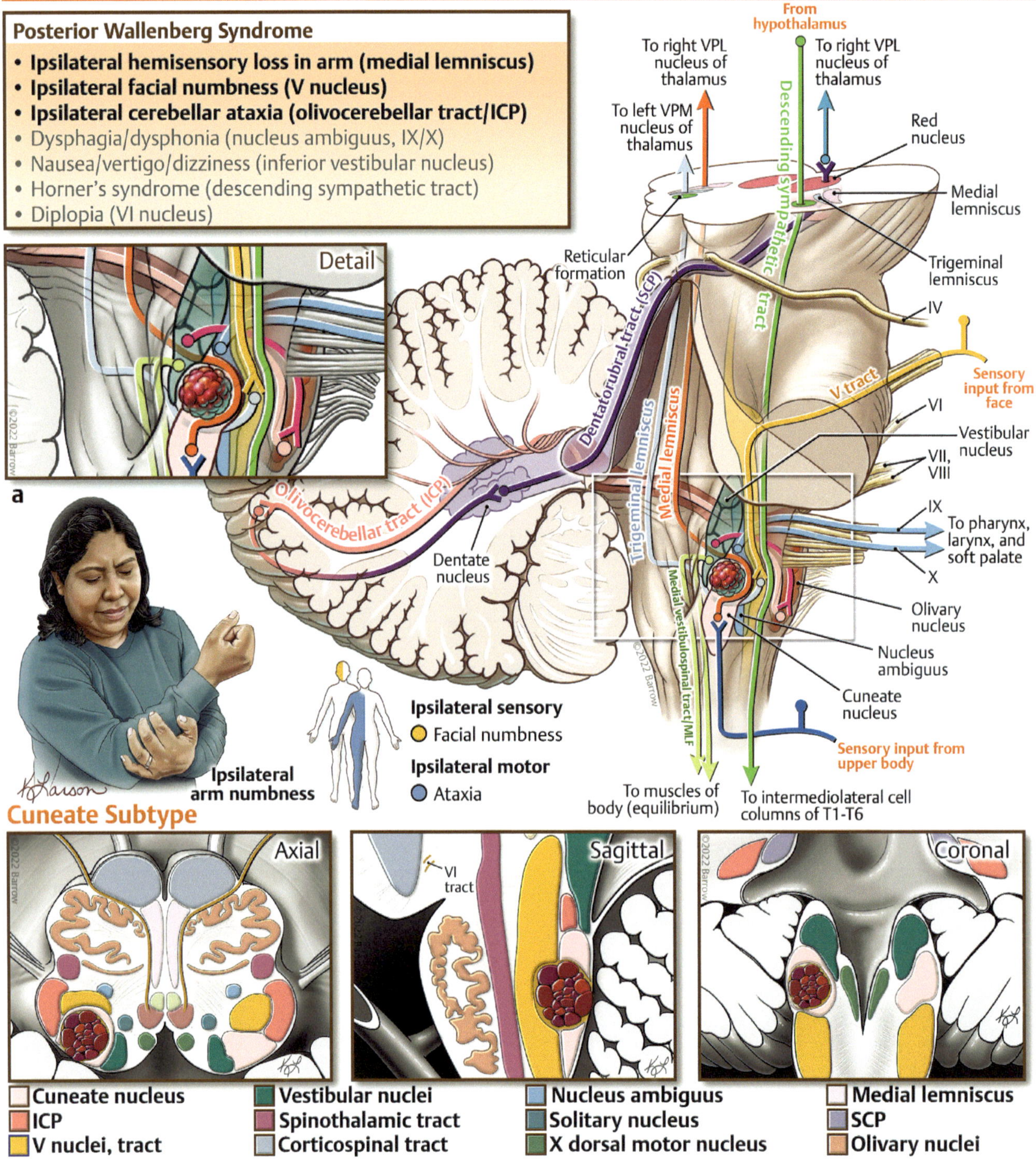

Fig. 16.6 Cuneate medullary clinical syndromes and surgical approaches. **(a)** Patients with cuneate CMs present with a posterior Wallenberg syndrome (ipsilateral loss of fine touch and proprioception in the arm, ipsilateral facial numbness, ipsilateral ataxia, dysphagia, dysphonia, nausea, vertigo, Horner's syndrome, and diplopia). The relationships between this right-sided medullary brainstem CM and the cuneate nucleus, medial lemniscus, trigeminal nuclei, olivocerebellar tract, ICP, nucleus ambiguus, inferior vestibular nucleus, descending sympathetic tract, and abducens nucleus are shown in axial, sagittal, and coronal views (*lower insets*).

(Continued)

Surgical Approach

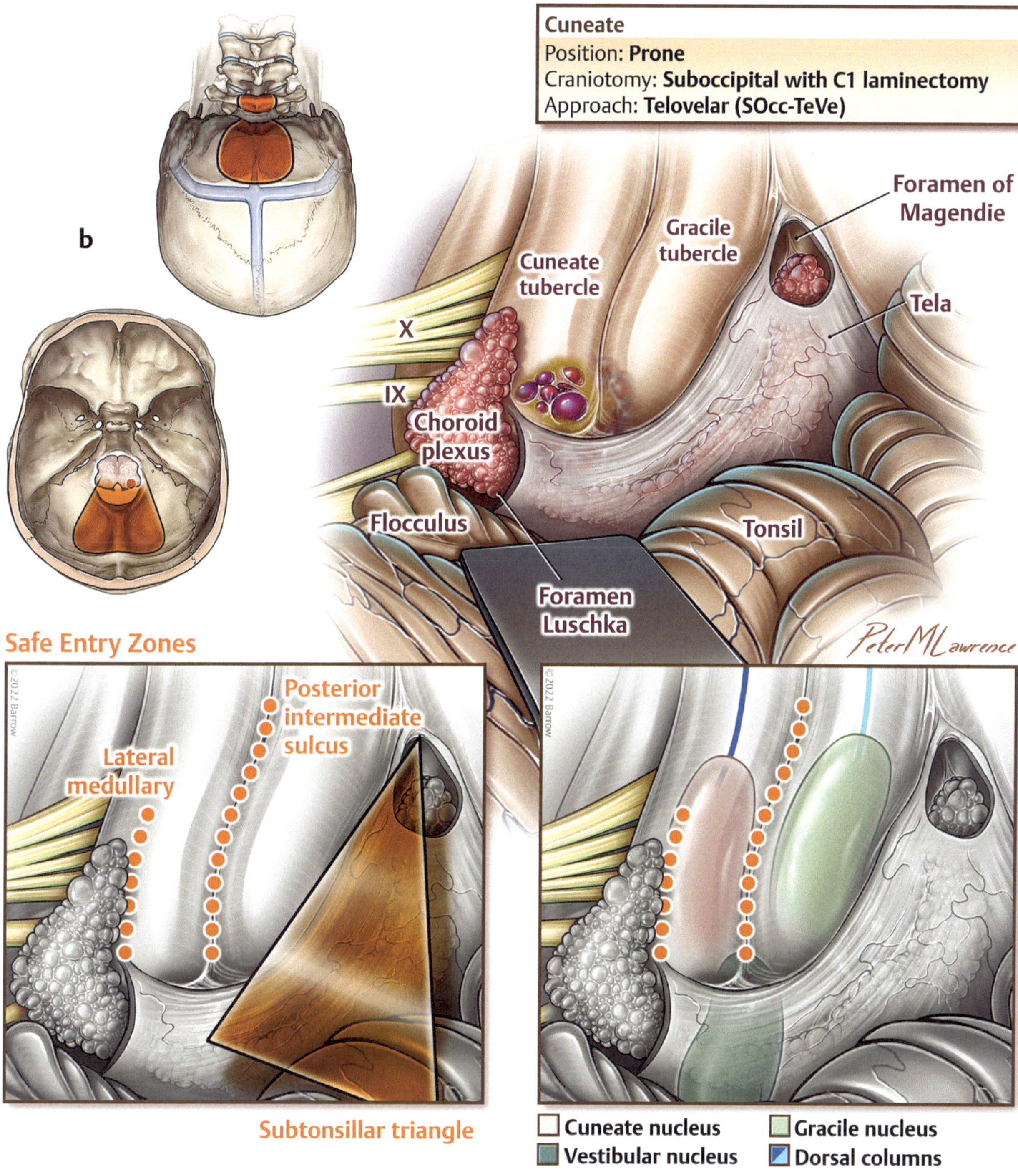

Fig. 16.6 *(Continued)* **(b)** Cuneate medullary CMs are exposed through a suboccipital craniotomy with C1 laminectomy (*upper left inset*) and telovelar approach (*middle left inset*; *orange circle*). The patient is placed in the prone position. Dissection of the PICA p3 (tonsillomedullary) segment in the cerebellomedullary cistern anterior to the tonsil and retraction of the tonsil opens the subtonsillar triangle formed by the midline, the medial border of the tonsil superolaterally, and insertion of the tela choroidea of the fourth ventricle inferolaterally (*lower left inset*). Incision of the inferior medullary velum visualizes the superomedial extent of the cuneate nucleus, and the rootlets of the vagus and accessory nerve mark the lateral extent. Superficial cuneate CMs are accessed through the lateral medullary SEZ (*lower left and right insets*; *orange dotted line*), and deep cuneate CMs are accessed through the posterior intermediate sulcus between the gracile and cuneate nuclei (*lower left and right insets*; *orange dotted line*). Entry through the posterior intermediate SEZ avoids the gracile and cuneate nuclei and dorsal columns. In contrast, the lateral medullary SEZ transgresses cuneate tissue (*lower right inset*; *ghosted structures*) (surgical cases; ▶ Video 16.6, ▶ Video 16.7, ▶ Video 16.8; QR codes). Roman numerals denote CNs. (Reproduced with permission from Barrow Neurological Institute, Phoenix, AZ.)

16

Surgical Case 16.6

MEDULLARY

Cavernoma Subtype: Cuneate

Position: Prone
Craniotomy: Suboccipital with C1 laminectomy
Approach: Telovelar (SOcc-TeVe)
Triangle: Subtonsillar
SEZ: None (exophytic)
Artery: Posterior spinal artery

Video: Resection of a right cuneate medullary cavernoma

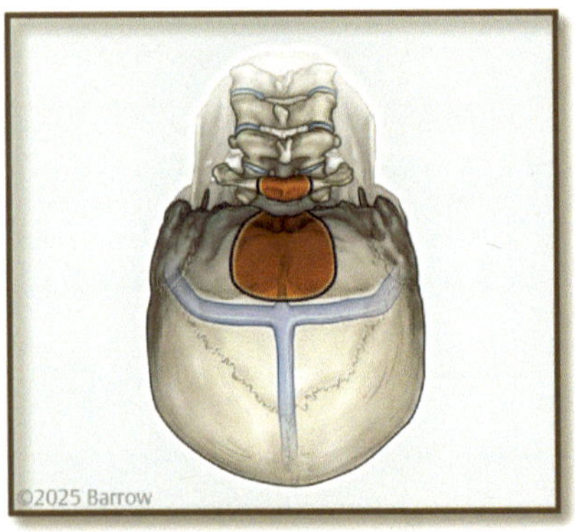

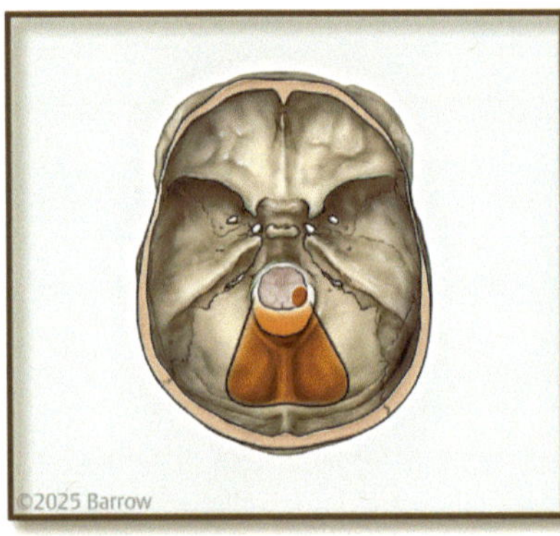

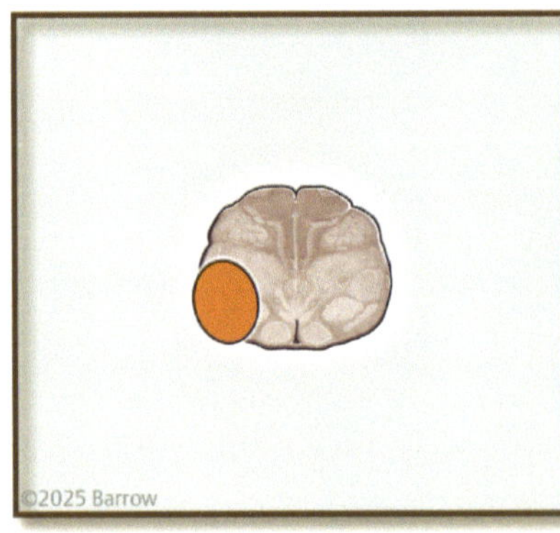

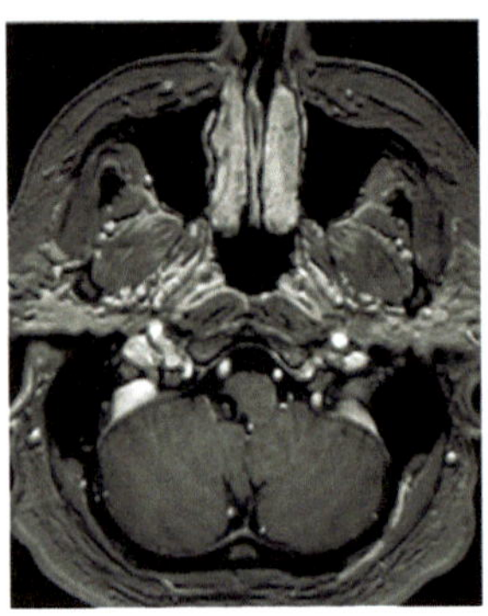

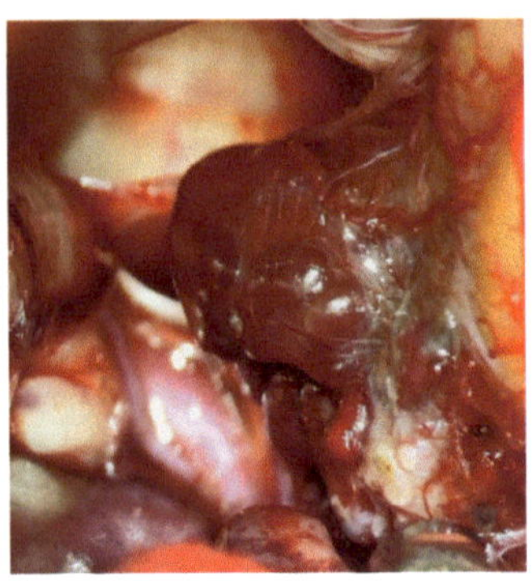

Video 16.6
Suboccipital Craniotomy with Telovelar Approach for Cuneate Medullary Cavernous Malformation Resection (Reproduced with permission from Barrow Neurological Institute, Phoenix, AZ.)

16

Surgical Case 16.7

MEDULLARY

Cavernoma Subtype: Cuneate

Position: Prone
Craniotomy: Suboccipital with C1 laminectomy
Approach: Telovelar (SOcc-TeVe)
Triangle: Subtonsillar
SEZ: None (exophytic)
Artery: Posterior spinal artery

Video: Resection of a right cuneate medullary cavernoma

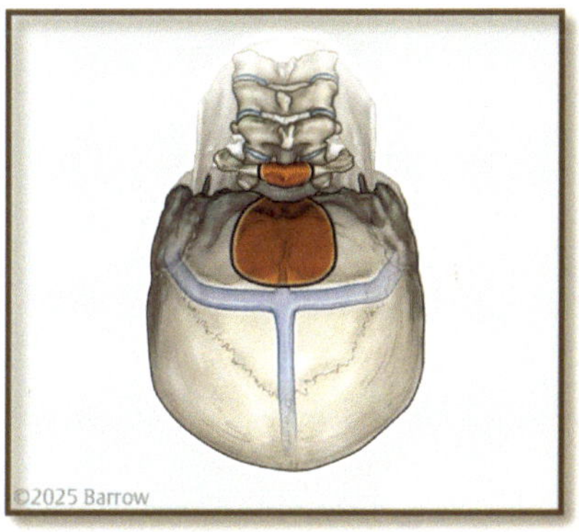

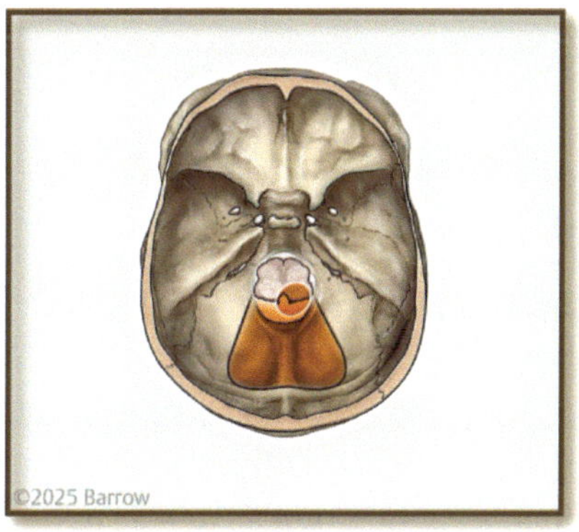

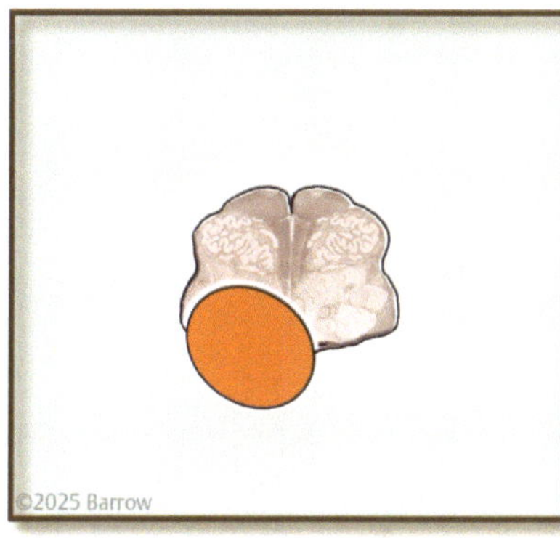

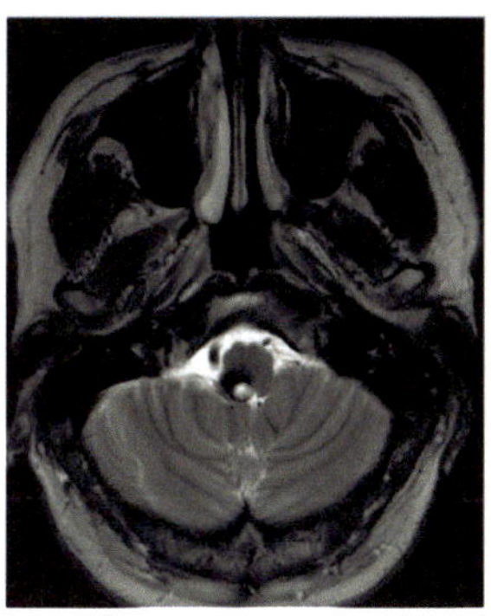

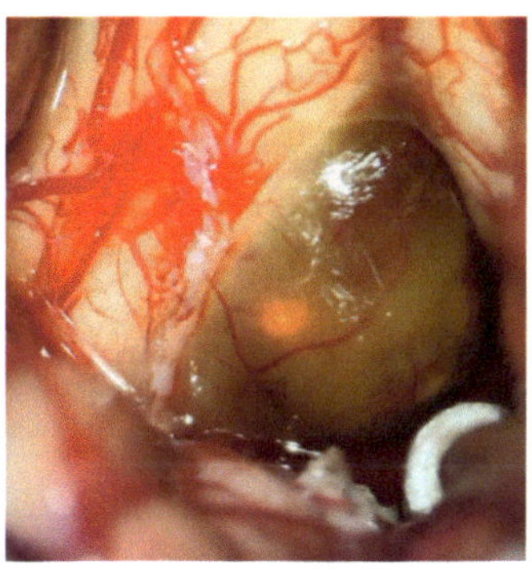

Video 16.7
Suboccipital Craniotomy with Telovelar Approach for Cuneate Medullary Cavernous Malformation Resection (Reproduced with permission from Barrow Neurological Institute, Phoenix, AZ.)

16

Surgical Case 16.8

MEDULLARY

Cavernoma Subtype: Cuneate

Position: Park bench (3/4 prone)
Craniotomy: Far lateral
Approach: Telovelar (FL-TeVe)
Triangle: Subtonsillar
SEZ: Posterior intermediate sulcus
Artery: Posterior spinal artery

Video: Resection of a left cuneate medullary cavernoma

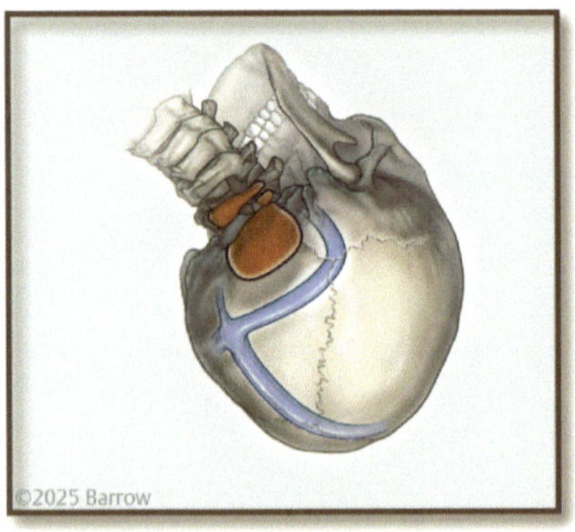

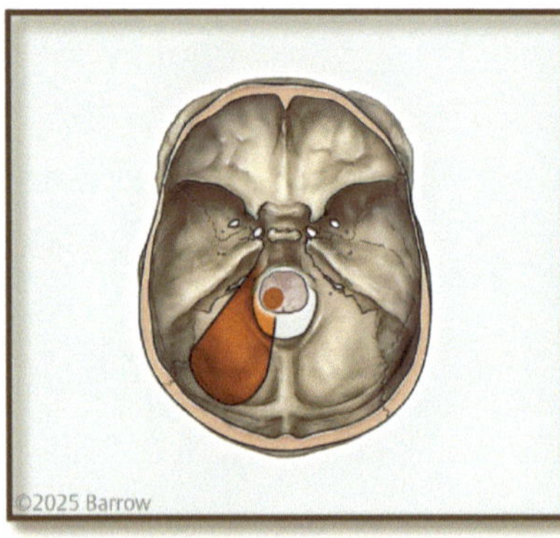

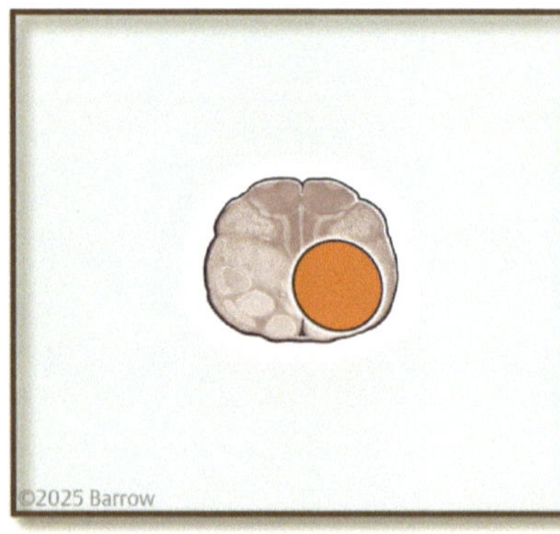

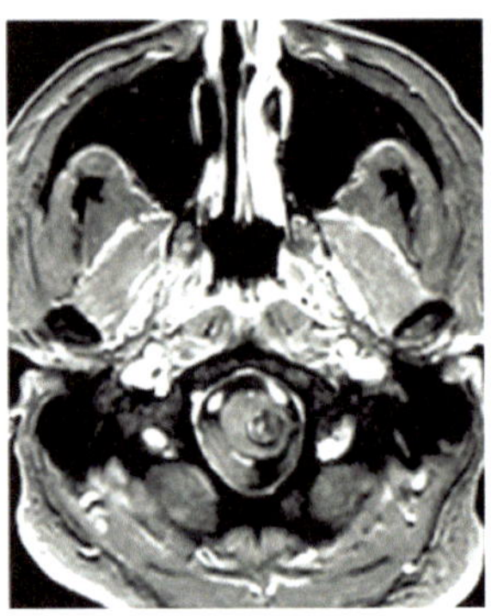

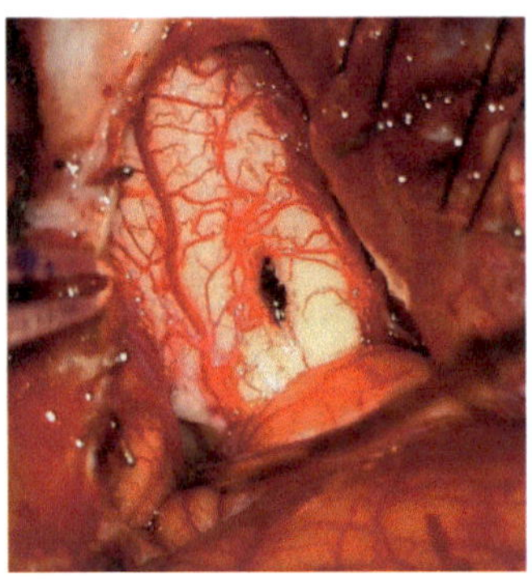

Video 16.8
Far Lateral Craniotomy with Telovelar Approach for Cuneate Medullary Cavernous Malformation Resection (Reproduced with permission from Barrow Neurological Institute, Phoenix, AZ.)

16

CMs present with hemisensory loss involving the ipsilateral leg (▶ Fig. 16.7a). They do not present with CN deficits because these lesions are outside the ventricle, below the level of CN nuclei. Bilateral lesions are associated with bilateral leg numbness.

The surgical approach to gracile CMs is a suboccipital craniotomy with C1 laminectomy for more inferior exposure of the lesion (▶ Fig. 16.7b; ▶ Video 16.9, ▶ Video 16.10). More inferiorly placed lesions require a linear dural incision rather than the standard Y-shaped incision. The gracile nuclei are located at or below the tonsils, which require mobilization or retraction. The caudal loop of the PICA often covered the lesion. These malformations were accessed directly or through the posterior median sulcus between the gracile nuclei. The posterior median sulcus may be opened 2 to 3 mm deep before transgressing tissue. This SEZ can be deepened to the level of the central canal and extended from the obex superiorly to the spinal cord inferiorly. The median posterior medullary vein overlies this sulcus and can be mobilized to one side. Separation and gentle displacement of the gracile nuclei and tracts provide access to these CMs without harming sensory function. The posterior intermediate sulcus SEZ is adjacent to this gracile nucleus, but entry from this midline suboccipital trajectory takes the dissection into the cuneate fasciculus.

16.4.5 Trigonal Subtype

The floor of the fourth ventricle forms the posterosuperior surface of the medulla, extending from the stria medullaris superiorly to the lateral recesses laterally and the obex inferiorly. This smaller, lower triangular part of the rhomboid fossa is defined by the calamus scriptorius and comprises the hypoglossal trigone, vagal trigone, and area postrema. The inferior fovea is a dimple in the sulcus limitans adjacent to the median eminence, just lateral to the hypoglossal trigone. Although the rhomboid fossa is described as the fourth ventricular floor, the rhomboid CM subtype refers only to pontine CMs in the larger, upper triangular part. Trigonal CMs are medullary ventricular lesions distinct from dorsal column CMs (gracile and cuneate), which are outside and below the fourth ventricle. The hypoglossal nucleus controls tongue movement, and the area postrema controls vomiting and autonomic functions. The vagal trigone, which consists of the dorsal motor nucleus of CN X, nucleus ambiguus, and solitary nucleus, collectively subserves visceral efferent motor activity, parasympathetic signals to the heart and lungs, parasympathetic signals to gastrointestinal smooth muscle and glands, chemoreception in numerous organ systems in the body, and sensory functions including taste. Patients with trigonal lesions present with tongue weakness, dysphagia, dysphonia, and severe nausea and vomiting, plus diplopia when lesions extend superiorly (▶ Fig. 16.8a). This constellation of trigonal signs and symptoms does not have an eponymous name.

Trigonal CMs were accessed through a suboccipital craniotomy with C1 laminectomy and the transventricular approach (▶ Fig. 16.8b; ▶ Video 16.11, ▶ Video 16.12). The inferior part of the fourth ventricular floor is easily exposed with tonsillar mobilization and widening of the vallecula. The cerebellar vallecular triangle is the space between the bilateral tonsils and the uvula of the inferior vermis superiorly. Occasionally, telovelar extension with incision of the inferior medullary velum is needed for laterally and superiorly located CMs. Unlike rhomboid CMs with multiple SEZs, trigonal lesions are accessed via the median sulcus SEZ. The medullary portion of the median sulcus lies inferior to the medial longitudinal fasciculi, making entry here less morbid than in its pontine portion. Five CM subtypes occur in or adjacent to the fourth ventricle. They include 2 subtypes in the pons (rhomboid and inferior peduncular), 3 in the medulla (trigonal, gracile, and cuneate), 2 in the fourth ventricle (rhomboid and trigonal), 2 around the lateral recess (inferior peduncular and cuneate), and 3 in or adjacent to the midline (rhomboid, trigonal, and gracile).

16

Gracile Medullary Cavernoma

Gracile Medullary Syndrome

- **Ipsilateral hemisensory loss in leg (gracile nucleus)**

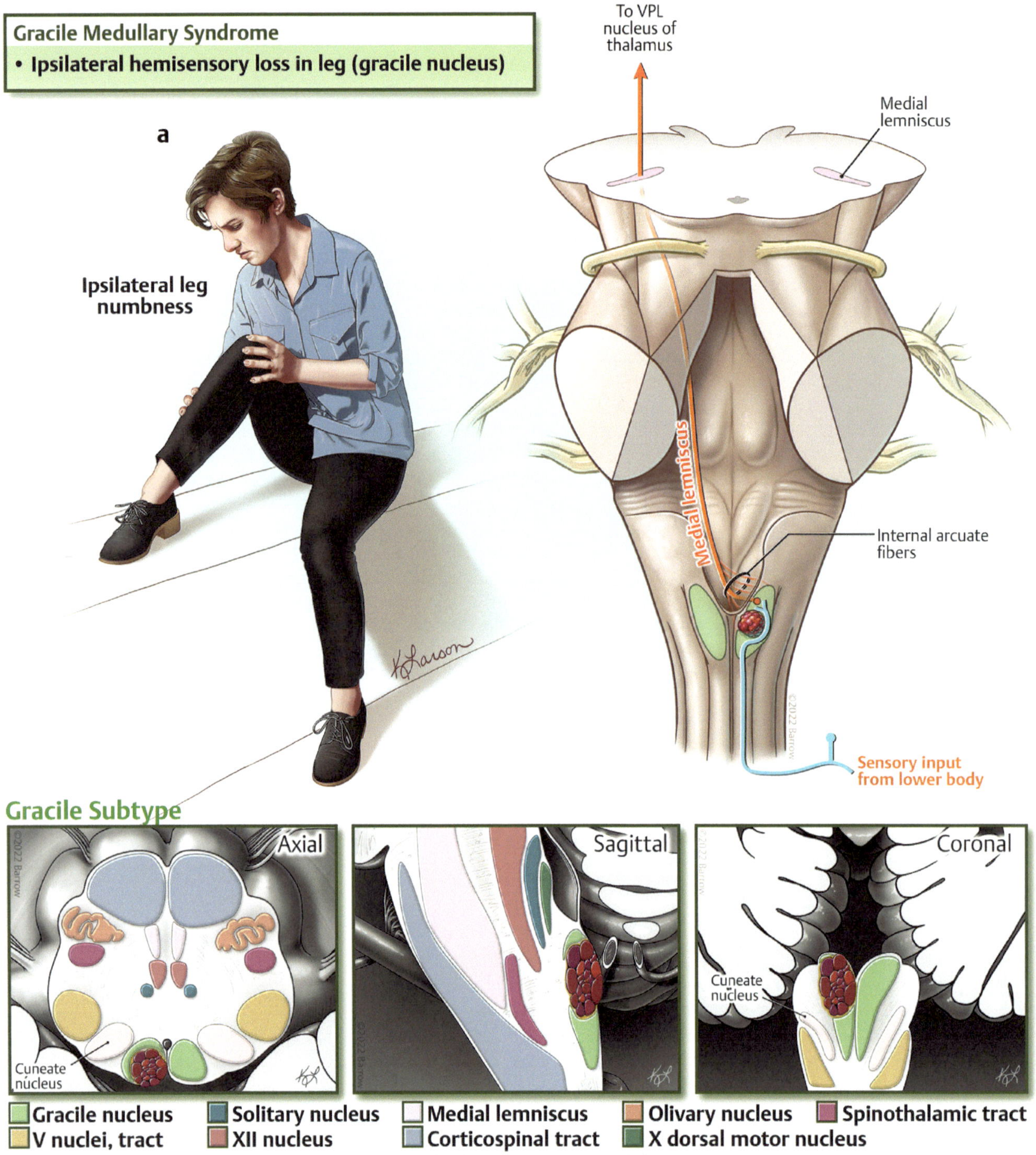

Fig. 16.7 Gracile medullary clinical syndromes and surgical approaches. **(a)** Patients with gracile CMs present with ipsilateral loss of fine touch and proprioception in the leg and bilateral sensory loss in cases with larger midline lesions. The relationships between this right-sided CM and the gracile nucleus, internal arcuate fibers, medial lemniscus, and dorsal columns are shown in axial, sagittal, and coronal views (*lower insets*).

(Continued)

Surgical Approach

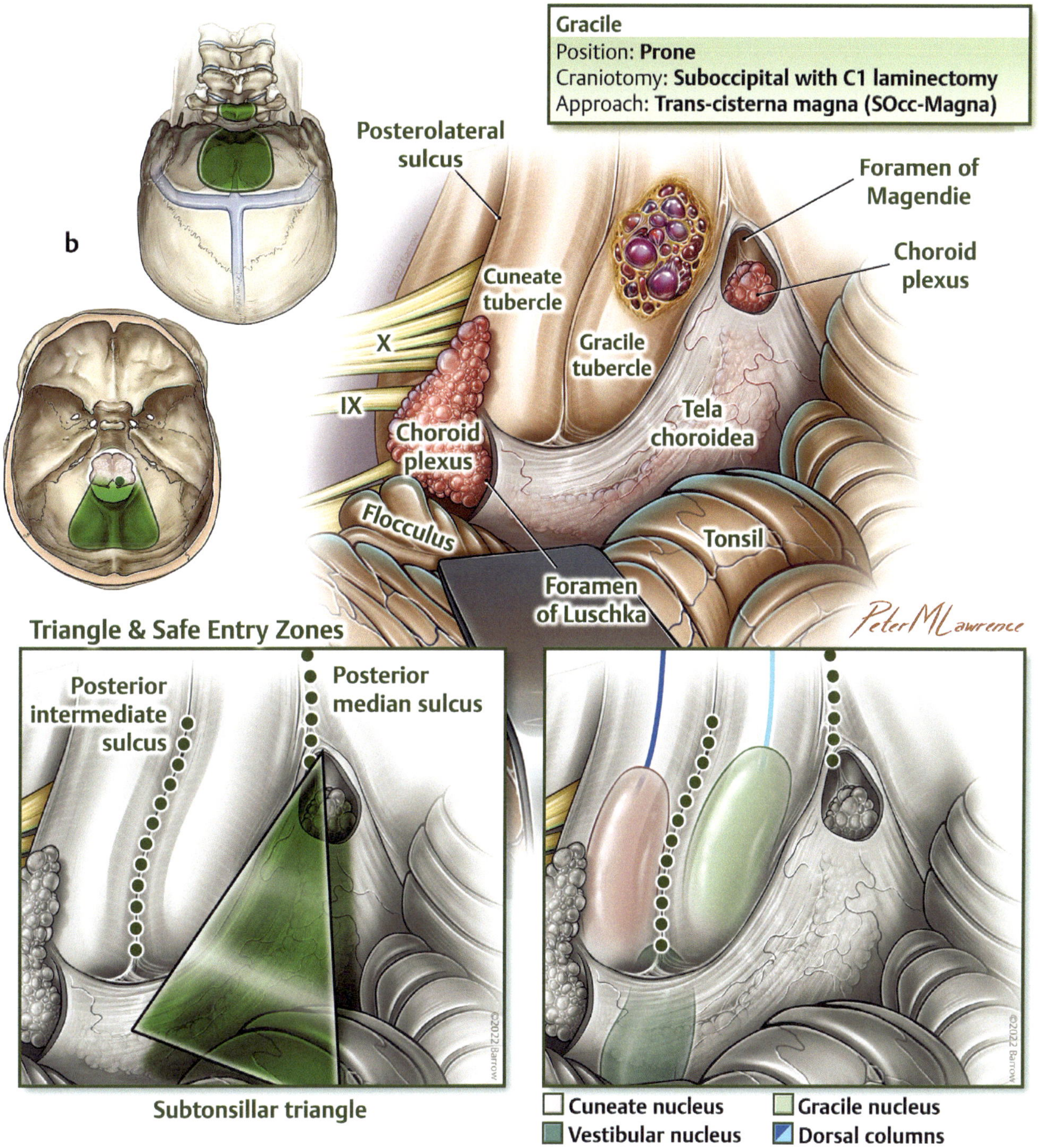

Fig. 16.7 *(Continued)* **(b)** Gracile CMs are exposed through a suboccipital craniotomy with C1 laminectomy (*upper left inset*) and are located within the cisterna magna (*middle left inset*; *green circle*). The patient is placed in the prone position. The gracile nuclei are located at or below the tonsils under the caudal loop (p3) of the PICA. These malformations are inferior to the subtonsillar triangle and accessed directly or through the posterior median sulcus. The posterior intermediate sulcus defines the lateral boundary of this subtype, but dissection through this SEZ leads laterally toward the cuneate CM (*lower left and right insets*; *green dotted line*). The posterior median sulcus SEZ is 2 to 3 mm deep and can be deepened to the level of the central canal, extending from the obex superiorly to the spinal cord inferiorly (*lower left and right insets*; *green dotted line*). Separation and gentle displacement of the gracile nuclei and tracts (*lower right inset*; *ghosted structures*) provide access to the lesion without harming sensory function (surgical cases; ▶ Video 16.9, ▶ Video 16.10; **QR codes**). Roman numerals denote CNs. (Reproduced with permission from Barrow Neurological Institute, Phoenix, AZ.)

Surgical Case 16.9

MEDULLARY

Cavernoma Subtype: Gracile

Position: Prone
Craniotomy: Suboccipital with C1 laminectomy
Approach: Trans-cisterna magna (SOcc-Magna)
Triangle: Vallecular
SEZ: Posterior median sulcus
Artery: p3 PICA

Video: Resection of a midline gracile medullary cavernoma

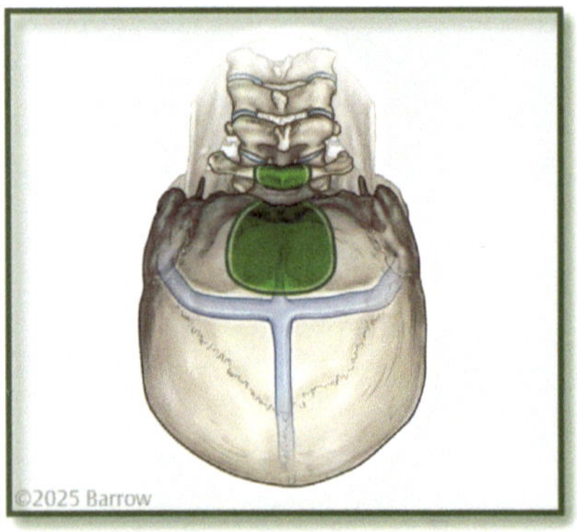

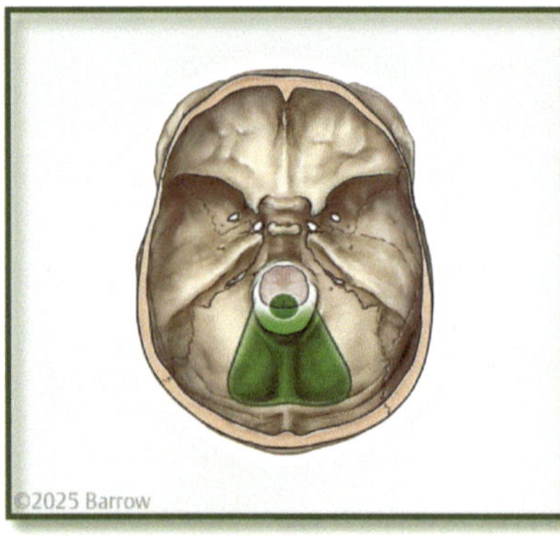

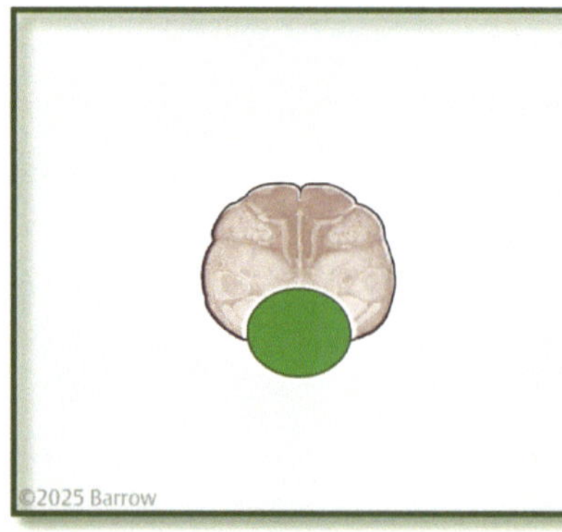

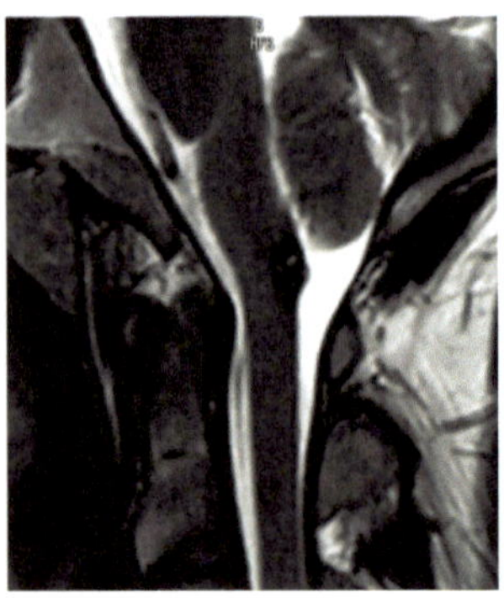

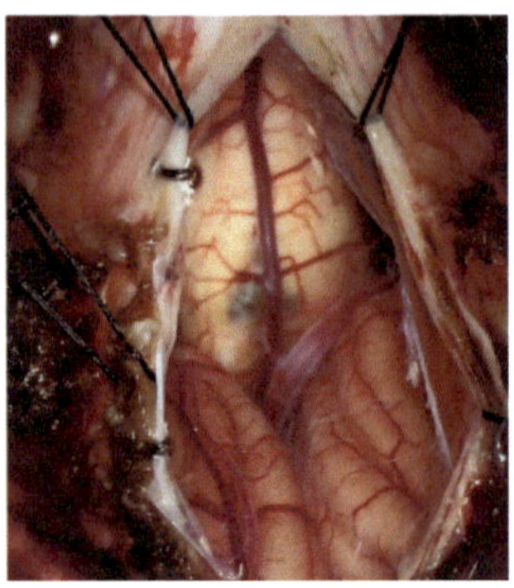

Video 16.9
Suboccipital Craniotomy with Trans-Cisterna Magna Approach for Gracile Medullary Cavernous Malformation Resection (Reproduced with permission from Barrow Neurological Institute, Phoenix, AZ.)

Surgical Case 16.10

MEDULLARY

Cavernoma Subtype: Gracile

Position: Prone
Craniotomy: Suboccipital with C1 laminectomy
Approach: Trans-cisterna magna (SOcc-Magna)
Triangle: Vallecular
SEZ: Posterior median sulcus
Artery: p3 PICA

Video: Resection of a midline gracile medullary cavernoma

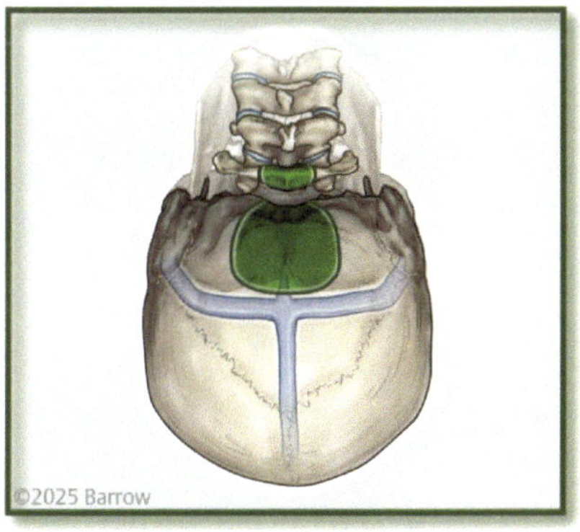

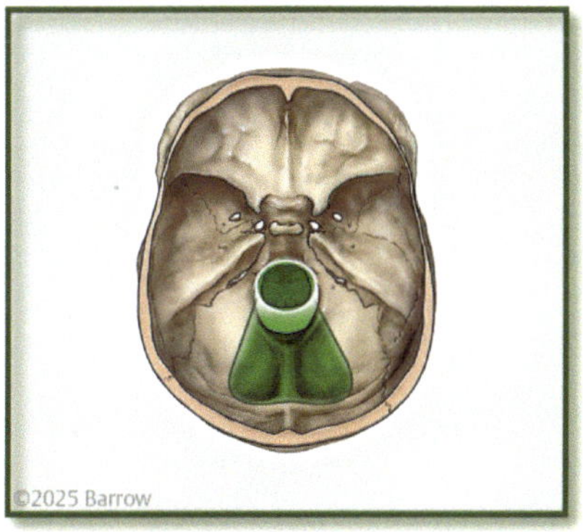

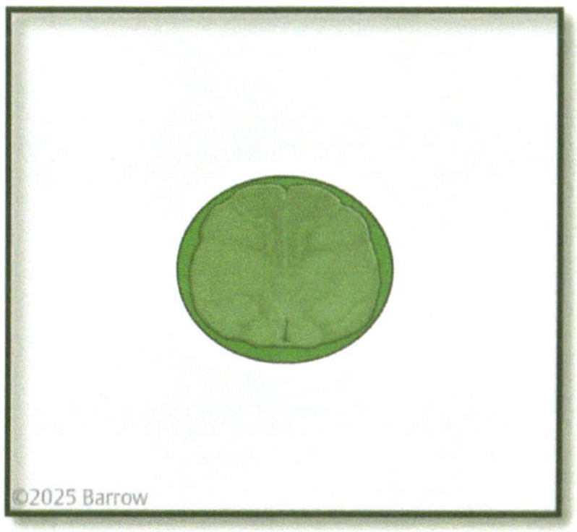

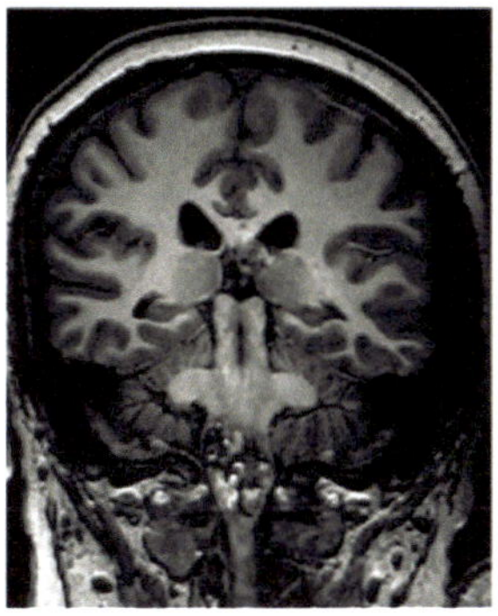

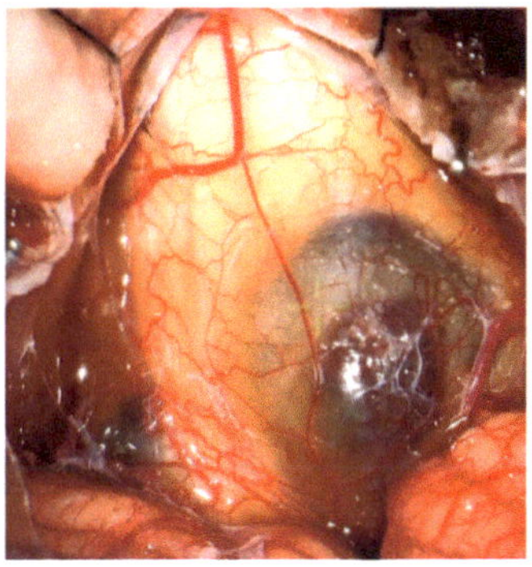

Video 16.10
Suboccipital Craniotomy with Trans-Cisterna Magna Approach for Gracile Medullary Cavernous Malformation Resection (Reproduced with permission from Barrow Neurological Institute, Phoenix, AZ.)

Trigonal Medullary Cavernoma

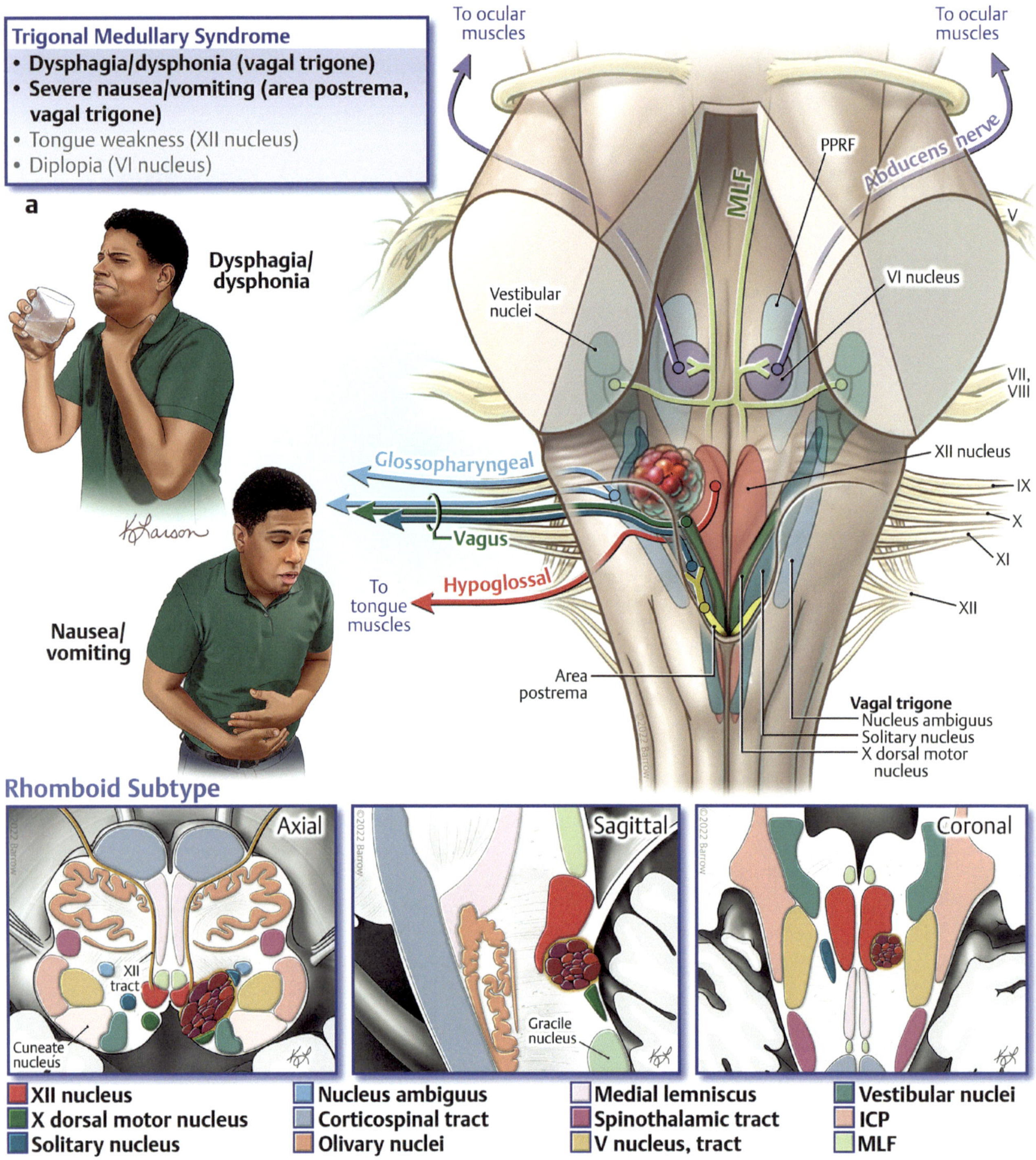

Fig. 16.8 Trigonal medullary clinical syndromes and surgical approaches. **(a)** Patients with trigonal CMs present with trigonal syndrome, consisting of dysphagia, dysphonia, nausea and vomiting, tongue weakness, and diplopia. The relationships between this left-sided CM and the nucleus ambiguus, solitary nucleus, dorsal motor nucleus of CN X, area postrema, hypoglossal nucleus, vestibular nuclei, and abducens nucleus are shown in axial, sagittal, and coronal views (*lower insets*).

(Continued)

Surgical Approach

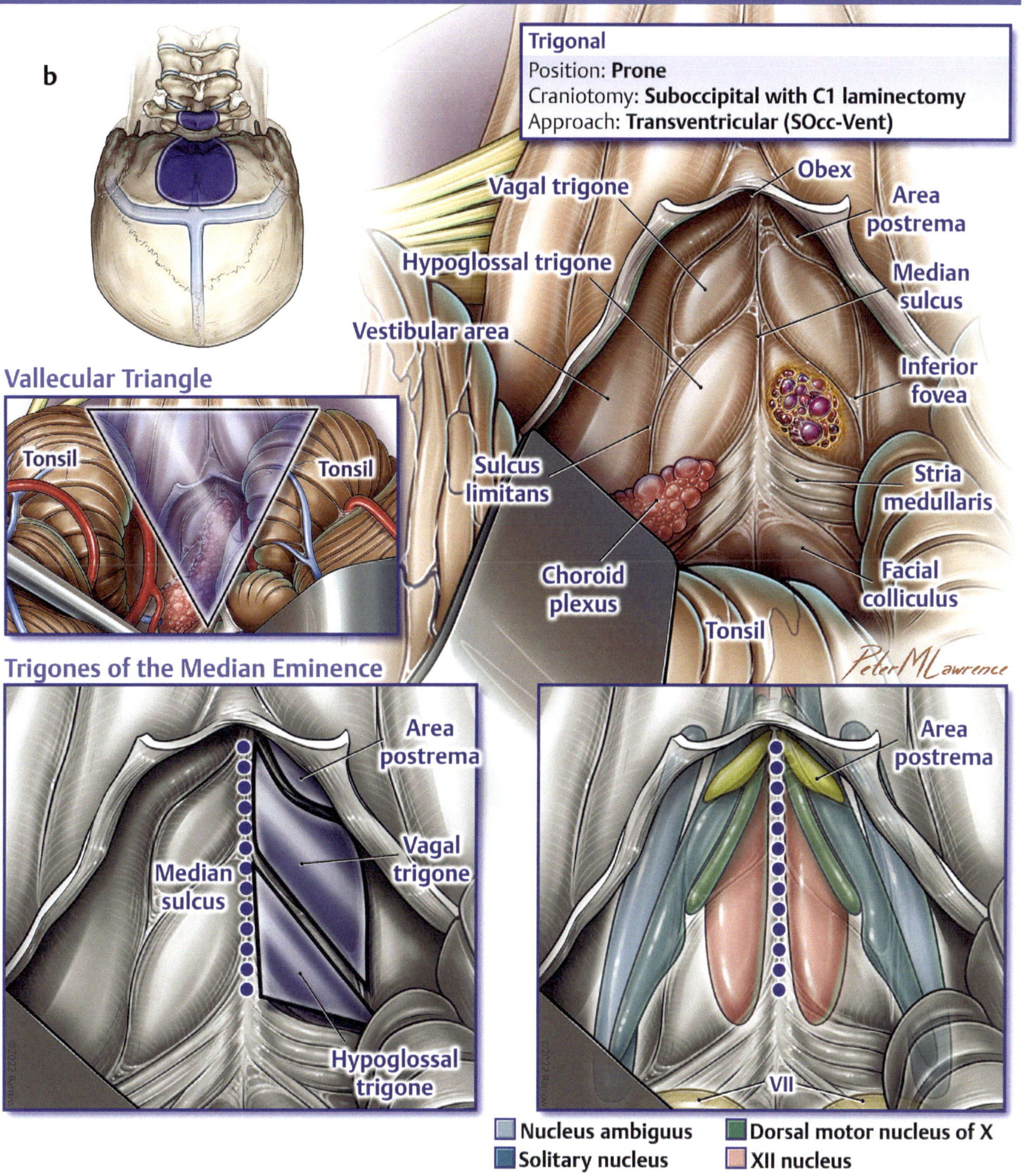

Fig. 16.8 *(Continued)* **(b)** Trigonal CMs are exposed through a suboccipital craniotomy with C1 laminectomy (*upper left inset*) and transventricular approach with the patient in the prone position. The inferior part of the fourth ventricular floor is exposed with tonsillar mobilization and opening of the cerebellar vallecular triangle, a potential space between the tonsils bilaterally and the uvula of the inferior vermis superiorly (*middle left inset*). Incision of the inferior medullary velum increases access to more laterally and superiorly placed lesions. The median sulcus SEZ accesses deep midline lesions (*lower left and right insets*; *purple dotted line*) and avoids trigonal structures adjacent to the midline (hypoglossal nucleus, dorsal motor nucleus of the vagus nerve, solitary nucleus, nucleus ambiguus, and area postrema [*lower right inset*; *ghosted structures*]). The infrafacial collicular SEZ is used for larger, high-riding lesions that extend beyond the medulla into the lower pons (surgical cases; ▸ Video 16.11, ▸ Video 16.12; QR codes). Roman numerals indicate CNs. (Reproduced with permission from Barrow Neurological Institute, Phoenix, AZ.)

Surgical Case 16.11

MEDULLARY

Cavernoma Subtype: Trigonal

Position: Prone
Craniotomy: Suboccipital with C1 laminectomy
Approach: Transventricular (SOcc-Vent)
Triangle: Vallecular
SEZ: Median sulcus
Artery: p3 PICA

Video: Resection of a midline trigonal medullary cavernoma

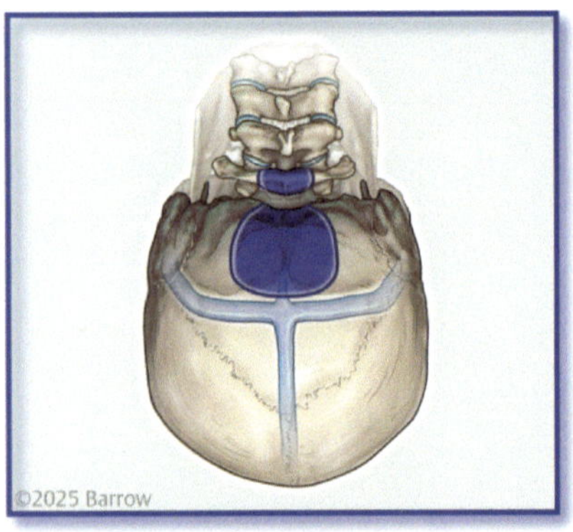

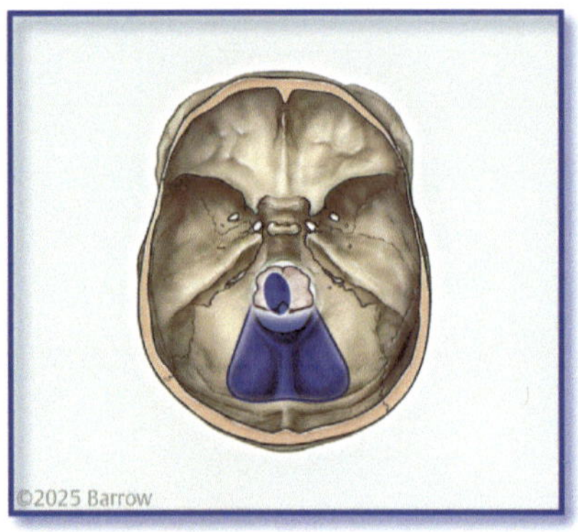

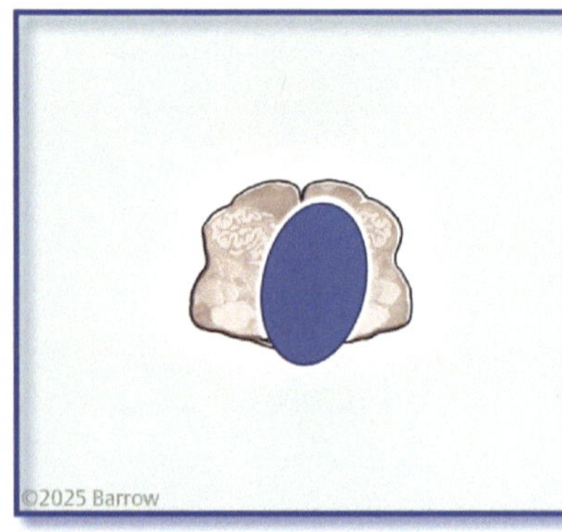

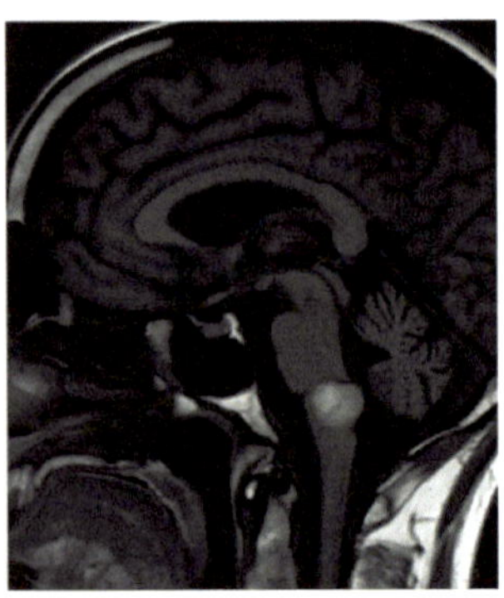

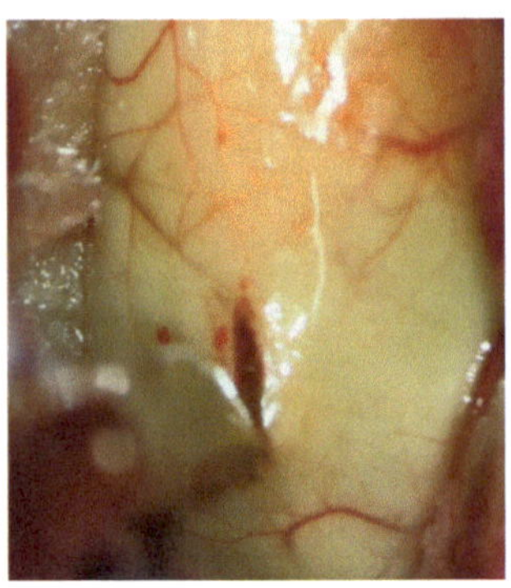

Video 16.11
Suboccipital Craniotomy with Transventricular Approach for Trigonal Medullary Cavernous Malformation Resection (Reproduced with permission from Barrow Neurological Institute, Phoenix, AZ.)

16

Surgical Case 16.12

MEDULLARY

Cavernoma Subtype: Trigonal

Position: Prone
Craniotomy: Suboccipital with C1 laminectomy
Approach: Transventricular (SOcc-Vent)
Triangle: Vallecular
SEZ: Median sulcus
Artery: p3 PICA

Video: Resection of a left trigonal medullary cavernoma

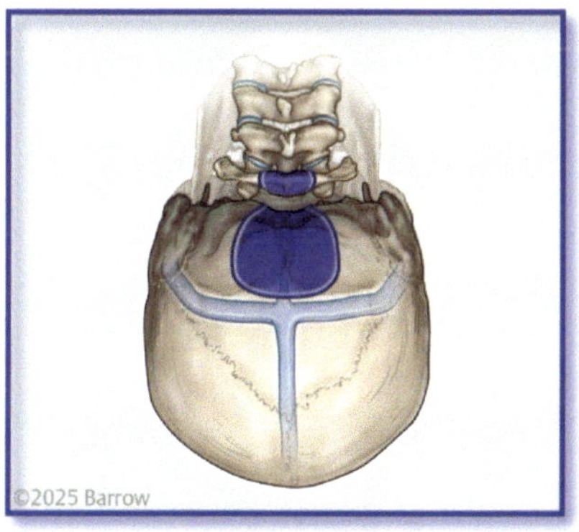

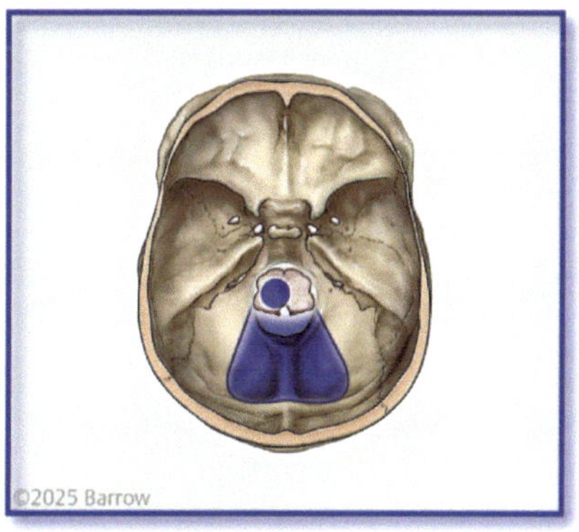

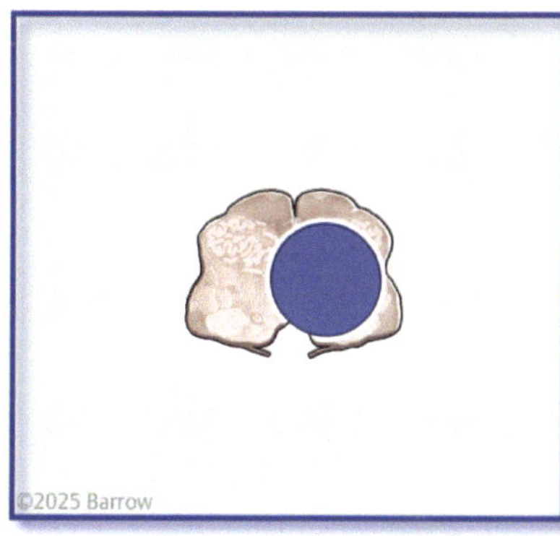

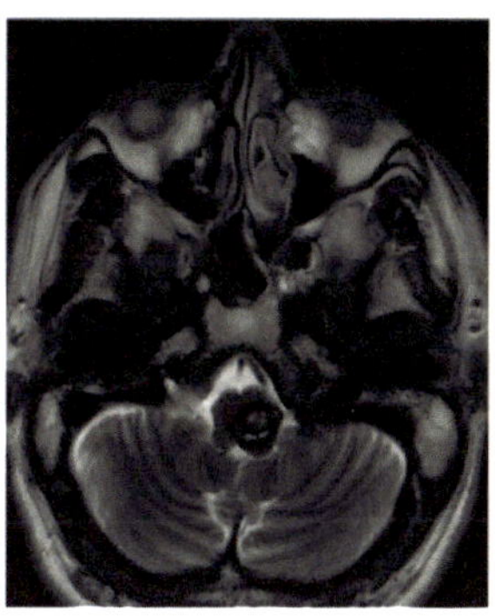

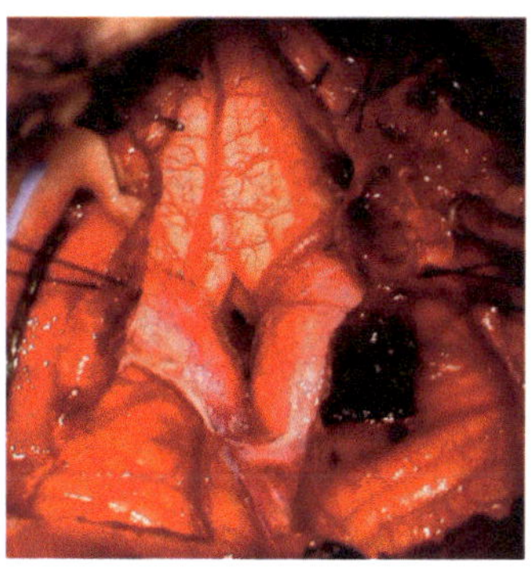

Video 16.12
Suboccipital Craniotomy with Transventricular Approach for Trigonal Medullary Cavernous Malformation Resection (Reproduced with permission from Barrow Neurological Institute, Phoenix, AZ.)

16.5 Conclusion

As with other brainstem CMs, the medullary taxonomy based on surface presentation (anterior, anterolateral, posterolateral, posteroinferior, and posterosuperior) guides the selection of surgical approach and resection strategy. Unlike CMs in the midbrain and pons that can be accessed from many trajectories through various approaches, medullary CMs are accessed posteriorly or laterally through suboccipital or far lateral approaches. The recommended surgical approach was selected in more than 90% of patients for a particular medullary subtype. In addition, the constellation of neurological signs and symptoms associated with a hemorrhagic medullary subtype defines it clinically as a neurological syndrome recognizable at the bedside. The taxonomy offers a useful scheme for classifying medullary CMs into subtypes, deciphering their clinical presentations at the bedside, and guiding surgical decision-making.

17 CEREBELLUM

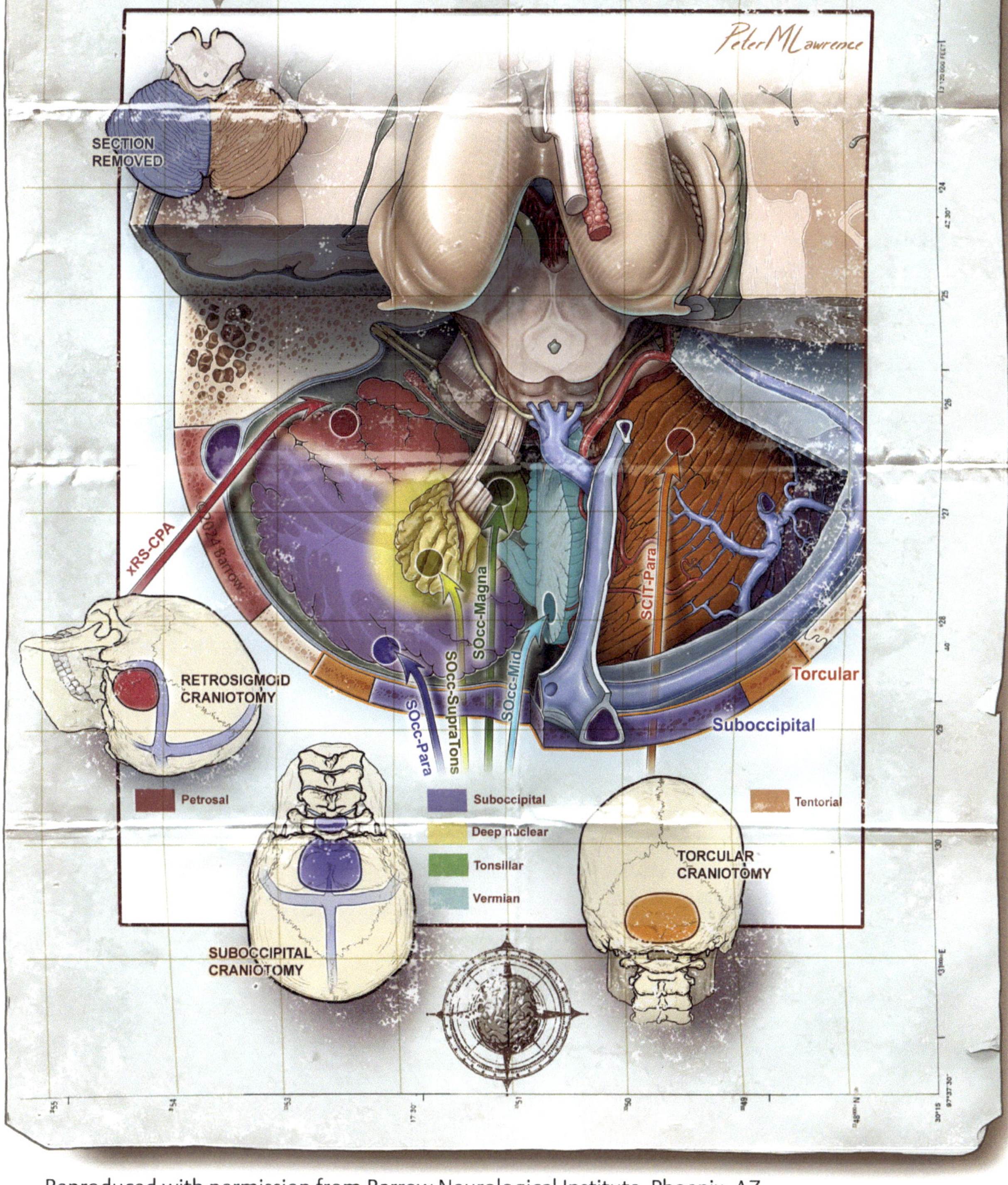

Reproduced with permission from Barrow Neurological Institute, Phoenix, AZ.

17 Cerebellar Cavernous Malformations

Summary

Cerebellar cavernous malformations (CMs) lie cortically in the cerebellar folia or subcortically in the underlying white matter, making them shallow and more accessible than brainstem CMs. The cerebellar taxonomy classifies CMs into six subtypes on the basis of their anatomical location relative to the cerebellar surfaces on preoperative magnetic resonance imaging (MRI). These subtypes are suboccipital, tentorial, petrosal, vermian, tonsillar, and deep nuclear. The cerebellar CM taxonomy was applied to 143 cases of microsurgically treated cerebellar CMs in 140 patients over a 25-year period. Of the 143 cases, 25 (17%) were suboccipital CMs, 13 (9%) were tentorial CMs, 62 (43%) were petrosal CMs, 18 (13%) were vermian CMs, 3 (2%) were tonsillar CMs, and 22 (15%) were deep nuclear CMs. The cerebellar CM subtypes guided the selection of the surgical approach. Suboccipital, vermian, and tonsillar CMs were exposed via suboccipital craniotomies. Petrosal CMs were exposed through retrosigmoid or extended retrosigmoid craniotomies. Tentorial CMs were approached via a torcular craniotomy, except when they reached the lateral tentorial surface, where they were exposed with a retrosigmoid craniotomy. Cerebellar CMs that presented to a cerebellar surface were resected without tissue transgression. Deep nuclear CMs are not associated with a cerebellar surface; therefore, translobular transgression was required to reach them, with or without a transsulcal component to shorten the distance through the tissue. Taxonomic subtyping is correlated with radiographic anatomy on MRI and can be associated with a constellation of symptoms and signs that help localize the lesion upon bedside examination. The taxonomy also describes cerebellar CMs precisely for clear clinical communications and publications.

Keywords: cavernoma, craniotomy, deep nuclear, fissure, peduncle, petrosal, suboccipital, subtype, taxonomy, tentorial, tonsillar, vermian

17.1 Introduction

The cerebellum, or *little brain*, is a mass of neural tissue attached to the posterior brainstem by the three pairs of cerebellar peduncles. The cerebellum comprises only 10% of the brain's volume, but its surface area is 80% of the cerebrum's, due to extensive folding of its folia, and it contains 80% of the brain's neurons. The cerebellum is involved in the planning of movement, influencing the output of the motor cortex. Inputs from the spinal cord, vestibular system, inferior olivary nuclei, and cerebral cortex enter the cerebellum and project to deep cerebellar nuclei and sites in the brainstem and thalamus. In addition to its motor role, the cerebellum is extensively involved in sensory processing.

Cerebellar cavernous malformations (CMs) are the seventh and final subtype described in seven cavernomas taxonomy. They lie cortically in the cerebellar folia or subcortically in the underlying white matter, making them shallow and more accessible than brainstem CMs. The craniotomies used for cerebellar CMs are the same as those used for some brainstem CMs. However, the approaches are transgyral through the lobules or transsulcal through the fissures, similar to those of superficial cerebral CMs. Therefore, cerebellar CM management is simpler from a strategic and technical point of view than brainstem or deep cerebral CMs. The taxonomy for cerebellar CMs completes the comprehensive system characterizing all CMs encountered in the brain.

17.2 Neuroanatomy of the Six Cerebellar Cavernous Malformation Subtypes

Cerebellar CMs were classified into six subtypes on the basis of their location relative to cerebellar surfaces (▶ Fig. 17.1, ▶ Fig. 17.2). The cerebellar CM subtypes are (1) suboccipital, (2) tentorial, (3) petrosal, (4) vermian, (5) tonsillar, and (6) deep nuclear. Each cerebellar hemisphere has three surfaces: suboccipital, tentorial, and petrosal. The vermis occupies the midline between the hemispheres, and vermian CMs are considered a unique subtype. The tonsils are caudal appendages, and tonsillar CMs comprise another subtype. Cortically located CMs were subtyped according to surface presentation, as were subcortical lesions located within 1 cm of the cerebellar surface. CMs in the deep cerebellum in or adjacent to the cerebellar nuclei (fastigial, globose, emboliform, and dentate) were classified as deep nuclear CMs (▶ Fig. 17.2).

17.2.1 Suboccipital

Suboccipital CMs are located on or beneath the hemispheric portion of the suboccipital surface of the cerebellum facing the occipital bone and located between the transverse sinuses superiorly and sigmoid sinuses laterally, excluding the vermis. This surface comprises the superior semilunar, inferior semilunar, gracile, and biventral lobules. The suboccipital (prebiventral) fissure is the major fissure on this surface, running between the gracile and biventral lobules and dividing this surface into superior and inferior parts. The postclival (posterior superior) fissure separating the simple and superior semilunar lobules forms the superior border of this subtype, and the tonsillobiventral fissure forms the inferior border. Although the petrosal (horizontal) fissure is the major fissure on the petrosal surface, it becomes a minor fissure as it extends onto the suboccipital surface and courses just below the transverse sinuses between the semilunar lobules. The medial border of the suboccipital territory is formed by the paramedian vermohemispheric fissure along the inferior vermis, which comprises the posterior cortical surface in the midline and lies in the posterior cerebellar incisura, a deep vertical depression in the suboccipital surface. The suboccipital surface has a close anatomical relationship with the p5 cortical segment of the posterior inferior cerebellar artery (PICA) because its branches supply the suboccipital surface.

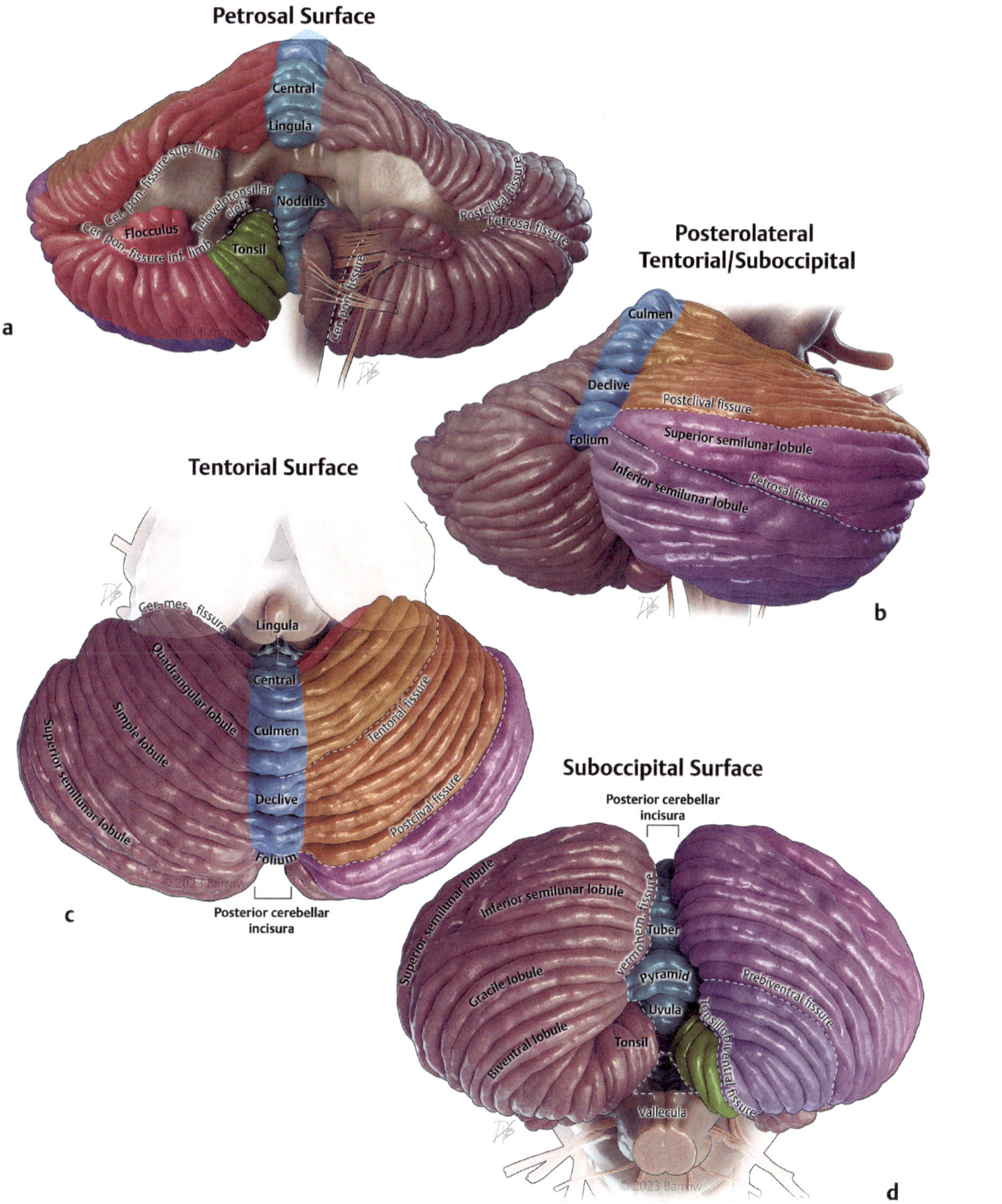

Fig. 17.1 Overview of cerebellar anatomy, surfaces, and subtypes. The cerebellar hemispheres are shown from **(a)** anterior (petrosal surface), **(b)** posterolateral oblique (tentorial and suboccipital surfaces), **(c)** superior (tentorial surface), and **(d)** inferior (suboccipital surface) views. The five superficial cerebellar subtypes consist of the petrosal (*red*), tentorial (*orange*), suboccipital (*purple*), vermian (*teal*), and tonsillar (*green*). The deep nuclear (*yellow*) subtypes (▶ Fig. 17.2) are the sixth cerebellar subtype. Key landmarks dividing the subtypes are the postclival fissure between the tentorial and suboccipital subtypes, the vermohemispheric fissure between the vermian and suboccipital subtypes, and the tonsillobiventral fissure between the tonsillar and suboccipital subtypes. The vallecula is located inferior to the vermis. (Reproduced with permission from Barrow Neurological Institute, Phoenix, AZ.)

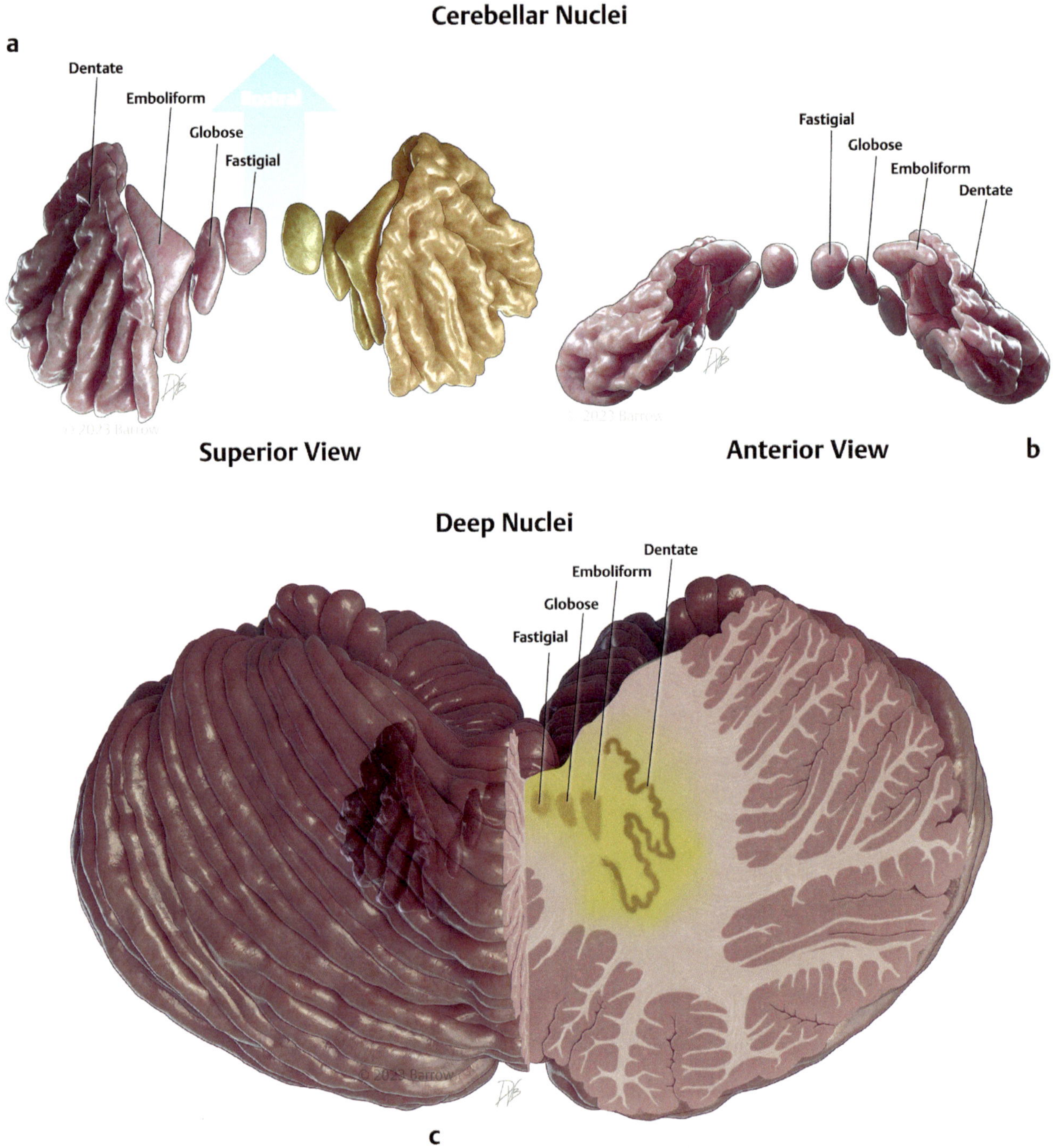

Fig. 17.2 Overview of deep nuclear subtype anatomy. The deep cerebellar nuclei consist of the dentate, emboliform, globose, and fastigial nuclei from laterally to medially, as seen from the **(a)** superior and **(b)** anterior views. **(c)** The relationships between these deep nuclei and the cerebellar surfaces are seen from above and in axial cross-section, with the fastigial nucleus located in the vermis, the globose and emboliform nuclei located in the paravermal or intermediate zone, and the dentate nucleus located deep within the cerebellar hemispheres. (Reproduced with permission from Barrow Neurological Institute, Phoenix, AZ.)

17.2.2 Tentorial

Tentorial CMs are located on or beneath the hemispheric portion of the tentorial surface facing the tentorium. The tentorial surface comprises the quadrangular and simple lobules, also called the anterior and posterior parts, respectively. The tentorial (primary) fissure separates these two lobules. The tentorial surface is bordered medially by the vermis (culmen and declive), with vermohemispheric fissures separating them. The postclival fissure is the posterior border of this tentorial territory, and the posterior cerebellar incisura is its anterior border. The tentorium surface is closely related to the s4 cortical segment of the superior cerebellar artery, running posteriorly from the cerebellomesencephalic fissure underneath the tentorial edge and supplying the tentorial surface lateral to the vermis.

17.2.3 Petrosal

Petrosal CMs are located on or beneath the petrosal surface of the cerebellum facing the posterior petrous bone. They involve the wings of the central lobule and the anterior surfaces of the quadrangular, simple, superior semilunar, inferior semilunar, gracile, and biventral lobules, as well as the flocculi. The petrosal surface is divided into superior and inferior parts by its major fissure, the petrosal fissure. CMs residing in the middle cerebellar peduncle (MCP) but not in the pons were included; CMs residing in the smaller superior and inferior cerebellar peduncles were not included in the cerebellar type but in the brainstem types (quadrigeminal midbrain and inferior peduncular pontine subtypes, respectively). The anterior inferior cerebellar artery courses through the cerebellopontine cistern and petrosal fissure to supply the petrosal surface.

17.2.4 Vermian

Vermian CMs are situated in the vermis, a midline structure spanning the suboccipital and tentorial cerebellar surfaces and joining the hemispheres. The inferior vermis on the suboccipital surface is delineated from the cerebellar hemispheres by vermohemispheric fissures in the posterior cerebellar incisura. In contrast, the superior vermis is the highest point on the tentorial surface and lacks a deep fissure separating it from the cerebellar hemisphere. CMs involving the suboccipital surface of the vermis are located in the folium, tuber, pyramid, uvula, and nodule. CMs involving the tentorial surface are located in the lingula, central lobule, culmen, and declive.

17.2.5 Tonsillar

Tonsillar CMs involve the cerebellar tonsils, two ovoid structures located bilaterally in the inferomedial part of the cerebellar hemispheres that attach superolaterally through the tonsillar peduncles. The lateral surface of each tonsil is covered by the biventral lobule and separated by the tonsillobiventral fissure. The remaining tonsillar surfaces (medial, anterior, superior) are free surfaces that are separated from adjacent neural structures by the vallecula medially, the cerebellomedullary fissure anteriorly, and the telovelotonsillar (also known as supratonsillar) cleft superiorly. The caudal loop of the p3 PICA wraps around the inferior pole of each tonsil and supplies it through p5 cortical arteries.

17.2.6 Deep Nuclear

CMs in the deep cerebellar nuclei reside within the white matter of the center of the cerebellum. Medially to laterally, there exist four deep cerebellar nuclei: the fastigial nuclei located in the vermis; the globose and emboliform nuclei, known as the interposed nuclei, residing in the paravermal or intermediate zone; and the dentate nuclei situated deep within the cerebellar hemispheres. The dentate nucleus is the largest of the cerebellar nuclei, receiving input from the spinocerebellar tract via the inferior cerebellar peduncle, as well as from neurons of the premotor and supplementary motor cortices. The dentate nucleus transmits output via the dentatorubrothalamic tract through the ipsilateral superior cerebellar peduncle. Dentate axons exit the cerebellum via the superior cerebellar peduncle, decussate in the caudal midbrain before joining the red nucleus, and subsequently ascend to the thalamus.

17.3 Clinical Evidence

The cerebellar CM taxonomy was applied to 143 cases of microsurgically treated cerebellar CMs in 140 patients that Robert F. Spetzler and I treated over a 25-year period (August 1997–December 2022). The cerebellar CMs were classified into six subtypes based on their anatomical location as identified on preoperative MRIs (▸ Table 17.1). Of the 143 CMs, 25 (17%) CMs were suboccipital, 13 (9%) were tentorial, 62 (43%) were petrosal, 18 (13%) were vermian, 3 (2%) were tonsillar, and 22 (15%) were deep nuclear. Petrosal cerebellar CMs were the most common subtype, with 49 of 62 located in the lateral MCP outside the pons and 13 in the cerebellar folia.

The cerebellar CM subtypes guided the selection of the surgical approach (▸ Fig. 17.3). Sixteen of 25 suboccipital CMs (64%)

Table 17.1 Clinical and radiographic outcomes after resection of cerebellar CMs by subtype

Variable	All subtypes	Tentorial	Suboccipital	Petrosal	Vermian	Tonsillar	Deep nuclear	*p*-value
All patients with data available[a]	140	13	25	59	18	3	22	
Number of CMs	143	13	25	62	18	3	22	
Preoperative mRS score								
Median (IQR)	2 (1–3)	2 (1–3)	2 (1–3)	2 (1–3)	2 (1–3)	2 (1–3)	1 (1–3)	0.07
>2	36 (25)	2 (15)	9 (36)	19 (31)	5 (28)	1 (33)	0 (0)	0.73
≤2	107 (75)	11 (85)	16 (64)	43 (69)	13 (72)	2 (67)	22 (100)	0.32

(Continued)

17

Table 17.1 (*Continued*) Clinical and radiographic outcomes after resection of cerebellar CMs by subtype

Variable	All subtypes	Tentorial	Suboccipital	Petrosal	Vermian	Tonsillar	Deep nuclear	*p*-value
Patients with clinical follow-up[b]	138	13	25	57	18	3	22	
No. of CMs	141	13	25	60	18	3	22	
Follow-up duration, mean (SD), mo	37 (54)	19 (25)	35 (50)	35 (48)	58 (77)	20 (30)	44 (64)	0.45
Follow-up mRS score								
Median (IQR)	1 (0–2)	1 (0–2)	1 (0–2)	1 (0–2)	1 (0–2)	1 (0–2)	1 (0–2)	**0.02**
>2	12 (9)	1 (8)	1 (4)	8 (13)	2 (11)	0 (0)	0 (0)	0.74
≤2	129 (91)	12 (92)	24 (96)	52 (87)	16 (89)	3 (100)	22 (100)	0.13
Worse	10 (7)	1 (8)	1 (4)	5 (8)	2 (11)	0 (0)	1 (5)	
Stable or improved	131 (93)	12 (92)	24 (96)	55 (92)	16 (89)	3 (100)	21 (95)	
Patients with radiographic follow-up	94	10	19	37	13	1	12	
Number of CMs	94	10	19	39	13	1	12	
Follow-up duration, mean (SD), mo	55 (59)	26 (27)	63 (66)	52 (56)	85 (81)	55 (0)	42 (41)	0.23
Recurrence	7 (7)	0 (0)	0 (0)	4 (10)	2 (15)	0 (0)	1 (8)	

Note: Data are reported as n (%) unless otherwise noted. Bold p-values indicate statistical significance.
[a]Three patients had 2 CMs each, underwent 2 separate operations, and were counted as patients twice, giving 143 patients in this analysis.
[b]Two patients in the group with petrosal subtype CMs did not have follow-up data available.

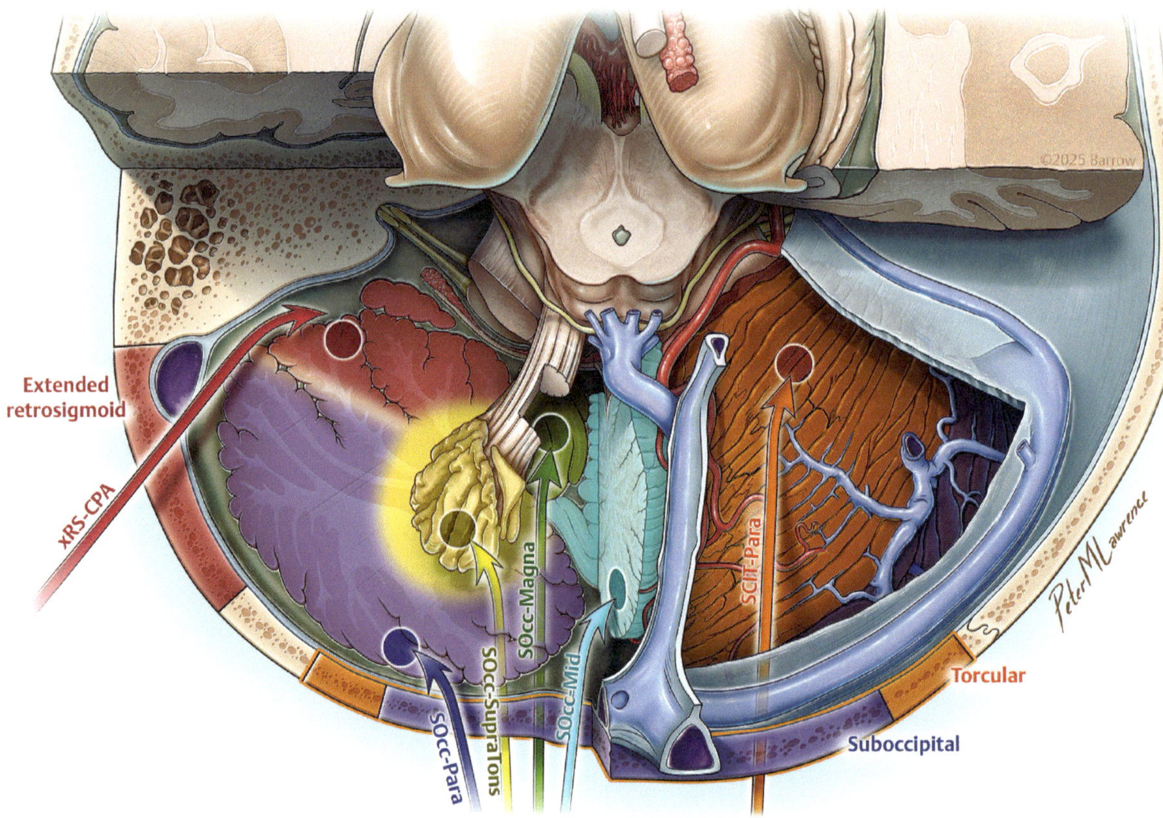

Fig. 17.3 Overview of surgical approaches to the six cerebellar CM subtypes shown in axial cross-section viewed from above (*colored arrows*). The SCIT-Para approach is recommended for tentorial CMs (*orange*), the SOcc-Para approach for suboccipital CMs (*purple*), the xRS-CPA approach for petrosal CMs (*red*), the SOcc-Mid approach for vermian CMs (*teal*), the SOcc-Magna approach for tonsillar CMs (*green*), and the SOcc-SupraTons approach for deep nuclear CMs (*yellow*). (Reproduced with permission from Barrow Neurological Institute, Phoenix, AZ.)

were resected through a midline suboccipital craniotomy. A lateral suboccipital craniotomy was used in 7 of 25 CMs (28%). Tentorial CMs required access to the tentorial surface through a torcular craniotomy in 4 of 13 patients (31%) or through suboccipital craniotomies extending up to but not across the transverse sinuses in 7 of 13 patients (54%). Petrosal CMs were exposed through a retrosigmoid or extended retrosigmoid craniotomy in 35 of 62 patients (56%) and a suboccipital craniotomy in 25 of 62 patients (40%). Vermian CMs were accessed through a midline suboccipital craniotomy in 17 of 18 patients (94%), even in those with CMs in the superior vermis. All three tonsillar CMs were exposed through a midline suboccipital craniotomy. Eleven of 22 deep nuclear CMs (50%) were exposed through midline suboccipital craniotomies, and the other half were reached via lateral suboccipital craniotomies. Eight other selected patients (6%) with various cerebellar subtypes underwent far lateral craniotomies.

Overall, 78 of 143 cerebellar CMs (55%) that presented to a cerebellar surface were resected without tissue transgression, and the remaining CMs (65/143, 45%) required translobular or transsulcal approaches. Complete resection was achieved in 134 patients (94%). Favorable outcomes (modified Rankin Scale [mRS] score ≤ 2) were achieved in 129 of 141 patients (91%) at late follow-up. Relative outcomes were unchanged or improved relative to the preoperative baseline in 131 of 141 patients (93%) and did not differ by subtype.

17.4 Resection Strategies for Cerebellar Cavernous Malformations

The cerebellar CM taxonomy guided the selection of approaches and resection strategies. Suboccipital, vermian, and tonsillar CMs were exposed via suboccipital craniotomies. Some tentorial CMs were also exposed through suboccipital craniotomies, along with some deep nuclear CMs. Petrosal CMs were exposed through retrosigmoid or extended retrosigmoid craniotomies. Cerebellar CMs that presented to a cerebellar surface were resected without tissue transgression, and the remaining CMs required translobular or transsulcal approaches.

17.4.1 Suboccipital, Vermian, and Tonsillar

As the largest and most accessible of the cerebellar surfaces, the suboccipital surface was exposed fully with a suboccipital craniotomy with C1 laminectomy, presenting the hemispheric convexity in full view, remote from the brainstem and skull base (▸ Fig. 17.4). Suboccipital, vermian (▸ Fig. 17.5), and tonsillar (▸ Fig. 17.6) CM subtypes reside on this surface and were exposed with the same craniotomy. Head flexion with the patient positioned prone opens the cranial-cervical angle. Midline suboccipital approaches with a linear midline incision were used for most of these CMs, but a more lateral approach with a linear paramedian incision or horseshoe incision extending from the midline to the mastoid bone was selected for CMs located laterally on the suboccipital surface. A Y-shaped incision in the posterior cervical fascia created an additional layer for watertight wound closure, and a T-shaped incision in the musculature below the superior nuchal line and along the midline nuchal ligament exposed the occipital bone. Two-thirds of suboccipital CMs and all vermian and tonsillar CMs were resected through midline craniotomies. Superior vermian CMs were exposed without extension across the torcula and transverse sinuses, but the craniotomy was immediately adjacent to these venous structures to optimize the upward view. Low-lying tonsillar CMs were accessible with a suboccipital craniotomy incorporating the foramen magnum. Minimal subarachnoid dissection is required for suboccipital CMs. Nonetheless, inferior vermian CMs require opening the arachnoid membrane of the cisterna magna, dissecting the posterior cerebellar incisura, and mobilizing the inferior vermian veins and p5 cortical segments of the PICA. Tonsillar CMs may also require widening the vallecula (vallecular triangle), opening the cerebellomedullary fissure, or splitting the tonsillobiventral fissure. The vermis is transgressed with caution, given the risks of cerebellar mutism reported after vermian disruption.

17.4.2 Tentorial

The tentorial surface is large, sloped, and viewed tangentially from the surgeon's perspective (▸ Fig. 17.7). Aggressive head flexion in patients positioned prone helped flatten this steep tentorial angle. A torcular craniotomy improved visibility and access by removing the ledge of overhanging bone often present after standard suboccipital craniotomy. Tacking sutures on the dural flap elevated the transverse sinuses and widened the supracerebellar-infratentorial corridor. The lateral exposure of a retrosigmoid craniotomy was more appropriate for CMs that reached the lateral tentorial surface. A torcular craniotomy uses the I-Y-T incision in the skin, fascia, and muscle, respectively, to create three layers for watertight closure. Arachnoid granulations and adhesions between the posterior border of the tentorial surface and the tentorium required release, and cerebrospinal fluid drainage from the cisterna magna relaxed the cerebellum. Bridging veins to the tentorium were preserved whenever possible, especially when associated with venous malformations. This tangential approach along the tentorial surface occasionally required a cortical incision into the simple or quadrangular lobules to visualize posterior and inferior margins, with the CM mobilized upward out of the hemisphere toward the tentorium to visualize deep planes.

17.4.3 Petrosal

Petrosal CMs were the most common of the cerebellar subtypes, which was surprising given the smaller size of this cerebellar surface. However, the MCP comprises the medial portion

Surgical Approach

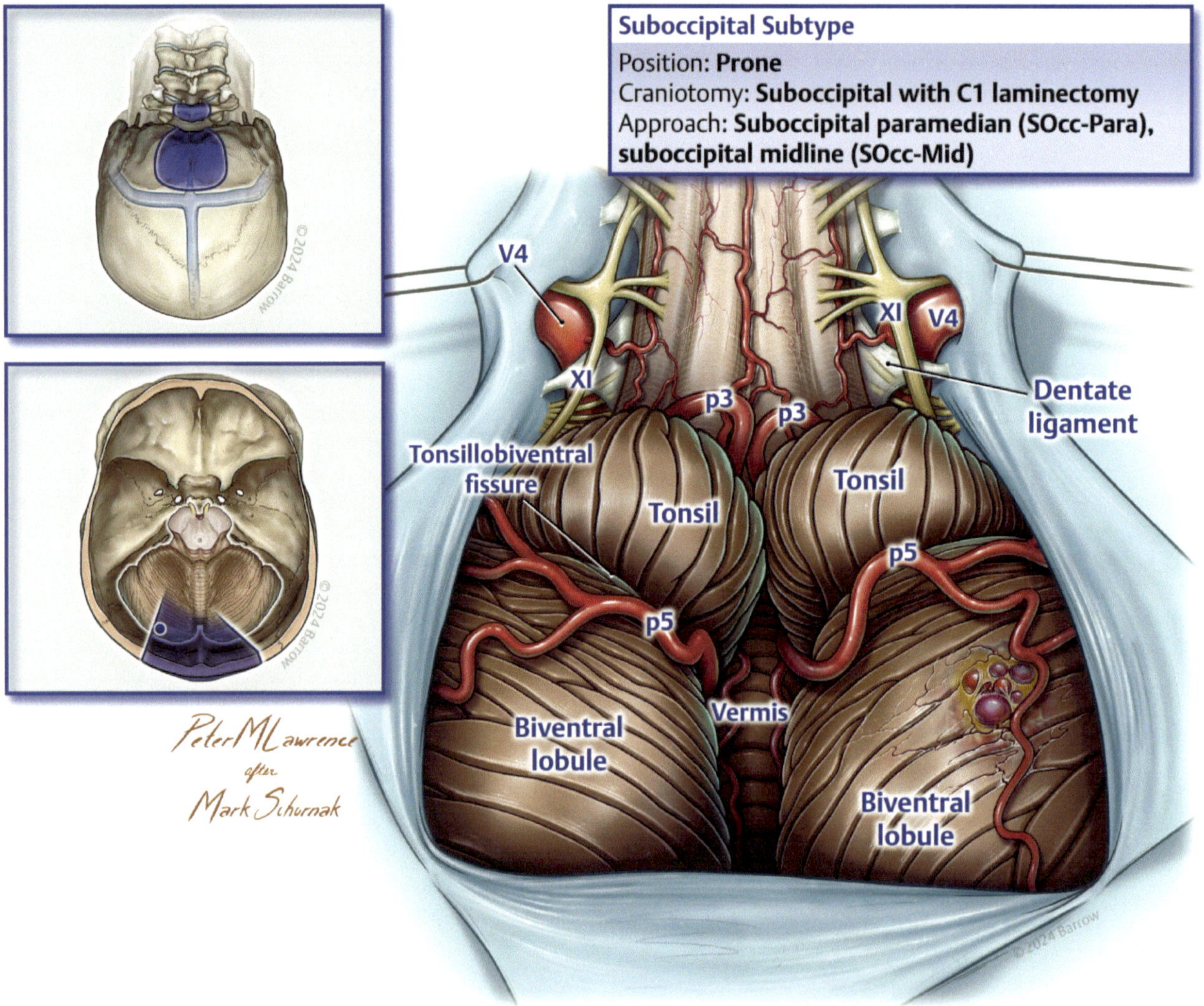

Fig. 17.4 Overview of approaches to suboccipital cerebellar CMs. Suboccipital CMs are accessed through a suboccipital craniotomy with C1 laminectomy (*upper left inset*) and SOcc-Para approach for lesions located laterally on the suboccipital surface, whereas lesions located along the midline (*lower left inset*; *purple circle*) are accessed through a SOcc-Mid approach. The bilateral PICAs are initially visualized as the caudal loops of the p3 tonsillomedullary segments that course below the tonsillar margin and, more distally, as the p5 cortical segments emerge from the tonsillobiventral fissure. The bilateral V4 intradural segments are visualized at the inferior aspect of the exposure as the vertebral arteries penetrate the posterior fossa dura, as are the spinal contributions of the accessory nerves (XI). Roman numerals denote CNs. (Reproduced with permission from Barrow Neurological Institute, Phoenix, AZ.)

Surgical Approach

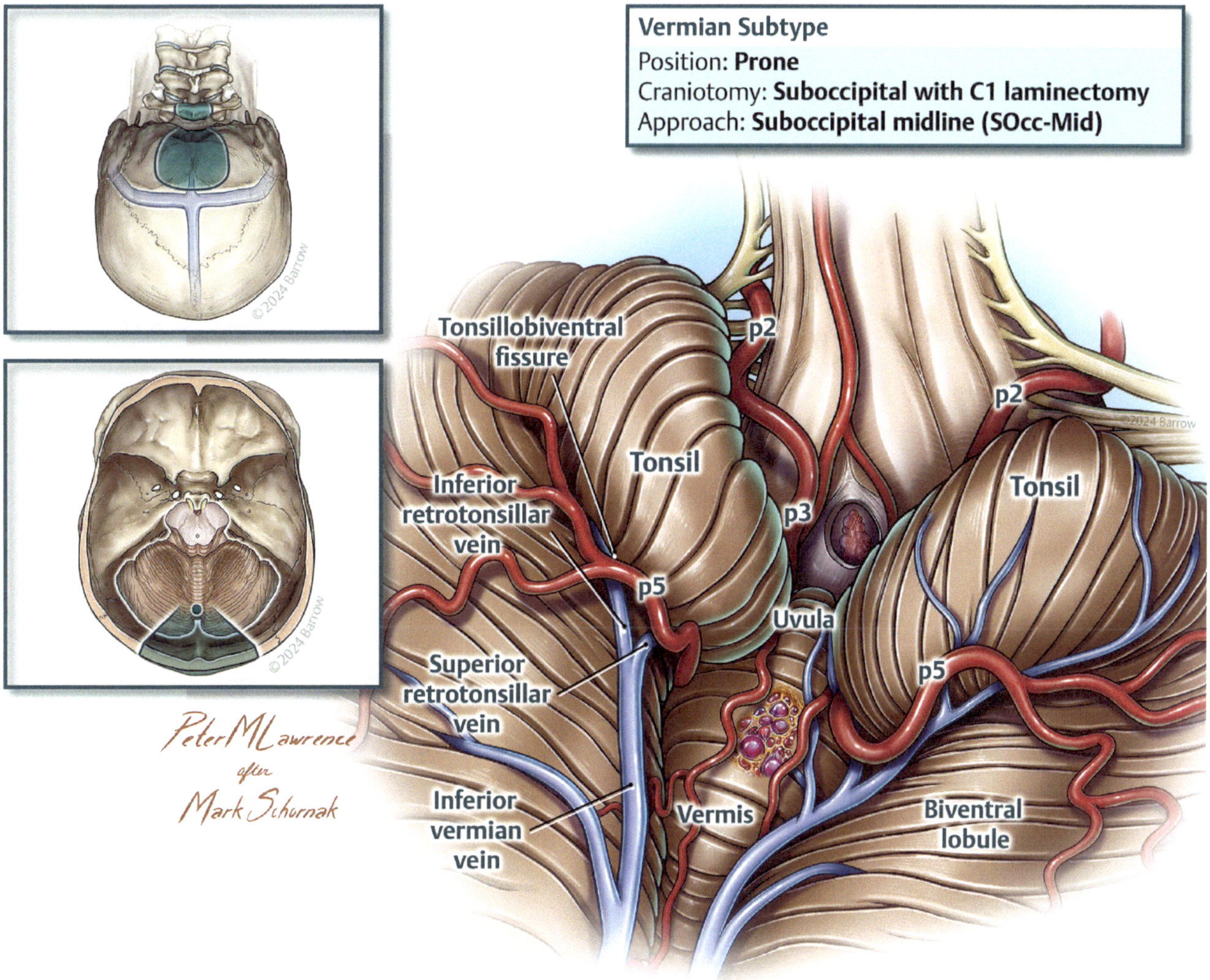

Fig. 17.5 Overview of approach to vermian cerebellar CMs. Vermian cerebellar CMs are accessed through a suboccipital craniotomy with C1 laminectomy (*upper left inset*) and SOcc-Mid approach (*lower left inset*; *teal circle*). Midline subarachnoid dissection separates the biventral lobules, revealing the bilateral p5 cortical segments of the PICA, as well as the dorsal midline cerebellar venous anatomy, including the inferior vermian and superior retrotonsillar veins. Deep dissection below the tonsils reveals the proximal PICA p2 lateral medullary and p3 tonsillomedullary segments, while the p4 telovelotonsillar segments remain obscured within the deep aspect of the tonsillobiventral fissures bilaterally. (Reproduced with permission from Barrow Neurological Institute, Phoenix, AZ.)

Surgical Approach

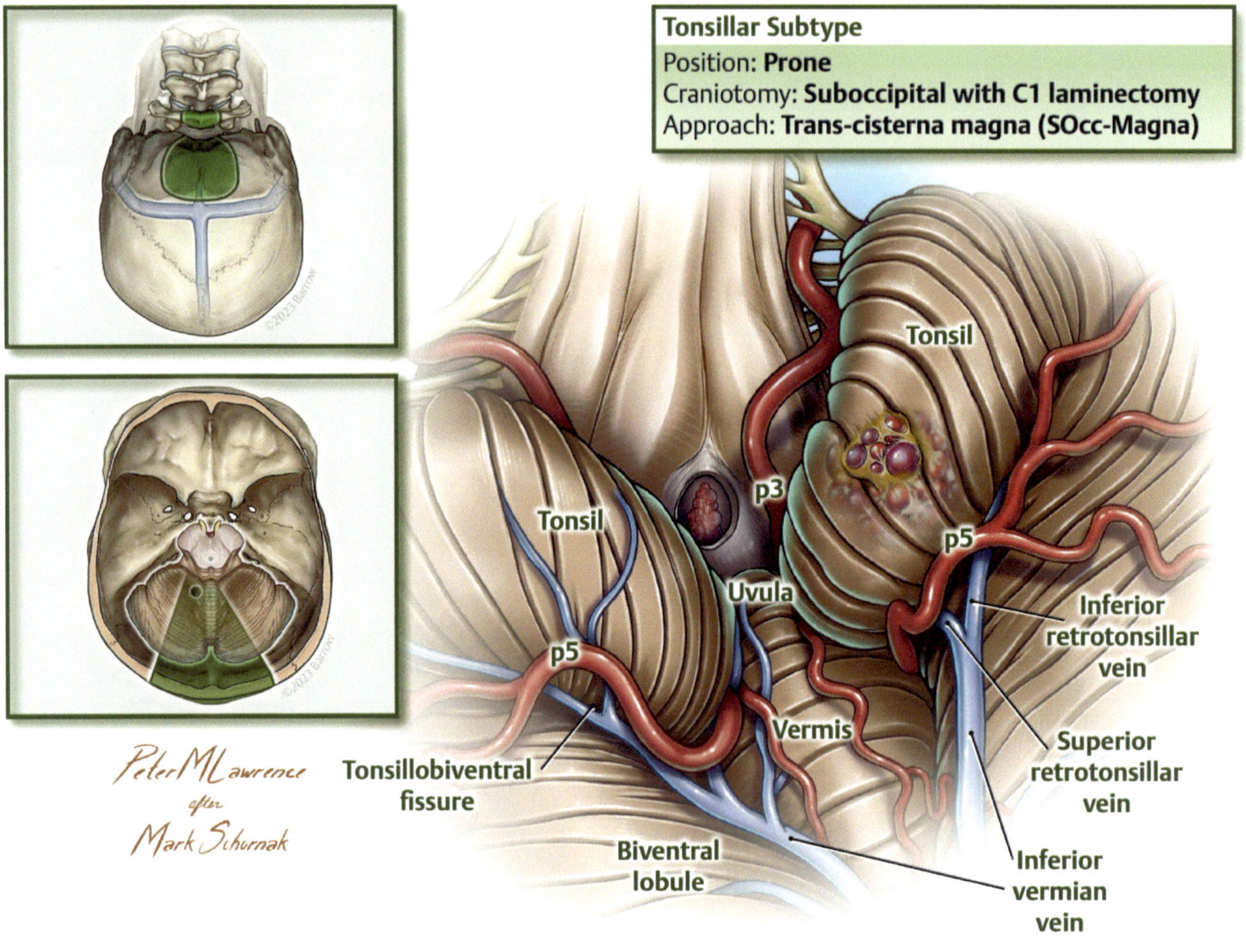

Fig. 17.6 Overview of approach to tonsillar cerebellar CMs. Tonsillar cerebellar CMs are accessed through a suboccipital craniotomy with C1 laminectomy (*upper left inset*) and trans-cisterna magna approach (*lower left inset*; *green circle*). p5 cortical segments of the PICAs are encountered superficially emerging from the tonsillobiventral fissures, where they cross the inferior and superior retrotonsillar veins. A lower dissection trajectory via the cisterna magna provides a more favorable approach to the cerebellar tonsils, with the extension of subarachnoid dissection incorporated as needed for access to deep-seated CMs. (Reproduced with permission from Barrow Neurological Institute, Phoenix, AZ.)

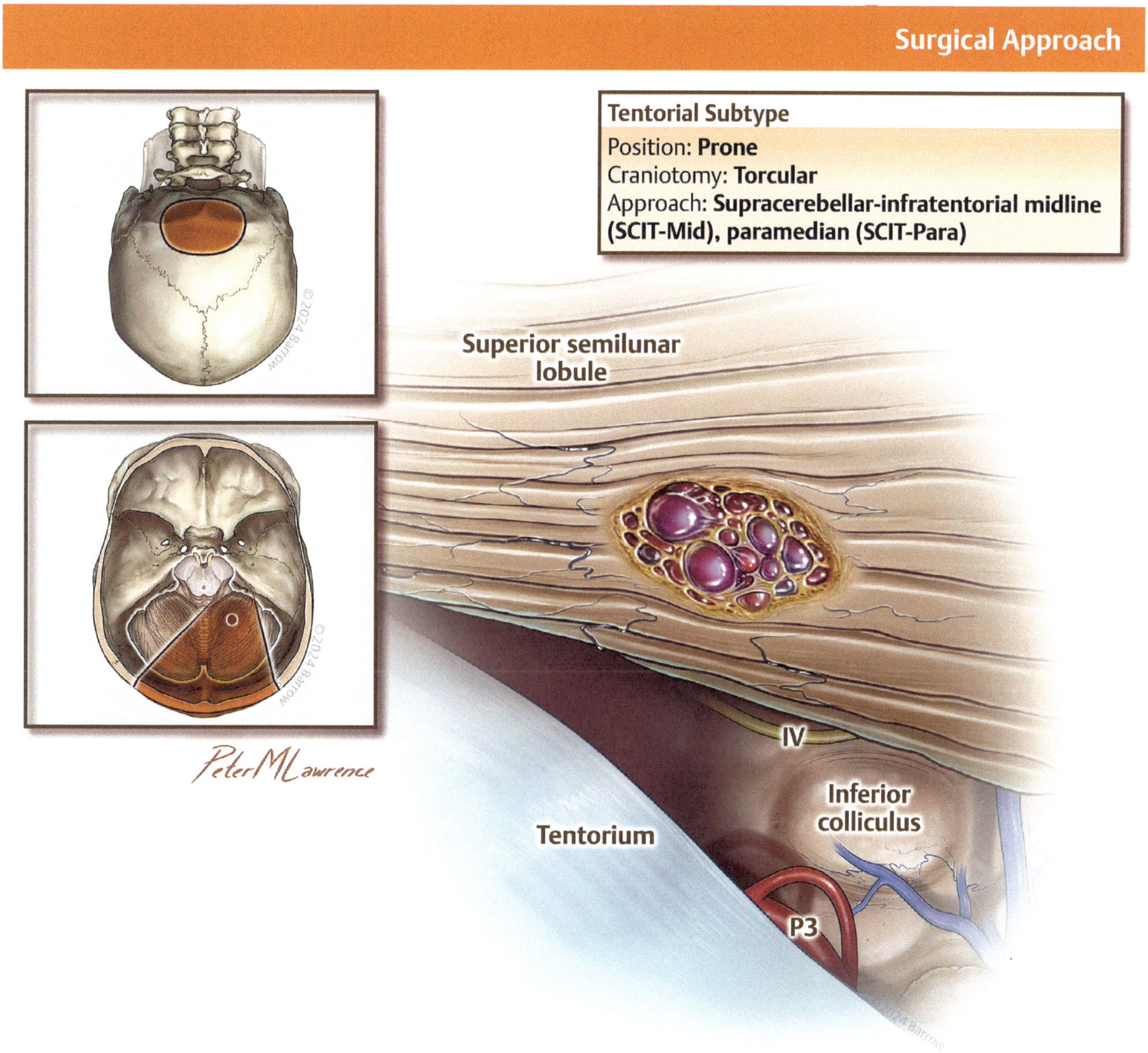

Fig. 17.7 Overview of approaches to tentorial cerebellar CMs. Tentorial cerebellar CMs are accessed through a torcular craniotomy (*upper left inset*) and SCIT-Mid or SCIT-Para approach, as dictated by the preferred cerebellar cortical entry point for the CM (*lower left inset*; *orange circle*). Deep dissection along the SCIT corridor reveals the inferior colliculus arising from the tectal plate of the posterior midbrain, with the trochlear nerve (IV) coursing below toward the ambient cistern. The distal P3 quadrigeminal segment of the PCA is visualized superior to the tentorial incisura coursing toward the ipsilateral occipital lobe. Roman numeral denotes CN. (Reproduced with permission from Barrow Neurological Institute, Phoenix, AZ.)

of this surface, and its proximity to the lateral pons made lesional hemorrhage more symptomatic in these patients than in patients with other subtypes, with a stronger indication for surgery. The incidences of vertigo (44%), gait imbalance (40%), ataxia (34%), and diplopia (29%) were higher with petrosal CMs than with other subtypes. Petrosal CMs were accessed through an extended retrosigmoid approach that skeletonizes the sigmoid sinus from the transverse–sigmoid junction to the jugular bulb, allowing the dural flap to pull the sinus anteriorly, maximize the opening into the cerebellopontine angle, and eliminate any fixed retraction (▶ Fig. 17.8; ▶ Video 17.1). Release of cerebrospinal fluid from the cerebellopontine

Surgical Approach

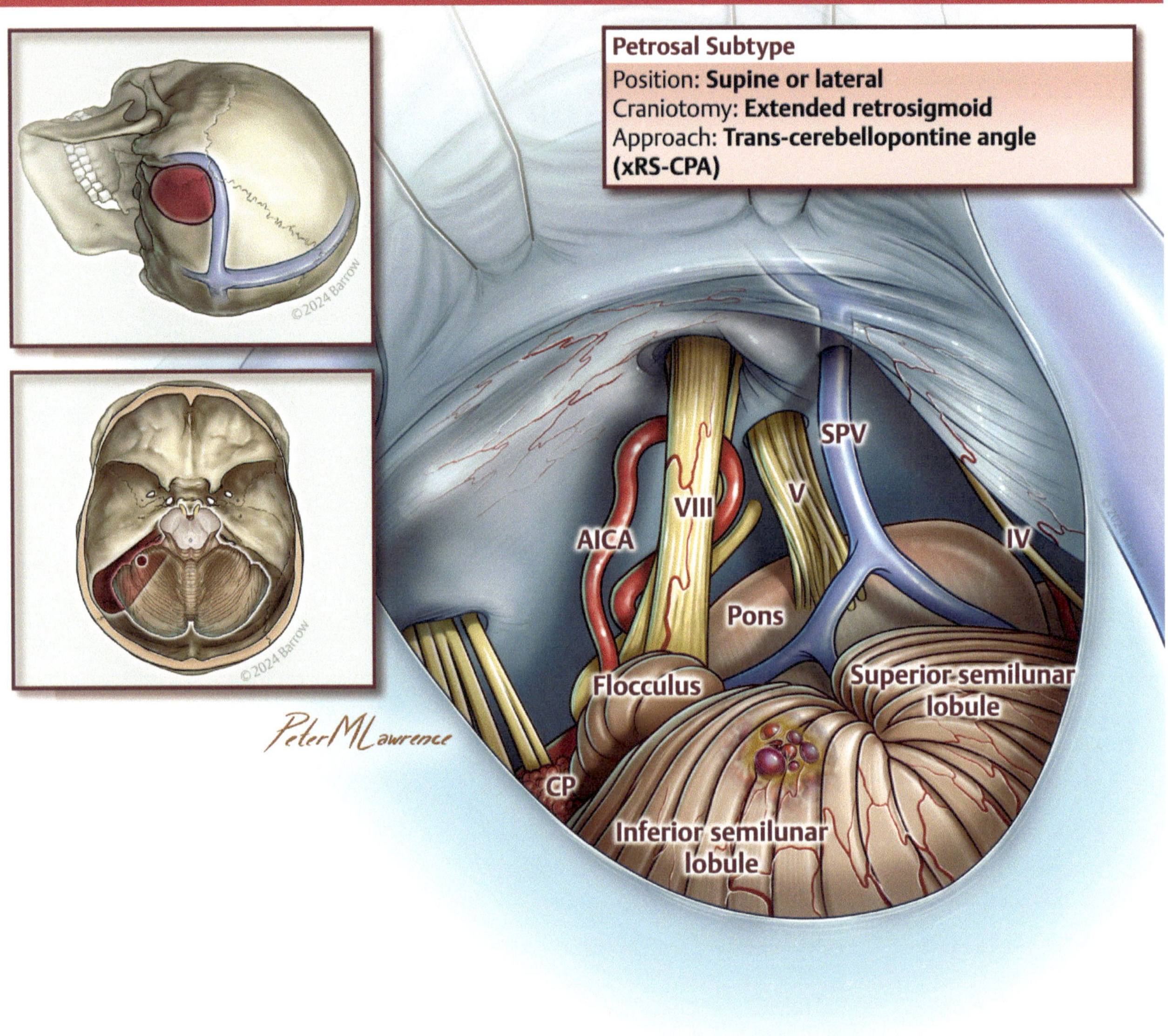

Fig. 17.8 Overview of approach to petrosal cerebellar CMs. Petrosal cerebellar CMs are accessed through an extended retrosigmoid craniotomy (*upper left inset*) and trans-cerebellopontine angle approach (*lower left inset*; *red circle*). This approach provides wide access to the CPA and its neurovascular structures. These structures include the trochlear (IV), trigeminal (V), and cochlear (VIII) nerves, as well as the lower CNs and the anterior inferior cerebellar artery, with its typically prominent loop at the level of the internal auditory canal. The SPV complex is encountered at the tentorial margin along the superior aspect of the petrous temporal bone (surgical case; ▶ Video 17.1; QR code). Roman numerals denote CNs. (Reproduced with permission from Barrow Neurological Institute, Phoenix, AZ.)

17

Surgical Case 17.1

CEREBELLAR & PONTINE

Cavernoma Subtype: Petrosal and Middle Peduncular

Position: Supine
Craniotomy: Extended retrosigmoid
Approach: Trans-cerebellopontine angle (xRS-CPA) and trans-middle cerebellar peduncle (xRS-MCP)
Triangle: Interlobular
SEZ: MCP (lateral pontine)
Artery: a4 and a3 AICA

Video: Resection of right middle peduncular pontine and right petrosal cerebellar cavernomas

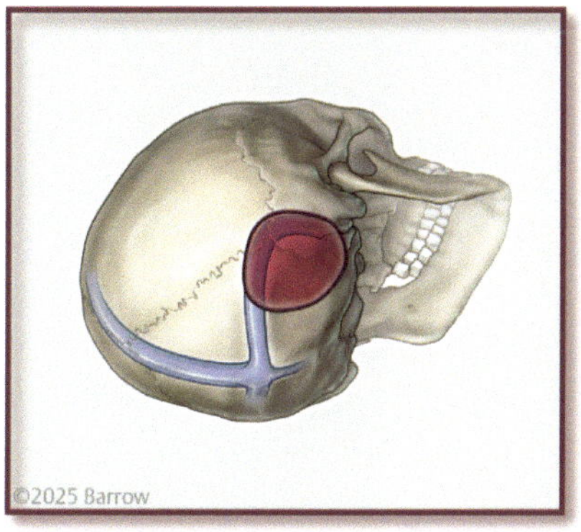

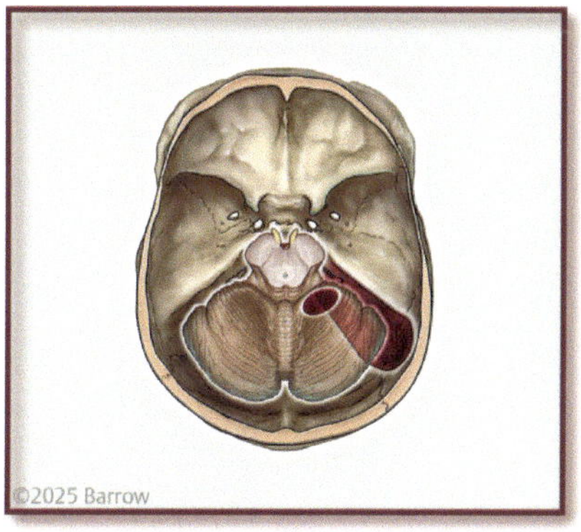

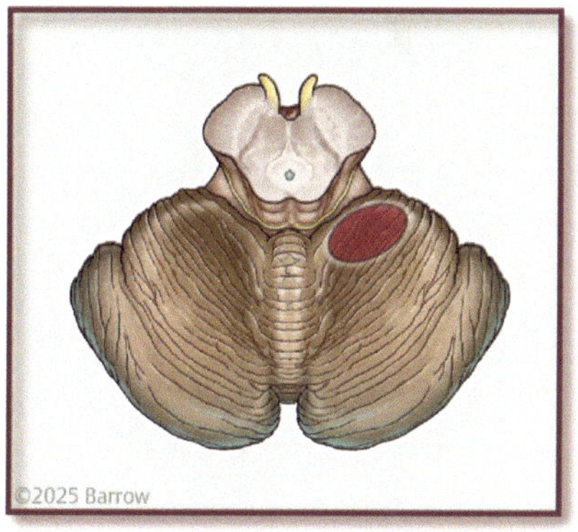

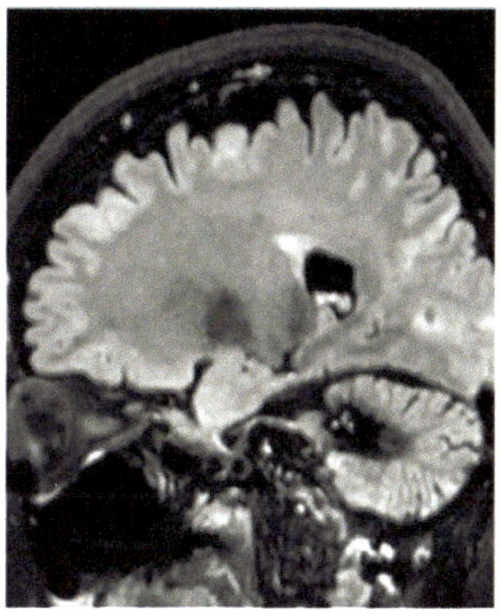

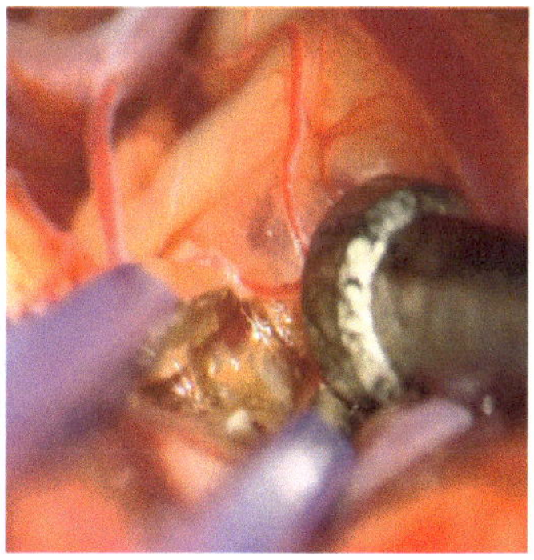

Video 17.1
Combined Trans-Cerebellopontine Angle and Trans-Middle Cerebellar Peduncle Approach for Middle Peduncular Pontine and Petrosal Cerebellar Cavernous Malformation Resections (Reproduced with permission from Barrow Neurological Institute, Phoenix, AZ.)

cistern and cisterna magna is necessary to relax the brain, but dissection around the lower cranial nerves and facial and vestibulocochlear nerves is not. MCP is accessed by splitting the petrosal (horizontal) fissure where the semilunar lobules wrap around the MCP from above (superior limb) and below (inferior limb). The anterior inferior cerebellar artery travels in the petrosal fissure. It is followed inward to separate the superior and inferior semilunar lobules, splitting the petrosal fissure, the so-called sylvian fissure of the cerebellum, and opening the interlobular triangle. Petrosal CMs in the MCP were accessible in the interlobular triangle, and mobilizing the flocculus inferiorly away from the vestibulocochlear nerve exposed the full extent of the MCP. Although petrosal CMs were lateral to the pons and outside the brainstem, their medial border often abutted the pons. A minority of petrosal CMs were located in the anterior surfaces of the quadrangular, simple, superior semilunar, inferior semilunar, gracile, and biventral lobules. These CMs did not require splitting the petrosal fissure.

17.4.4 Deep Nuclear

Deep nuclear CMs are not associated with a cerebellar surface. Translobular transgression was required to reach these lesions with or without a transsulcal component to shorten the distance through tissue. The fissures around the superior tonsil provided access to the deep nuclei in the form of a telovelar approach for medial CMs in the fastigial, globose, and emboliform nuclei or a supratonsillar approach for lateral CMs in the dentate nuclei (▶ Fig. 17.9; ▶ Video 17.2). The telovelar approach progresses from the medial side of the tonsil, through the inferior medullary velum toward the lateral recess of the fourth ventricle, and over the superior tonsillar surface between the uvula and the tonsil. The supratonsillar approach progresses from the lateral side of the tonsil through the tonsillobiventral (or *secondary*) fissure toward the tonsillar peduncle, inferior cerebellar peduncle, and dentate nucleus. This fissure becomes prominent and recognizable laterally where the folia of the biventral lobule and tonsil intersect at an acute angle rather than in parallel, as folia do elsewhere, to form a chevron along the fissure. In addition, the p5 cortical segments of the PICA emerge from this fissure and radiate as medial vermian and lateral hemispheric branches, serving as clear landmarks that identify the fissure and help open it during the dissection. The tonsillar peduncle lies at the depths of the fissure and marks the extent of transulcal reach, after which tissue transgression is needed to reach the target. Both approaches are performed through a standard suboccipital craniotomy. The original report of the supratonsillar approach described a three-quarter prone position. We transitioned to a fully prone position and linear incision, with a C1 laminectomy to steepen the ascent over the tonsil.

Surgical Approach

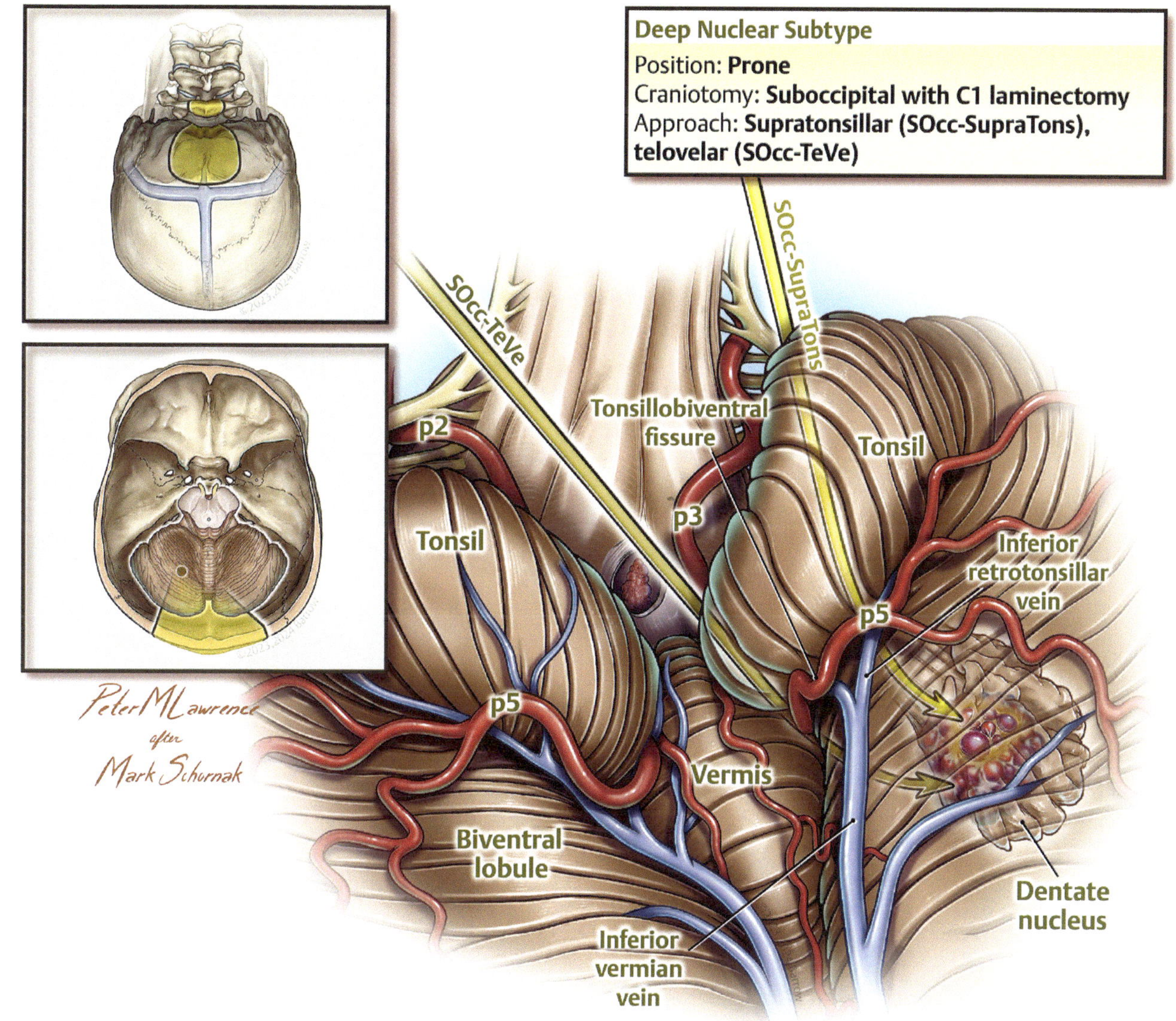

Fig. 17.9 Overview of approaches to deep nuclear cerebellar CMs. Deep nuclear cerebellar CMs are accessed through a suboccipital craniotomy with C1 laminectomy (*upper left inset*) and supratonsillar approach for lateral lesions, or the telovelar approach for medial lesions (*lower left inset*; *yellow circle*). The SOcc-SupraTons approach traces the p5 cortical segment of the PICA distally to proximally, as the tonsillobiventral fissure is split to provide a dissection corridor for laterally seated deep nuclear CMs. The SOcc-TeVe approach mobilizes the tonsil superiorly together with the ipsilateral biventral lobule, allowing dissection of the tela choroidea from the inferior medullary velum and opening of an inferior-to-superior corridor that is optimal for medially seated deep nuclear CMs (surgical case; ▸ Video 17.2; QR code). (Reproduced with permission from Barrow Neurological Institute, Phoenix, AZ.)

Surgical Case 17.2

CEREBELLAR

Cavernoma Subtype: Deep Nuclear

Position: Prone
Craniotomy: Suboccipital with a C1 laminectomy
Approach: Supratonsillar (SOcc-SupraTons)
Triangle: None
SEZ: None
Artery: p4 PICA

Video: Resection of a left deep nuclear cerebellar cavernoma

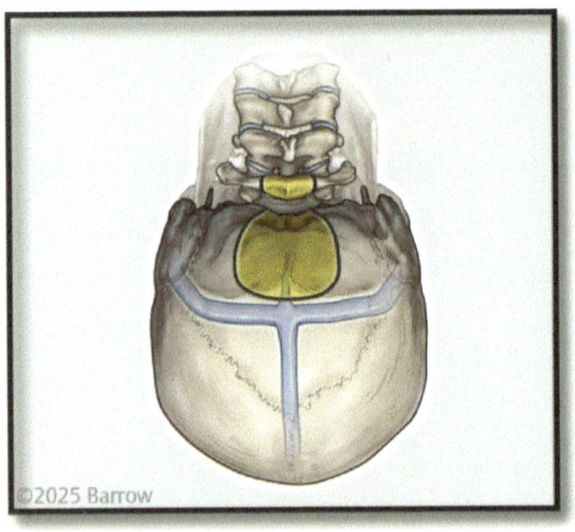

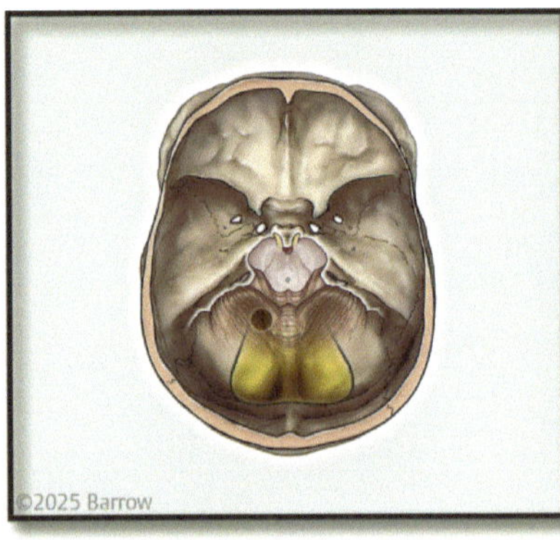

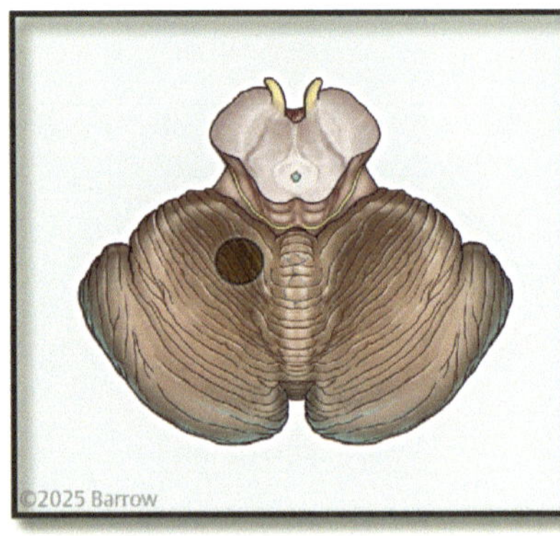

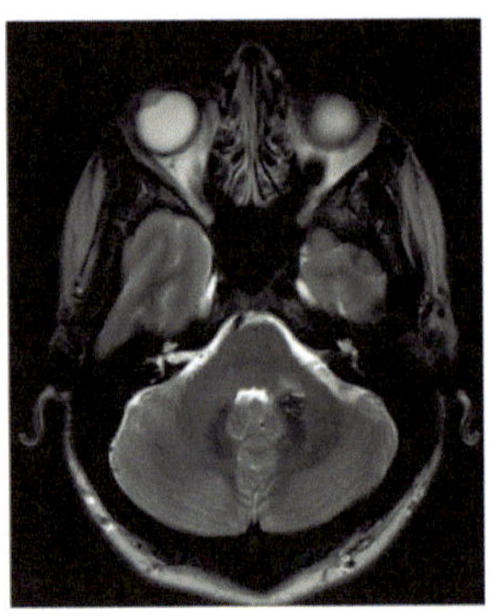

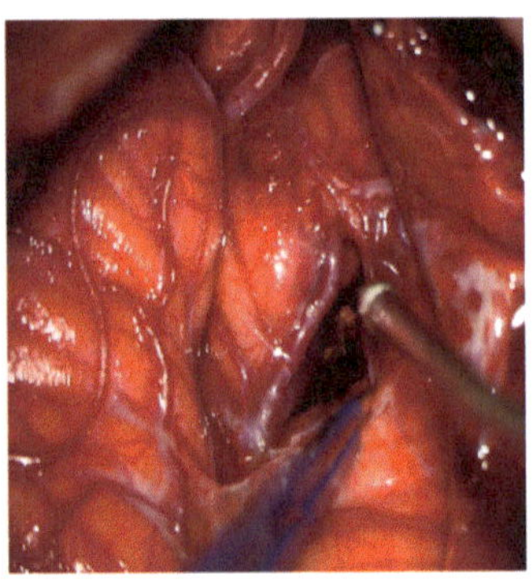

Video 17.2
Suboccipital Craniotomy with Supratonsillar Approach for Deep Nuclear Cerebellar Cavernous Malformation Resection (Reproduced with permission from Barrow Neurological Institute, Phoenix, AZ.)

17

17.5 Conclusion

The taxonomy for cerebellar CMs completes the comprehensive system characterizing all CMs we have encountered in the brain, with seven types, including the cerebrum, basal ganglia, thalamus, midbrain, pons, medulla, and cerebellum. Multiple subtypes are associated with each CM type, as defined by the anatomical surfaces on which the lesions present (anterior, lateral, posterior, anterolateral, or posterolateral). Overall, 35 CM subtypes have been defined, including 16 subtypes in the brainstem, 9 deep cerebral subtypes, 4 superficial cerebral subtypes, and 6 subtypes in the cerebellum. With this taxonomy, a particular CM's anatomical location is uniquely defined by its type and subtype, analogous to the binomial nomenclature that classifies plants and animals by genus and species. Additionally, taxonomic subtyping is correlated with radiographic anatomy on MRI. The subtype can be associated with a constellation of symptoms and signs that localize the lesion with bedside examination findings, and it describes CMs precisely for clear clinical communications and publications.

The taxonomy for brainstem CMs and deep cerebral CMs succeeded in defining specific neurological syndromes and informing microsurgical management by associating each subtype with a specific craniotomy, approach, dissection triangle, and safe entry zone. In contrast, taxonomy for cerebellar CMs was less impactful because specific syndromes were not apparent, and the selection of craniotomy and approach reduced to a choice between three craniotomies (suboccipital, torcular, or retrosigmoid) and two approaches (translobular or transsulcal).

Despite the many cranial nerves and the skull base anatomy in the posterior fossa, cerebellar CMs are primarily convexity lesions that do not require dissection triangles or safe entry zones for exposure. When CMs were located beneath the cerebellar surface, we minimized tissue transgression to preserve associated function and reduce morbidity, exploiting transsulcal approaches through major and minor fissures like the petrosal and tonsillobiventral fissures. These fissures were prominent in patients with atrophy, but unlike cerebral fissures that transmit arteries defining separation planes, cerebellar fissures might not have such arteries, and the folia can be more difficult to separate. Outcomes after cerebellar CM resection are excellent, with most operations achieving complete resection without a new deficit. The proposed taxonomy for cerebellar CMs (suboccipital, tentorial, petrosal, vermian, tonsillar, and deep nuclear) can guide the selection of craniotomy and approach to enhance patient safety and optimize neurological outcomes.

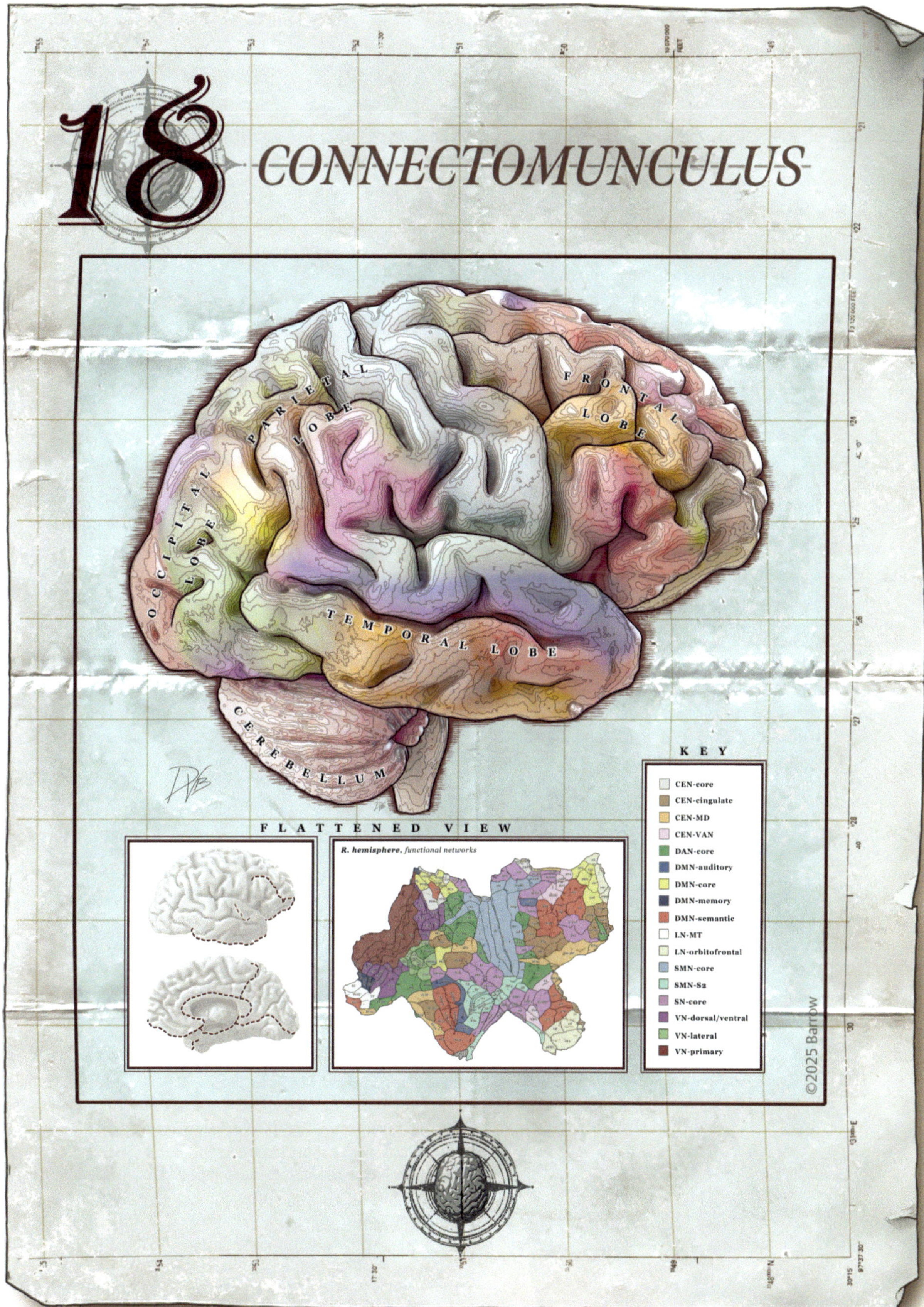

Reproduced with permission from Barrow Neurological Institute, Phoenix, AZ.

18 Seven Cavernomas: Project Connectomunculus and the Mind

Summary

One of the goals of *Seven Cavernomas* was to develop a taxonomy to guide the surgical management of cavernous malformations (CMs) in the brain. A classification system of lesion locations and surface presentations was developed, comprising 7 types and 35 subtypes. This systematic approach served as a roadmap to guide neurosurgeons safely to targeted lesions. Thus, cartography became a recurring theme. Cartography for brainstem CMs mapped the special relationships of craniotomy to approach to anatomical triangles, safe entry zones, and arteries as vascular waypoints. These relationships provide heuristics to help with approach selection and surgical rehearsal. The taxonomic framework inspires confidence, improves patient outcomes, and provides a consistent nomenclature for discussion. Cartography for cerebral cavernomas was distinctly more complex, drawing on different organizational paradigms such as somatotopy, tonotopy, and retinotopy. Thus, Penfield created the homunculus to map cognition and movement to somatotopic brain parcels. Modern neuroimaging and connectomics have now progressed to more sophisticated systems of brain connectivity. Modern heuristics must now account for intelligence, creativity, memory, and reason on the basis of *eloquent* and *eloquent noneloquent* brain parcellations. When the brain's surface was flattened for mapping, network triads clustered in certain lobes. Three primary network triads (central executive network-core, default mode network [DMN]-core, and DMN-semantic) are positioned between crucial motor and sensory networks in the frontal, parietal, and temporal lobes. This positioning enables access to afferent and efferent information, relays it to centers involved in internal and external cognitive tasks, and communicates that activity through language. Thus, the idea of the connectomunculus was created. We have a basic knowledge of motor, sensory, and visual systems, but we do not yet understand emotion, memory, neural plasticity, intelligence, and consciousness. These amazing facets of the mind make us human, and nothing is more important than understanding that. If we can conceive a future where our neurosurgical specialty is the vehicle for voyaging to this final frontier, then the future of neurosurgery is transformative and thrilling. This goal of exploring the mind to unravel these mysteries is the most exciting way to conclude this *Seven Cavernomas* book.

Keywords: brainstem, cartography, cavernous malformation, cerebrum, connectome, craniotomy, homunculus, maps, microsurgical approach

18.1 Seven Cavernomas Cartography

Cartography is the chosen metaphor in *Seven Cavernomas*, and one of the objectives of this project was to create maps that synthesize the book's content. *Seven Cavernomas* embodies a framework for the classification and surgical management of cavernomas in the brain. A taxonomy was constructed that classified lesions according to their location and surface presentation into 7 types and 35 subtypes (▶ Fig. 18.1). This taxonomy established optimal or preferred surgical approaches to reach and resect each target cavernoma safely. The framework prioritized safe and elegant approaches through natural corridors for free passage within the brain's subarachnoid space. The framework was designed to lead neurosurgeons through decision-making to select the best approach to targeted cavernomas, better prepare for surgery, and improve patient outcomes. Analyses of cavernoma subtypes revealed associated clinical syndromes, which could increase bedside acumen. Significant tools like the brainstem cavernous malformation (CM) grading scale and the definition of giant-sized cavernomas were provided to help guide patient selection. The right-angle method was introduced to identify residual pathology before closure to ensure complete resection. Ultimately, the *Seven Cavernomas* framework was created, which genuinely enhances the conceptualization, surgical management, and discussion of these lesions.

Cartography for brainstem cavernomas was successful, with maps that incorporated the taxonomy and the triangle concept, with its relationship of craniotomy to approach to anatomical triangles, safe entry zones, and arteries as vascular waypoints (▶ Fig. 18.2). The complex skull base anatomy and intricate neural circuitry of the brainstem make these maps robust. The maps are heuristics that help with approach selection, surgical rehearsal, intraoperative dissection, neurosurgeon confidence, and patient outcomes. They can also educate the next generation of neurosurgeons, who have limitless enthusiasm but limited experience, and help them gain the surgical competence needed to begin treating patients. The maps can motivate their learning and whet their appetite for treating cavernomas. These maps can inspire the trailblazers among us to explore remote territories and discover new paths, expanding the neurosurgical armamentarium in ways we cannot envision today.

Building robust maps for cerebral cavernomas proved more elusive. Although it is possible to describe a set of approaches, as we have done, it is unclear whether these approaches are sufficient to optimize patient outcomes. Cerebral and cerebellar approaches are either transgyral or transsulcal, making them simpler, shallower, and less informed by cartography. More significantly, the cerebrum's complexity is staggering and becomes ever more complicated as we study it.

Anatomical organization paradigms, such as somatotopy, tonotopy, and retinotopy, provide learnable and intellectually pleasing frameworks to explain complex brain anatomy in understandable and actionable ways. Penfield's homunculus (▶ Fig. 18.3) made sense when cognition was conceived as parcels of the brain arranged somatotopically, acting individually to move, feel, or see. The homunculus made sense when only certain parts of the cerebrum were considered eloquent, and

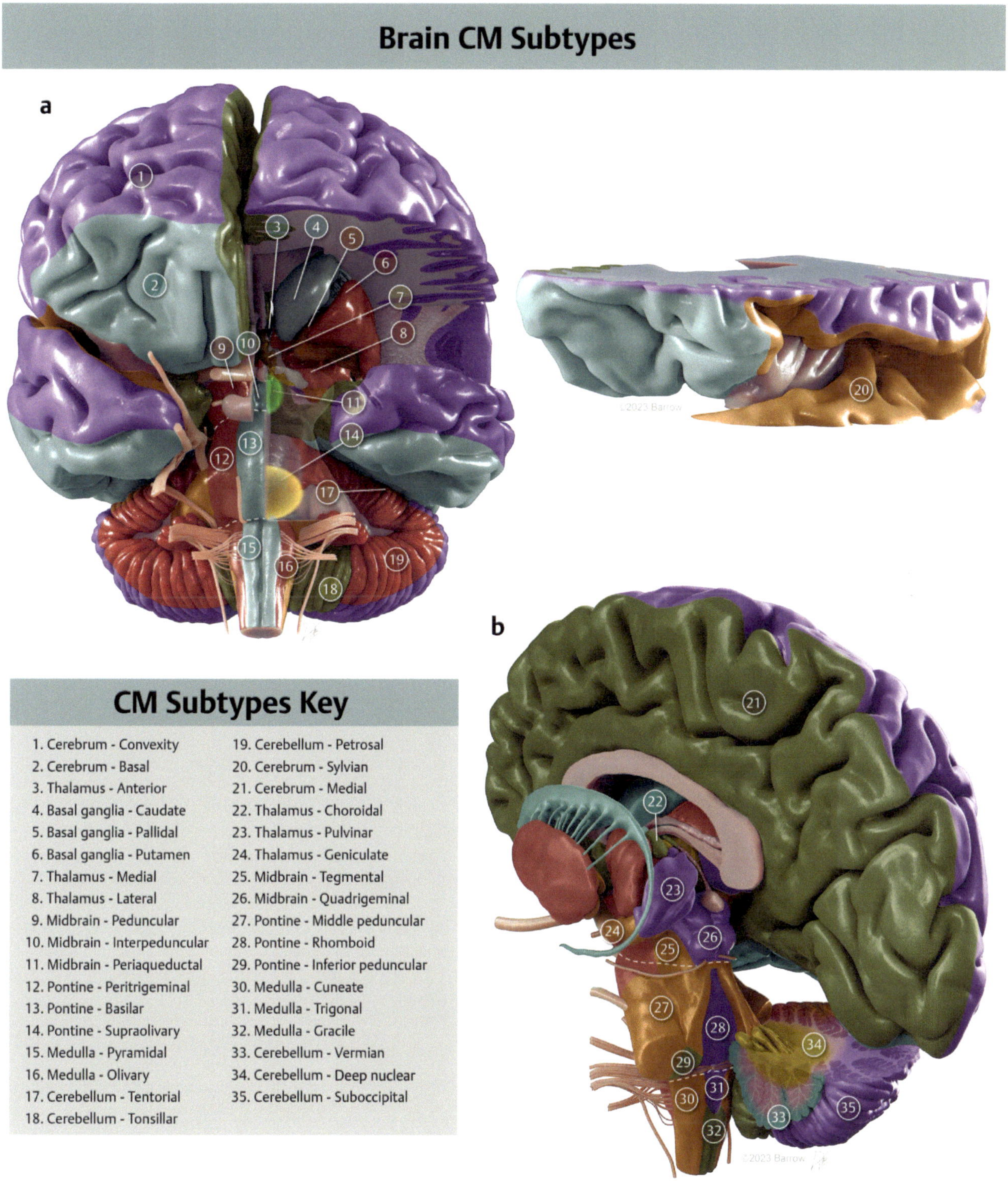

Fig. 18.1 Summary of the comprehensive taxonomy of 7 types and 35 subtypes of CMs in the brain that categorize the spectrum of pathology into specific and recognizable entities, leading to unique recommendations for microsurgical management. **(a)** Anterior view of the brain, with anterolateral view of a section of the brain. **(b)** Posterolateral view of the right hemisphere, left basal ganglia, left thalamus, and brainstem. (Reproduced with permission from Barrow Neurological Institute, Phoenix, AZ.)

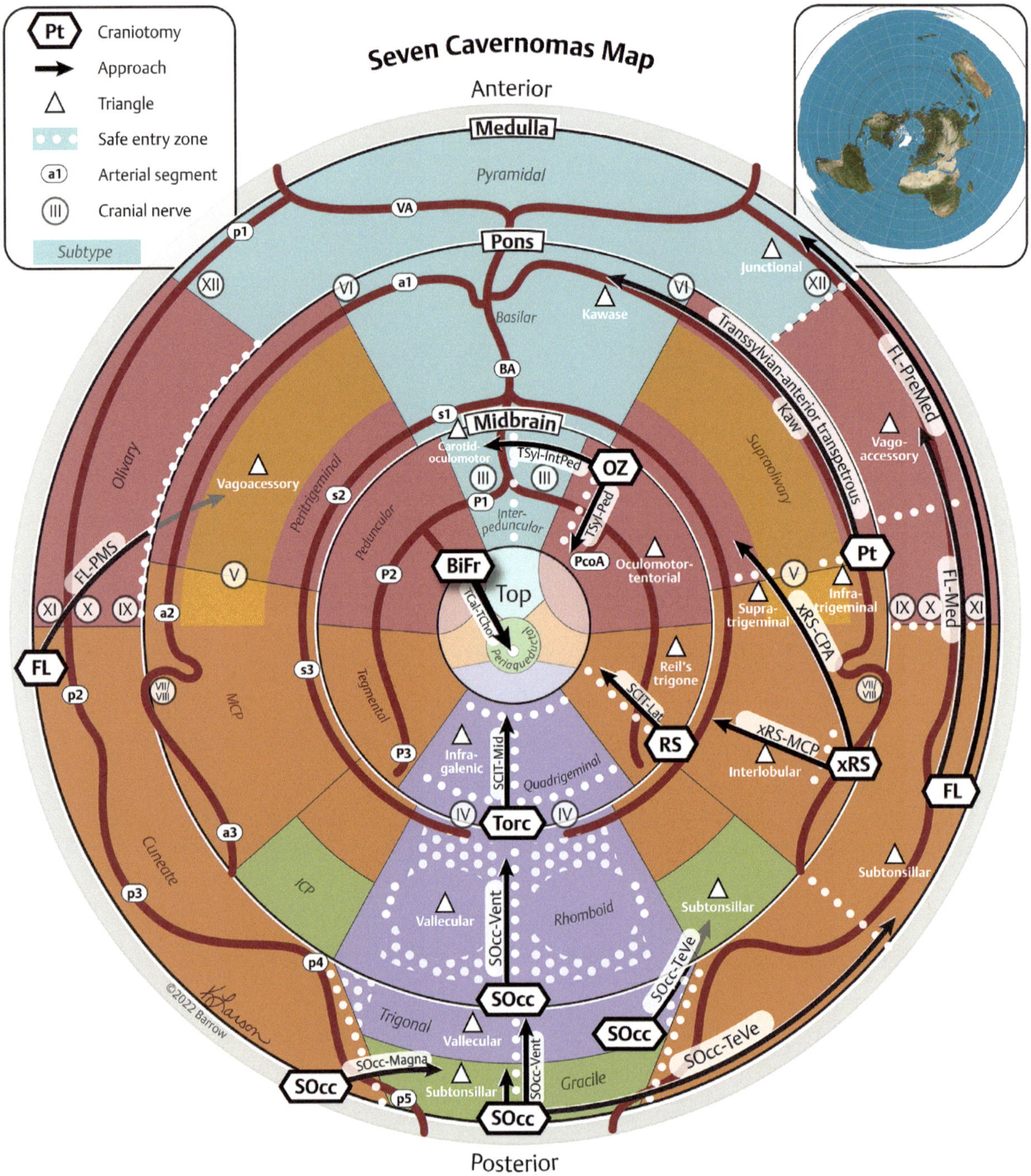

Fig. 18.2 Example of cartography summarizing the taxonomy of cavernoma types and subtypes, craniotomies, approaches, anatomical triangles, arterial waypoints, SEZs, and CNs associated with the 16 brainstem cavernomas. This map is based on an azimuthal equidistant projection (*inset*). Roman numerals denote CNs. (Reproduced with permission from Barrow Neurological Institute, Phoenix, AZ.)

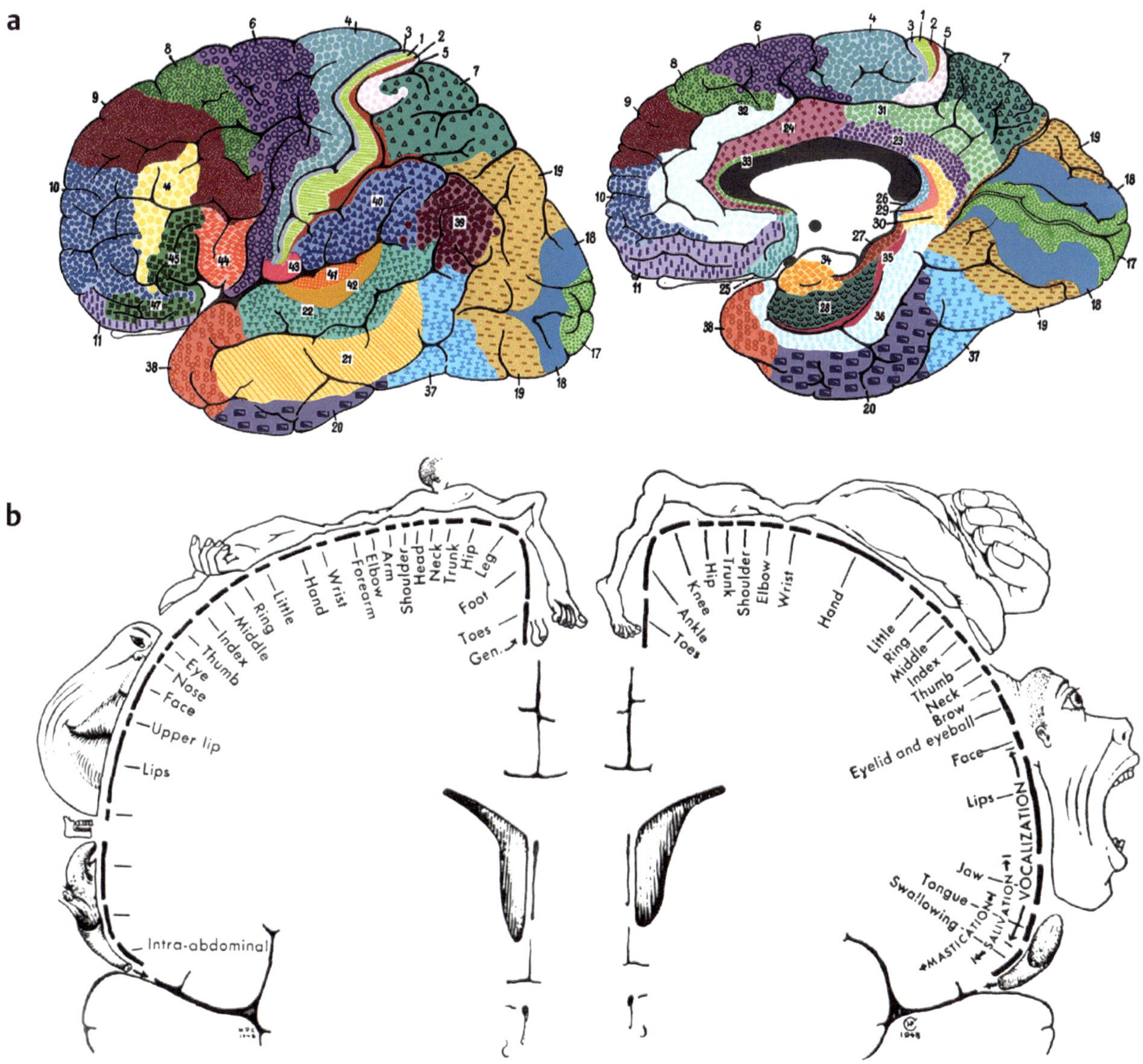

Fig. 18.3 Mapping brain function. **(a)** Brodmann areas define 52 distinct regions based on cytoarchitecture and correspond to discrete brain functions (lateral [*left*] and medial [*right*] views). However, the gaps in the numerical sequence from 13 to 16 and from 48 to 51 are not shown on the human map because Brodmann described them in primate brains and could not find corresponding areas in the human brain. **(b)** Classic illustration of Wilder Penfield's homunculus showing the somatotopic organization of sensation on the left and motor function on the right of this coronal transection through the cerebrum, with neurological representation proportionate to the size of the figures. (Image **a** is modified from public domain: https://commons.wikimedia.org/wiki/File:Human_Brodmann_areas_(K._Brodmann,_1909,_p._131,_Fig._85-86).jpg. Image **b** is provided courtesy of Osler Library of the History of Medicine, McGill University.)

the rest were considered silent or transitional from an evolutionary perspective.

However pleasing this idea is, it is now evident that the higher cognitive systems of the brain are not organized in this simple, easily understandable way. Modern neuroimaging and human connectomics now inform our understanding of the brain as a sophisticated system of seemingly unrelated brain parcels interconnected through white matter tracts and synchronized electrically with spikes and oscillations of variable amplitudes, frequencies, and phases. The wiring of 86 billion neurons and signaling among 100 trillion synapses is so bewildering that armies of neuroengineers, computer scientists, cognitive neuroscientists, functional neurosurgeons, and neurologists struggle to understand the brain's orchestrated interactivity. A mysterious language underlies the brain's relationship to human cognition and mental ability, and we are barely able to hear, much less decipher, this language. The ability to decode and encode this language seems remote now and would be transformative. From this perspective, heuristics like the homunculus are antiquated or anachronistic, and modern heuristics must account for higher functions like intelligence, creativity, memory, and reason. Given this context, creating a map to suitably represent the human cerebrum is a vexing challenge, and it will require concerted, multidisciplinary action to solve this puzzle. Defining the scope of future efforts is a critical first step.

18.2 The Connectomunculus

The code name for our cerebral map was *Connectomunculus*. I initially envisioned it as an update to the homunculus that would incorporate human connectomics and large-scale brain networks formed by interconnected cortical parcellations to create a contemporary heuristic to guide surgery in eloquent and *eloquent noneloquent* cerebral parcels. ▸ Fig. 18.3, ▸ Fig. 18.4, ▸ Fig. 18.5, ▸ Fig. 18.6 show the progression from Brodmann areas and Penfield's homunculus to the immense surface area of cerebral convolutions, Glasser's 180 parcellations in each hemisphere, the dense wiring of interconnecting white matter tracts, and the large-scale brain networks that consist of these parcels and tracts. We attempted to simplify the bewildering number of parcellations by dividing them into regional clusters that might make large-scale brain networks more memorable or intuitive (▸ Fig. 18.7, ▸ Fig. 18.8). However, these gyral-parcellation-sulcal maps, or *gypsum* maps, yielded what might be characterized as subway art or brain graffiti. Finding a simple way to describe the cognitive systems of the brain is not so simple.

Next, we attempted to flatten the cerebrum's three dimensions into two, in the same manner that maps flatten the spherical Earth. Surface cuts allowed the cortex to unfurl into flat maps (▸ Fig. 18.9, ▸ Fig. 18.10), and a pattern among the parcellations revealed a clue to the brain's logic. We noticed network triads where parcellations from three networks clustered in multiple lobes of the brain: the central executive network (CEN)-core, the default mode network (DMN)-core, and the DMN-semantic. The DMN is one of the largest and most significant networks because it runs the internal activity of the mind to process sensory information, filter memories, and ruminate. In contrast, the CEN performs functions such as engaging in external tasks, thinking through problems, making decisions, and planning actions. Semantic cognition allows humans to understand the meaning of words, objects, places, and people to guide thoughts and actions. Language is a unique human capacity that enables us to understand ideas, draw inferences, maintain coherence, and conduct conversation. The CEN-core,

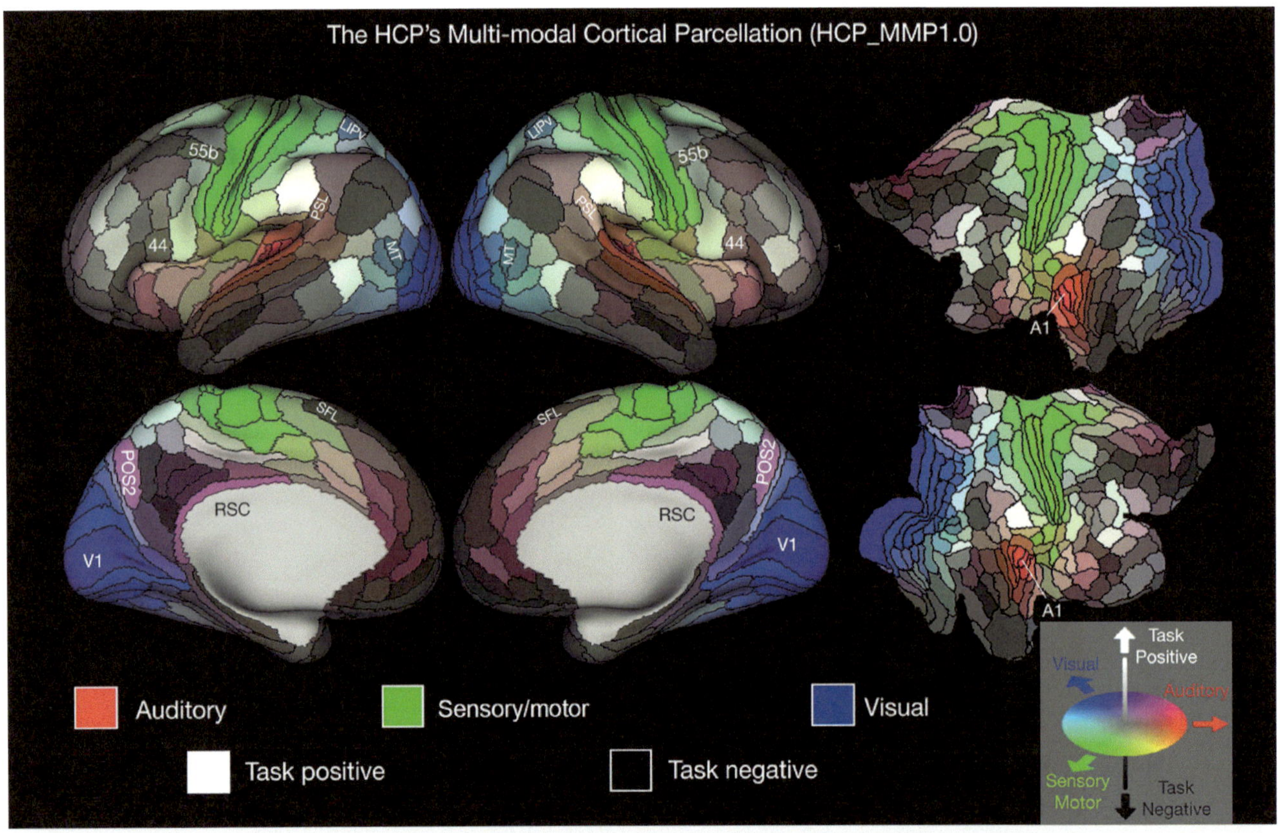

Fig. 18.4 Mapping brain function. Glasser delineated 180 parcels per hemisphere in the human cerebral cortex bounded by sharp changes in cortical architecture, function, connectivity, and topography based on multimodal MRI from the Human Connectome Project. (Reproduced with permission from Glasser MF, Coalson TS, Robinson EC, et al. A multi-modal parcellation of human cerebral cortex. Nature 2016;536(7615):171–178).

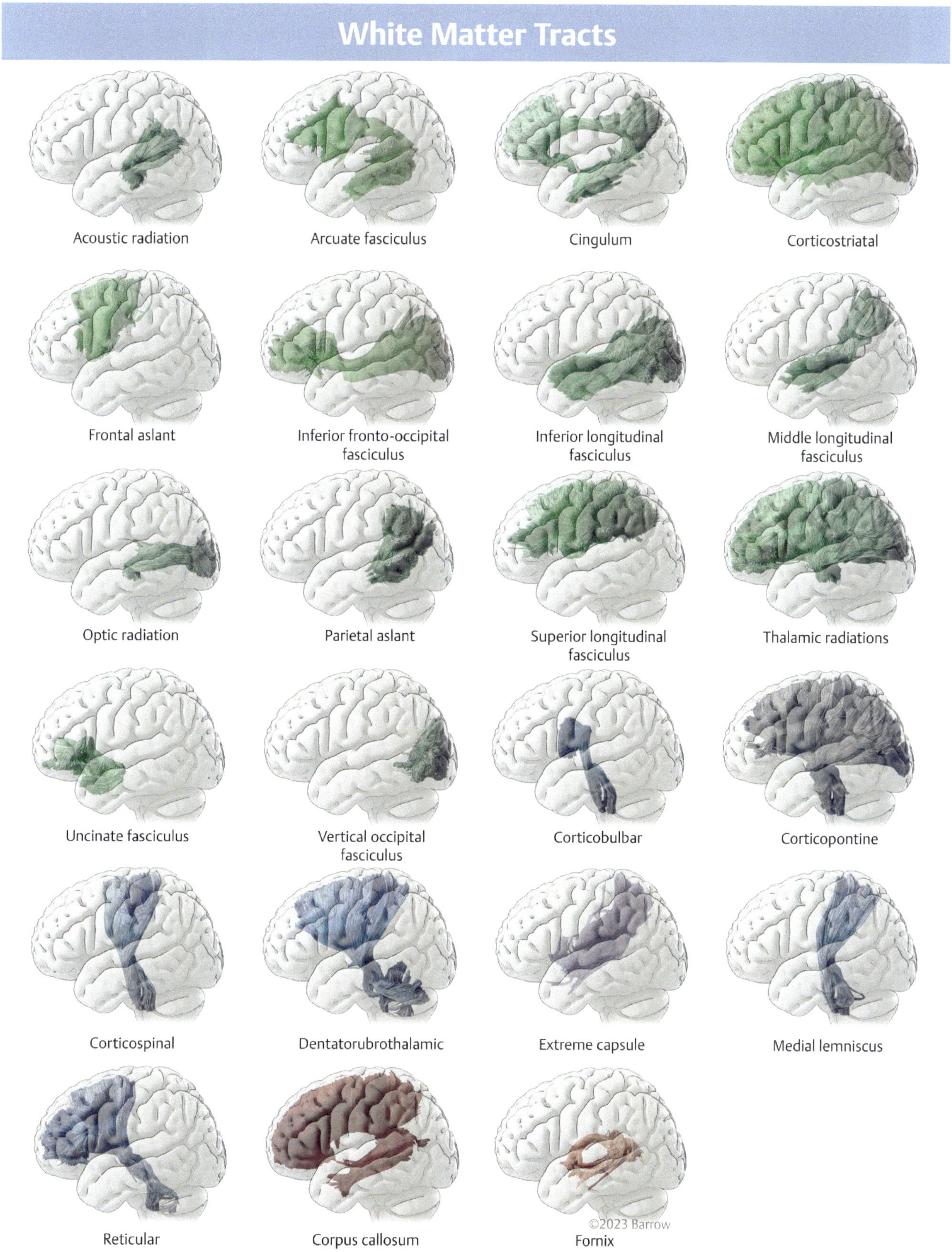

Fig. 18.5 Summary of 23 tracts in the cerebral white matter connecting cortical parcels, deep nuclei, and brainstem areas. (Reproduced with permission from Barrow Neurological Institute, Phoenix, AZ.)

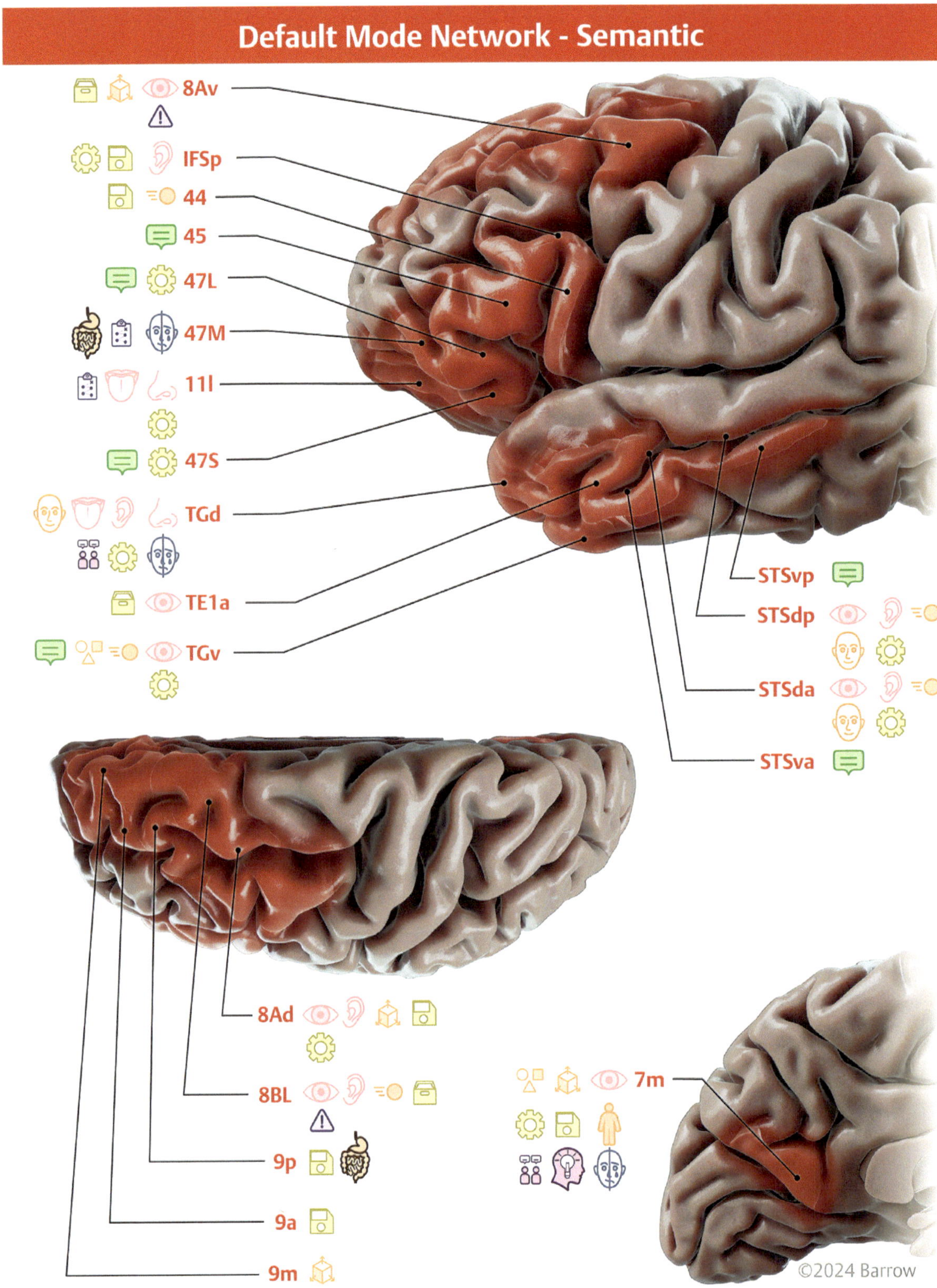

Fig. 18.6 Illustration of the DMN-semantic and the cortical parcels that it comprises. DMN-semantic is one of 17 large-scale brain networks that include the sensorimotor network, CEN, visual network, salience network, limbic network, and ventral and dorsal attention networks. A key to the icons depicting a parcel's function can be found in the network gallery at the end of this chapter. (Reproduced with permission from Barrow Neurological Institute, Phoenix, AZ.)

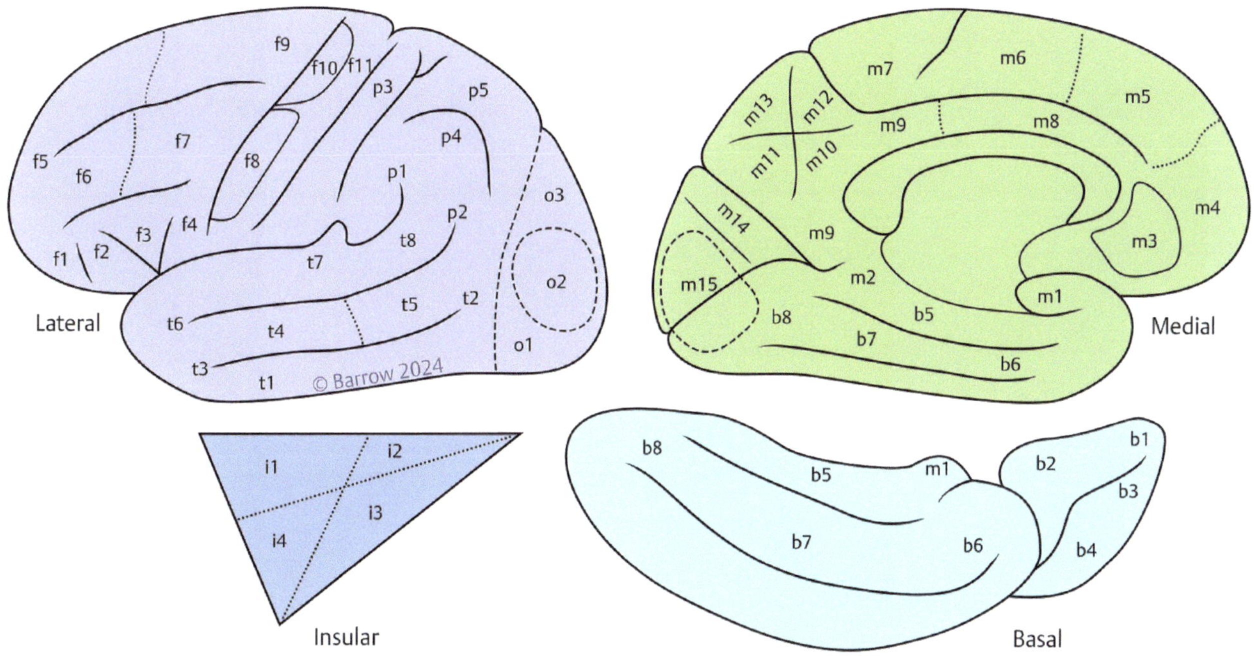

Fig. 18.7 Mapping gyral and sulcal networks. Gyral-parcellation-sulcal maps, or *gypsum* maps, condense multiple parcels into larger clusters and are labeled alphanumerically as b, basal; f, frontal; i, insular; m, medial; o, occipital; p, parietal; t, temporal. (Reproduced with permission from Lawton MT, Tayebi Meybodi A, Sughrue ME, et al. Seven Cavernomas, Project "Connectomunculus," and the mind. J Neurosurg 2025;142(5):1498–1516.)

DMN-core, and DMN-semantic triads are positioned between other important motor and sensory networks in the frontal, parietal, and temporal lobes. This positioning apparently enables access to afferent and efferent information, feeds it forward to centers involved in internal and external cognitive tasks, and communicates that activity through language.

What is the point of this pattern of repetition? Evolutionary and developmental study is frequently helpful in deducing organ function, especially when a structure first appeared in the evolutionary process. Although few detailed connectome-level comparisons have been performed using neuroimaging, a wealth of detailed cytoarchitectural work spans decades. A reasonable inference can be made that cytoarchitecturally similar regions in the cortex in similar anatomic areas are likely to perform similar network functions. This assumption is under study with comparative neuroimaging.

When we compared the network anatomy of human, primate, and rat brains, there was a clear pattern of triadic expansion during mammalian evolution, notably during primate evolution (▶ Fig. 18.11). Triads, limited in lower mammals like felines and rats, begin to emerge phylogenetically in primates and are concentrated in the neocortical areas that are evolutionarily newer. This observation suggests that higher cognitive function in humans might be due to the hardwiring that drives broader and faster dissemination of neuronal activity across brain networks. Creativity, intelligence, insight, and wisdom may translate to the extent or speed of intercommunication between the parcellations composing the cerebrum. In other words, triads likely help the brain assume complex brain states, coordinating numerous regions in unique ways. These changes underlie our emergence as cognitively flexible beings.

Embryologic studies suggest that brain networks, rather than being a random hodgepodge of regions, follow a pattern strongly rooted in the developmental patterning of the neural tube before folding and cortical maturation. The fetal cerebrum begins as a spherical telencephalon with the basic networks (i.e., sensorimotor, visual, auditory, and attention) arranged territorially in proximity to one another (▶ Fig. 18.12; ▶ Video 18.1). As the brain develops, the ever-increasing cortical surface area is confined within a fixed cranial volume. This confinement triggers expansion into lobules and lobes, rotation of lobes to conform to the skull shape, and convolutional infoldings to form sulci and fissures. The basic networks appear static in size throughout fetal development. In contrast, the triads associated

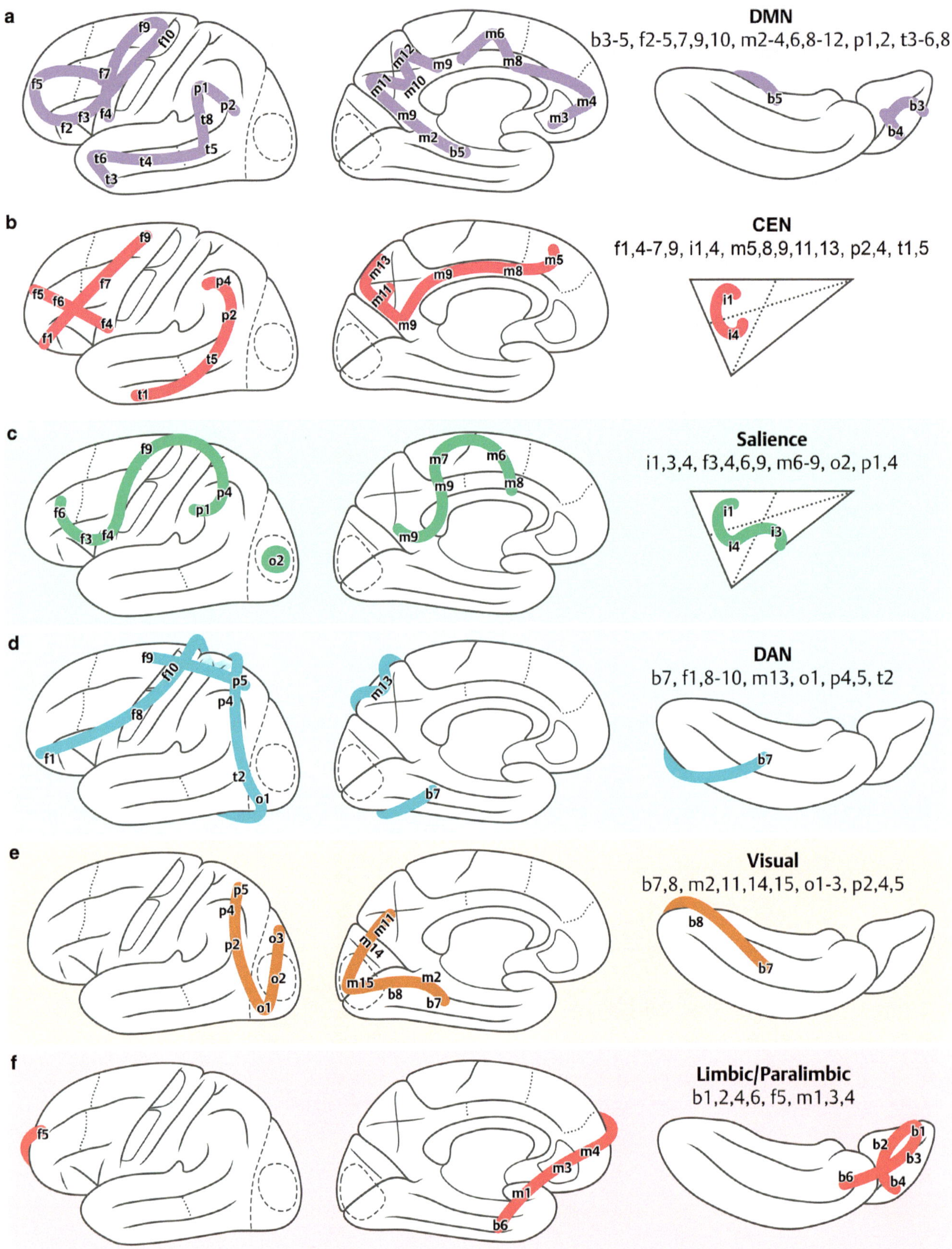

Fig. 18.8 Mapping gyral and sulcal networks. The clusters involved in the **(a)** DMN, **(b)** CEN, **(c)** salience, **(d)** DAN, **(e)** visual, and **(f)** limbic networks are joined by the colored letters, which reflect the acronyms of these networks. (Reproduced with permission from Lawton MT, Tayebi Meybodi A, Sughrue ME, et al. Seven Cavernomas, Project "Connectomunculus," and the mind. J Neurosurg 2025;142(5):1498–1516.)

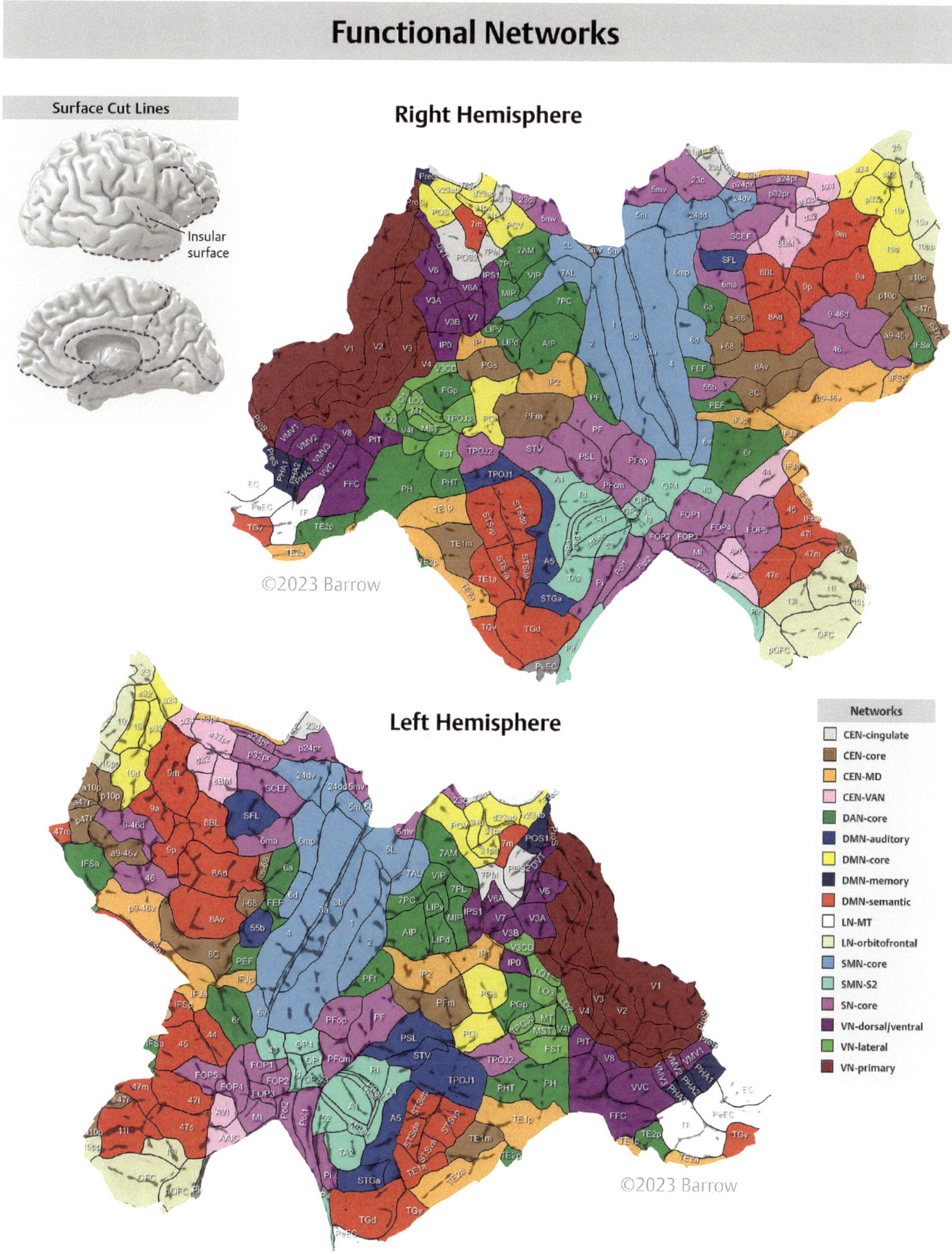

Fig. 18.9 Mapping functional networks and triads. Flat map showing the right cerebrum's parcellations and the 17 large-scale brain networks associated with these parcels. Cuts are made in various places in the lateral and medial cortex (*inset, dashed lines*) to convert the three-dimensional hemisphere into two-dimensional flat maps. (Reproduced with permission from Barrow Neurological Institute, Phoenix, AZ.)

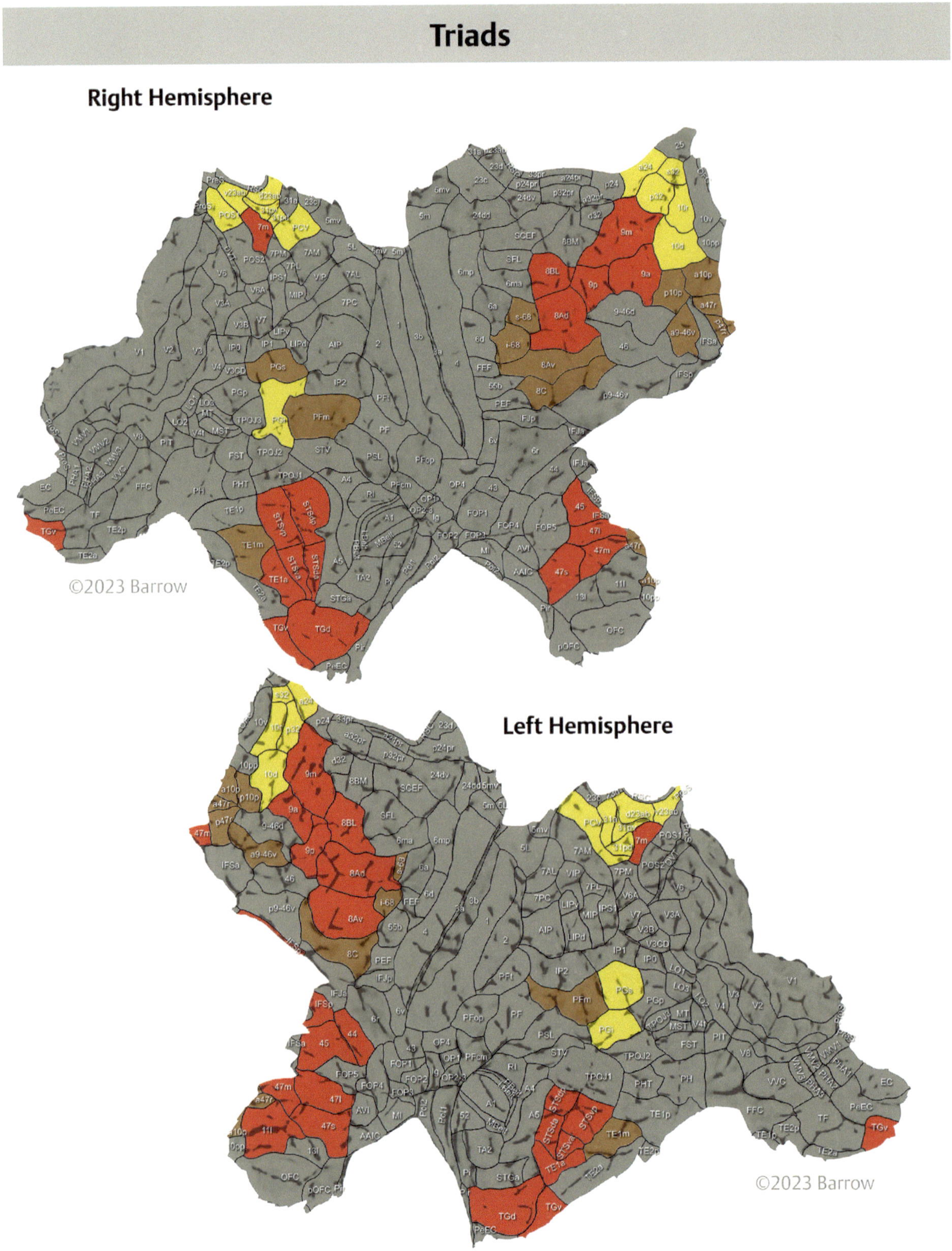

Fig. 18.10 Mapping functional networks and triads. Parcellations from three networks clustered as triads in multiple lobes of the brain: the CEN-core (*brown*), the DMN-core (*yellow*), and the DMN-semantic (*red*). These triads are located between other important motor and sensory networks (*gray*) to access afferent and efferent information, feed that information to centers involved in cognitive tasks, and communicate that activity through language. (Reproduced with permission from Barrow Neurological Institute, Phoenix, AZ.)

Rat, Macaque, and Human Functional Networks

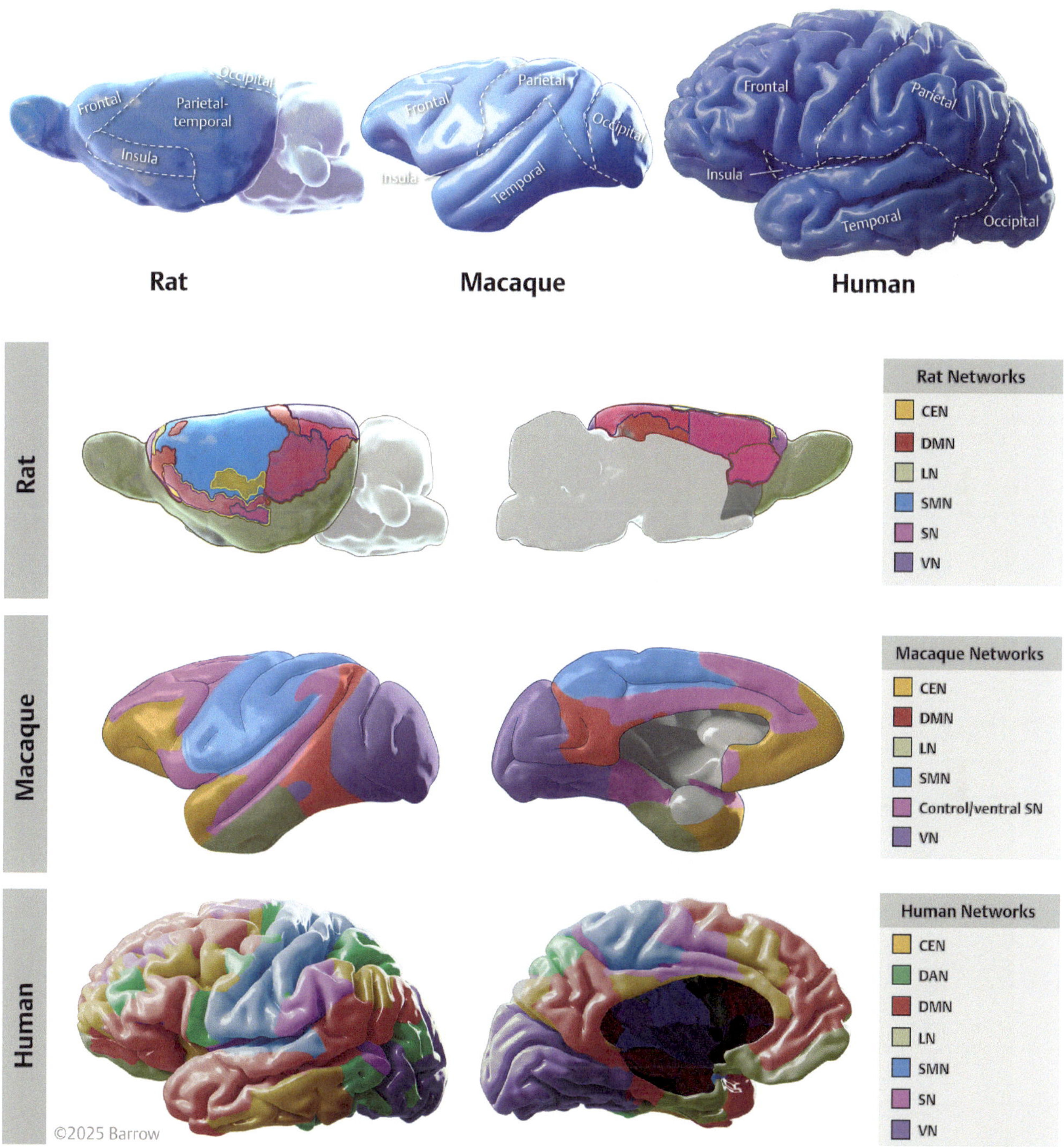

Fig. 18.11 Comparison of functional networks in rat, macaque, and human brains. Gross anatomy demonstrates evolutionary increases in overall brain volume, with enlargement of the frontal, parietal, and temporal lobes and increasing convolutions of the cortical surface (*first row*). Importantly, limited areas of the DMN and CEN are seen in rats (*second row*), with progressive expansion of triads in macaques (*third row*) and humans (*fourth row*) and concentrations of triads in evolutionarily newer neocortical areas. (Reproduced with permission from Barrow Neurological Institute, Phoenix, AZ.)

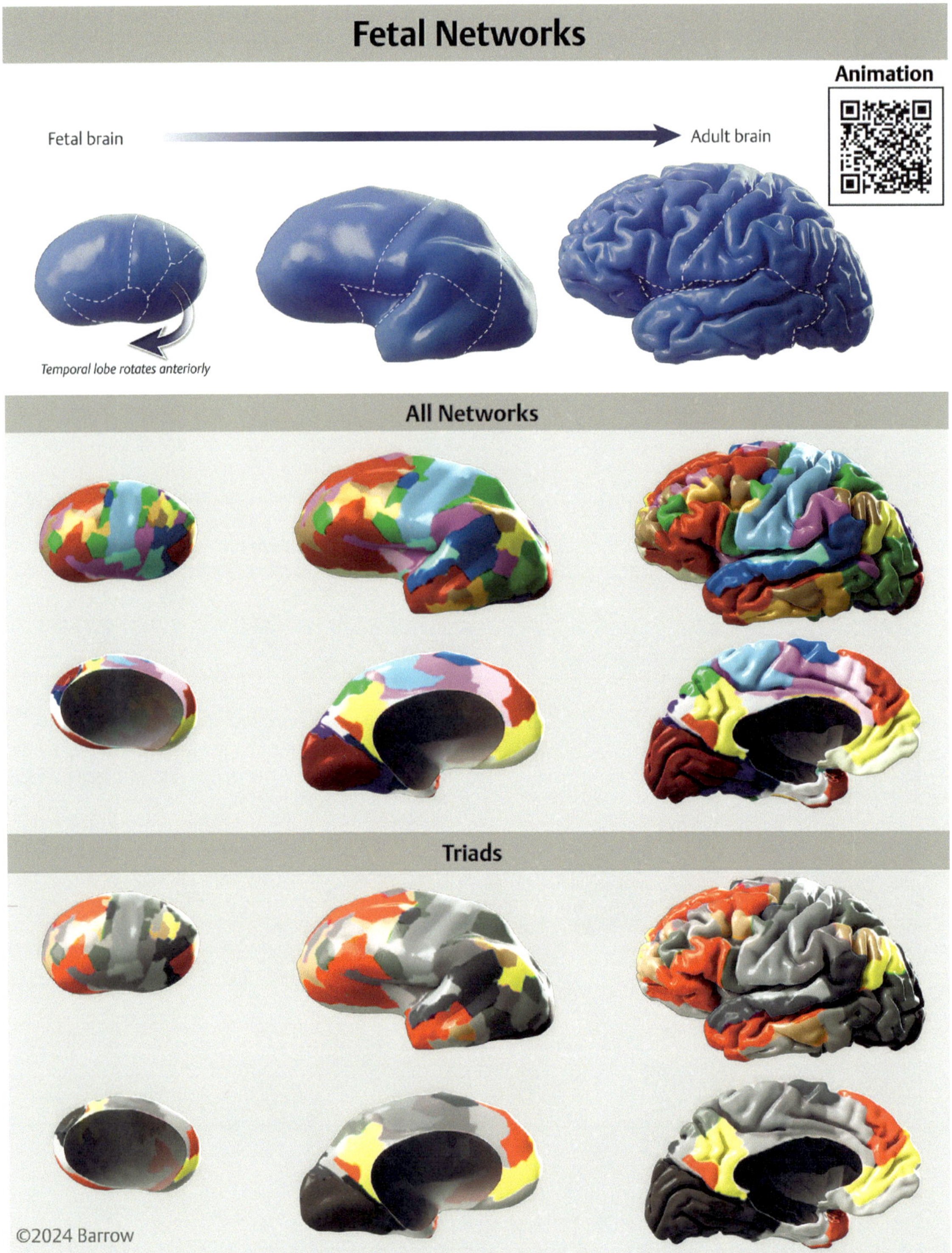

Fig. 18.12 Embryologically, the brain begins as a spherical telencephalon, expands into lobules and lobes (outlined with *dashed lines*), rotates to conform to skull confines, and convolutes to form sulci and fissures (*upper panel*). Basic networks including the sensorimotor, visual, auditory, and attention networks appear static in size throughout fetal development (*middle panel*). Lateral (*middle panel, upper row*) and medial (*middle panel, lower row*) views of the developing brain are shown, with all networks highlighted. In contrast, the CEN-core, DMN-core, and DMN-semantic triads associated with higher cognitive function appear to enlarge and displace the basic networks (*lower panel*). Lateral (*lower panel, upper row*) and medial (*lower panel, lower row*) views of the developing brain are shown, with triads highlighted (animation; ▶ Video 18.1, Lateral and medial views of the developing brain; QR code). (Reproduced with permission from Barrow Neurological Institute, Phoenix, AZ.)

with higher cognitive function appear to enlarge and displace the basic networks in a manner akin to continental drift in geology. About 200 million years ago, the continents on Earth were one huge supercontinent surrounded by ocean, and this Pangaea (▶ Fig. 18.13) broke apart and spread out as the tectonic plates migrated over time to form the seven continents we know today. Similarly, the basic networks seen across animal species break apart and separate as the triads of networks found only in higher species expand. This neuroanatomy may be one explanation of our cognitive gifts.

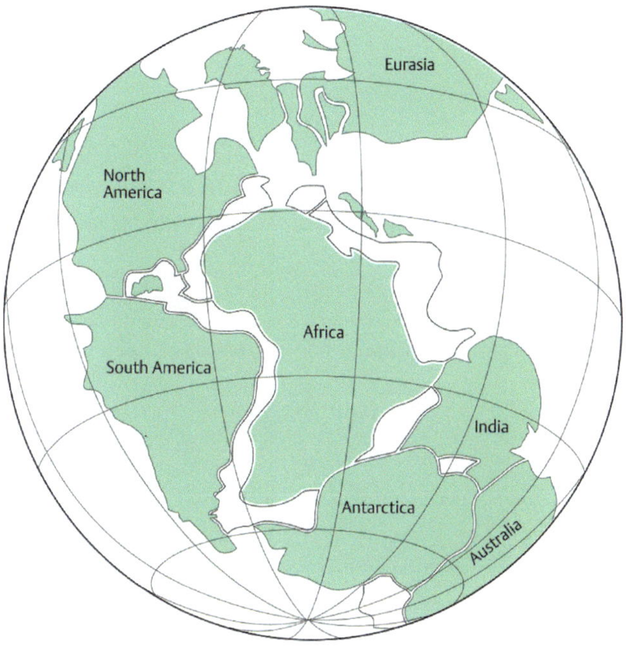

Fig. 18.13 Pangaea was a supercontinent that broke apart about 200 million years ago and spread out to form the seven continents. Basic brain networks are analogous to Pangaea, and the triads (CEN-core, DMN-core, and DMN-semantic) associated with higher species and higher cortical function displace these networks with evolution and fetal development in a manner analogous to continental drift. (Copyright made available under Creative Commons CC BY-SA 3.0; https://creativecommons.org/licenses/by-sa/3.0.)

These musings around a connectomunculus were intended to define cortical safe entry zones analogous to the brainstem safe entry zones that meaningfully guide the neurosurgeon's entrance into and through critical tissues. ▶ Fig. 18.14 and ▶ Fig. 18.15 depict traditional eloquence and new eloquent noneloquence based on classical anatomy and our superficial cerebral cavernoma experience. With the addition of the seven cerebral hotspots of eloquent noneloquence and the triads coordinating cognitive activity, the amount of unsafe, unenterable cortex has nearly doubled. Substantial areas of safe entry still exist in the cortical landscape, but this reduction heralds an important shift in the conduct of transcerebral surgery. Given the complexity of large-scale brain networks and the importance of white matter interconnections to intelligence and creativity, one might argue that the cortical safe entry zones are still too generous. These so-called safe areas are more likely to reflect the lack of neuropsychological outcome data to demonstrate the eloquence of this brain tissue. However, the figures serve as a conclusion of our work thus far. They are crude at best and difficult to apply intuitively. Although I had hoped to arrive at the definitive connectomunculus for generations to come, I have submitted these figures as a work in progress from my team.

Many people have worked to grasp the intricacies of the cerebrum, thus far with only partial success. Our evolving understanding of the cerebrum is analogous to our understanding of the astronomical universe. When humans first looked skyward with the naked eye, stars were organized into constellations and recorded on celestial maps (▶ Fig. 18.16). The invention of the optical telescope magnified light, enabling deeper views and the discovery of galaxies. The Hubble space telescope was positioned beyond Earth's atmosphere to see even deeper, unobscured by clouds and pollution, and the Webb telescope measured infrared light to see more of the electromagnetic spectrum. With composites of visible and infrared light, what once were dots on the celestial map are

Eloquent Cortex

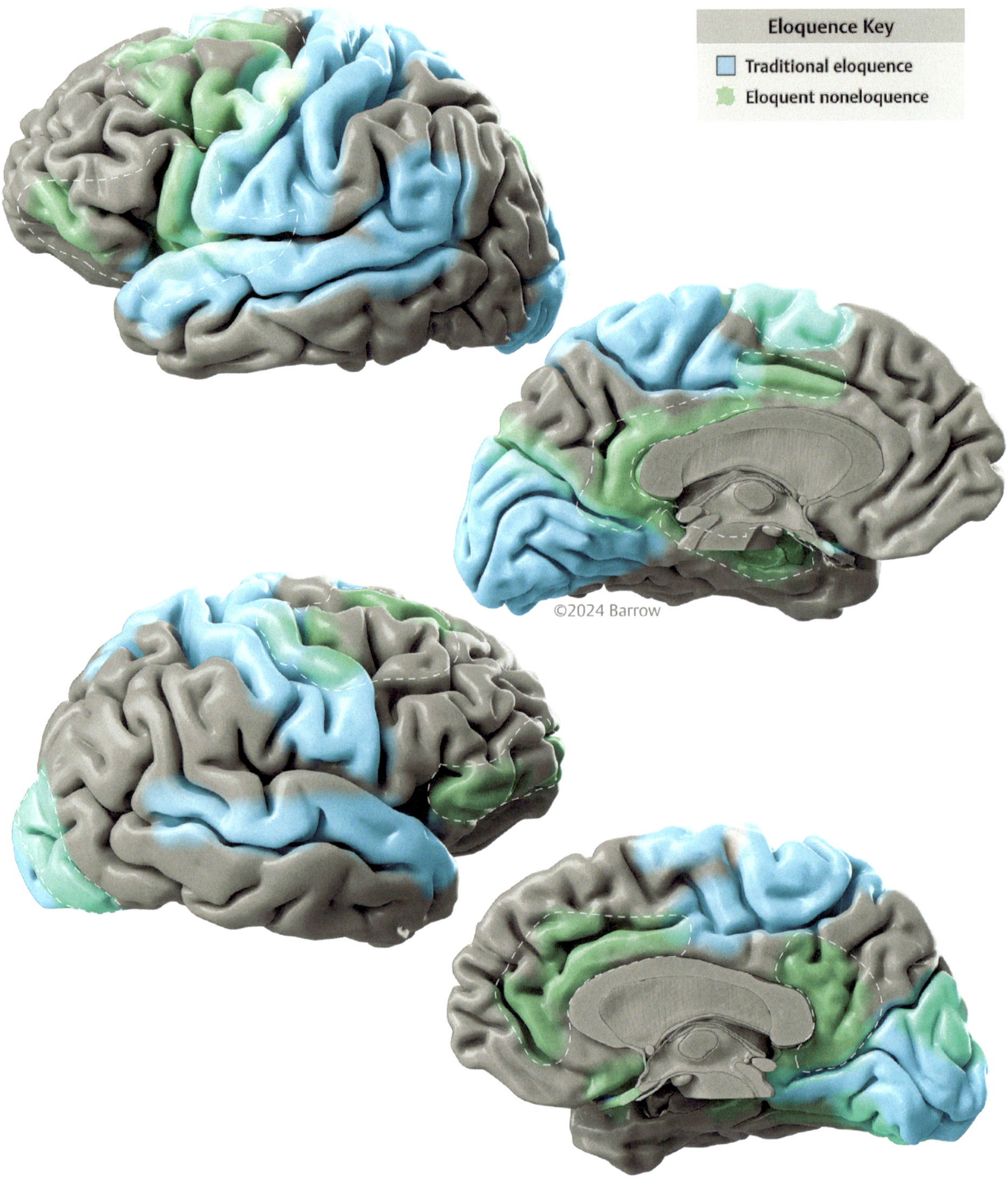

Fig. 18.14 Traditional and contemporary eloquence of the brain. Eloquent cortex includes traditional areas (*in blue*) such as motor, somatosensory, visual, auditory, and language cortices as well as hotspots of eloquent noneloquence (*in green*) determined by our superficial cerebral cavernoma experience (left and right hemispheres are shown in lateral and medial views, respectively). (Reproduced with permission from Barrow Neurological Institute, Phoenix, AZ.)

Eloquent Cortex

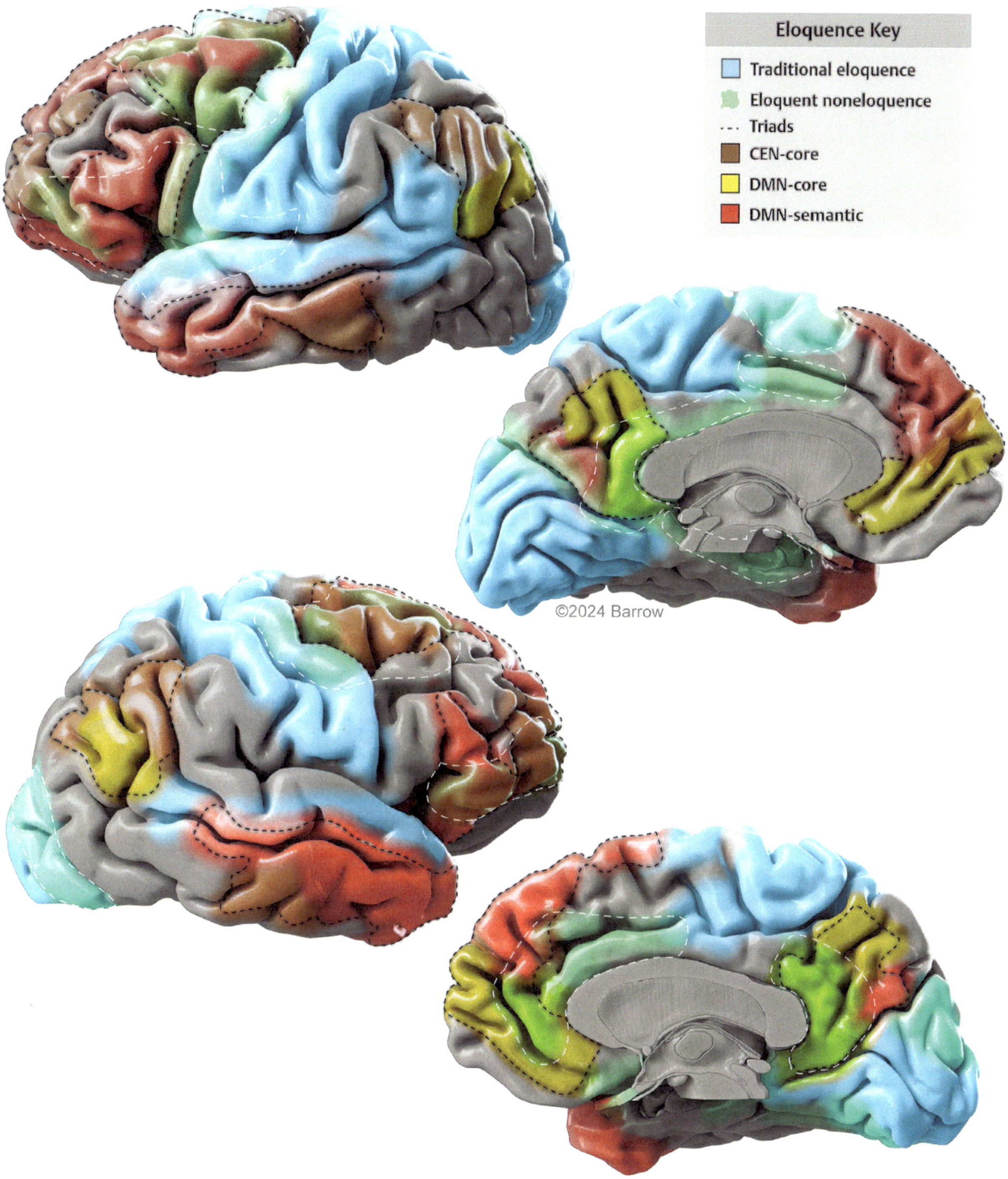

Fig. 18.15 Traditional and contemporary eloquence of the brain. With the addition of triads (CEN-core, DMN-core, and DMN-semantic), the amount of unsafe, unenterable cortex has increased dramatically, heralding an important shift in the conduct of transcerebral surgery. (Reproduced with permission from Barrow Neurological Institute, Phoenix, AZ.)

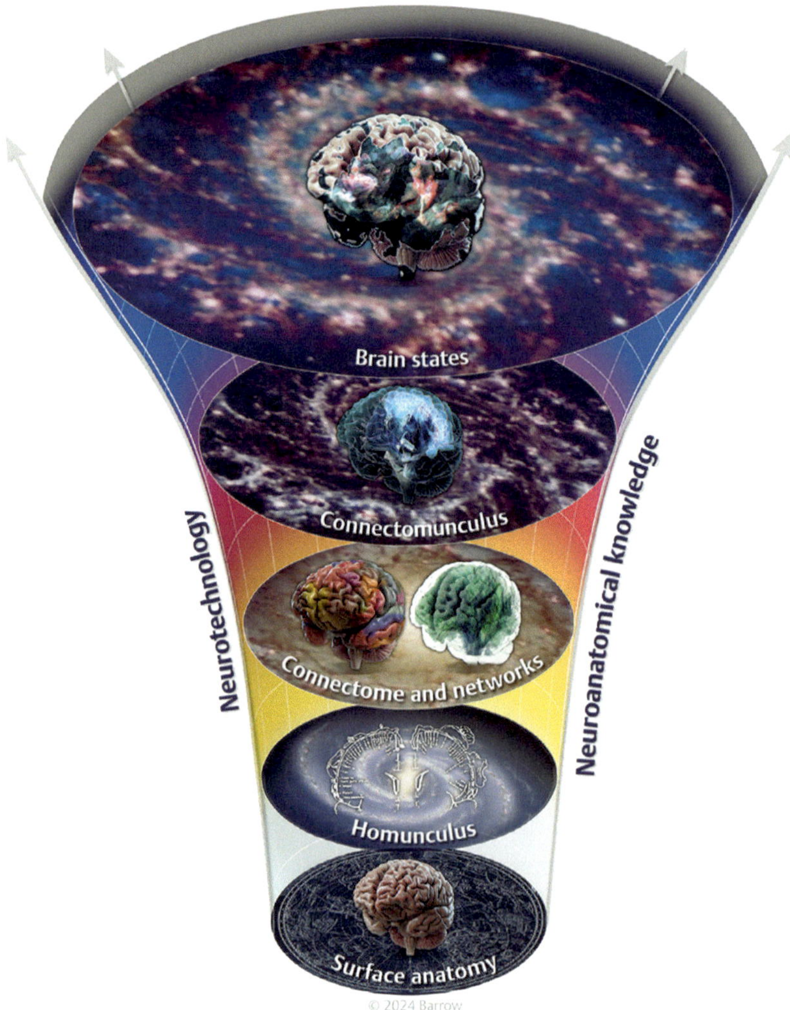

Fig. 18.16 The cerebral map is analogous to the celestial map. Just as our understanding of the astronomical universe progressed from constellations on a celestial map to galaxies seen through optical, space, and infrared space telescopes, our understanding of the cerebrum progressed from surface anatomy to the homunculus to connectomics and the connectomunculus. Human cognition can be understood as the ever-changing synchrony of neurons and networks firing simultaneously at the same frequency in complex patterns distributed across the brain, leading to various brain states. (Reproduced with permission from Barrow Neurological Institute, Phoenix, AZ.)

now galaxies within the heavens. Similarly, the brain observed with the unaided eye was understood on the basis of its surface anatomy, and neurophysiology informed the homunculus. With connectomics and brain networks, cognition can be understood as the ever-changing synchrony of neurons and networks firing simultaneously at the same frequency in complex patterns distributed across the brain, leading to various brain states (▶ Fig. 18.16). And, just like celestial maps, cerebral maps will deepen and evolve with new instruments, neuroanatomical knowledge, and insight. The upward arrows on our cerebral map depict this dynamic state of neurotechnology and neuroanatomical knowledge, ever increasing the comprehension of brain function.

18.3 The Mind

The *Seven Cavernomas* journey has been special because it has changed my view on neurosurgery. This textbook embodies my core values as a vascular neurosurgeon: (1) it introduces a taxonomic construct that brings order to a chaotic discipline; (2) it adds structure to the decision-making process; (3) it emphasizes the use of natural subarachnoid corridors to navigate and dissect CMs in the deepest structures of the brain; (4) it presents new concepts and ideas, like the triangle concept and right-angle method, to make neurosurgeons better in the operating room; (5) it discusses predictive models and grading systems to improve patient selection; (6) it incorporates arteries as

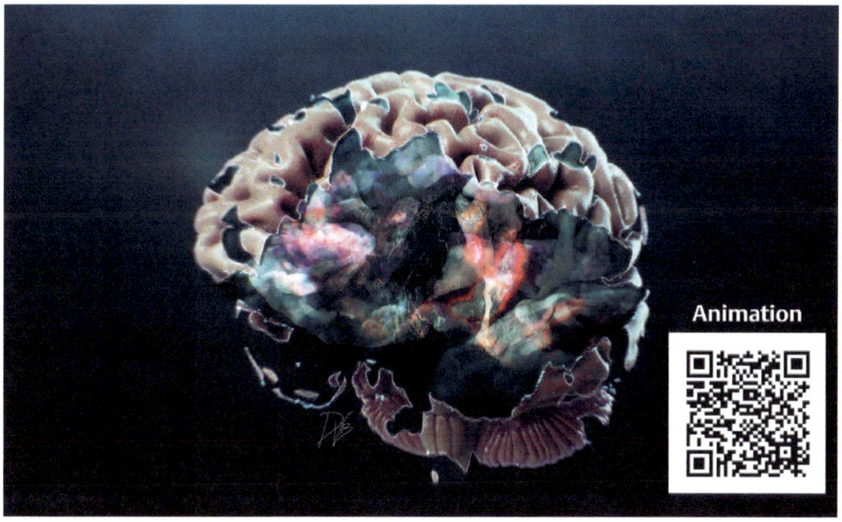

Fig. 18.17 A still image from a three-dimensional animation of the brain depicting brain states during higher cognitive function. This function involves the simultaneous electrochemical activity of seemingly unrelated cortical parcels and multiple brain networks interconnected through white matter tracts. These interconnections fire in sophisticated and synchronized sequences, with spikes and oscillations of variable amplitudes, frequencies, and phases (animation; ▶ Video 18.2, Brain states during higher cognitive function; QR code). (Reproduced with permission from Barrow Neurological Institute, Phoenix, AZ.)

valuable landmarks and guideposts; and (7) it improves discourse about cavernomas with specific and standardized terminology (e.g., subtypes and size categories). Nonetheless, our efforts in the cerebrum made me realize that vascular neurosurgeons deliberately avoid brain parenchyma. We operate outside of it and avoid transgressing it at all costs, and our vascular research interests focus on supplying it rather than understanding its function. *Seven Cavernomas* reawakened the feeling that we should seek to understand how the brain works as an organ system rather than delight in its surface anatomy and subarachnoid corridors. As specialists, we should use our exclusive access to the brain to understand how it functions in relation to the mind, regarding it expansively and holistically instead of treating it as simply the setting for neurosurgery.

In 1982, I was in college and majoring in biomedical engineering when Robert Jarvik built an entirely artificial heart. Dr. William Devries implanted it in Barney Clark to extend his life for almost a year. I was amazed that our understanding of cardiac physiology enabled engineers to design and fabricate the Jarvik-7 and was inspired to attend medical school to become a surgeon who could implant these devices. My journey to cardiac surgery was derailed in medical school, and my journey to vascular neurosurgery instead turned out to be for the best. However, while writing this book, I rediscovered the desire to understand the brain as thoroughly as cardiac surgeons understand the heart. I realized that, as neurosurgeons, we do not have a comparable understanding of the organ in which we specialize. We do not fully understand how the brain corresponds to the mind. We have a basic knowledge of motor, sensory, and visual systems, but we do not understand emotion, memory, neural plasticity, intelligence, and consciousness. These amazing facets of the mind make us human, and nothing is more important than understanding that.

Understanding the brain and these higher cognitive functions is the way forward to safer and more elegant neurosurgery, among the other benefits that such understanding will bring (▶ Fig. 18.17; ▶ Video 18.2; and the network gallery [▶ Fig. 18.18, ▶ Fig. 18.19, ▶ Fig. 18.20, ▶ Fig. 18.21, ▶ Fig. 18.22, ▶ Fig. 18.23, ▶ Fig. 18.24, ▶ Fig. 18.25, ▶ Fig. 18.26, ▶ Fig. 18.27, ▶ Fig. 18.28, ▶ Fig. 18.29, ▶ Fig. 18.30, ▶ Fig. 18.31, ▶ Fig. 18.32, ▶ Fig. 18.33, ▶ Fig. 18.34, ▶ Fig. 18.35]). As this *Seven Cavernomas* book concludes, I have a newfound respect for neural circuits and minimally invasive techniques. We are on an evolutionary continuum from contemporary neurosurgery with open techniques and manual craftsmanship to completely closed techniques and robotics, with or without neurosurgeon involvement. We need to drive this evolution by innovating new operative techniques that are less invasive and safer and by better understanding the mind. We are good at the former, but the latter is embryonic. That said, we have a unique opportunity to turn our operating rooms into laboratories and discern the brain's inner workings. Whether through awake surgery, stereoelectroencephalography, outcome research, or innovative technology, we can transform our neurosurgical tools and this window of opportunity to revolutionize our knowledge of brain and mind functions. This goal of exploring the mind is the most exciting way to conclude this book. If we can come to a future where our neurosurgical specialty is the vehicle for voyaging to this final frontier, then the future of neurosurgery is exciting and transformative. The challenges to understanding the mind have yet to be solved. We are finally developing the prowess and creating the tools and techniques to unravel these mysteries.

18.4 Gallery of Functional Networks

The functional network gallery includes maps of the seven primary networks, the CEN, DAN, limbic and paralimbic, sensorimotor, salience, and visual networks. The icons in ▶ Fig. 18.18 depict brain functions at the alphanumeric regional addresses by network.

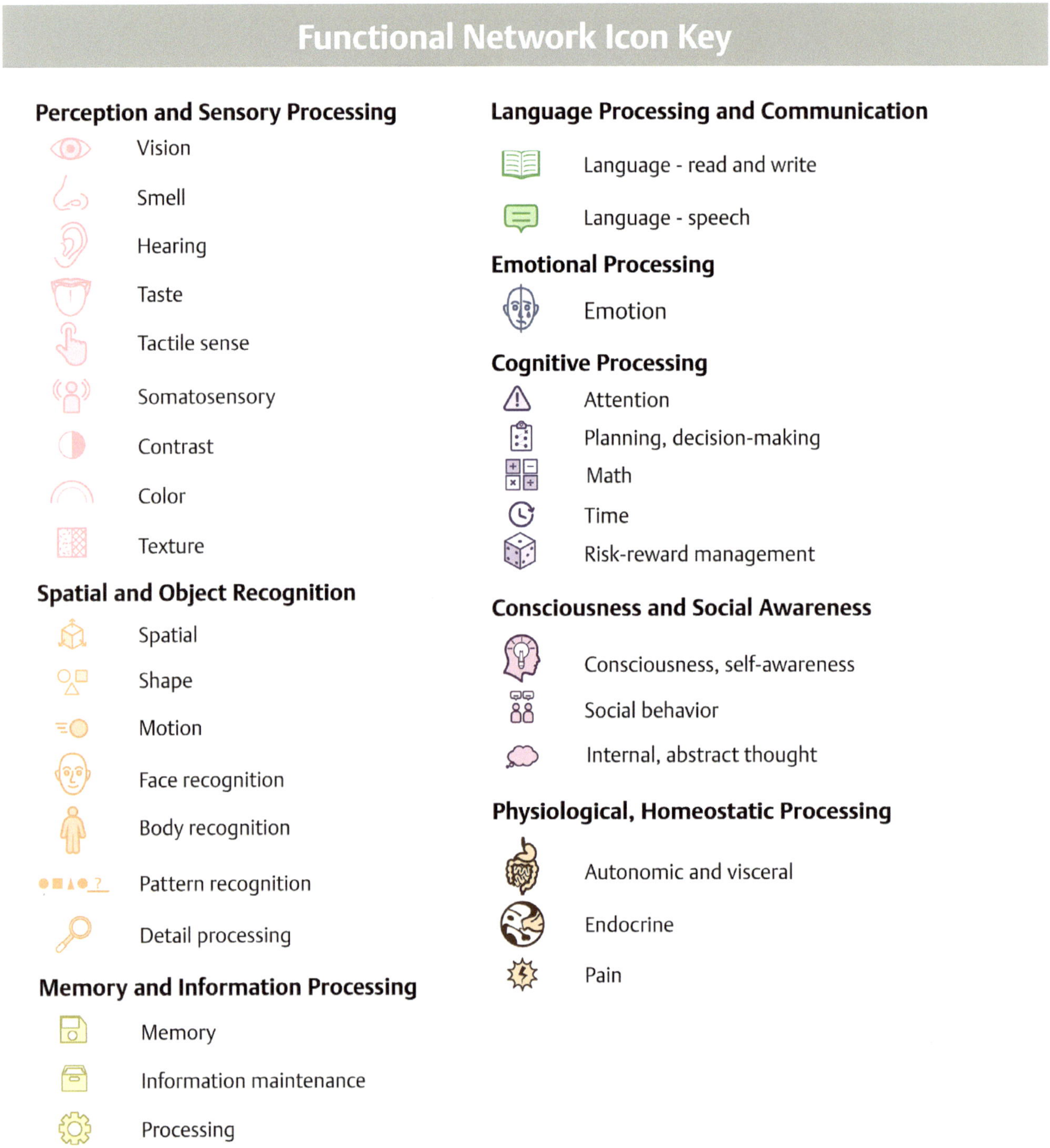

Fig. 18.18 Network gallery. This icon key defines the parcel functions in the gallery of figures that follow. The gallery of large-scale networks in the human brain, depict the parcellations (acronyms and alphanumerics) that make up the network as well as the specific functions (graphic icons) of each parcel. (Reproduced with permission from Barrow Neurological Institute, Phoenix, AZ.)

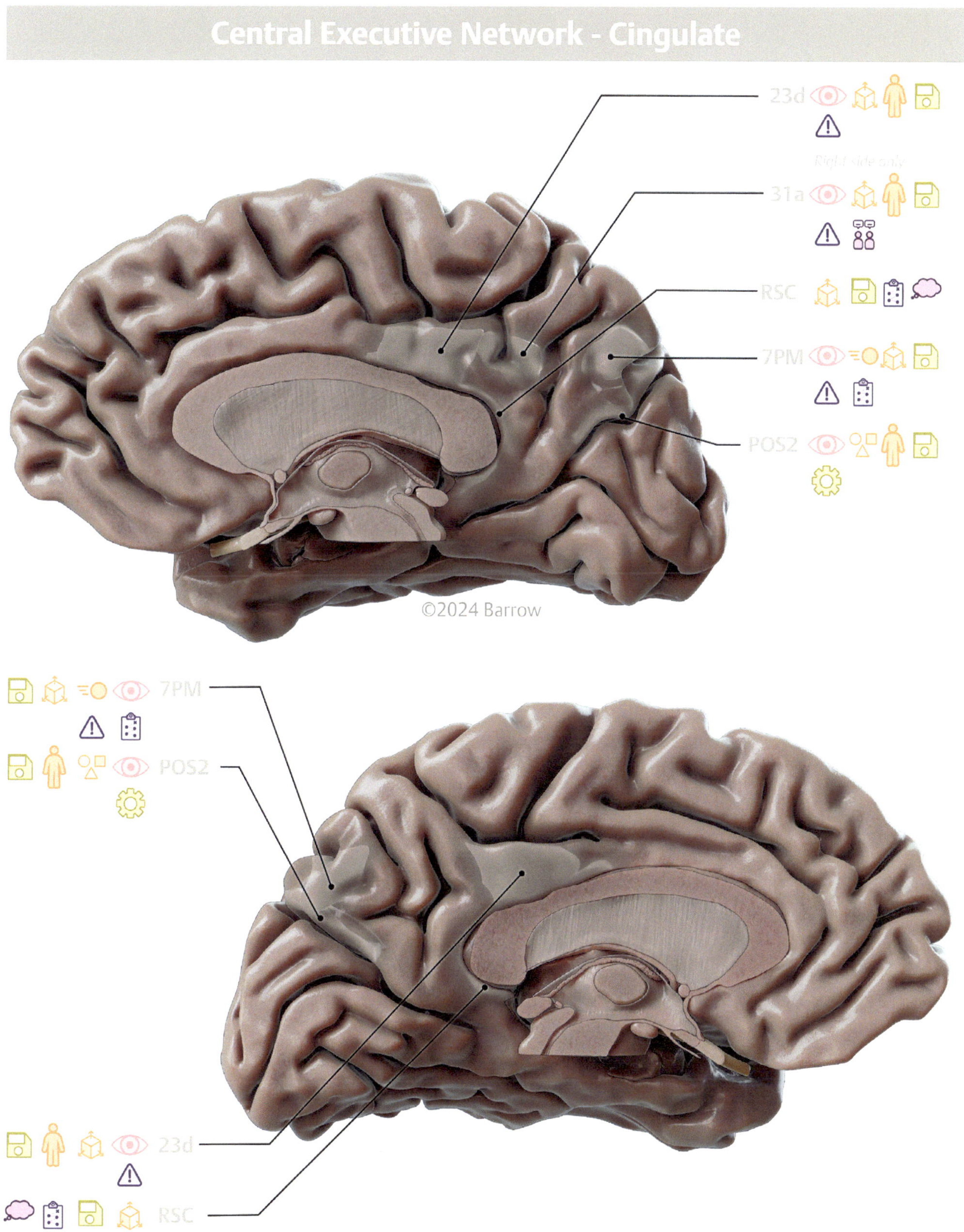

Fig. 18.19 Central executive network - cingulate. (Reproduced with permission from Barrow Neurological Institute, Phoenix, AZ.)

Central Executive Network - Core

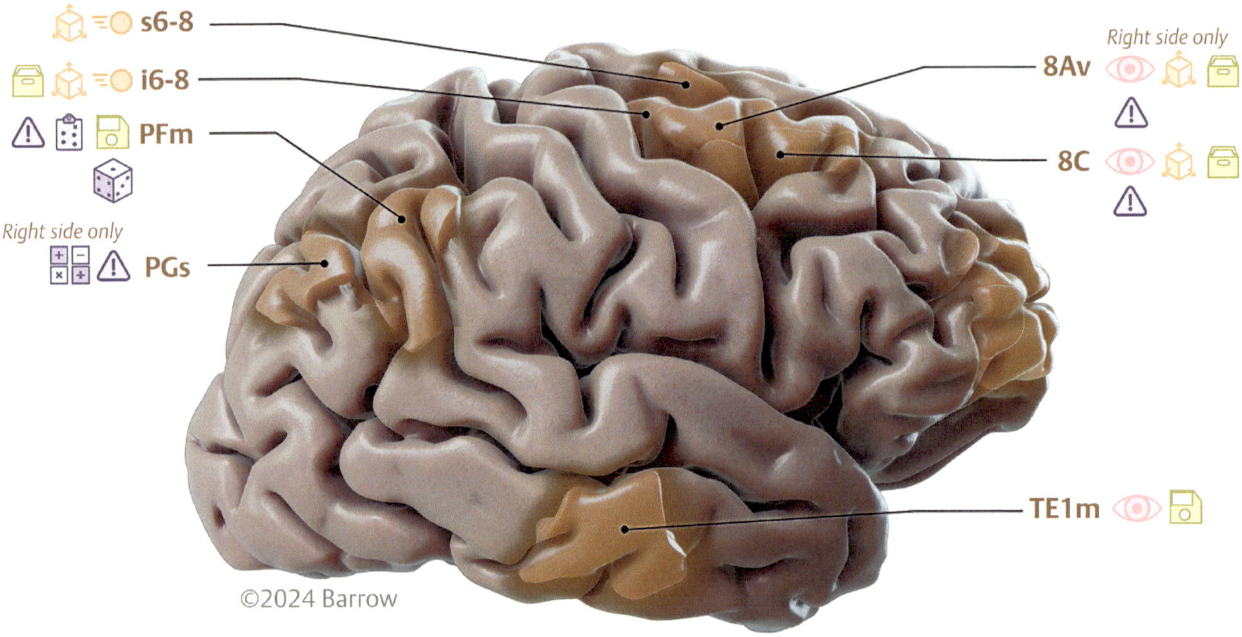

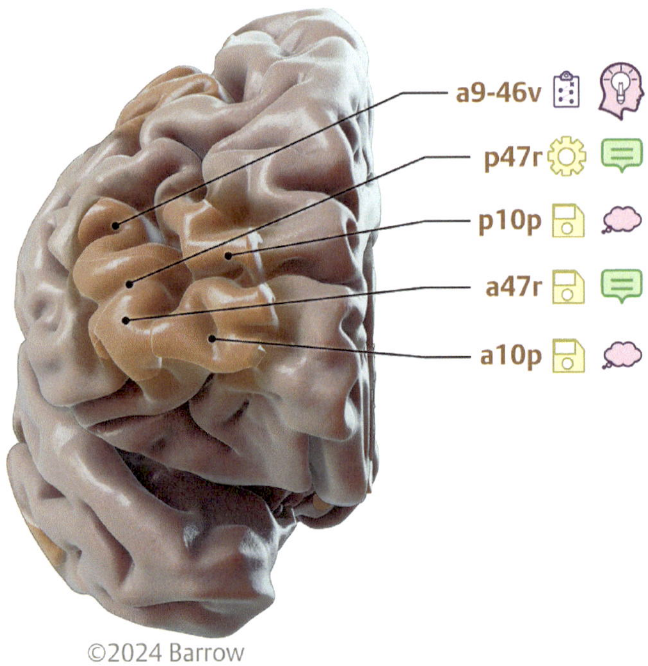

Fig. 18.20 Central executive network - core. (Reproduced with permission from Barrow Neurological Institute, Phoenix, AZ.)

Central Executive Network - Multiple Demand

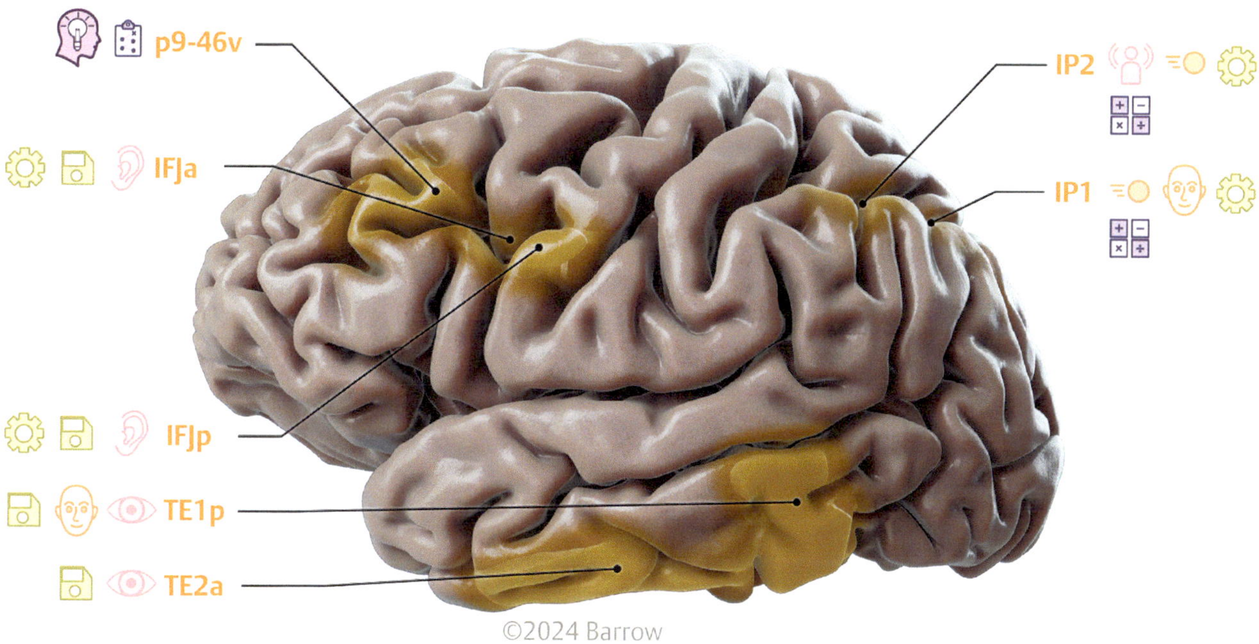

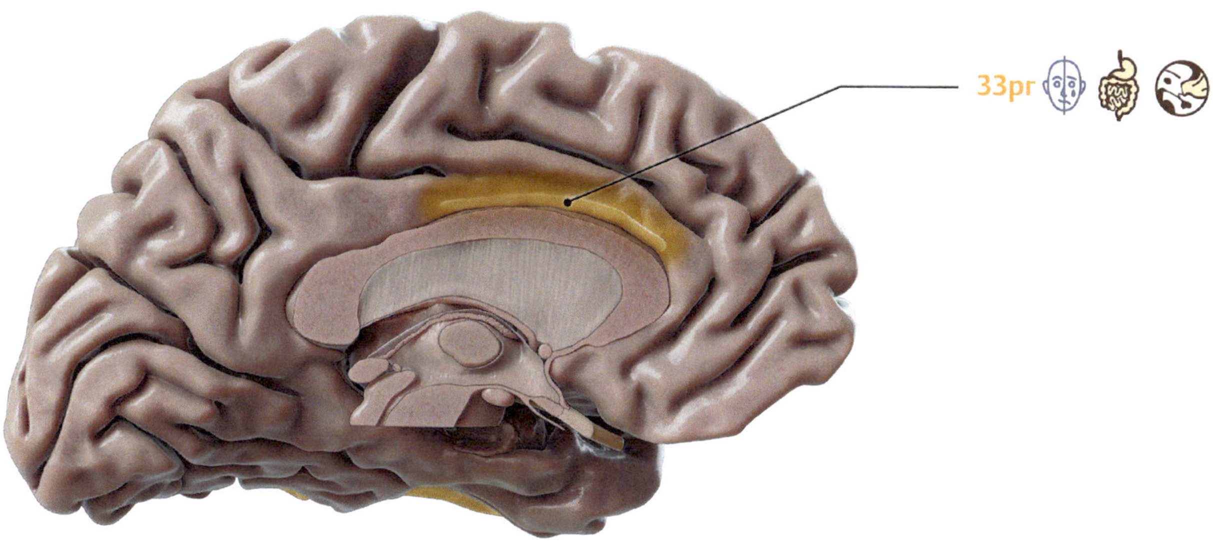

Fig. 18.21 Central executive network - multiple demand. (Reproduced with permission from Barrow Neurological Institute, Phoenix, AZ.)

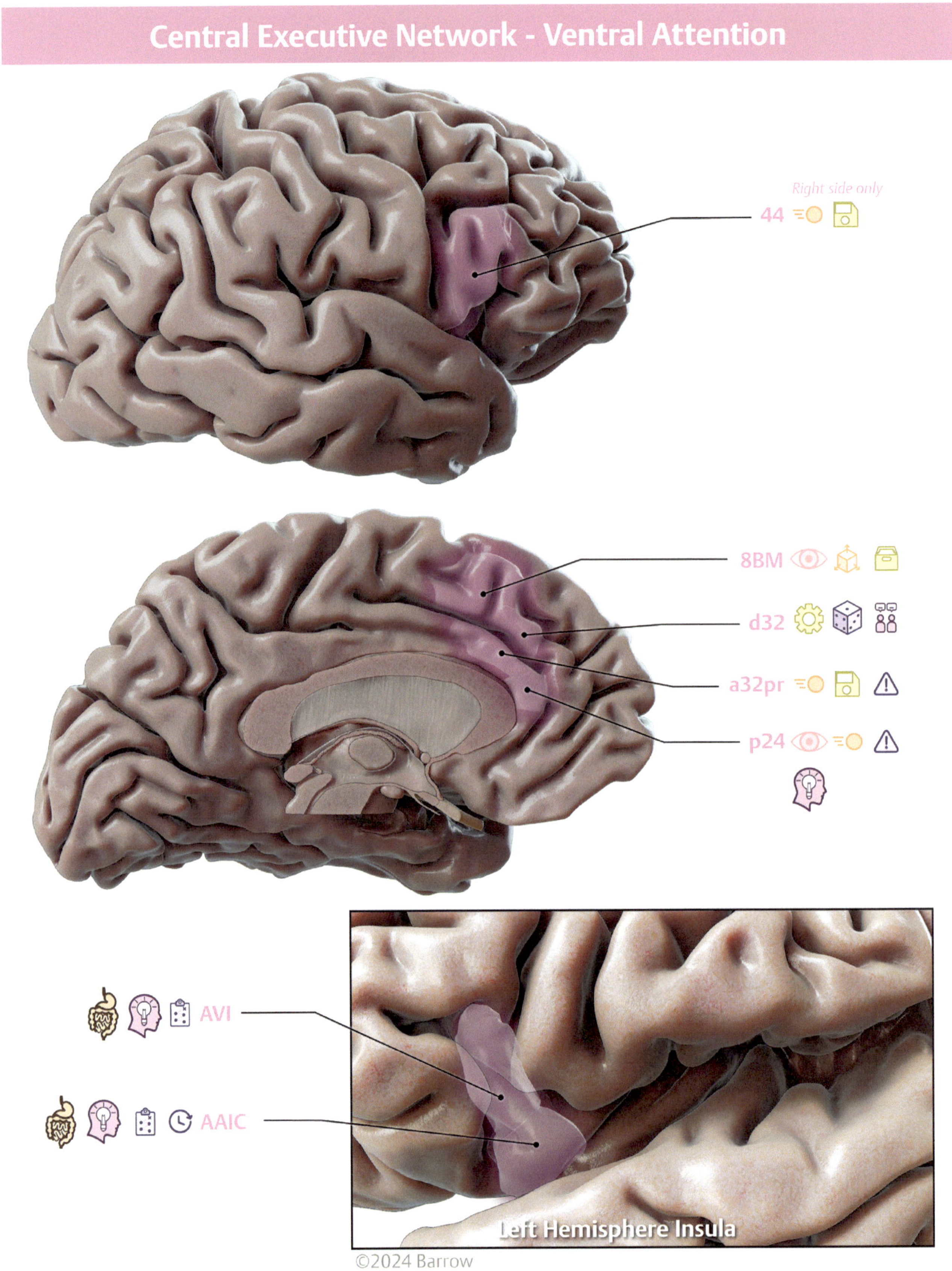

Fig. 18.22 Central executive network - ventral attention. Enlarged view of the central executive network - ventral attention (*inset*). (Reproduced with permission from Barrow Neurological Institute, Phoenix, AZ.)

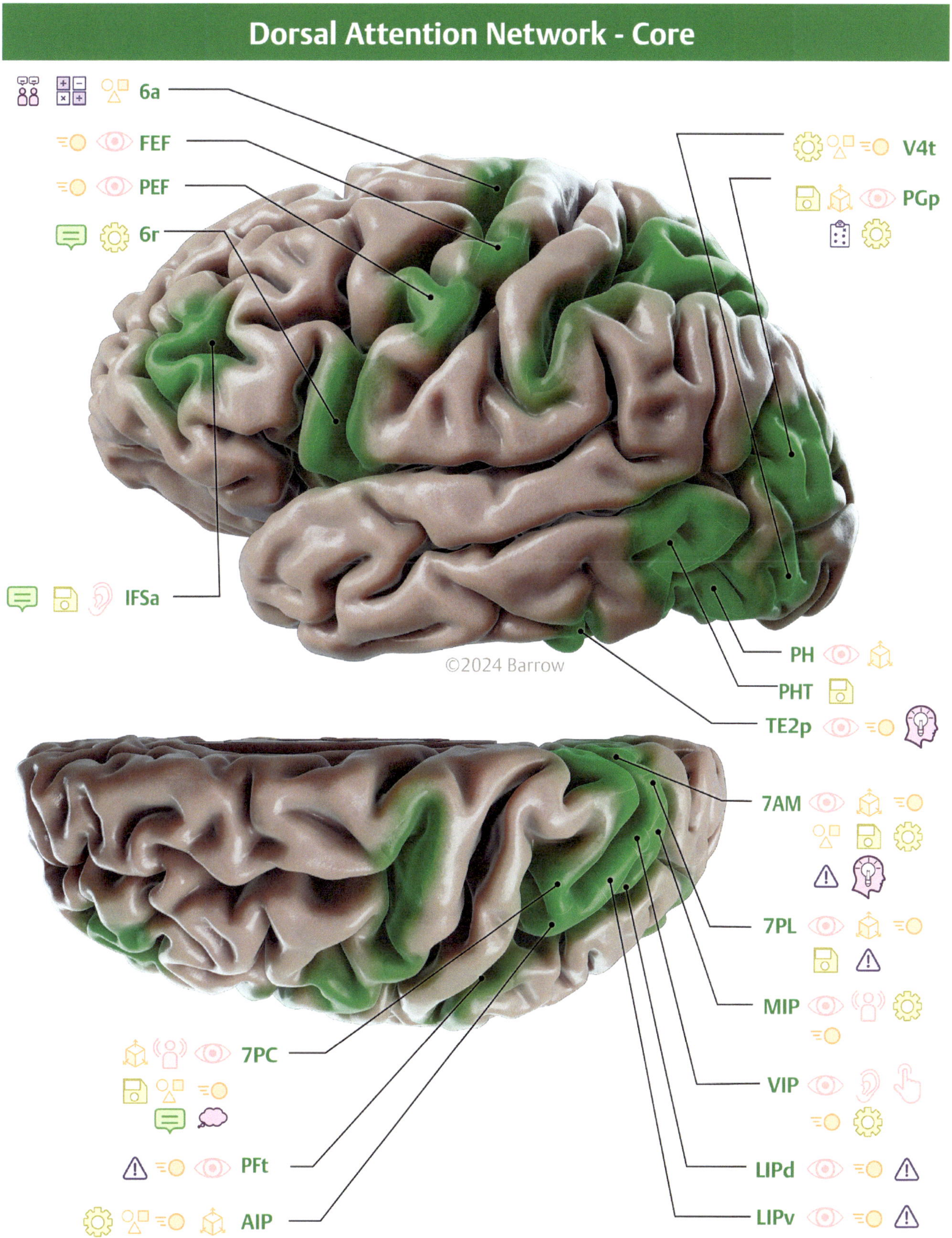

Fig. 18.23 Dorsal attention network - core. (Reproduced with permission from Barrow Neurological Institute, Phoenix, AZ.)

Default Mode Network - Auditory

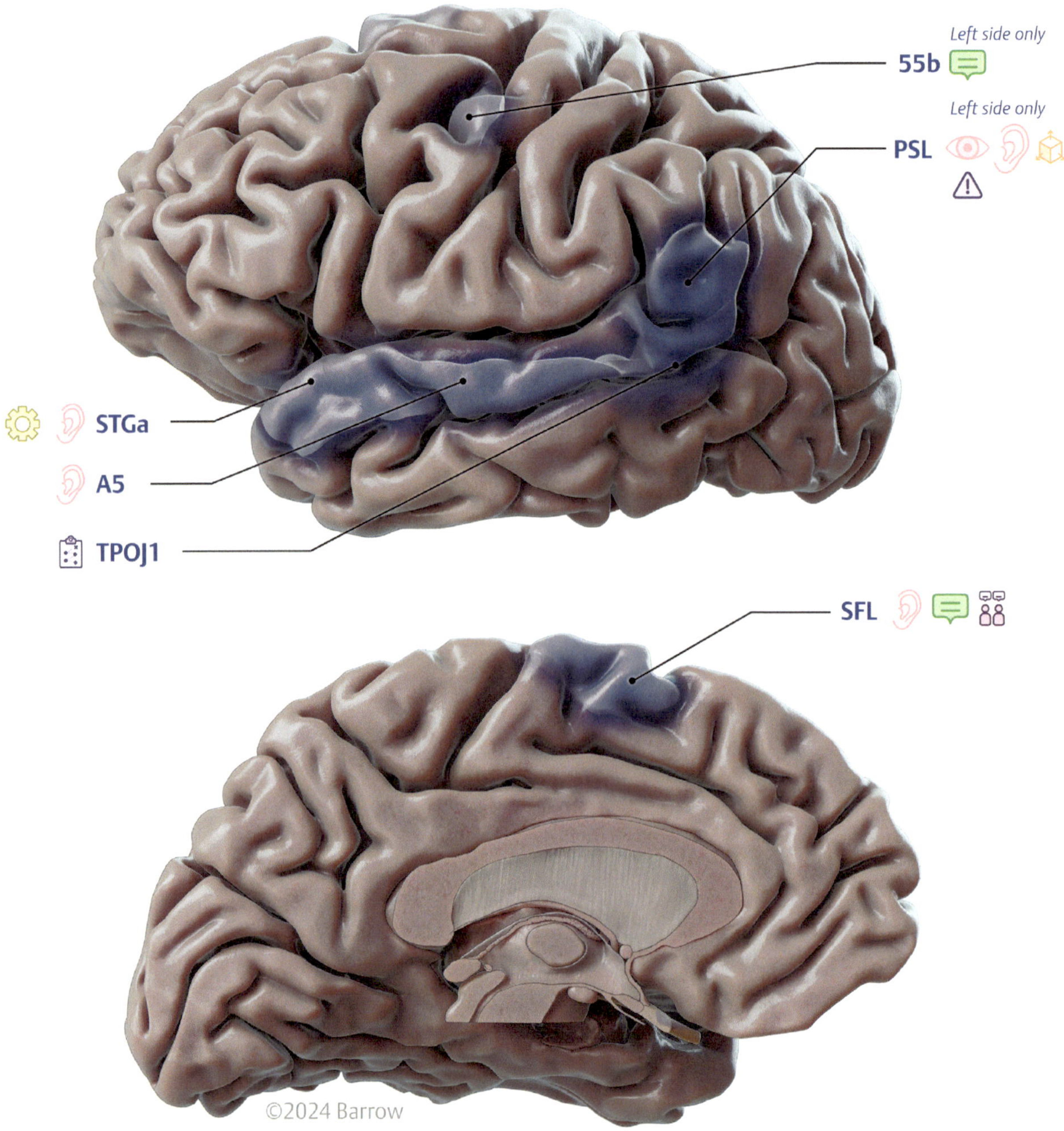

Fig. 18.24 Default mode network - auditory. (Reproduced with permission from Barrow Neurological Institute, Phoenix, AZ.)

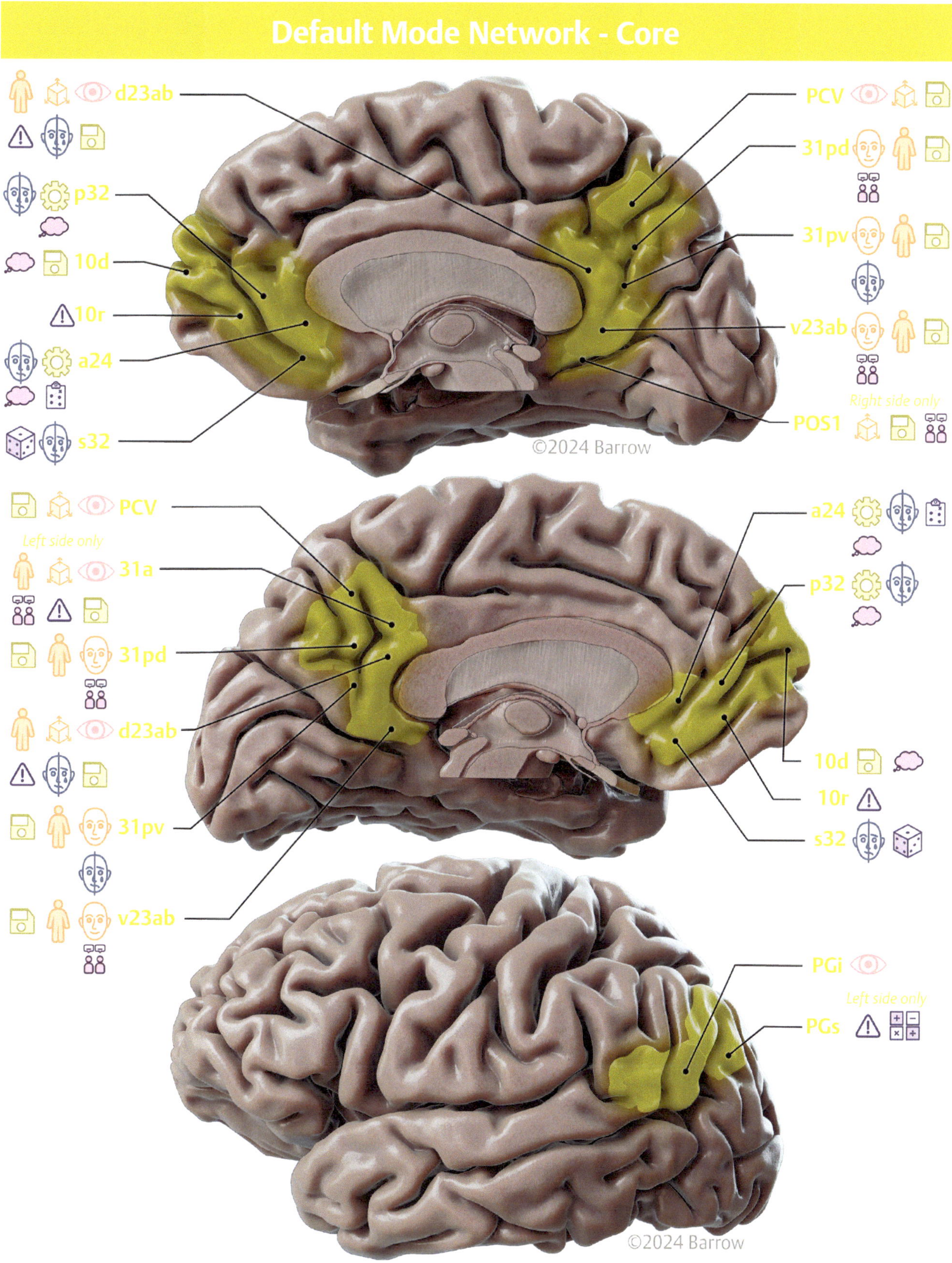

Fig. 18.25 Default mode network - core. (Reproduced with permission from Barrow Neurological Institute, Phoenix, AZ.)

Default Mode Network - Memory

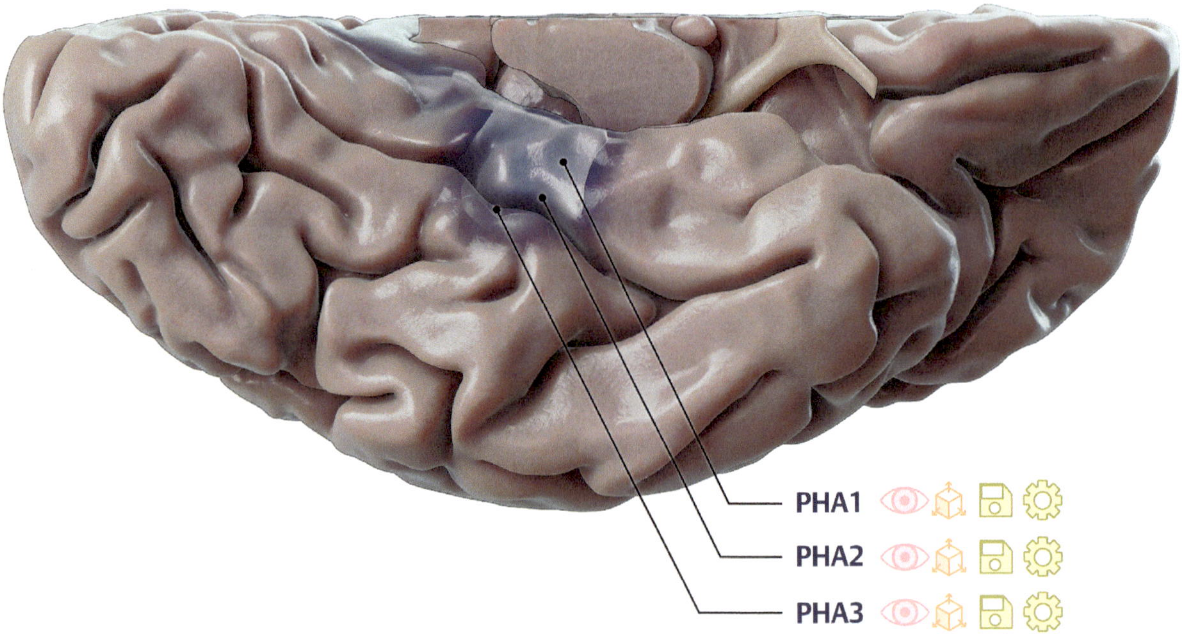

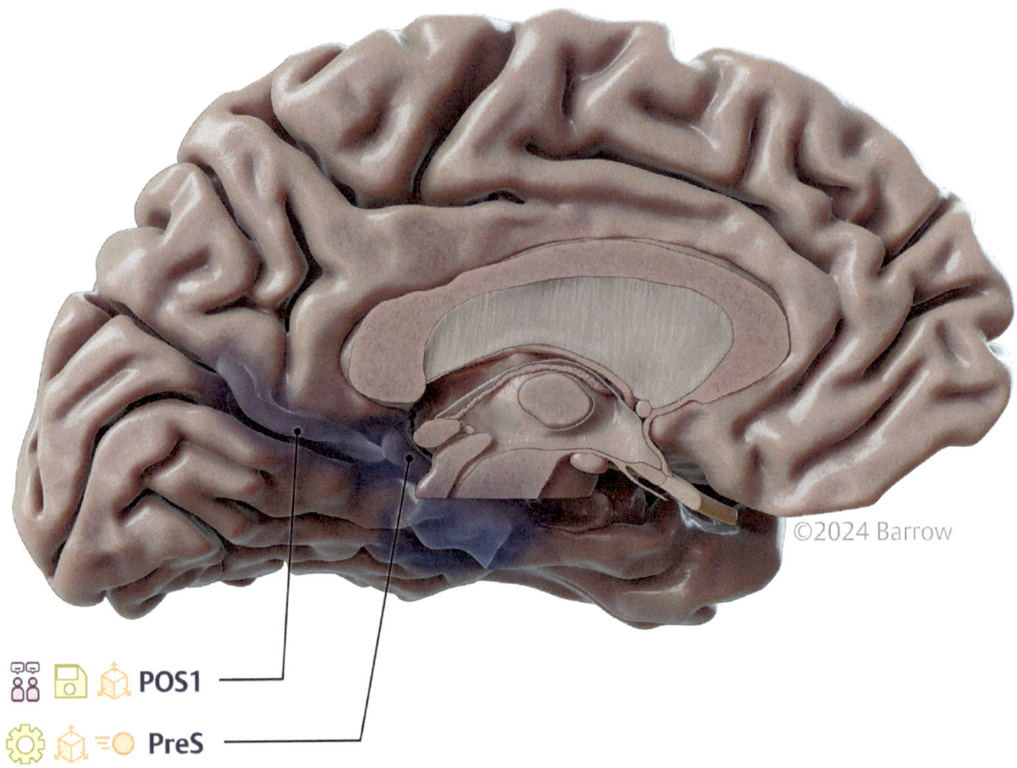

Fig. 18.26 Default mode network - memory. (Reproduced with permission from Barrow Neurological Institute, Phoenix, AZ.)

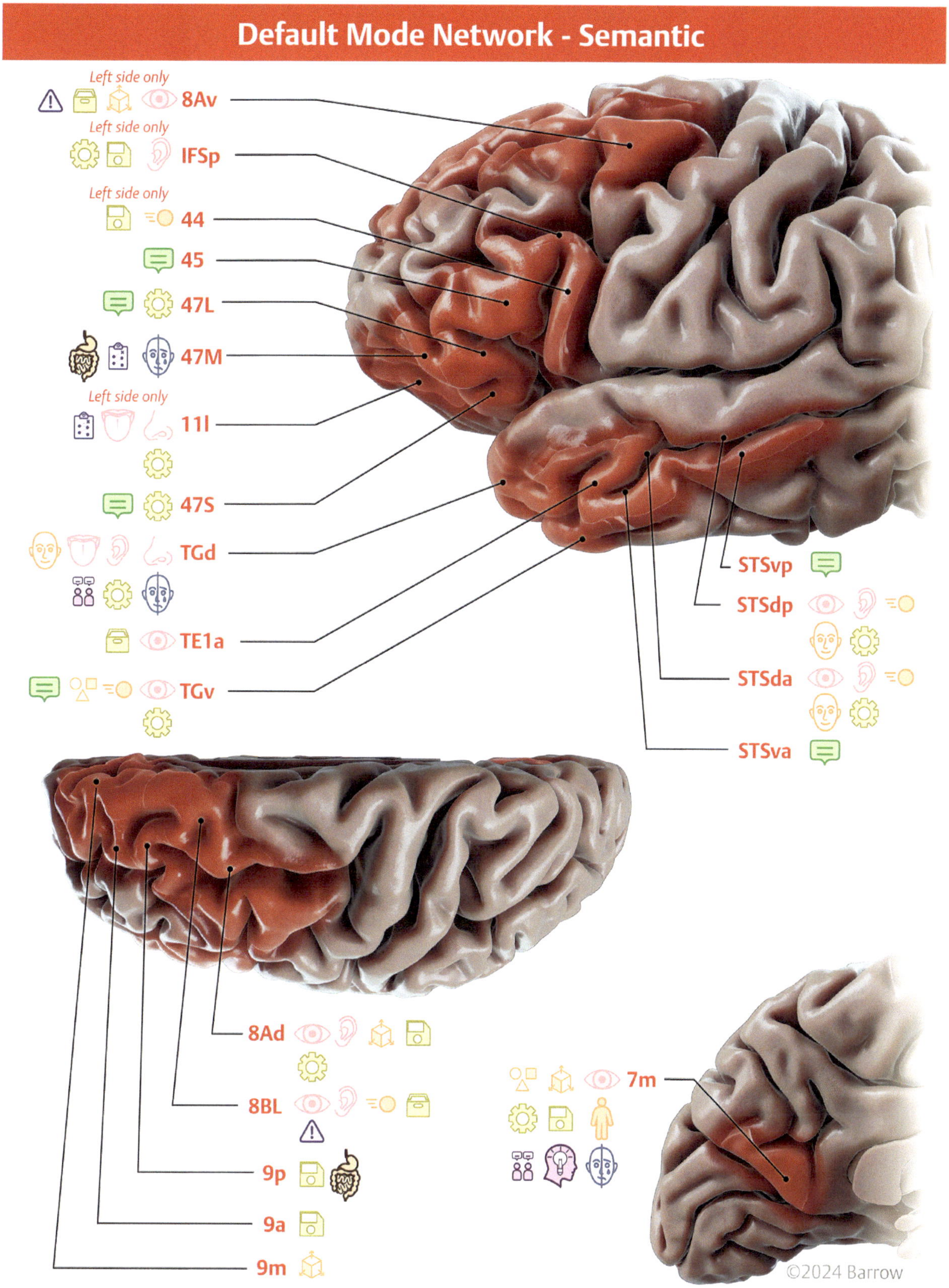

Fig. 18.27 Default mode network - semantic. (Reproduced with permission from Barrow Neurological Institute, Phoenix, AZ.)

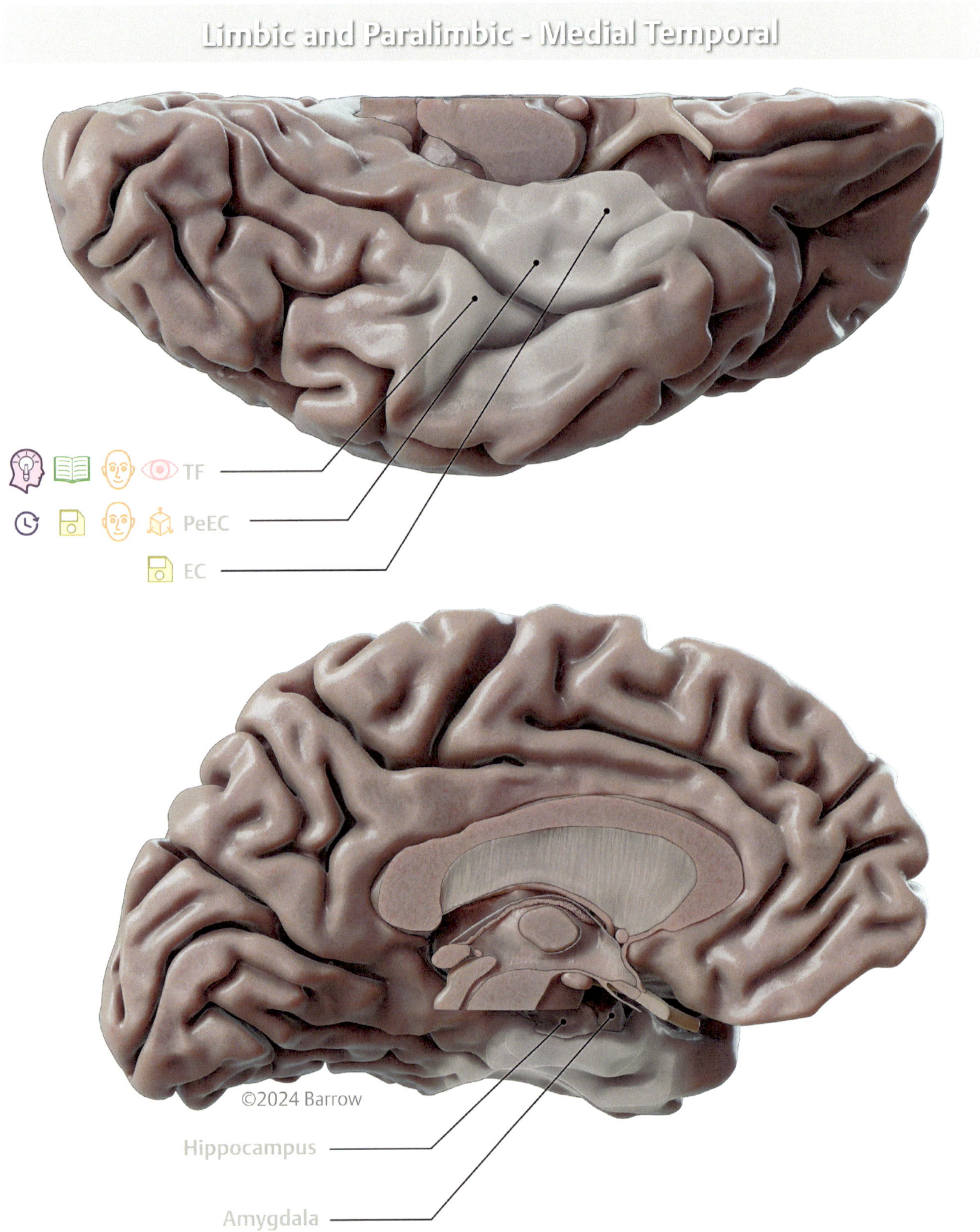

Fig. 18.28 Limbic and paralimbic network - medial temporal. (Reproduced with permission from Barrow Neurological Institute, Phoenix, AZ.)

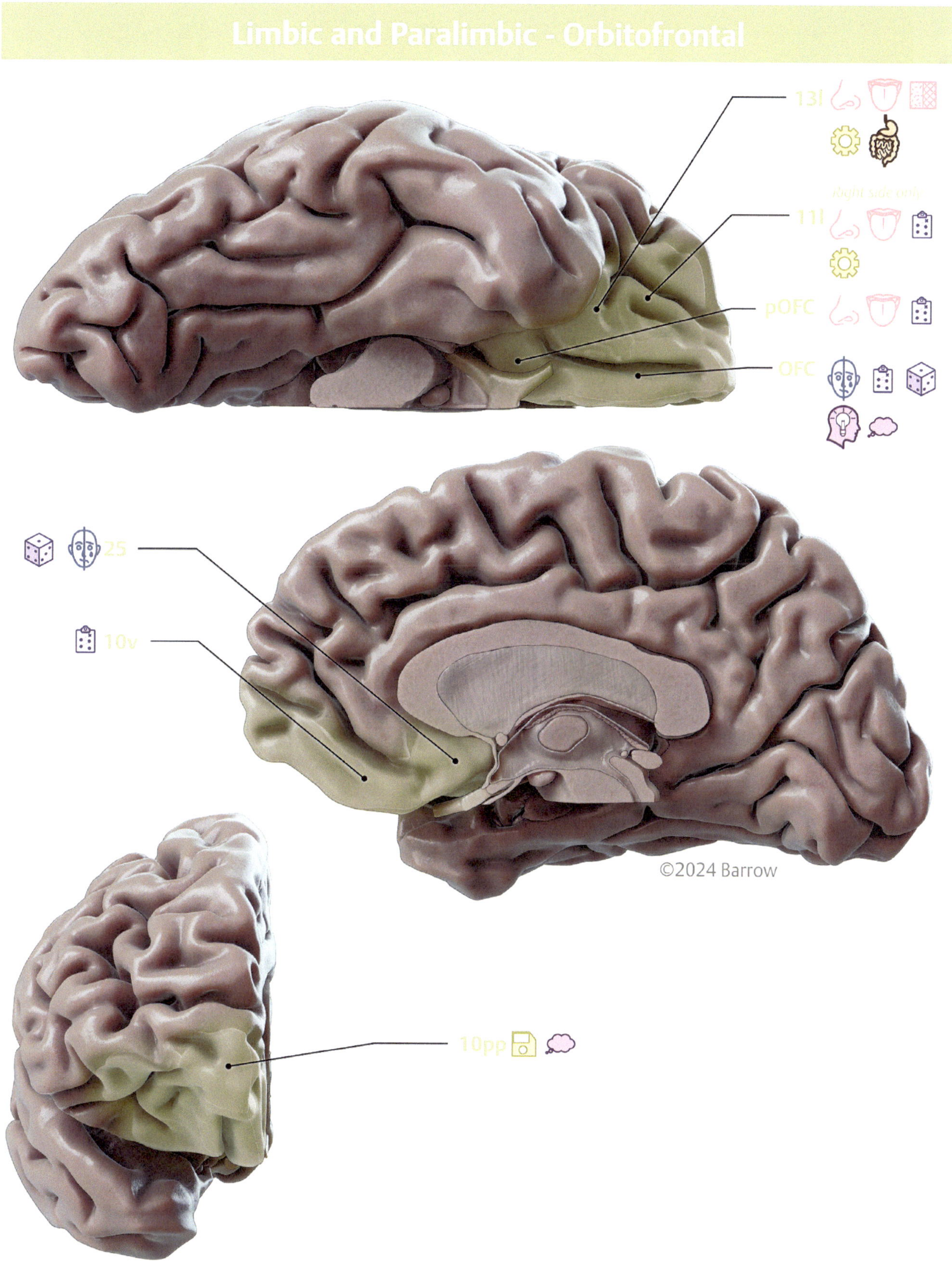

Fig. 18.29 Limbic and paralimbic network - orbitofrontal. (Reproduced with permission from Barrow Neurological Institute, Phoenix, AZ.)

Sensorimotor Network - Core

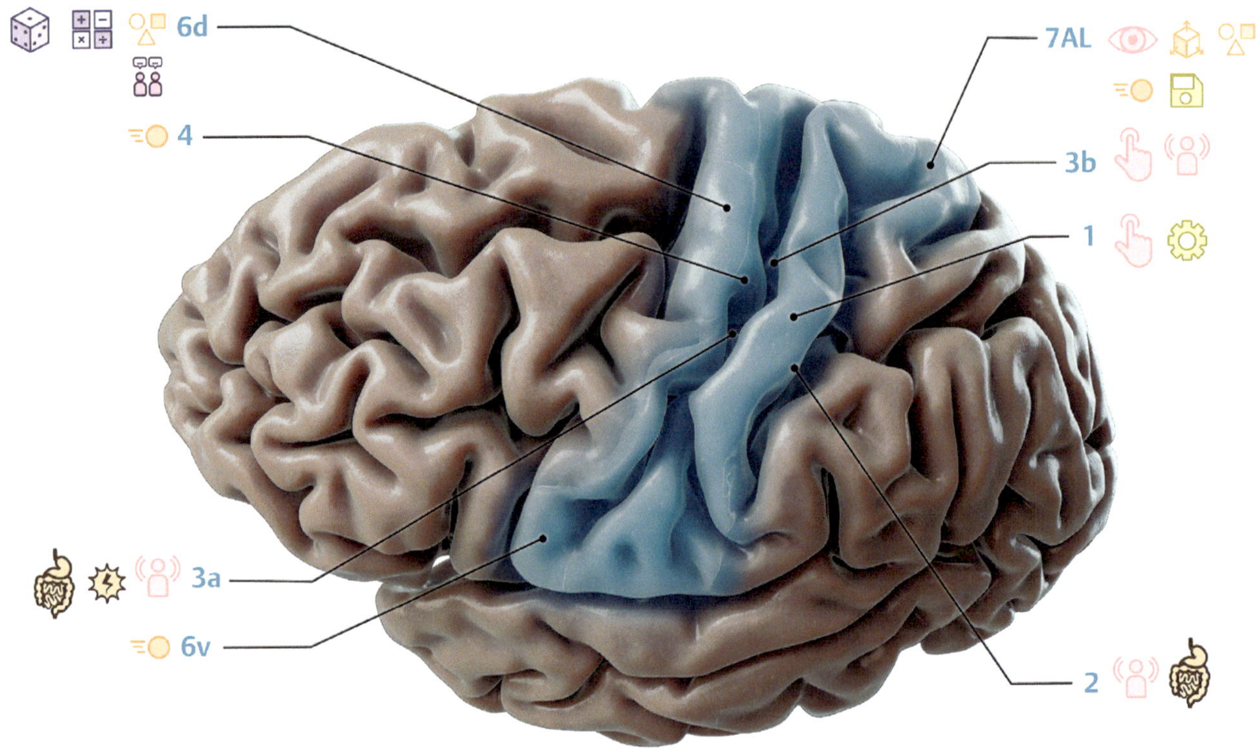

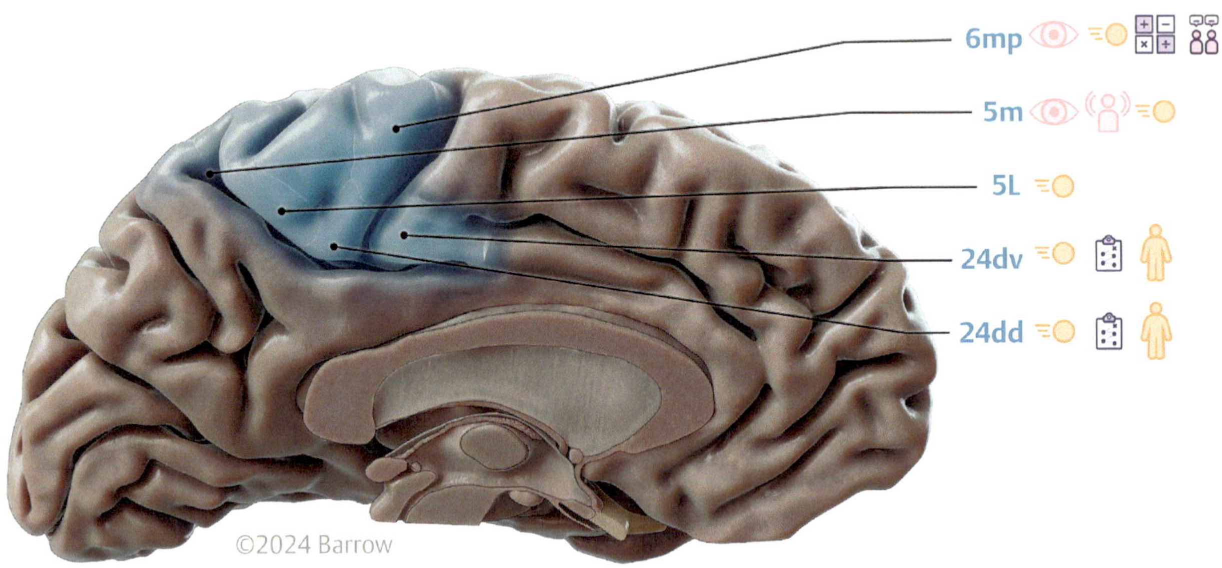

Fig. 18.30 Sensorimotor network - core. (Reproduced with permission from Barrow Neurological Institute, Phoenix, AZ.)

Sensorimotor Network - S2

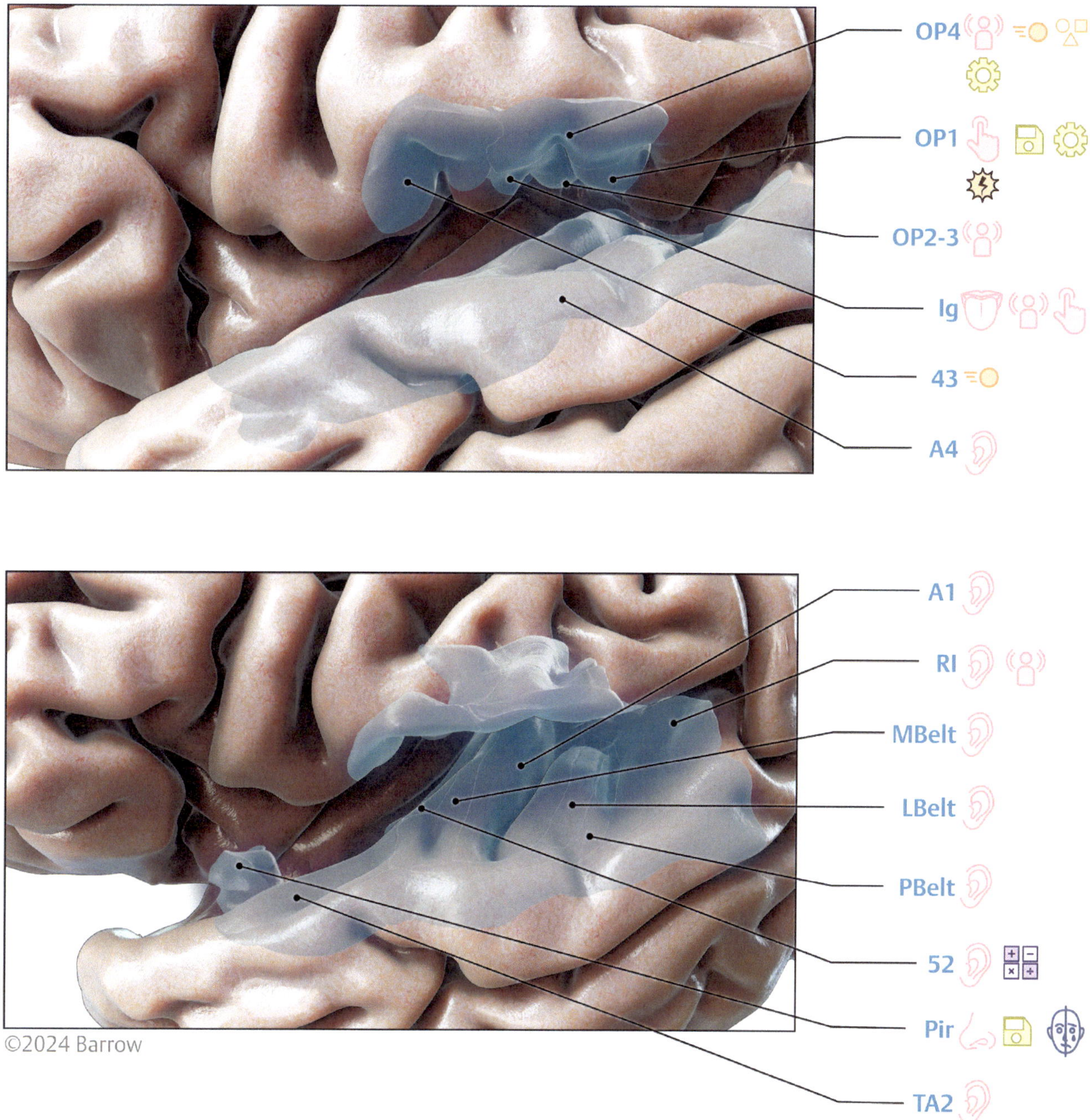

Fig. 18.31 Sensorimotor network - S2, enlarged view. (Reproduced with permission from Barrow Neurological Institute, Phoenix, AZ.)

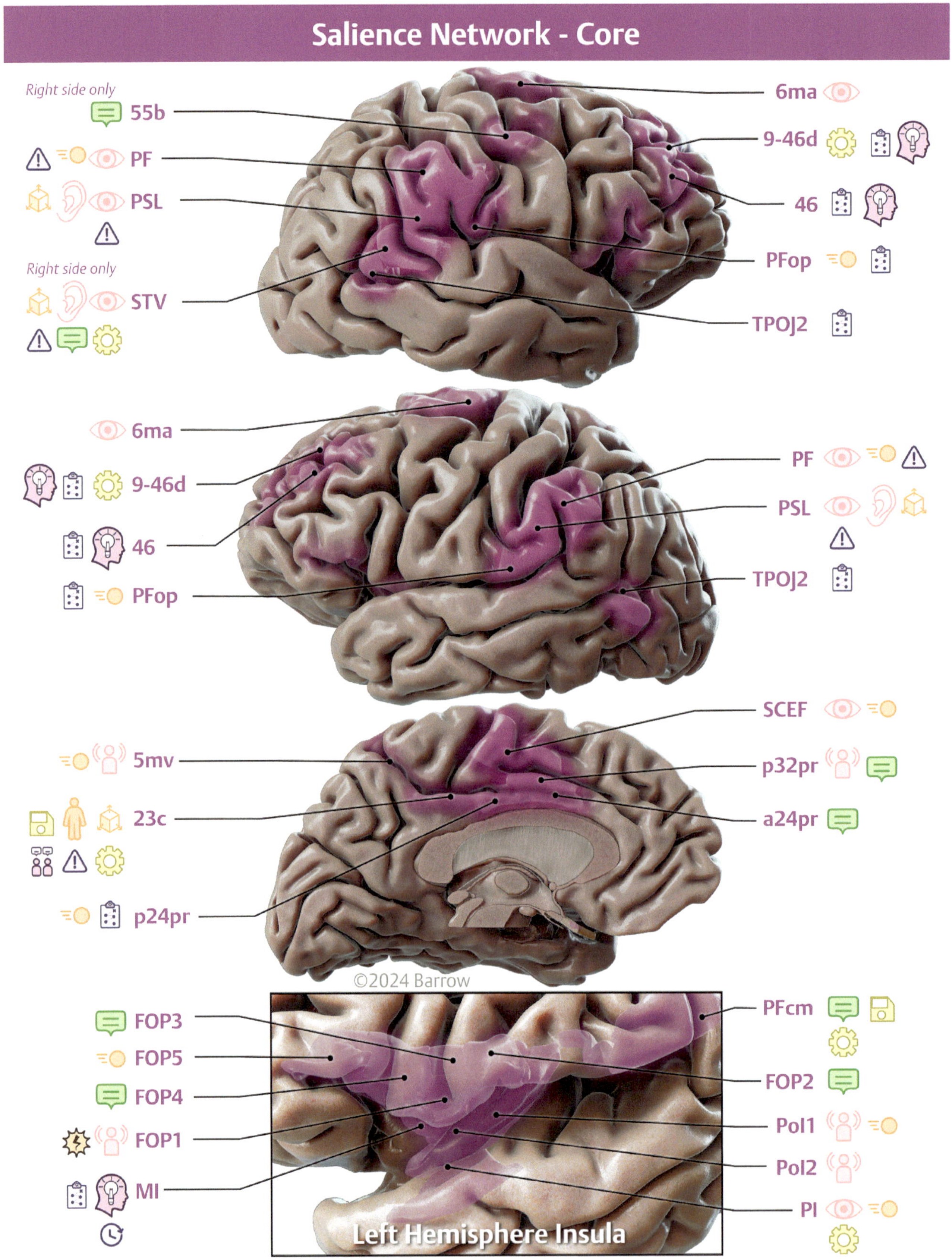

Fig. 18.32 Salience network - core. Enlarged view of the salience network - core (*inset*). (Reproduced with permission from Barrow Neurological Institute, Phoenix, AZ.)

Visual Network - Lateral

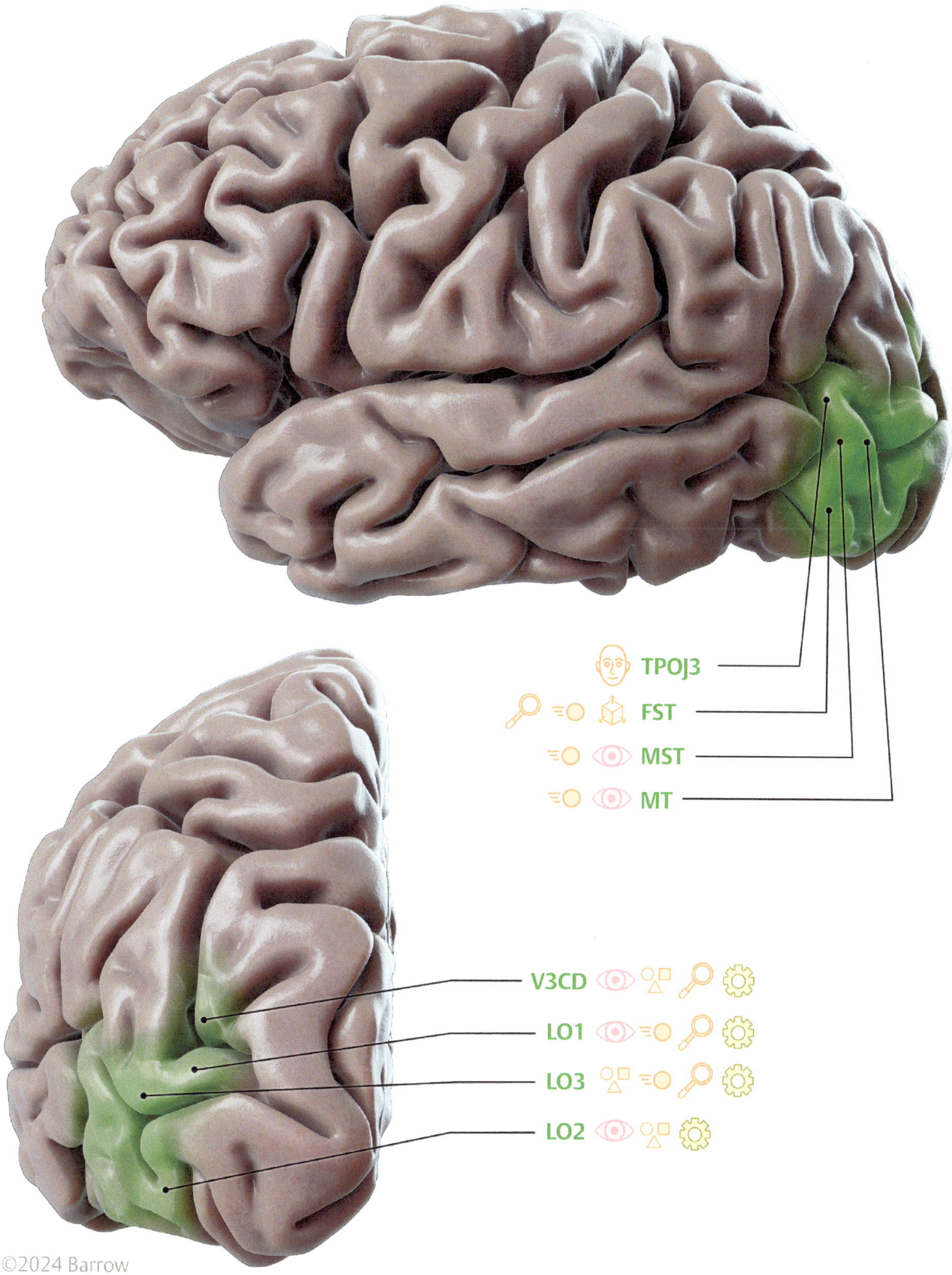

Fig. 18.33 Visual network - lateral. (Reproduced with permission from Barrow Neurological Institute, Phoenix, AZ.)

Visual Network - Primary

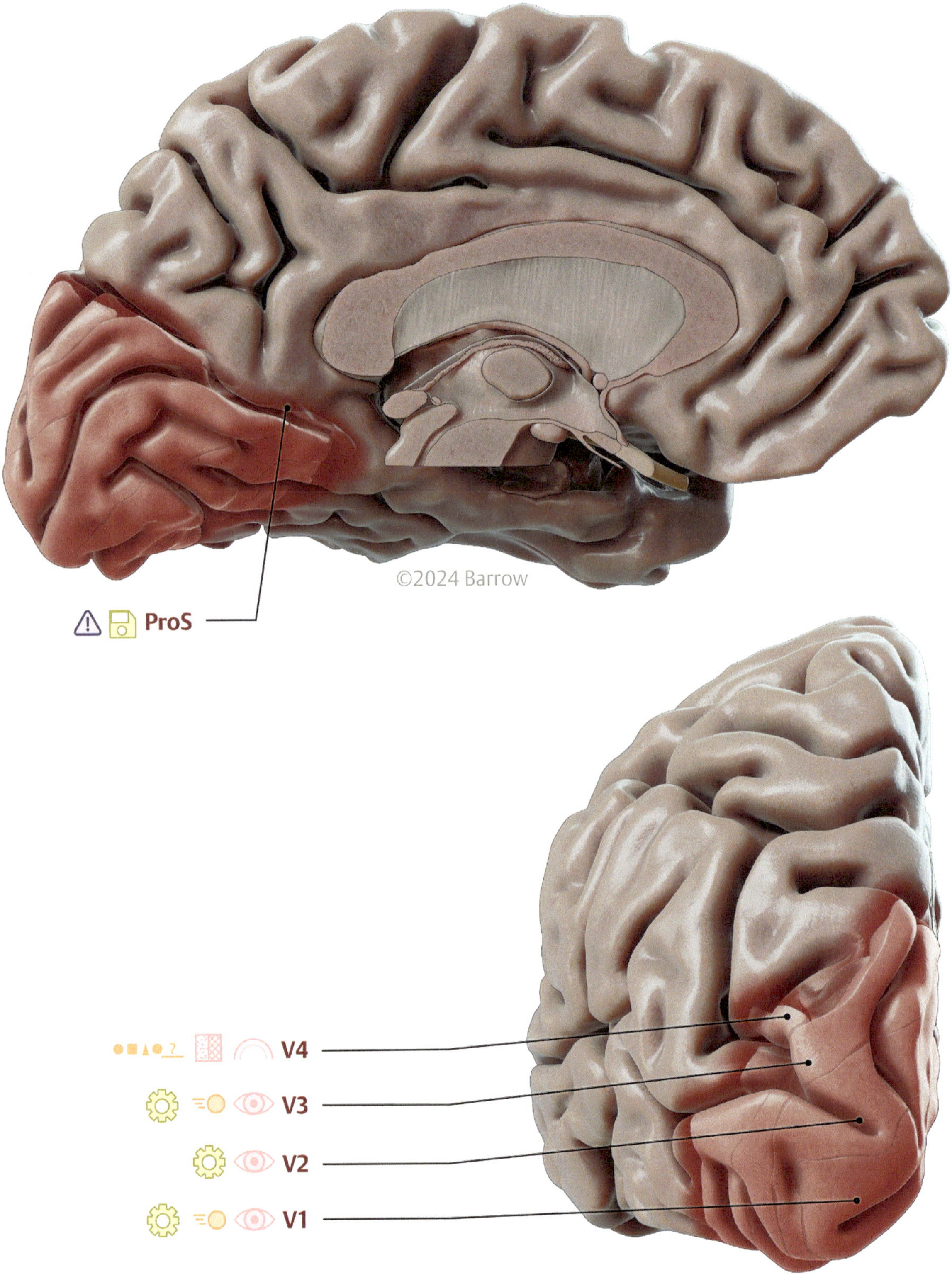

Fig. 18.34 Visual network - primary. (Reproduced with permission from Barrow Neurological Institute, Phoenix, AZ.)

Visual Network - Dorsal and Ventral Streams

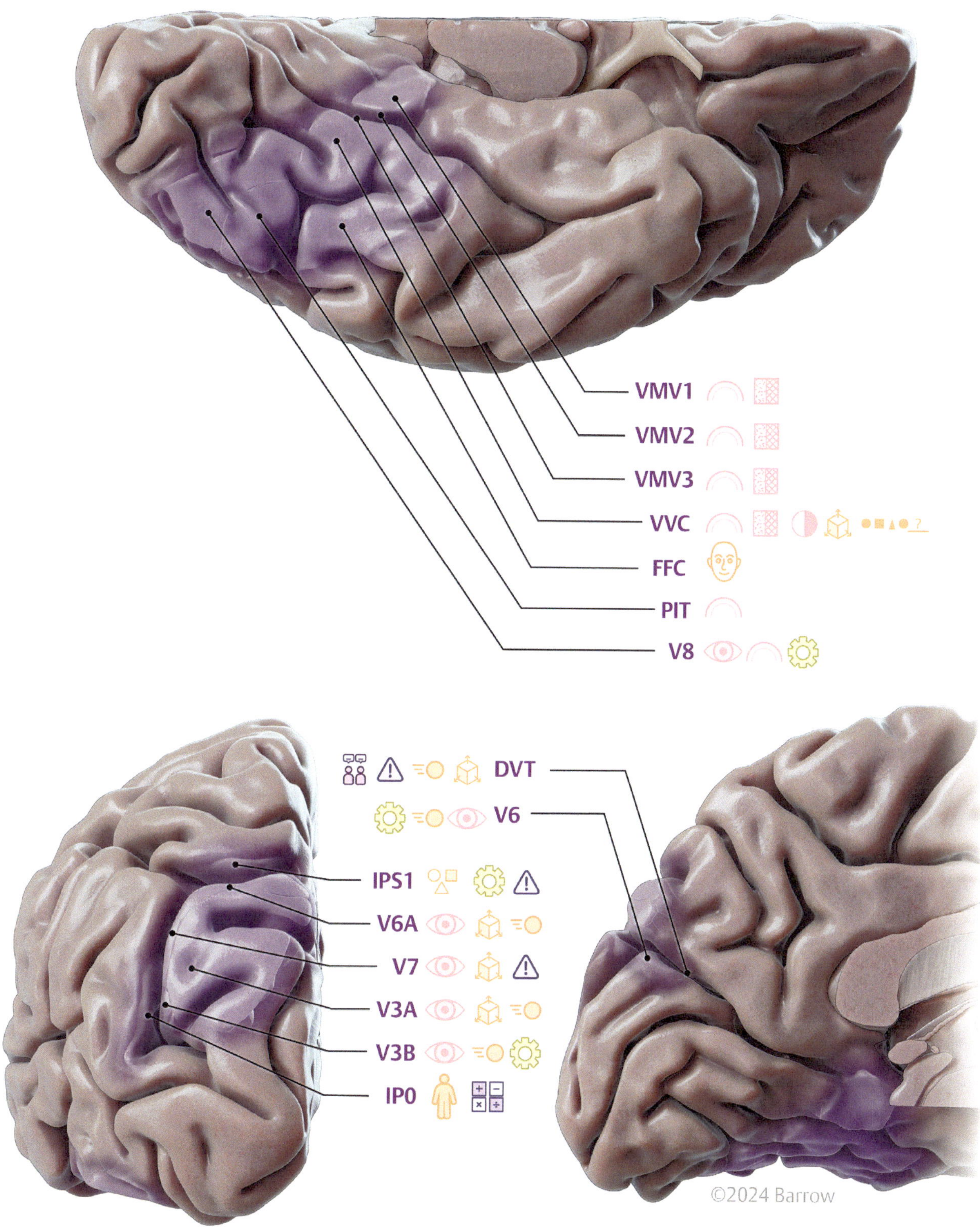

Fig. 18.35 Visual network - dorsal and ventral streams. (Reproduced with permission from Barrow Neurological Institute, Phoenix, AZ.)

Suggested Readings

Abla AA, Benet A, Lawton MT. The far lateral transpontomedullary sulcus approach to pontine cavernous malformations: technical report and surgical results. Neurosurgery. 2014; 10 Suppl 3:472–480

Abla AA, Clark AJ, Lawton ML. Resection of pontine cavernous malformation through the pontomedullary sulcus. Neurosurg Focus. 2014; 36(1) Suppl:1

Abla AA, Lekovic GP, Garrett M, et al. Cavernous malformations of the brainstem presenting in childhood: surgical experience in 40 patients. Neurosurgery. 2010; 67(6):1589–1598, discussion 1598–1599

Abla AA, Lekovic GP, Turner JD, de Oliveira JG, Porter R, Spetzler RF. Advances in the treatment and outcome of brainstem cavernous malformation surgery: a single-center case series of 300 surgically treated patients. Neurosurgery. 2011; 68(2): 403–414, discussion 414–415

Abla AA, Spetzler RF. Brainstem cavernoma surgery: the state of the art. World Neurosurg. 2013; 80(1–2):44–46

Abla AA, Spetzler RF, Albuquerque FC. Trans-striatocapsular contralateral interhemispheric resection of anterior inferior basal ganglia cavernous malformation. World Neurosurg. 2013; 80(6):e397–e399

Abla AA, Turner JD, Mitha AP, Lekovic G, Spetzler RF. Surgical approaches to brainstem cavernous malformations. Neurosurg Focus. 2010; 29(3):E8

Aboud E, Abolfotoh M, Pravdenkova S, Gokoglu A, Gokden M, Al-Mefty O. Giant intracranial epidermoids: is total removal feasible? J Neurosurg. 2015; 122(4): 743–756

Abramov I, Labib MA, Houlihan LM, et al. Volumetric three-dimensional analysis of the retrosigmoid, extended retrosigmoid, and presigmoid-retrolabyrinthine transpetrosal fissure approaches to the middle cerebellar peduncle. J Neurol Surg B Skull Base. 2022; 83(S01):P158

Abramov I, Scherschinski L, Labib MA, et al. Supracerebellar infratentorial approach for a malignant pineal region tumor mimicking a cavernous malformation. World Neurosurg. 2022; 167:122

Adeeb N, Mortazavi MM, Tubbs RS, Cohen-Gadol AA. The cranial dura mater: a review of its history, embryology, and anatomy. Childs Nerv Syst. 2012; 28(6): 827–837

Akakin A, Peris-Celda M, Kilic T, Seker A, Gutierrez-Martin A, Rhoton A, Jr. The dentate nucleus and its projection system in the human cerebellum: the dentate nucleus microsurgical anatomical study. Neurosurgery. 2014; 74(4):401–424, discussion 424–425

Akiyama O, Matsushima K, Gungor A, et al. Microsurgical and endoscopic approaches to the pulvinar. J Neurosurg. 2017; 127(3):630–645

Akpolat YT, İnceoğlu S, Kinne N, Hunt D, Cheng WK. Fatigue performance of cortical bone trajectory screw compared with standard trajectory pedicle screw. Spine. 2016; 41(6):E335–E341

Al-Shahi Salman R, Berg MJ, Morrison L, Awad IA, Angioma Alliance Scientific Advisory Board. Hemorrhage from cavernous malformations of the brain: definition and reporting standards. Stroke. 2008; 39(12):3222–3230

Albalkhi I, Shafqat A, Bin-Alamer O, et al. Long-term functional outcomes and complications of microsurgical resection of brainstem cavernous malformations: a systematic review and meta-analysis. Neurosurg Rev. 2023; 46(1):252

Allan PG, Briggs RG, Conner AK, et al. Parcellation-based tractographic modeling of the dorsal attention network. Brain Behav. 2019; 9(10):e01365

Allan PG, Briggs RG, Conner AK, et al. Parcellation-based tractographic modeling of the ventral attention network. J Neurol Sci. 2020; 408:116548

American Association of Neurological Surgeons. ENRICH Trial Findings Debuts at the 2023 American Association of Neurological Surgeons Annual Scientific Meeting. April 22, 2023. Accessed May 24, 2023 at: https://www.aans.org/en/Media/Press-Releases

Asakawa H, Yanaka K, Nose T. MRI of Claude's syndrome. Neurology. 2003; 61(4):575

Atalar M, Kars Z, Egilmez R, Egilmez H. Giant cavernous angioma mimicking cerebellar neoplasm with major bleed: a case report. Tip Arastirmalari Dergisi. 2007; 5(3):153–156

Baker CM, Burks JD, Briggs RG, et al. A connectomic atlas of the human cerebrum-chapter 8: the posterior cingulate cortex, medial parietal lobe, and parieto-occipital sulcus. Oper Neurosurg (Hagerstown). 2018; 15 suppl_1:S350–S371

Baker CM, Burks JD, Briggs RG, et al. A connectomic atlas of the human cerebrum-chapter 5: the insula and opercular cortex. Oper Neurosurg (Hagerstown). 2018; 15 suppl_1:S175–S244

Baker CM, Burks JD, Briggs RG, et al. A connectomic atlas of the human cerebrum chapter 4: the medial frontal lobe, anterior cingulate gyrus, and orbitofrontal cortex. Oper Neurosurg (Hagerstown). 2018; 15 suppl_1:S122–S174

Baker CM, Burks JD, Briggs RG, et al. A connectomic atlas of the human cerebrum chapter 9: the occipital lobe. Oper Neurosurg (Hagerstown). 2018; 15 suppl_1:S372–S406

Baker CM, Burks JD, Briggs RG, et al. A connectomic atlas of the human cerebrum-chapter 1: introduction, methods, and significance. Oper Neurosurg (Hagerstown). 2018; 15 suppl_1:S1–S9

Baker CM, Burks JD, Briggs RG, et al. A connectomic atlas of the human cerebrum-chapter 7: the lateral parietal lobe. Oper Neurosurg (Hagerstown). 2018; 15 suppl_1:S295–S349

Baker CM, Burks JD, Briggs RG, et al. A connectomic atlas of the human cerebrum-chapter 6: the temporal lobe. Oper Neurosurg (Hagerstown). 2018; 15 suppl_1: S245–S294

Baker CM, Burks JD, Briggs RG, et al. A connectomic atlas of the human cerebrum-chapter 3: the motor, premotor, and sensory cortices. Oper Neurosurg (Hagerstown). 2018; 15 suppl_1:S75–S121

Baker CM, Burks JD, Briggs RG, et al. A connectomic atlas of the human cerebrum chapter 2: the lateral frontal lobe. Oper Neurosurg (Hagerstown). 2018; 15 suppl_1:S10–S74

Balaev V, Orlov I, Petrushevsky A, Martynova O. Functional connectivity between salience, default mode and frontoparietal networks in post-stroke depression. J Affect Disord. 2018; 227:554–562

Balami JS, Chen RL, Buchan AM. Stroke syndromes and clinical management. QJM. 2013; 106(7):607–615

Baranoski JF, Bajaj A, Przybylowski CJ, et al. Clip retraction of the tentorium: application of a novel technique for tentorial retraction during supracerebellar transtentorial approaches. J Neurosurg. 2020; 134(3):1198–1202

Baranoski JF, Koester SW, Przybylowski CJ, et al. The glossopharyngo-cochlear triangle-part II: case series highlighting the clinical application to high-riding posterior inferior cerebellar artery aneurysms exposed through the extended retrosigmoid approach. Oper Neurosurg (Hagerstown). 2021; 20(3):252–259

Barrow DL, Schuette AJ. Cavernous malformations: a paradigm for progress. Clin Neurosurg. 2011; 58:27–41

Belotti F, Tengattini F, Mattavelli D, et al. Transclival approaches for intradural pathologies: historical overview and present scenario. Neurosurg Rev. 2021; 44 (1):279–287

Belykh E, Yağmurlu K, Lei T, et al. Quantitative anatomical comparison of the ipsilateral and contralateral interhemispheric transcallosal approaches to the lateral ventricle. J Neurosurg. 2018; 128(5):1492–1502

Benarroch EE. Periaqueductal gray: an interface for behavioral control. Neurology. 2012; 78(3):210–217

Benet A, Bang JS, Tabani H, Meybodi AT, Lawton MT. Supratonsillar approach to deep cerebellar cavernous malformations near the dentate nucleus: 3-dimensional operative video. Oper Neurosurg (Hagerstown). 2017; 13(6):759

Benet A, Tabani H, Griswold D, Yousef S, Rubio RR, Lawton MT. Supracerebellar-infratentorial approach for resection of tectal and thalamic cavernous malformations: 3-dimensional operative video. Oper Neurosurg (Hagerstown). 2018; 14(3):316

Benner D, Hendricks BK, Benet A, et al. A system of anatomical triangles defining dissection routes to brainstem cavernous malformations: definitions and application to a cohort of 183 patients. J Neurosurg. 2022; 138(3):768–784

Benner D, Hendricks BK, Preul MC, Lawton MT. A skull base surgeon's GPS: 27 anatomical triangles of the anterior, posterior and middle fossae. J Neurol Surg B Skull Base. 2020; 81(S01):P022

Bertalanffy H, Gilsbach JM, Eggert HR, Seeger W. Microsurgery of deep-seated cavernous angiomas: report of 26 cases. Acta Neurochir (Wien). 1991; 108(3–4): 91–99

Bhardwaj RD, Auguste KI, Kulkarni AV, Dirks PB, Drake JM, Rutka JT. Management of pediatric brainstem cavernous malformations: experience over 20 years at the hospital for sick children. J Neurosurg Pediatr. 2009; 4(5):458–464

Bhatia KP, Marsden CD. The behavioural and motor consequences of focal lesions of the basal ganglia in man. Brain. 1994; 117(Pt 4):859–876

Bhatia S, O'Neill BR, Pu F, Aziz K. Giant tentorial cavernous hemangioma: case report and review of literature. Clin Neurol Neurosurg. 2011; 113(10):937–942

Bonnelle V, Ham TE, Leech R, et al. Salience network integrity predicts default mode network function after traumatic brain injury. Proc Natl Acad Sci U S A. 2012; 109(12):4690–4695

Boord P, Madhyastha TM, Askren MK, Grabowski TJ. Executive attention networks show altered relationship with default mode network in PD. Neuroimage Clin. 2016; 13:1–8

Boschi A, Consoli A, Buccoliero A, Barbagli G, Mangiafico S, Ammannati F. Left deep frontal cavernous angioma mimicking a glioma in an adult patient. Asian J Neurosurg. 2018; 13(4):1233–1235

Bozkurt B, Yağmurlu K, Belykh E, et al. Quantitative anatomic analysis of the transcallosal-transchoroidal approach and the transcallosal-subchoroidal approach to the floor of the third ventricle: an anatomic study. World Neurosurg. 2018; 118:219–229

Bricolo A. Surgical management of intrinsic brain stem gliomas. Oper Tech Neurosurg. 2000; 3(2):137–154

Briggs RG, Allan PG, Poologaindran A, et al. The frontal aslant tract and supplementary motor area syndrome: moving towards a connectomic initiation axis. Cancers (Basel). 2021; 13(5):1116

Briggs RG, Conner AK, Baker CM, et al. A connectomic atlas of the human cerebrum-chapter 18: the connectional anatomy of human brain networks. Oper Neurosurg (Hagerstown). 2018; 15 suppl_1:S470–S480

Briggs RG, Conner AK, Rahimi M, et al. A connectomic atlas of the human cerebrum-chapter 14: tractographic description of the frontal aslant tract. Oper Neurosurg (Hagerstown). 2018; 15 suppl_1:S444–S449

Briggs RG, Conner AK, Sali G, et al. A connectomic atlas of the human cerebrum chapter 17: tractographic description of the cingulum. Oper Neurosurg (Hagerstown). 2018; 15 suppl_1:S462–S469

Briggs RG, Conner AK, Sali G, et al. A connectomic atlas of the human cerebrum-chapter 16: tractographic description of the vertical occipital fasciculus. Oper Neurosurg (Hagerstown). 2018; 15 suppl_1:S456–S461

Briggs RG, Rahimi M, Conner AK, et al. A connectomic atlas of the human cerebrum-chapter 15: tractographic description of the uncinate fasciculus. Oper Neurosurg (Hagerstown). 2018; 15 suppl_1:S450–S455

Briggs RG, Young IM, Dadario NB, et al. Parcellation-based tractographic modeling of the salience network through meta-analysis. Brain Behav. 2022; 12(7):e2646

Broadley SA, Taylor J, Waddy HM, Thompson PD. The clinical and MRI correlate of ischaemia in the ventromedial midbrain: Claude's syndrome. J Neurol. 2001; 248 (12):1087–1089

Brodmann K. Vergleichende Lokalisationslehre der Grosshirnrinde in ihren Prinzipien dargestellt auf Grund des Zellenbaues. Leipzig: Johann Ambrosius Barth Verlag; 1909

Brown AP, Thompson BG, Spetzler RF. The two-point method: evaluating brain stem lesions. BNI Q. 1996; 12(1):20–24

Brown P, Eusebio A. Paradoxes of functional neurosurgery: clues from basal ganglia recordings. Mov Disord. 2008; 23(1):12–20, quiz 158

Brüggemann N. Contemporary functional neuroanatomy and pathophysiology of dystonia. J Neural Transm (Vienna). 2021; 128(4):499–508

Bruneau M, Bijlenga P, Reverdin A, et al. Early surgery for brainstem cavernomas. Acta Neurochir (Wien). 2006; 148(4):405–414

Buckner RL. The cerebellum and cognitive function: 25 years of insight from anatomy and neuroimaging. Neuron. 2013; 80(3):807–815

Buckner RL, Andrews-Hanna JR, Schacter DL. The brain's default network: anatomy, function, and relevance to disease. Ann N Y Acad Sci. 2008; 1124:1–38

Burkhardt JK, Gandhi S, Tabani H, Benet A, Lawton MT. Left transsylvian-transinsular approach for radiation-induced cavernous malformation: 3-dimensional operative video. Oper Neurosurg (Hagerstown). 2019; 17(2):E62–E63

Butts T, Green MJ, Wingate RJ. Development of the cerebellum: simple steps to make a 'little brain'. Development. 2014; 141(21):4031–4041

Calvert GC, Lawrence BD, Abtahi AM, Bachus KN, Brodke DS. Cortical screws used to rescue failed lumbar pedicle screw construct: a biomechanical analysis. J Neurosurg Spine. 2015; 22(2):166–172

Cannizzaro D, Sabatino G, Mancarella C, et al. Management and surgical approaches of brainstem cavernous malformations: our experience and literature review. Asian J Neurosurg. 2019; 14(1):131–139

Cantu C, Murillo-Bonilla L, Arauz A, Higuera J, Padilla J, Barinagarrementeria F. Predictive factors for intracerebral hemorrhage in patients with cavernous angiomas. Neurol Res. 2005; 27(3):314–318

Catalino MP, Yao S, Green DL, Laws ER, Golby AJ, Tie Y. Mapping cognitive and emotional networks in neurosurgical patients using resting-state functional magnetic resonance imaging. Neurosurg Focus. 2020; 48(2):E9

Catapano JS, Benner D, Rhodenhiser EG, et al. Safety of brainstem safe entry zones: comparison of microsurgical outcomes associated with superficial, exophytic, and deep brainstem cavernous malformations. J Neurosurg. 2022; 139(1):113–123

Catapano JS, Koester SW, Rumalla K, et al. Microsurgical resection of brainstem cavernous malformations in older adults: a multicenter, 30-year experience. Neurosurgery. 2024; 95(3):669–675

Catapano JS, Rumalla K, Srinivasan VM, et al. A taxonomy for deep cerebral cavernous malformations: subtypes of thalamic lesions. J Neurosurg. 2023; 139 (6):1681–1696

Catapano JS, Rumalla K, Srinivasan VM, Lawrence PM, Larson Keil K, Lawton MT. A taxonomy for brainstem cavernous malformations: subtypes of midbrain lesions. J Neurosurg. 2021; 136(6):1667–1686

Catapano JS, Rumalla K, Srinivasan VM, Lawrence PM, Larson Keil K, Lawton MT. A taxonomy for brainstem cavernous malformations: subtypes of medullary lesions. J Neurosurg. 2022; 138(1):128–146

Catapano JS, Rumalla K, Srinivasan VM, Lawrence PM, Larson Keil K, Lawton MT. A taxonomy for brainstem cavernous malformations: subtypes of pontine lesions. Part 1: basilar, peritrigeminal, and middle peduncular. J Neurosurg. 2022; 137 (5):1462–1476

Catapano JS, Rumalla K, Srinivasan VM, Lawrence PM, Larson Keil K, Lawton MT. A taxonomy for brainstem cavernous malformations: subtypes of pontine lesions. Part 2: inferior peduncular, rhomboid, and supraolivary. J Neurosurg. 2022; 137 (5):1477–1490

Catapano JS, Rutledge C, Rumalla K, et al. External validation of the Lawton brainstem cavernous malformation grading system in a cohort of 277 microsurgical patients. J Neurosurg. 2021; 136(5):1231–1239

Catapano JS, Rumalla K, Srinivasan VM, et al. A taxonomy for deep cerebral cavernous malformations: subtypes of basal ganglia lesions. J Neurosurg. 2023; 140(5):1312–1327

Cavalcanti DD, Preul MC, Kalani MY, Spetzler RF. Microsurgical anatomy of safe entry zones to the brainstem. J Neurosurg. 2016; 124(5):1359–1376

Cavalheiro S, Yagmurlu K, da Costa MD, et al. Surgical approaches for brainstem tumors in pediatric patients. Childs Nerv Syst. 2015; 31(10):1815–1840

Cenzato M, Colistra D, Iacopino G, et al. Holmes tremor: a delayed complication after resection of brainstem cavernomas. J Neurosurg. 2020; 135(3):693–703

Cenzato M, Stefini R, Ambrosi C, Giovanelli M. Post-operative remnants of brainstem cavernomas: incidence, risk factors and management. Acta Neurochir (Wien). 2008; 150(9):879–886, discussion 887

Chaichana K, Quinones-Hinojosa A. Comprehensive Overview of Modern Surgical Approaches to Intrinsic Brain Tumors. Philadelphia, PA: Elsevier; 2019

Chang EF, Gabriel RA, Potts MB, Berger MS, Lawton MT. Supratentorial cavernous malformations in eloquent and deep locations: surgical approaches and outcomes. Clinical article. J Neurosurg. 2011; 114(3):814–827

Chang EF, Gabriel RA, Potts MB, Garcia PA, Barbaro NM, Lawton MT. Seizure characteristics and control after microsurgical resection of supratentorial cerebral cavernous malformations. Neurosurgery. 2009; 65(1):31–37, discussion 37–38

Chang EF, Raygor KP, Berger MS. Contemporary model of language organization: an overview for neurosurgeons. J Neurosurg. 2015; 122(2):250–261

Chang YT, Lu CH, Wu MK, et al. Salience network and depressive severities in Parkinson's disease with mild cognitive impairment: a structural covariance network analysis. Front Aging Neurosci. 2018; 9:417

Chen AC, Oathes DJ, Chang C, et al. Causal interactions between fronto-parietal central executive and default-mode networks in humans. Proc Natl Acad Sci U S A. 2013; 110(49):19944–19949

Chen L, Zhao Y, Zhou L, Zhu W, Pan Z, Mao Y. Surgical strategies in treating brainstem cavernous malformations. Neurosurgery. 2011; 68(3):609–620, discussion 620–621

Chen LH, Zhang HT, Chen L, Liu LX, Xu RX. Minimally invasive resection of brainstem cavernous malformations: surgical approaches and clinical experiences with 38 patients. Clin Neurol Neurosurg. 2014; 116:72–79

Cheng YK, Weng HH, Yang JT, Lee MH, Wang TC, Chang CN. Factors affecting graft infection after cranioplasty. J Clin Neurosci. 2008; 15(10):1115–1119

Child ND, Benarroch EE. Anterior nucleus of the thalamus: functional organization and clinical implications. Neurology. 2013; 81(21):1869–1876

Choquet H, Pawlikowska L, Lawton MT, Kim H. Genetics of cerebral cavernous malformations: current status and future prospects. J Neurosurg Sci. 2015; 59 (3):211–220

Clark AJ, Wang DD, Lawton MT. Spinal cavernous malformations. Handb Clin Neurol. 2017; 143:303–308

Clatterbuck RE, Bernardo A, Spetzler RF. Discovering the novel surgical approach. Clin Neurosurg. 2003; 50:36–44

Claude H. Syndrome pedonculaire de la region du noyau rouge. Rev Neurol (Paris). 1912; 23:311–313

Cofano F, Marengo N, Ajello M, et al. The era of cortical bone trajectory screws in spine surgery: a qualitative review with rating of evidence. World Neurosurg. 2020; 134:14–24

Collins L. MNI Average Brain (305 MRI) Stereotaxic Registration Model. McConnell Brain Imaging Centre, Montreal Neurological Institute, McGill University. Accessed August 25, 2021 at: https://www.bic.mni.mcgill.ca/ServicesAtlases/MNI305

Conner AK, Briggs RG, Rahimi M, et al. A connectomic atlas of the human cerebrum-chapter 10: tractographic description of the superior longitudinal fasciculus. Oper Neurosurg (Hagerstown). 2018; 15 suppl_1:S407–S422

Conner AK, Briggs RG, Rahimi M, et al. A connectomic atlas of the human cerebrum-chapter 12: tractographic description of the middle longitudinal fasciculus. Oper Neurosurg (Hagerstown). 2018; 15 suppl_1:S429–S435

Conner AK, Briggs RG, Sali G, et al. A connectomic atlas of the human cerebrum-chapter 13: tractographic description of the inferior fronto-occipital fasciculus. Oper Neurosurg (Hagerstown). 2018; 15 suppl_1:S436–S443

Consales A, Piatelli G, Ravegnani M, et al. Treatment and outcome of children with cerebral cavernomas: a survey on 32 patients. Neurol Sci. 2010; 31(2): 117–123

Corbetta M, Shulman GL. Spatial neglect and attention networks. Annu Rev Neurosci. 2011; 34:569–599

Dadario NB, Brahimaj B, Yeung J, Sughrue ME. Reducing the cognitive footprint of brain tumor surgery. Front Neurol. 2021; 12:711646

Dadario NB, Sughrue ME. Should neurosurgeons try to preserve non-traditional brain networks? A systematic review of the neuroscientific evidence. J Pers Med. 2022; 12(4):587

Dammann P, Abla AA, Al-Shahi Salman R, et al. Surgical treatment of brainstem cavernous malformations: an international Delphi consensus. J Neurosurg. 2021; 136(5):1220–1230

Dammann P, Wrede K, Jabbarli R, et al. Of bubbles and layers: which cerebral cavernous malformations are most difficult to dissect from surrounding eloquent brain tissue? Neurosurgery. 2017; 81(3):498–503

Dao I, Akhaddar A, El-Mostarchid B, Boucetta M. Giant cerebral cavernoma. Case report with literature review. Neurosciences (Riyadh). 2012; 17(1):69–73

Darby RR, Joutsa J, Burke MJ, Fox MD. Lesion network localization of free will. Proc Natl Acad Sci U S A. 2018; 115(42):10792–10797

Das KK, Singh S, Deora H, et al. Microsurgical excision of giant dominant lobe insular cavernoma presenting acutely: sometimes you win, sometimes you learn. Interdiscip Neurosurg. 2019; 18:100475

Davies J, Tawk RG, Lawton MT. The contralateral transcingulate approach: operative technique and results with vascular lesions. Neurosurgery. 2012; 71(1) Suppl Operative:4–13, discussion 13–14

Davies JM, Kim H, Lawton MT. Surgical treatment of cerebral cavernous malformations. J Neurosurg Sci. 2015; 59(3):255–270

Day JD, Fukushima T, Giannotta SL. Microanatomical study of the extradural middle fossa approach to the petroclival and posterior cavernous sinus region: description of the rhomboid construct. Neurosurgery. 1994; 34(6):1009–1016, discussion 1016

de Oliveira E, Tedeschi H, Siqueira MG, Ono M, Rhoton AL, Jr. Arteriovenous malformations of the basal ganglia region: rationale for surgical management. Acta Neurochir (Wien). 1997; 139(6):487–506

Dejerine J. Semiologie des affections du système nerveux. Paris: Masson; 1914:226–230

Delgado-Fernandez J, García-Pallero MÁ, Blasco G, Pulido-Rivas P, Sola RG. Review of cortical bone trajectory: evidence of a new technique. Asian Spine J. 2017; 11(5): 817–831

Delgado-Fernández J, Pulido Rivas P, Gil-Simoes R, de Sola RG. How I do it? Lumbar cortical bone trajectory fixation with image-guided neuronavigation. Acta Neurochir (Wien). 2019; 161(12):2423–2428

Deshmukh VR, Rangel-Castilla L, Spetzler RF. Lateral inferior cerebellar peduncle approach to dorsolateral medullary cavernous malformation. J Neurosurg. 2014; 121(3):723–729

Devia DA, Graffeo CS, Benner D, et al. Experience and balance: long-term trends in preferred skull base approach for a case series of cavernous malformation resections. Oper Neurosurg (Hagerstown). 2023; 25(1):33–40

Dick AS, Garic D, Graziano P, Tremblay P. The frontal aslant tract (FAT) and its role in speech, language and executive function. Cortex. 2019; 111:148–163

Ding D, Starke RM, Crowley RW, Liu KC. Surgical approaches for symptomatic cerebral cavernous malformations of the thalamus and brainstem. J Cerebrovasc Endovasc Neurosurg. 2017; 19(1):19–35

Diogo M, Fragata I, Castanho P, Ramalho J, Mafra M, Reis J. Cerebellar giant cystic cavernoma mimicking neoplasia (abstract P-1.2). IInd Joint Meeting of the Portuguese Society of Neuroradiology (SPNR) and of the Spanish Society of Neuroradiology (SENR): (IX National Congress of the SPNR and XLII Annual Meeting of the SENR) 17–19 October 2013, Lisbon, Portugal. Neuroradiol. 2013; 55(12):1455–1511

Dolenc VV. Anatomy and Surgery of the Cavernous Sinus. Vienna: Springer; 1989

Doucet GE, Lee WH, Frangou S. Evaluation of the spatial variability in the major resting-state networks across human brain functional atlases. Hum Brain Mapp. 2019; 40(15):4577–4587

Drake CG, Peerless SJ, Hernesniemi JA, Hernesniemi J. Surgery of Vertebrobasilar Aneurysms: London, Ontario Experience on 1767 Patients. New York, NY: Springer; 1996

Drazin D, Wang JM, Alonso F, et al. Intracranial anatomical triangles: a comprehensive illustrated review. Cureus. 2017; 9(10):e1741

Dukatz T, Sarnthein J, Sitter H, et al. Quality of life after brainstem cavernoma surgery in 71 patients. Neurosurgery. 2011; 69(3):689–695

Eickhoff SB, Yeo BTT, Genon S. Imaging-based parcellations of the human brain. Nat Rev Neurosci. 2018; 19(11):672–686

Ellard KK, Zimmerman JP, Kaur N, et al. Functional connectivity between anterior insula and key nodes of frontoparietal executive control and salience networks distinguish bipolar depression from unipolar depression and healthy control subjects. Biol Psychiatry Cogn Neurosci Neuroimaging. 2018; 3(5):473–484

"Eloquence." Merriam-Webster.com. Accessed May 24, 2023 at: https://www.merriam-webster.com/dictionary/eloquence

Englot DJ, Han SJ, Lawton MT, Chang EF. Predictors of seizure freedom in the surgical treatment of supratentorial cavernous malformations. J Neurosurg. 2011; 115 (6):1169–1174

Espinosa PS. Teaching NeuroImage: one-and-a-half syndrome. Neurology. 2008; 70 (5):e20

Etminan N, Brown RD, Jr, Beseoglu K, et al. The unruptured intracranial aneurysm treatment score: a multidisciplinary consensus. Neurology. 2015; 85(10):881–889

Ferroli P, Schiariti M, Cordella R, et al. The lateral infratrigeminal transpontine window to deep pontine lesions. J Neurosurg. 2015; 123(3):699–710

Ferroli P, Sinisi M, Franzini A, Giombini S, Solero CL, Broggi G. Brainstem cavernomas: long-term results of microsurgical resection in 52 patients. Neurosurgery. 2005; 56(6):1203–1212, discussion 1212–1214

Figueiredo EG, Beer-Furlan A, Welling LC, et al. Microsurgical approaches to the ambient cistern region: an anatomic and qualitative study. World Neurosurg. 2016; 87:584–590

Firbank M, Kobeleva X, Cherry G, et al. Neural correlates of attention-executive dysfunction in lewy body dementia and Alzheimer's disease. Hum Brain Mapp. 2016; 37(3):1254–1270

Forsting M. Intracranial Vascular Malformations and Aneurysms: From Diagnostic Work-up to Endovascular Therapy. Berlin: Springer; 2006

Foster BL, Parvizi J. Resting oscillations and cross-frequency coupling in the human posteromedial cortex. Neuroimage. 2012; 60(1):384–391

François P, Ben Ismail M, Hamel O, Bataille B, Jan M, Velut S. Anterior transpetrosal and subtemporal transtentorial approaches for pontine cavernomas. Acta Neurochir (Wien). 2010; 152(8):1321–1329, discussion 1329

Freeman JB, Ambady N. MouseTracker: software for studying real-time mental processing using a computer mouse-tracking method. Behav Res Methods. 2010; 42(1):226–241

Frisoli FA, Baranoski JF, Catapano JS, Lang MJ, Lawton MT. Contralateral supracerebellar-transtentorial approach for posterior mediobasal temporal cavernous malformation resection. World Neurosurg. 2022; 158:166

Frisoli FA, Catapano JS, Baranoski JF, Lawton MT. The middle communicating artery: a novel fourth-generation bypass for revascularizing trapped middle cerebral artery bifurcation aneurysms in 2 cases. J Neurosurg. 2020; 134(6):1879–1886

Fritschi JA, Reulen HJ, Spetzler RF, Zabramski JM. Cavernous malformations of the brain stem. A review of 139 cases. Acta Neurochir (Wien). 1994; 130(1–4):35–46

Gandhi S, Chen T, Mascitelli JR, et al. Contralateral supracerebellar transtentorial approach for a thalamic cavernous malformation resection: operative video. Neurosurg Focus Video. 2019; 1(1):V21

Garcia RM, Ivan ME, Lawton MT. Brainstem cavernous malformations: surgical results in 104 patients and a proposed grading system to predict neurological outcomes. Neurosurgery. 2015; 76(3):265–277, discussion 277–278

Garcia RM, Oh T, Cole TS, Hendricks BK, Lawton MT. Recurrent brainstem cavernous malformations following primary resection: blind spots, fine lines, and the right-angle method. J Neurosurg. 2020; 135(3):671–682

Garin CM, Hori Y, Everling S, et al. An evolutionary gap in primate default mode network organization. Cell Rep. 2022; 39(2):110669

Georgieva VB, Krastev ED. Surgical treatment of brainstem cavernous malformation with concomitant developmental venous anomaly. Asian J Neurosurg. 2019; 14 (2):557–560

Giliberto G, Lanzino DJ, Diehn FE, Factor D, Flemming KD, Lanzino G. Brainstem cavernous malformations: anatomical, clinical, and surgical considerations. Neurosurg Focus. 2010; 29(3):E9

Glasser MF, Coalson TS, Robinson EC, et al. A multi-modal parcellation of human cerebral cortex. Nature. 2016; 536(7615):171–178

Glassock ME, III, Jackson CG, Dickins JR, Wiet RJ. Panel discussion: glomus jugulare tumors of the temporal bone. The surgical management of glomus tumors. Laryngoscope. 1979; 89(10, Pt 1):1640–1654

Gondim JA, Almeida JP, Albuquerque LA, Gomes EF, Schops M. Giant pituitary adenomas: surgical outcomes of 50 cases operated on by the endonasal endoscopic approach. World Neurosurg. 2014; 82(1–2):e281–e290

Gonzalez LF, Crawford NR, Horgan MA, Deshmukh P, Zabramski JM, Spetzler RF. Working area and angle of attack in three cranial base approaches: pterional, orbitozygomatic, and maxillary extension of the orbitozygomatic approach. Neurosurgery. 2002; 50(3):550–555, discussion 555–557

Gonzalez LF, Lekovic GP, Eschbacher J, Coons S, Porter RW, Spetzler RF. Are cavernous sinus hemangiomas and cavernous malformations different entities? Neurosurg Focus. 2006; 21(1):e6

Graffeo CS, Hanalioglu S, Baranoski JF, Srinivasan VM, Lawton MT. Orbitozygomatic craniotomy and transsylvian approach for resection of an interpeduncular midbrain cavernous malformation: 2-dimensional operative video. Oper Neurosurg (Hagerstown). 2023; 24(5):e366–e367

Graffeo CS, Link MJ, Lawton MT. Complex cranial surgery and the future of open cerebrovascular training. J Neurosurg. 2022; 137(5):1554–1561

Graffeo CS, Scherschinski L, Baranoski JF, Srinivasan VM, Lawton MT. Resection of quadrigeminal midbrain cavernous malformation using the supracollicular safe entry zone. World Neurosurg. 2023; 169:51

Graffeo CS, Scherschinski L, Baranoski JF, Srinivasan VM, Lawton MT. Microsurgical resection of a lateral pontine arteriovenous malformation masquerading as a cavernous malformation: 2-dimensional operative video. Oper Neurosurg (Hagerstown). 2024; 27(3):386

Graffeo CS, Scherschinski L, Benner D, et al. Approach selection strategies for repeat resection of brain cavernous malformations: cohort study. Oper Neurosurg (Hagerstown). 2023; 24(6):590–601

Graffeo CS, Srinivasan VM, Scherschinski L, et al. Expanding the reach of the trans-middle cerebellar peduncle approach: pontine cavernous malformations, tissue transgression beyond the safe entry zone, and the invisible triangle. J Neurosurg. 2023; 140(5):1344–1356

Grant SW, Collins GS, Nashef SAM. Statistical primer: developing and validating a risk prediction model. Eur J Cardiothorac Surg. 2018; 54(2):203–208

Gratton C, Sun H, Petersen SE. Control networks and hubs. Psychophysiology. 2018; 55(3):e13032

Grodd W, Kumar VJ, Schüz A, Lindig T, Scheffler K. The anterior and medial thalamic nuclei and the human limbic system: tracing the structural connectivity using diffusion-weighted imaging. Sci Rep. 2020; 10(1):10957

Gross BA, Batjer HH, Awad IA, Bendok BR. Brainstem cavernous malformations. Neurosurgery. 2009; 64(5):E805–E818, discussion E818

Gross BA, Batjer HH, Awad IA, Bendok BR, Du R. Brainstem cavernous malformations: 1390 surgical cases from the literature. World Neurosurg. 2013; 80(1–2):89–93

Gross BA, Du R. Hemorrhage from cerebral cavernous malformations: a systematic pooled analysis. J Neurosurg. 2017; 126(4):1079–1087

Gross BA, Lin N, Du R, Day AL. The natural history of intracranial cavernous malformations. Neurosurg Focus. 2011; 30(6):E24

Gruters KG, Groh JM. Sounds and beyond: multisensory and other non-auditory signals in the inferior colliculus. Front Neural Circuits. 2012; 6:96

Guillery RW, Sherman SM. Thalamic relay functions and their role in corticocortical communication: generalizations from the visual system. Neuron. 2002; 33(2): 163–175

Guiot G, Derome P. Surgical problems of pituitary adenomas. In: Krayenbühl H, Brihaye J, Loew F, et al, eds. Advances and Technical Standards in Neurosurgery. Vienna: Springer; 1976:3–33

Guo X, Tabani H, Griswold D, et al. Hearing preservation during anterior petrosectomy: the "cochlear safety line." World Neurosurg. 2017; 99:618–622

Gupta S, Mends F, Hagiwara M, Fatterpekar G, Roehm PC. Imaging the facial nerve: a contemporary review. Radiol Res Pract. 2013; 2013:248039

Guyatt GH, Oxman AD, Vist GE, et al. GRADE Working Group. GRADE: an emerging consensus on rating quality of evidence and strength of recommendations. BMJ. 2008; 336(7650):924–926

Haciyakupoglu E, Yilmaz DM, Kinali B, Akbas T, Haciyakupoglu S. Analysis of cavernous malformations: experience with 18 cases. Turk Neurosurg. 2019; 29(3):340–348

Haines DE. Fundamental Neuroscience for Basic and Clinical Applications. 4th ed. Philadelphia, PA: Elsevier; 2013

Hakuba A. Surgical approaches to the cavernous sinus: repair of a C-C fistula at the C5 portion of the internal carotid artery]. No Shinkei Geka. 1986; 14(5):601–607

Hakuba A, Tanaka K, Suzuki T, Nishimura S. A combined orbitozygomatic infratemporal epidural and subdural approach for lesions involving the entire cavernous sinus. J Neurosurg. 1989; 71(5, Pt 1):699–704

Han SJ, Englot DJ, Kim H, Lawton MT. Brainstem arteriovenous malformations: anatomical subtypes, assessment of "occlusion in situ" technique, and microsurgical results. J Neurosurg. 2015; 122(1):107–117

Hart MG, Romero-Garcia R, Price SJ, Santarius T, Suckling J. Connections, tracts, fractals, and the rest: a working guide to network and connectivity studies in neurosurgery. World Neurosurg. 2020; 140:389–400

Hauck EF, Barnett SL, White JA, Samson D. Symptomatic brainstem cavernomas. Neurosurgery. 2009; 64(1):61–70, discussion 70–71

Hebb MO, Spetzler RF. Lateral transpeduncular approach to intrinsic lesions of the rostral pons. Neurosurgery. 2010; 66(3) Suppl Operative:26–29, discussion 29

Hendricks BK, Benet A, Lawrence PM, Benner D, Preul MC, Lawton MT. Anatomical triangles for use in skull base surgery: a comprehensive review. World Neurosurg. 2022; 164:79–92

Hendricks BK, Rumalla K, Benner D, Lawton MT. Cavernous malformations and artificial intelligence: machine learning applications. Neurosurg Clin N Am. 2022; 33(4):461–467

Hendricks BK, Scherschinski L, Jubran JH, et al. A taxonomy for superficial cerebral cavernous malformations: subtypes of cortical and subcortical lesions. J Neurosurg. 2024; 141(1):123–137

Hendricks BK, Scherschinski L, Jubran JH, et al. Eloquent noneloquence: redefinition of cortical eloquence based on outcomes of superficial cerebral cavernous malformation resection. J Neurosurg. 2024; 141(2):291–305

Heus P, Damen JAAG, Pajouheshnia R, et al. Poor reporting of multivariable prediction model studies: towards a targeted implementation strategy of the TRIPOD statement. BMC Med. 2018; 16(1):120

Hoffman JE, Ryan M, Wittenberg B, Armstrong J, Greenan K, Wilkinson C. Successful treatment of hemorrhagic brainstem cavernous malformation with hematoma evacuation and postoperative propranolol. Childs Nerv Syst. 2020; 36(9):2109–2112

Honnold A. Alone on the Wall (Expanded Edition). New York, NY: WW Norton & Company; 2018

Horne MA, Flemming KD, Su IC, et al. Cerebral Cavernous Malformations Individual Patient Data Meta-analysis Collaborators. Clinical course of untreated cerebral cavernous malformations: a meta-analysis of individual patient data. Lancet Neurol. 2016; 15(2):166–173

Hosmer DW, Lemeshow S. Applied Logistic Regression. New. York, NY: Wiley; 2000

Huang AP, Chen JS, Yang CC, et al. Brain stem cavernous malformations. J Clin Neurosci. 2010; 17(1):74–79

Huang C, Bertalanffy H, Kar S, Tsuji Y. Microsurgical management of midbrain cavernous malformations: does lesion depth influence the outcome? Acta Neurochir (Wien). 2021; 163(10):2739–2754

Hustwit G. The New York Subway Map Debate. New York, NY: Standards Manual; 2021:140

Hyodo A, Yanaka K, Higuchi O, Tomono Y, Nose T. Giant interdural cavernous hemangioma at the convexity. Case illustration. J Neurosurg. 2000; 92(3):503

Ichinose T, Goto T, Morisako H, Takami T, Ohata K. Microroll retractor for surgical resection of brainstem cavernomas. World Neurosurg. 2010; 73(5):520–522

Ivan ME, Lawton MT. Mini supraorbital approach to inferior frontal lobe cavernous malformations: case series. J Neurol Surg A Cent Eur Neurosurg. 2013; 74(3): 187–191

Ivan ME, Safaee MM, Martirosyan NL, et al. Anatomical triangles defining routes to anterior communicating artery aneurysms: the junctional and precommunicating triangles and the role of dome projection. J Neurosurg. 2019; 132(5):1517–1528

Jacobs DA, Galetta SL. Neuro-ophthalmology for neuroradiologists. AJNR Am J Neuroradiol. 2007; 28(1):3–8

James W. The energies of men. Science. 1907; 25(635):321–332

Kalani MY, Yagmurlu K, Martirosyan NL, Cavalcanti DD, Spetzler RF. Approach selection for intrinsic brainstem pathologies. J Neurosurg. 2016; 125(6):1596–1607

Kalani MY, Yagmurlu K, Martirosyan NL, Spetzler RF. The retrosigmoid petrosal fissure transpeduncular approach to central pontine lesions. World Neurosurg. 2016; 87:235–241

Kalani MYS, Yagmurlu K, Martirosyan NL, Spetzler RF. Transsylvian, transanterior sulcus approach to basal ganglia cavernous malformations. Oper Neurosurg (Hagerstown). 2017; 13(6):756

Kalani MYS, Yağmurlu K, Spetzler RF. The interpeduncular fossa approach for resection of ventromedial midbrain lesions. J Neurosurg. 2018; 128(3): 834–839

Kanzaki J, Kawase T, Sano K, Shiobara R, Toya S. A modified extended middle cranial fossa approach for acoustic tumors. Arch Otorhinolaryngol. 1977; 217 (1):119–121

Karas PJ, Mikell CB, Christian E, Liker MA, Sheth SA. Deep brain stimulation: a mechanistic and clinical update. Neurosurg Focus. 2013; 35(5):E1

Kawase T, Shiobara R, Toya S. Anterior transpetrosal-transtentorial approach for sphenopetroclival meningiomas: surgical method and results in 10 patients. Neurosurgery. 1991; 28(6):869–875, discussion 875–876

Kawase T, Toya S, Shiobara R, Mine T. Transpetrosal approach for aneurysms of the lower basilar artery. J Neurosurg. 1985; 63(6):857–861

Keane JR. The pretectal syndrome: 206 patients. Neurology. 1990; 40(4):684–690

Kearns KN, Chen CJ, Tvrdik P, Park MS, Kalani MYS. Outcomes of surgery for brainstem cavernous malformations: a systematic review. Stroke. 2019; 50(10): 2964–2966

Keleş A, Harput MV, Türe U. Microneurosurgical removal of a globus pallidus tumor with cottonoid-guided intraoperative ultrasonography: 2-dimensional operative video. Oper Neurosurg (Hagerstown). 2020; 19(2):E154

Keorochana G, Pairuchvej S, Trathitephun W, Arirachakaran A, Predeeprompan P, Kongtharvonskul J. Comparative outcomes of cortical screw trajectory fixation and pedicle screw fixation in lumbar spinal fusion: systematic review and meta-analysis. World Neurosurg. 2017; 102:340–349

Kerchner GA, Smith W, Lawton MT, Singh V. Co-occurrence of a cavernous malformation and contralateral moyamoya. Neurology. 2006; 66(10): 1601–1602

Kim H, Abla AA, Nelson J, et al. Validation of the supplemented Spetzler-Martin grading system for brain arteriovenous malformations in a multicenter cohort of 1009 surgical patients. Neurosurgery. 2015; 76(1):25–31, discussion 31–32, quiz 32–33

Kim JS, Han YS. Medial medullary infarction: clinical, imaging, and outcome study in 86 consecutive patients. Stroke. 2009; 40(10):3221–3225

Kimball MM, Lewis SB, Werning JW, Mocco JD. Resection of a pontine cavernous malformation via an endoscopic endonasal approach: a case report. Neurosurgery. 2012; 71(1) Suppl Operative:186–193, discussion 193–194

Kivelev J, Laakso A, Niemelä M, Hernesniemi J. A proposed grading system of brain and spinal cavernomas. Neurosurgery. 2011; 69(4):807–813, discussion 813–814

Koester SW, Rhodenhiser EG, Dabrowski SJ, et al. Radiation-induced cerebral cavernous malformations: a single-center experience and systematic literature review. World Neurosurg. 2023; 179:222–232.e2

Koester SW, Scherschinski L, Srinivasan VM, et al. Radiation-induced cavernous malformations in the spine: patient series. J Neurosurg Case Lessons. 2023; 5 (23):CASE22482

Kolz JM, Pinter ZW, Bydon M, Sebastian AS. Controversies in spine surgery: is a cortical bone trajectory superior to traditional pedicle screw trajectory? Clin Spine Surg. 2022; 35(6):225–228

Kuiper JJ, Lin YH, Young IM, et al. A parcellation-based model of the auditory network. Hear Res. 2020; 396:108078

Kumar KK, Parikh B, Jabarkheel R, Dirlikov B, Singh H. Fluoroscopic versus CT-guided cortical bone trajectory pedicle screw fixation: comparing trajectory related complications. J Clin Neurosci. 2021; 89:354–359

La Corte E, Eldahaby D, Greco E, et al. The frontal aslant tract: a systematic review for neurosurgical applications. Front Neurol. 2021; 12:641586

Lang J, Jr, Ohmachi N, Lang J, Sr. Anatomical landmarks of the rhomboid fossa (floor of the 4th ventricle), its length and its width. Acta Neurochir (Wien). 1991; 113 (1–2):84–90

Lang MJ, Lawton MT. Brainstem tumors. In: Jallo GI, Noureldine MHA, Shimony N, eds. Surgery for vascular lesions of the brainstem. Cham: Springer; 2020:195–215

Lashkarivand A, Ringstad G, Eide PK. Surgery for brainstem cavernous malformations: association between preoperative grade and postoperative quality of life. Oper Neurosurg (Hagerstown). 2020; 18(6):590–598

Lawton MT. Basilar apex aneurysms: surgical results and perspectives from an initial experience. Neurosurgery. 2002; 50(1):1–8, discussion 8–10

Lawton MT. Seven Aneurysms: Tenets and Techniques for Clipping. New York, NY: Thieme; 2011

Lawton MT. Seven AVMs: Tenets and Techniques for Resection. New York, NY: Thieme; 2014

Lawton MT. Seven Bypasses: Tenets and Techniques for Revascularization. New York, NY: Thieme; 2018

Lawton MT, Golfinos JG, Spetzler RF. The contralateral transcallosal approach: experience with 32 patients. Neurosurgery. 1996; 39(4):729–734, discussion 734–735

Lawton MT, Graffeo CS, Srinivasan VM, et al. Seven cavernomas and neurosurgical cartography, with an assessment of vascular waypoints. J Neurosurg. 2022; 138 (4):1148–1162

Lawton MT, Kim H, McCulloch CE, Mikhak B, Young WL. A supplementary grading scale for selecting patients with brain arteriovenous malformations for surgery. Neurosurgery. 2010; 66(4):702–713, discussion 713

Lawton MT, Lang MJ. The future of open vascular neurosurgery: perspectives on cavernous malformations, AVMs, and bypasses for complex aneurysms. J Neurosurg. 2019; 130(5):1409–1425

Lawton MT, Quiñones-Hinojosa A, Jun P. The supratonsillar approach to the inferior cerebellar peduncle: anatomy, surgical technique, and clinical application to cavernous malformations. Neurosurgery. 2006; 59(4) Suppl 2:ONS244–ONS251, discussion ONS251–ONS252

Lawton MT, Tayebi Meybodi A, Sughrue ME, et al. Seven Cavernomas, Project "Connectomunculus," and the mind. J Neurosurg. 2025; 142(5):1498–1516

Lawton MT, Vates GE, Quinones-Hinojosa A, McDonald WC, Marchuk DA, Young WL. Giant infiltrative cavernous malformation: clinical presentation, intervention, and genetic analysis: case report. Neurosurgery. 2004; 55(4):979–980

Le XF, Shi Z, Wang QL, Xu YF, Zhao JW, Tian W. Rate and risk factors of superior facet joint violation during cortical bone trajectory screw placement: a comparison of robot-assisted approach with a conventional technique. Orthop Surg. 2020; 12 (1):133–140

Lee GW, Son JH, Ahn MW, Kim HJ, Yeom JS. The comparison of pedicle screw and cortical screw in posterior lumbar interbody fusion: a prospective randomized noninferiority trial. Spine J. 2015; 15(7):1519–1526

Leksell L. The stereotaxic method and radiosurgery of the brain. Acta Chir Scand. 1951; 102(4):316–319

Li H, Ju Y, Cai BW, Chen J, You C, Hui XH. Experience of microsurgical treatment of brainstem cavernomas: report of 37 cases. Neurol India. 2009; 57(3):269–273

Li H-M, Zhang R-J, Gao H, et al. Biomechanical fixation properties of the cortical bone trajectory in the osteoporotic lumbar spine. World Neurosurg. 2018; 119: e717–e727

Li Y, Khahera A, Kim J, Mandel M, Han SS, Steinberg GK. Basal ganglia cavernous malformations: case series and systematic review of surgical management and long-term outcomes. J Neurosurg. 2021; 135(4):1113–1121

Liu GT, Crenner CW, Logigian EL, Charness ME, Samuels MA. Midbrain syndromes of Benedikt, Claude, and Nothnagel: setting the record straight. Neurology. 1992; 42(9):1820–1822

Locksley HB. Natural history of subarachnoid hemorrhage, intracranial aneurysms and arteriovenous malformations. Based on 6368 cases in the cooperative study. J Neurosurg. 1966; 25(2):219–239

London D, Lieberman S, Tanweer O, Pacione D. Transclival approach for resection of a pontine cavernous malformation: 2-dimensional operative video. Oper Neurosurg (Hagerstown). 2020; 19(4):E413

Lowe LH, Marchant TC, Rivard DC, Scherbel AJ. Vascular malformations: classification and terminology the radiologist needs to know. Semin Roentgenol. 2012; 47(2):106–117

Lu DC, Lawton MT. Clinical presentation and surgical management of intramedullary spinal cord cavernous malformations. Neurosurg Focus. 2010; 29(3):E12

Mao Y, Zhao Y, Zhou LF, et al. A novel gene mutation (1292 deletion) in a Chinese family with cerebral cavernous malformations. Neurosurgery. 2005; 56(5): 1149–1153, discussion 1149–1153

Marengo N, Matsukawa K, Monticelli M, et al. Cortical bone trajectory screw placement accuracy with a patient-matched 3-dimensional printed guide in lumbar spinal surgery: a clinical study. World Neurosurg. 2019; 130:e98–e104

Martin S. How graphic design legend Massimo Vignelli cracked the NYC subway system. Accessed May 23, 2022 at: https://www.ceros.com/inspire/originals/massimo-vignelli-nyc-subway/

Martinez JA, de Oliveira E, Tedeschi H, Wen HT, Rhoton AL. Microsurgical anatomy of the brain stem. Operative Techniques in Neurosurgery. 2000; 3(2):80–86

Mascitelli J, Burkhardt JK, Gandhi S, Lawton MT. Contralateral supracerebellar-infratentorial approach for resection of thalamic cavernous malformations. Oper Neurosurg (Hagerstown). 2018; 15(4):404–411

Mascitelli J, Gandhi S, Wright E, Lawton MT. Transsylvian-transinsular approach for an insular cavernous malformation resection: 3-dimensional operative video. Oper Neurosurg (Hagerstown). 2019; 16(2):50

Mascitelli JR, Gandhi S, Cavallo C, Nanaszko MJ, Wright EJ, Lawton MT. Right pretemporal-transsylvian approach for resection of a midbrain cavernous malformation: 3-dimensional operative video. Oper Neurosurg (Hagerstown). 2019; 16(4):E113

Mascitelli JR, Gandhi S, Tayebi Meybodi A, Lawton MT. The oculomotor-tentorial triangle. Part 2: a microsurgical workspace for vascular lesions in the crural and ambient cisterns. J Neurosurg. 2018; 130(5):1435–1445

Matsukawa K, Kato T, Yato Y, et al. Incidence and risk factors of adjacent cranial facet joint violation following pedicle screw insertion using cortical bone trajectory technique. Spine. 2016; 41(14):E851–E856

Matsukawa K, Yanai Y, Fujiyoshi K, Kato T, Yato Y. Depth of vertebral screw insertion using a cortical bone trajectory technique in lumbar spinal fusion: radiological significance of a long cortical bone trajectory. J Neurosurg Spine. 2021; 35(5): 601–606

Matsuno H, Rhoton AL, Jr, Peace D. Microsurgical anatomy of the posterior fossa cisterns. Neurosurgery. 1988; 23(1):58–80

Matsushima K, Yagmurlu K, Kohno M, Rhoton AL, Jr. Anatomy and approaches along the cerebellar-brainstem fissures. J Neurosurg. 2016; 124(1):248–263

Mazziotta J, Toga A, Evans A, et al. A probabilistic atlas and reference system for the human brain: International Consortium for Brain Mapping (ICBM). Philos Trans R Soc Lond B Biol Sci. 2001; 356(1412):1293–1322

Mazziotta J, Toga A, Evans A, et al. A four-dimensional probabilistic atlas of the human brain. J Am Med Inform Assoc. 2001; 8(5):401–430

Mazziotta JC, Toga AW, Evans A, Fox P, Lancaster J, The International Consortium for Brain Mapping (ICBM). A probabilistic atlas of the human brain: theory and rationale for its development. Neuroimage. 1995; 2(2):89–101

McCormick WF. The pathology of vascular ("arteriovenous") malformations. J Neurosurg. 1966; 24(4):807–816

McMillan JJ, Williams B. Aqueduct stenosis. Case review and discussion. J Neurol Neurosurg Psychiatry. 1977; 40(6):521–532

Mendelow AD, Gregson BA, Rowan EN, Murray GD, Gholkar A, Mitchell PM, STICH II Investigators. Early surgery versus initial conservative treatment in patients with spontaneous supratentorial lobar intracerebral haematomas (STICH II): a randomised trial. Lancet. 2013; 382(9890):397–408

Menon G, Gopalakrishnan CV, Rao BR, Nair S, Sudhir J, Sharma M. A single institution series of cavernomas of the brainstem. J Clin Neurosci. 2011; 18(9): 1210–1214

Miao HL, Zhang DY, Wang T, Jiao XT, Jiao LQ. Clinical importance of the posterior inferior cerebellar artery: a review of the literature. Int J Med Sci. 2020; 17(18): 3005–3019

Mirzadeh Z, Sanai N, Lawton MT. The azygos anterior cerebral artery bypass: double reimplantation technique for giant anterior communicating artery aneurysms. J Neurosurg. 2011; 114(4):1154–1158

Mishima K, Sasaki T, Ojima T, Mukasa A, Kirino T. Multilobular cavernous malformation: report of two cases. Acta Neurochir (Wien). 1998; 140(1):20–25

Moeller S, Yacoub E, Olman CA, et al. Multiband multislice GE-EPI at 7 tesla, with 16-fold acceleration using partial parallel imaging with application to high spatial and temporal whole-brain fMRI. Magn Reson Med. 2010; 63(5):1144–1153

Moher D, Liberati A, Tetzlaff J, Altman DG, PRISMA Group. Preferred reporting items for systematic reviews and meta-analyses: the PRISMA statement. PLoS Med. 2009; 6(7):e1000097

Moons KG, Altman DG, Reitsma JB, et al. Transparent Reporting of a multivariable prediction model for Individual Prognosis or Diagnosis (TRIPOD): explanation and elaboration. Ann Intern Med. 2015; 162(1):W1–W73

Moore DR. Anatomy and physiology of binaural hearing. Audiology. 1991; 30(3): 125–134

Morez J, Sijbers J, Vanhevel F, Jeurissen B. Constrained spherical deconvolution of nonspherically sampled diffusion MRI data. Hum Brain Mapp. 2021; 42 (2):521–538

Morley TP, Barr HW. Giant intracranial aneurysms: diagnosis, course, and management. Clin Neurosurg. 1969; 16:73–94

Nagata S, Rhoton AL, Jr, Barry M. Microsurgical anatomy of the choroidal fissure. Surg Neurol. 1988; 30(1):3–59

Narayan V, Bir SC, Mohammed N, Savardekar AR, Patra DP, Nanda A. Surgical management of giant intracranial meningioma: operative nuances, challenges, and outcome. World Neurosurg. 2018; 110:e32–e41

Nathal E, Patiño-Rodriguez HM, Arauz A, et al. Risk factors for unfavorable outcomes in surgically treated brainstem cavernous malformations. World Neurosurg. 2018; 111:e478–e484

Neuroimaging Informatics Tools and Resources Clearinghouse (NITRC). Dictionary learning based functional atlases in four primate species (mouse lemurs, marmosets, macaques, and humans). NITRC. Accessed March 1, 2024 at: https://www.nitrc.org/projects/prim_func_2020/

Nico E, Adereti CO, Hackett AM, et al. Assessing the relationship between surgical timing and postoperative seizure outcomes in cavernoma-related epilepsy: a single-institution retrospective analysis of 63 patients with a review of the literature. Brain Sci. 2024; 14(5):494

Niehues JE, Blevins J. The Man Behind the Maps: Legendary Ski Artist James Niehues. Seattle, WA: Open Road Ski Company; 2019

Noll KR, Chen HS, Wefel JS, et al. Alterations in functional connectomics associated with neurocognitive changes following glioma resection. Neurosurgery. 2021; 88 (3):544–551

Obeso JA, Rodriguez-Oroz MC, Stamelou M, Bhatia KP, Burn DJ. The expanding universe of disorders of the basal ganglia. Lancet. 2014; 384(9942):523–531

Ohue S, Fukushima T, Friedman AH, Kumon Y, Ohnishi T. Retrosigmoid suprafloccular transhorizontal fissure approach for resection of brainstem cavernous malformation. Neurosurgery. 2010; 66(6) Suppl Operative:306–312, discussion 312–313

Ohue S, Fukushima T, Kumon Y, Ohnishi T, Friedman AH. Surgical management of brainstem cavernomas: selection of approaches and microsurgical techniques. Neurosurg Rev. 2010; 33(3):315–322, discussion 323–324

Pandey P, Westbroek EM, Gooderham PA, Steinberg GK. Cavernous malformation of brainstem, thalamus, and basal ganglia: a series of 176 patients. Neurosurgery. 2013; 72(4):573–589, discussion 588–589

Parkinson D. A surgical approach to the cavernous portion of the carotid artery. Anatomical studies and case report. J Neurosurg. 1965; 23(5):474–483

Párraga RG, Possatti LL, Alves RV, Ribas GC, Türe U, de Oliveira E. Microsurgical anatomy and internal architecture of the brainstem in 3D images: surgical considerations. J Neurosurg. 2016; 124(5):1377–1395

Penfield W, Boldrey E. Somatic motor and sensory representation in the cerebral cortex of man as studied by electrical stimulation. Brain. 1937; 60(4):389–443

Penfield W, Roberts L. Speech and Brain: Mechanisms. Princeton, NJ: Princeton University Press; 1959

Phan K, Ramachandran V, Tran TM, et al. Systematic review of cortical bone trajectory versus pedicle screw techniques for lumbosacral spine fusion. J Spine Surg. 2017; 3(4):679–688

Porter PJ, Willinsky RA, Harper W, Wallace MC. Cerebral cavernous malformations: natural history and prognosis after clinical deterioration with or without hemorrhage. J Neurosurg. 1997; 87(2):190–197

Porter RW, Detwiler PW, Spetzler RF, et al. Cavernous malformations of the brainstem: experience with 100 patients. J Neurosurg. 1999; 90(1):50–58

Potts MB, Chang EF, Young WL, Lawton MT, UCSF Brain AVM Study Project. Transsylvian-transinsular approaches to the insula and basal ganglia: operative techniques and results with vascular lesions. Neurosurgery. 2012; 70 (4):824–834, discussion 834

Quiñones-Hinojosa A, Chang EF, Lawton MT. The extended retrosigmoid approach: an alternative to radical cranial base approaches for posterior fossa lesions. Neurosurgery. 2006; 58(4) Suppl 2:ONS-208–ONS-214, discussion ONS-214

Quiñones-Hinojosa A, Lyon R, Du R, Lawton MT. Intraoperative motor mapping of the cerebral peduncle during resection of a midbrain cavernous malformation: technical case report. Neurosurgery. 2005; 56(2) Suppl:E439–, discussion E439

Rahman M, Tadi P. Neuroanatomy, Pons. Treasure Island, FL: StatPearls Publishing; 2021

Ramina R, Mattei TA, de Aguiar PH, et al. Surgical management of brainstem cavernous malformations. Neurol Sci. 2011; 32(6):1013–1028

Rangel-Castilla L, Spetzler RF. The 6 thalamic regions: surgical approaches to thalamic cavernous malformations, operative results, and clinical outcomes. J Neurosurg. 2015; 123(3):676–685

Rasmussen T, Penfield W. Further studies of the sensory and motor cerebral cortex of man. Fed Proc. 1947; 6(2):452–460

Rauschenbach L, Santos AN, Engel A, et al. Functional neurological outcome of spinal cavernous malformation surgery. Eur Spine J. 2023; 32(5):1714–1720

Rauscher S, Santos AN, Gull HH, et al. Modifiable vascular risk factors in patients with cerebral and spinal cavernous malformations: a complete 10-year follow-up study. Eur J Neurol. 2023; 30(5):1346–1351

Rees A. Aligning maps of visual and auditory space. Sensory maps. Curr Biol. 1996; 6 (8):955–958

Ren AA, Snellings DA, Su YS, et al. PIK3CA and CCM mutations fuel cavernomas through a cancer-like mechanism. Nature. 2021; 594(7862):271–276

Ren H, Zhu J, Su X, et al. Application of structural and functional connectome mismatch for classification and individualized therapy in Alzheimer disease. Front Public Health. 2020; 8:584430

Rhoton A. Rhoton: Cranial Anatomy and Surgical Approaches: Neurosurgery. Philadelphia, PA: Lippincott Williams & Wilkins; 2008

Rhoton AL, Jr. The cerebellar arteries. Neurosurgery. 2000; 47(3) Suppl:S29–S68

Rhoton AL, Jr. Cerebellum and fourth ventricle. Neurosurgery. 2000; 47(3) Suppl: S7–S27

Rhoton AL, Jr. The cerebral veins. Neurosurgery. 2002; 51(4) Suppl:S159–S205

Rhoton AL Jr; Congress of Neurological Surgeons (CNS). Rhoton's Cranial Anatomy and Surgical Approaches. Oxford: Oxford University Press; 2019

Ribas EC, Yağmurlu K, de Oliveira E, Ribas GC, Rhoton A. Microsurgical anatomy of the central core of the brain. J Neurosurg. 2018; 129(3):752–769

Rigamonti D, Drayer BP, Johnson PC, Hadley MN, Zabramski J, Spetzler RF. The MRI appearance of cavernous malformations (angiomas). J Neurosurg. 1987; 67(4): 518–524

Rodríguez-Hernández A, Lawton MT. Anatomical triangles defining surgical routes to posterior inferior cerebellar artery aneurysms. J Neurosurg. 2011; 114(4): 1088–1094

Rodríguez-Hernández A, Lawton MT. Contralateral transcallosal approach to basal ganglia cavernous malformation: 3-dimensional operative video. Neurosurgery. 2013; 72(2) Suppl Operative:ons182

Ruchalski K, Hathout GM. A medley of midbrain maladies: a brief review of midbrain anatomy and syndromology for radiologists. Radiol Res Pract. 2012; 2012: 258524

Rumalla K, Srinivasan VM, Gaddis M, et al. Cavernous Malformation Surgery in the United States: Validation of a Novel International Classification of Disease, 10th Edition, Clinical Modification Code Search Algorithm and Volume-Driven Surgical Outcomes. World Neurosurg. 2021; 150:e66–e73

Rutledge C, Raper DMS, Rodriguez Rubio R, Winkler EA, Abla AA. Supracerebellar infratentorial infratrochlear trans-quadrangular lobule approach to pontine cavernous malformations. Oper Neurosurg (Hagerstown). 2021; 20(3):268–275

Rutledge C, Tonetti DA, Raygor KP, Abla AA. How I do it: horizontal fissure approach to the middle cerebellar peduncle. Acta Neurochir (Wien). 2022; 164(3):763–766

Sacco RL, Freddo L, Bello JA, Odel JG, Onesti ST, Mohr JP. Wallenberg's lateral medullary syndrome. Clinical-magnetic resonance imaging correlations. Arch Neurol. 1993; 50(6):609–614

Sacks D, Baxter B, Campbell BCV, et al. From the American Association of Neurological Surgeons (AANS), American Society of Neuroradiology (ASNR), Cardiovascular and Interventional Radiology Society of Europe (CIRSE), Canadian Interventional Radiology Association (CIRA), Congress of Neurological Surgeons (CNS), European Society of Minimally Invasive Neurological Therapy (ESMINT), European Society of Neuroradiology (ESNR), European Stroke Organization (ESO), Society for Cardiovascular Angiography and Interventions (SCAI), Society of Interventional Radiology (SIR), Society of NeuroInterventional Surgery (SNIS), and World Stroke Organization (WSO). Multisociety Consensus Quality Improvement Revised Consensus Statement for Endovascular Therapy of Acute Ischemic Stroke. Int J Stroke. 2018; 13(6):612–632

Sali G, Briggs RG, Conner AK, et al. A connectomic atlas of the human cerebrum-chapter 11: tractographic description of the inferior longitudinal fasciculus. Oper Neurosurg (Hagerstown). 2018; 15 suppl_1:S423–S428

Sanai N, Mirzadeh Z, Lawton MT. Supracerebellar-supratrochlear and infratentorial-infratrochlear approaches: gravity-dependent variations of the lateral approach over the cerebellum. Neurosurgery. 2010; 66(6) Suppl Operative:264–274, discussion 274

Sansur CA, Caffes NM, Ibrahimi DM, et al. Biomechanical fixation properties of cortical versus transpedicular screws in the osteoporotic lumbar spine: an in vitro human cadaveric model. J Neurosurg Spine. 2016; 25(4):467–476

Santos AN, Rauschenbach L, Darkwah Oppong M, et al. Assessment and validation of proposed classification tools for brainstem cavernous malformations. J Neurosurg. 2020; 135(2):410–416

Scherschinski L, Eberle AT, Saggi S, et al. A taxonomy for cerebellar cavernous malformations: subtypes of cerebellar lesions. J Neurosurg. 2024; 142(2): 380–393

Schneider JR, Chiluwal AK, Nouri M, Prashant GN, Dehdashti AR. Retrosigmoid transhorizontal fissure approach to lateral pontine cavernous malformation: comparison to transpetrosal presigmoid retrolabyrinthine approach. J Neurosurg. 2021; 136(1):205–214

Schnurman Z, Nakamura A, McQuinn MW, Golfinos JG, Roland JT, Kondziolka D. Volumetric growth rates of untreated vestibular schwannomas. J Neurosurg. 2019; 133(3):742–748

Scott BB, Seeger JF, Schneider RC. Successful evacuation of a pontine hematoma secondary to rupture of a pathologically diagnosed "cryptic" vascular malformation. Case report. J Neurosurg. 1973; 39(1):104–108

Sereno MI, Diedrichsen J, Tachrount M, Testa-Silva G, d'Arceuil H, De Zeeuw C. The human cerebellum has almost 80% of the surface area of the neocortex. Proc Natl Acad Sci U S A. 2020; 117(32):19538–19543

Serrato-Avila JL, Paz Archila JA, Silva da Costa MD, et al. Three-dimensional quantitative analysis of the brainstem safe entry zones based on internal structures. World Neurosurg. 2022; 158:e64–e74

Shah AS, Sylvester PT, Yahanda AT, et al. Intraoperative MRI for newly diagnosed supratentorial glioblastoma: a multicenter-registry comparative study to conventional surgery. J Neurosurg. 2020; 135(2):505–514

Sheets JR, Briggs RG, Bai MY, et al. Parcellation-based modeling of the dorsal premotor area. J Neurol Sci. 2020; 415:116907

Sheets JR, Briggs RG, Dadario NB, et al. A cortical parcellation based analysis of ventral premotor area connectivity. Neurol Res. 2021; 43(7):595–607

Silverman IE, Liu GT, Volpe NJ, Galetta SL. The crossed paralyses. The original brain-stem syndromes of Millard-Gubler, Foville, Weber, and Raymond-Cestan. Arch Neurol. 1995; 52(6):635–638

Simić G, Hof PR. In search of the definitive Brodmann's map of cortical areas in human. J Comp Neurol. 2015; 523(1):5–14

Simonin A, Passaplan C, Sancho S, Rusconi A, Otten P. Giant extra-axial cavernous angioma of the falx: case report. Neurosurgery. 2019; 84(3):E211–E214

Singh R, Srinivasan VM, Lawton MT. Minipterional transsylvian approach for resection of a cavernous malformation in the optic chiasm. World Neurosurg. 2021; 152:152–153

Sotiropoulos SN, Moeller S, Jbabdi S, et al. Effects of image reconstruction on fiber orientation mapping from multichannel diffusion MRI: reducing the noise floor using SENSE. Magn Reson Med. 2013; 70(6):1682–1689

Spetzler RF, Kalani MY, Nakaji P. Neurovascular Surgery. 2nd ed. New York, NY: Thieme Medical Publishers; 2015

Spetzler RF, Kalani MY, Nakaji P, Yagmurlu K. Color Atlas of Brainstem Surgery. New York, NY: Thieme; 2017

Spetzler RF, Martin NA. A proposed grading system for arteriovenous malformations. J Neurosurg. 1986; 65(4):476–483

Spetzler RF, Sanai N. The quiet revolution: retractorless surgery for complex vascular and skull base lesions. J Neurosurg. 2012; 116(2):291–300

Spiller WG. The symptom-complex of a lesion of the uppermost portion of the anterior spinal and adjoining portion of the vertebral arteries. J Nerv Ment Dis. 1908; 35:775–777

Srinivasan VM, Karahalios K, Reddy VP, et al. Back to basal: contemporary cerebrovascular cohort study of the supratentorial-infraoccipital approach. J Neurosurg. 2022; 138(3):793–803

Srinivasan VM, Karahalios K, Rumalla K, et al. Giant cerebral cavernous malformations: redefinition based on surgical outcomes and systematic review of the literature. J Neurosurg. 2022; 137(6):1733–1741

Srinivasan VM, Karahalios K, Shlobin NA, et al. Residual and recurrent spinal cord cavernous malformations: outcomes and techniques to optimize resection and a systematic review of the literature. Oper Neurosurg (Hagerstown). 2023; 24(1): 44–54

Srinivasan VM, Koester SW, Wang MS, et al. Cavernous malformations of the optic nerve and optic pathway: a case series and systematic review of the literature. Oper Neurosurg (Hagerstown). 2021; 21(5):291–302

Srinivasan VM, Labib MA, Furey CG, Catapano JS, Lawton MT. The "binder ring" bypass: transection, rerouting, and reanastomosis as an alternative to macrovascular decompression of a dolichoectatic vertebral artery. Oper Neurosurg (Hagerstown). 2022; 22(4):224–230

Srinivasan VM, Lee KE, Catapano JS, Lawton MT. Suboccipital craniotomy and transventricular resection of a trigonal medullary cavernous malformation: 2-dimensional operative video. Oper Neurosurg (Hagerstown). 2022; 23(1):e66

Srinivasan VM, Singh R, Godzik J, Catapano JS, Lawton MT. Supracerebellar transtentorial approach for resection of a recurrent geniculate thalamic cavernous malformation: 2-dimensional operative video. Oper Neurosurg (Hagerstown). 2022; 22(3):e132

Stalcup ST, Tuan AS, Hesselink JR. Intracranial causes of ophthalmoplegia: the visual reflex pathways. Radiographics. 2013; 33(5):E153–E169

Steiger HJ, Markwalder TM, Reulen HJ. Clinicopathological relations of cerebral cavernous angiomas: observations in eleven cases. Neurosurgery. 1987; 21(6): 879–884

Steinberg GK, Chang SD, Gewirtz RJ, Lopez JR. Microsurgical resection of brainstem, thalamic, and basal ganglia angiographically occult vascular malformations. Neurosurgery. 2000; 46(2):260–270, discussion 270–271

Steinmetz H, Seitz RJ. Functional anatomy of language processing: neuroimaging and the problem of individual variability. Neuropsychologia. 1991; 29(12): 1149–1161

Steňo J, Bízik I, Steňová J, Timárová G. Subtemporal transtentorial resection of cavernous malformations involving the pyramidal tract in the upper pons and mesencephalon. Acta Neurochir (Wien). 2011; 153(10):1955–1962, discussion 1962

Sterne JA, Hernán MA, Reeves BC, et al. ROBINS-I: a tool for assessing risk of bias in non-randomised studies of interventions. BMJ. 2016; 355:i4919

Sughrue ME, Saloner D, Rayz VL, Lawton MT. Giant intracranial aneurysms: evolution of management in a contemporary surgical series. Neurosurgery. 2011; 69(6):1261–1270, discussion 1270–1271

Sun Q, Zhao X, Gandhi S, et al. Quantitative analysis of ipsilateral and contralateral supracerebellar infratentorial and occipital transtentorial approaches to the cisternal pulvinar: laboratory anatomical investigation. J Neurosurg. 2019; 133 (4):1172–1181

Sundt TM, III, Sundt TM, Jr. Principles of preparation of vein bypass grafts to maximize patency. J Neurosurg. 1987; 66(2):172–180

Surek CC, Van Ess M, Stephens R. Acousticofacial-glossopharyngeal triangle: an anatomic model for rapid surgical orientation. Skull Base. 2010; 20(3): 139–142

Symon L, Jakubowski J, Kendall B. Surgical treatment of giant pituitary adenomas. J Neurol Neurosurg Psychiatry. 1979; 42(11):973–982

Tan T, Tee JW, Trost N, McKelvie P, Wang YY. Anterior visual pathway cavernous malformations. J Clin Neurosci. 2015; 22(2):258–267

Tan Z, McLachlin S, Whyne C, Finkelstein J. Validation of a freehand technique for cortical bone trajectory screws in the lumbar spine. J Neurosurg Spine. 2019; 31 (2):201–208

Tanaka S, Takanashi J, Fujii K, Ujiie H, Hori T. Motor evoked potential mapping and monitoring by direct brainstem stimulation. Technical note. J Neurosurg. 2007; 107(5):1053–1057

Tanglay O, Young IM, Dadario NB, et al. Anatomy and white-matter connections of the precuneus. Brain Imaging Behav. 2022; 16(2):574–586

Tayebi Meybodi A, Borba Moreira L, Zhao X, Preul MC, Lawton MT. Anatomical analysis of the vagoaccessory triangle and the triangles within: the suprahypoglossal, infrahypoglossal, and hypoglossal-hypoglossal triangles. World Neurosurg. 2019; 126:e463–e472

Tayebi Meybodi A, Gadhiya A, Borba Moreira L, Lawton MT. Coding cerebral bypasses: a proposed nomenclature to better describe bypass constructs and revascularization techniques. J Neurosurg. 2021; 136(1):163–174

Tayebi Meybodi A, Gandhi S, Mascitelli J, et al. The oculomotor-tentorial triangle. Part 1: microsurgical anatomy and techniques to enhance exposure. J Neurosurg. 2018; 130(5):1426–1434

Tayebi Meybodi A, Lawton MT, Tabani H, Benet A. Tonsillobiventral fissure approach to the lateral recess of the fourth ventricle. J Neurosurg. 2017; 127(4):768–774

Terao H, Hori T, Matsutani M, Okeda R. Detection of cryptic vascular malformations by computerized tomography. Report of two cases. J Neurosurg. 1979; 51(4):546–551

Tufte ER. The Visual Display of Quantitative Information. Cheshire, CT: Graphics Press; 2001

Valli D, Zhao X, Belykh E, Sun Q, Lawton MT, Preul MC. Partial gyrus rectus resection as a technique to improve the exposure to the anterior communicating artery complex through the junctional triangle: a quantitative study. J Neurol Surg B Skull Base. 2021; 82 Suppl 3:e211–e216

Van Essen DC. A tension-based theory of morphogenesis and compact wiring in the central nervous system. Nature. 1997; 385(6614):313–318

Van Essen DC. Surface-based atlases of cerebellar cortex in the human, macaque, and mouse. Ann N Y Acad Sci. 2002; 978:468–479

Van Essen DC, Donahue CJ, Glasser MF. Development and evolution of cerebral and cerebellar cortex. Brain Behav Evol. 2018; 91(3):158–169

Van Essen DC, Ugurbil K, Auerbach E, et al. WU-Minn HCP Consortium. The Human Connectome Project: a data acquisition perspective. Neuroimage. 2012; 62(4): 2222–2231

van Swieten JC, Koudstaal PJ, Visser MC, Schouten HJ, van Gijn J. Interobserver agreement for the assessment of handicap in stroke patients. Stroke. 1988; 19 (5):604–607

Ventral Attention Network (VAN). Accessed May 24, 2023 at: https:// quicktome.o8t.com/guide/network/ventral-attention-network

Vertes RP, Linley SB, Hoover WB. Limbic circuitry of the midline thalamus. Neurosci Biobehav Rev. 2015; 54:89–107

Villalonga JF, Saenz A, Campero A. Surgical treatment of an asymptomatic giant supratentorial cavernous hemangioma. Case report. J Clin Neurosci. 2019; 62: 231–234

Virgo JD, Plant GT. Internuclear ophthalmoplegia. Pract Neurol. 2017; 17(2):149–153

Voelker JL, Stewart DH, Schochet SS, Jr. Giant intracranial and extracranial cavernous malformation. Case report. J Neurosurg. 1998; 89(3):465–469

Walcott BP, Breshears JD, Choudhri O, Lawton MT. Transcallosal-transchoroidal fissure approach for resection of third ventricle cavernous malformation: 3-dimensional operative video. Oper Neurosurg (Hagerstown). 2017; 13(3):398

Walcott BP, Choudhri O, Lawton MT. Brainstem cavernous malformations: natural history versus surgical management. J Clin Neurosci. 2016; 32:164–165

Waldron JS, Lawton MT. The supracarotid-infrafrontal approach: surgical technique and clinical application to cavernous malformations in the anteroinferior basal ganglia. Neurosurgery. 2009; 64(3) Suppl:ons86–ons95, discussion ons95

Wang C, Zhao M, Wang J, Wang S, Zhang D, Zhao J. Giant cavernous malformations: a single center experience and literature review. J Clin Neurosci. 2018; 56:108–113

Wang CC, Liu A, Zhang JT, Sun B, Zhao YL. Surgical management of brain-stem cavernous malformations: report of 137 cases. Surg Neurol. 2003; 59(6):444–454, discussion 454

Wang J, He X, Sun T. Comparative clinical efficacy and safety of cortical bone trajectory screw fixation and traditional pedicle screw fixation in posterior lumbar fusion: a systematic review and meta-analysis. Eur Spine J. 2019; 28(7): 1678–1689

Wangsawatwong P, Sawa AGU, de Andrada Pereira B, et al. Adjacent-segment effects of lumbar cortical screw-rod fixation versus pedicle screw-rod fixation with and without interbody support. J Neurosurg Spine. 2021; 35 (3):263–269

Weinsheimer S, Nelson J, Abla AA, et al. Brain Vascular Malformation Consortium Cerebral Cavernous Malformation Investigator Group. Intracranial hemorrhage rate and lesion burden in patients with familial cerebral cavernous malformation. J Am Heart Assoc. 2023; 12(3):e027572

Welker WI. The significance of foliation and fissuration of cerebellar cortex. The cerebellar folium as a fundamental unit of sensorimotor integration. Arch Ital Biol. 1990; 128(2–4):87–109

Weyand TG. The multifunctional lateral geniculate nucleus. Rev Neurosci. 2016; 27 (2):135–157

Winkler EA, Lawton MT. Transcallosal-transchoroidal fissure approach for midbrain and thalamic cavernous malformations: 2-dimensional operative video. Oper Neurosurg (Hagerstown). 2024; 26(3):347–348

Winter F, Blair L, Buchfelder M, Roessler K. Risk factors for poor postoperative outcome and epileptic symptoms in patients diagnosed with cerebral cavernous malformations. J Neurol Surg A Cent Eur Neurosurg. 2021; 82(1):59–63

Woodall MN, Catapano JS, Lawton MT, Spetzler RF. Cavernous malformations in and around the third ventricle: indications, approaches, and outcomes. Oper Neurosurg (Hagerstown). 2020; 18(6):736–746

Xu N, LaGrow TJ, Anumba N, et al. Functional connectivity of the brain across rodents and humans. Front Neurosci. 2022; 16:816331

Xu T, Sturgeon D, Ramirez JSB, et al. Interindividual variability of functional connectivity in awake and anesthetized rhesus macaque monkeys. Biol Psychiatry Cogn Neurosci Neuroimaging. 2019; 4(6):543–553

Yağmurlu K, Kalani MYS, Preul MC, Spetzler RF. The superior fovea triangle approach: a novel safe entry zone to the brainstem. J Neurosurg. 2017; 127(5): 1134–1138

Yağmurlu K, Rhoton AL, Jr, Tanriover N, Bennett JA. Three-dimensional microsurgical anatomy and the safe entry zones of the brainstem. Neurosurgery. 2014; 10(4) Suppl 4:602–619, discussion 619–620

Yang Y, van Niftrik B, Ma X, et al. Analysis of safe entry zones into the brainstem. Neurosurg Rev. 2019; 42(3):721–729

Yarkoni T, Poldrack RA, Nichols TE, Van Essen DC, Wager TD. Large-scale automated synthesis of human functional neuroimaging data. Nat Methods. 2011; 8(8): 665–670

Yaşargil MG, Kasdaglis K, Jain KK, Weber HP. Anatomical observations of the subarachnoid cisterns of the brain during surgery. J Neurosurg. 1976; 44(3):298–302

Yeh FC. Population-based tract-to-region connectome of the human brain and its hierarchical topology. Nat Commun. 2022; 13(1):4933

Yeo BT, Krienen FM, Sepulcre J, et al. The organization of the human cerebral cortex estimated by intrinsic functional connectivity. J Neurophysiol. 2011; 106(3): 1125–1165

Yoshita M, Yamada M. Allodynia in the flank after thalamic stroke. J Clin Neurosci. 2006; 13(2):288–291

Youssef AS, Abdel Aziz KM, Kim EY, Keller JT, Zuccarello M, van Loveren HR. The carotid-oculomotor window in exposure of upper basilar artery aneurysms: a cadaveric morphometric study. Neurosurgery. 2004; 54(5):1181–1187, discussion 1187–1189

Zabramski JM, Kalani MYS, Filippidis AS, Spetzler RF. Propranolol treatment of cavernous malformations with symptomatic hemorrhage. World Neurosurg. 2016; 88:631–639

Zabramski JM, Kiriş T, Sankhla SK, Cabiol J, Spetzler RF. Orbitozygomatic craniotomy. Technical note. J Neurosurg. 1998; 89(2):336–341

Zabramski JM, Wascher TM, Spetzler RF, et al. The natural history of familial cavernous malformations: results of an ongoing study. J Neurosurg. 1994; 80(3): 422–432

Zafar A, Quadri SA, Farooqui M, et al. Familial cerebral cavernous malformations. Stroke. 2019; 50(5):1294–1301

Zaidi HA, Mooney MA, Levitt MR, Dru AB, Abla AA, Spetzler RF. Impact of timing of intervention among 397 consecutively treated brainstem cavernous malformations. Neurosurgery. 2017; 81(4):620–626

Zhang R-J, Li H-M, Gao H, et al. Cortical bone trajectory screws used to save failed traditional trajectory screws in the osteoporotic lumbar spine and vice versa: a human cadaveric biomechanical study. J Neurosurg Spine. 2019; 30(6):759–766

Zhao X, Tayebi Meybodi A, Naeem K, et al. The glossopharyngo-cochlear triangle--part I: quantitative anatomic analysis of high-riding posterior inferior cerebellar artery aneurysms exposed through the extended retrosigmoid approach. Oper Neurosurg (Hagerstown). 2021; 20(3):242–251

Zubricky RD, Das JM. Neuroanatomy, Superior Colliculus. Treasure Island, FL: StatPearls Publishing; 2021

Index

Note: Page numbers set **bold** or *italic* indicate headings or figures, respectively.

V

W

X